Structural Heart Disease Interventions

Editors

John D. Carroll, MD, FACC, FSCAI

Professor of Medicine
University of Colorado Denver
Director, Interventional Cardiology
Medical Director, Cardiac and Vascular Center
University of Colorado Hospital
Aurora, Colorado

John G. Webb, MD, FACC

McLeod Professor of Heart Valve Intervention
University of British Columbia
Director, Cardiac Catheterization and Interventional Cardiology
St. Paul's Hospital
Vancouver, British Columbia, Canada

 Wolters Kluwer | Lippincott Williams & Wilkins
Health

Philadelphia · Baltimore · New York · London
Buenos Aires · Hong Kong · Sydney · Tokyo

Acquisitions Editor: Frances DeStefano
Product Manager: Leanne Vandetty
Production Manager: Alicia Jackson
Senior Manufacturing Manager: Benjamin Rivera
Marketing Manager: Kimberly Schonberger
Design Coordinator: Stephen Druding
Production Service: Absolute Service, Inc.

Printed in China

Library of Congress Cataloging-in-Publication Data

Structural heart disease interventions/editors, John D. Carroll, John G. Webb.
    p. ; cm.
  Includes bibliographical references and index.
   ISBN 978-1-60913-710-6 (hardback)
  I. Carroll, John D. II. Webb, John G. (John Graydon), 1954-
   [DNLM: 1. Heart Diseases—therapy. 2. Adult. 3. Balloon Dilation—methods. 4. Cardiac Surgical Procedures—methods. 5. Heart Catheterization—methods. 6. Heart Valve Prosthesis Implantation—methods. WG 166]
  LC classification not assigned
  616.1'20754—dc23

                                                                                  2011031527

Care has been taken to confirm the accuracy of the information presented and to describe generally accepted practices. However, the authors, editors, and publisher are not responsible for errors or omissions or for any consequences from application of the information in this book and make no warranty, expressed or implied, with respect to the currency, completeness, or accuracy of the contents of the publication. Application of the information in a particular situation remains the professional responsibility of the practitioner.

The authors, editors, and publisher have exerted every effort to ensure that drug selection and dosage set forth in this text are in accordance with current recommendations and practice at the time of publication. However, in view of ongoing research, changes in government regulations, and the constant flow of information relating to drug therapy and drug reactions, the reader is urged to check the package insert for each drug for any change in indications and dosage and for added warnings and precautions. This is particularly important when the recommended agent is a new or infrequently employed drug.

Some drugs and medical devices presented in the publication have Food and Drug Administration (FDA) clearance for limited use in restricted research settings. It is the responsibility of the health care provider to ascertain the FDA status of each drug or device planned for use in their clinical practice.

To purchase additional copies of this book, call our customer service department at (800) 638-3030 or fax orders to (301) 223-2320. International customers should call (301) 223-2300.

Visit Lippincott Williams & Wilkins on the Internet: at LWW.com. Lippincott Williams & Wilkins customer service representatives are available from 8:30 AM to 6 PM, EST.

10 9 8 7 6 5 4 3 2 1

To my wife, Eugenia; my children, Ian, Nick, Adam, and Grace; and my parents, Marjorie and James Carroll.

John Carroll

For my wife Jennifer, my sons Geoffrey and Rory, and my parents Don and Marilyn Webb.

John Webb

CONTENTS

Section III: Closure of Congenital and Acquired Cardiac Defects in Adults

Section IV: Transcatheter Therapy for Valvular Disease

Section V: Specialized Procedures

PREFACE

Structural heart disease (SHD) interventions are a diverse group of novel treatments that have grown in the last decade from a small number of interventions to an impressive array of novel approaches to diseases that have been traditionally managed by surgery and medical therapy. Some interventions are actually to prevent clinical manifestations, whereas others reduce symptoms and increase the quality of life. The field is young, has a high level of investigative activity, and is seen as the third wave of interventional cardiology activity after coronary and noncoronary vascular interventions. The knowledge, skills, clinical outcomes, and adjunctive techniques used in SHD interventions are unique and have become well established with numerous publications. Thus, we believe this knowledge is ready to be presented in a practical manual format. In addition, a substantial number of devices have been recently approved in Europe and many are approved or close to approval in the United States. Clinicians are building their own SHD interventional programs and have a practical need for a timely publication from the experts around the world.

This book has been prepared for use by physicians and nonphysicians who have an interest in SHD interventions in adults and desire a practical, comprehensive, clinical, and compact summary of established and emerging percutaneous interventions. The chapters are authored by recognized experts from around the world and we greatly appreciate their efforts in creating these chapters despite the heavy demands on their time and other commitments to developing this field.

There are five major sections including: I, Core Knowledge in Structural Heart Disease Intervention; II, Specialized Skills for the Interventionalist; III, Closure of Congenital and Acquired Cardiac Defects in Adults; IV, Transcatheter Therapy for Valvular Disease; and V, Specialized Procedures.

Authors have used graphics content that have enhanced the educational value of the book with an emphasis of clinically practical knowledge. Interactive three-dimensional (3D) graphics are a special feature developed by Adam Hansgen of the 3D Lab at the University of Colorado and augment the educational impact of the text, especially in regard to understanding the 3D anatomy of various forms of SHD.

ACKNOWLEDGMENTS

We would like to acknowledge the many people who are part of the SHD programs at each of our institutions. These included personnel in the cardiac catheterization but also the echocardiography lab, the operating room, the intensive care units, and the other areas responsible for caring for these patients. In addition, we thank our colleagues in cardiac imaging, surgery, anesthesiology, and other specialties who have been so important in the development of this field. We finally want to acknowledge the patients who often have participated in the investigative phase of many of these treatments and only through their willingness have these treatments been brought to the many patients around the world.

Adam Hansgen is acknowledged for his graphic ability in creating the cover images.

Wail Alkashkari, MD
Congenital/Structural Heart Disease Intervention
Rush Center for Congenital & Structural Heart Disease
Rush University Medical Center
Chicago, Illinois

Anita W. Asgar, MD, FRCPC
Associate Professor
Department of Medicine
Université de Montréal
Director, Transcatheter Valve Therapy Clinic
Department of Cardiology
Institut de Cardiologie de Montréal
Montreal, Quebec, Canada

Lee N. Benson, MD, FRCP(C), FACC, FSCAI
Professor of Pediatrics (Cardiology)
Department of Pediatrics
University of Toronto School of Medicine
Director, The Cardiac Diagnostic and Interventional Unit
Department of Pediatrics
The Hospital for Sick Children
Toronto, Ontario, Canada

Stefan Bertog, MD, FACC, FSCAI
Codirector, Cardiac Catheterization Laboratory
Department of Cardiology
Minneapolis Veterans Affairs Medical Center
Minneapolis, Minnesota
CardioVascular Center
Frankfurt, Germany

Klaudija Bijuklic, MD
Fellow
Medical Care Center Prof. Mathey, Prof. Schofer
Hamburg University Cardiovascular Center
Hamburg, Germany

Raoul Bonan, MD
Associate Professor
Department of Medicine
University of Montreal
Interventional Cardiologist
Department of Medicine
Institut de Cardiologie de Montréal
Montreal, Quebec, Canada

Philipp Bonhoeffer, MD
Professor of Cardiology
London, England

Stephen J.D. Brecker, MD, FACC
Honorary Senior Lecturer
Cardiac and Vascular Sciences
St. George's, University of London
Consultant Cardiologist
Department of Cardiology
St. George's Hospital
London, England

Eric Brochet, MD
Department of Cardiology
Hôpital Bichat
Paris, France

Quang T. Bui, MD
Assistant Professor of Medicine
Department of Medicine
David Geffen School of Medicine at UCLA
Director, Structural Heart Disease Program
Department of Medicine
Division of Cardiology
Harbor-UCLA Medical Center
Torrance, California

Qi-Ling Cao, MD
Research Scientist
Department of Pediatrics
Rush University
Chicago, Illinois

John D. Carroll, MD, FACC, FSCAI
Professor of Medicine
University of Colorado Denver
Director, Interventional Cardiology
Medical Director, Cardiac and Vascular Center
University of Colorado Hospital
Aurora, Colorado

Ivan P. Casserly, MB, BCh
Assistant Professor
Division of Cardiology
University of Colorado School of Medicine
Interventional Cardiologist
Cardiac and Vascular Center
University of Colorado Hospital
Aurora, Colorado

Mehmet Cilingiroglu, MD, FESC, FACC, FSCAI
Director, Structural Heart Interventions
Division of Cardiovascular Diseases
Department of Medicine
University of Maryland Medical Center
Baltimore, Maryland

Alain Cribier, MD
Head, Department of Cardiology
Rouen University Hospital Charles Nicolle
Rouen, France

Yuriy Dudiy, MD
Research Associate
Department of Interventional Cardiology
Lenox Hill Hospital
New York, New York

Helene Eltchaninoff, MD
Professor
Department of Cardiology
Rouen University Hospital Charles Nicolle
Rouen, France

Ted Feldman, MD
Director, Cardiac Catheterization Laboratory
Evanston Hospital
Evanston, Illinois

Jennifer Franke, MD
CardioVascular Center Frankfurt
Frankfurt, Germany

Philippe Généreux, MD
Department of Interventional Cardiology
Columbia University Medical Center
Department of Medicine/Cardiology
The Presbyterian Hospital
New York, New York

Adam R. Hansgen, BS
Senior Professional Research Assistant
Medicine/Cardiology
University of Colorado Denver
Aurora, Colorado

William E. Hellenbrand, MD
Professor of Pediatrics
Department of Pediatric Cardiology
Columbia University
Chief of Pediatric Cardiology
Department of Pediatric Cardiology
Children's Hospital of New York-Presbyterian
New York, New York

Thomas J. Helton, DO
Chief Fellow, Interventional Cardiology
Department of Cardiovascular Medicine
Cleveland Clinic
Cleveland, Ohio

Howard C. Herrmann, MD
Professor of Medicine
University of Pennsylvania School of Medicine
Director, Interventional Cardiology and Cardiac
    Catheterization Labs
Hospital of the University of Pennsylvania
Philadelphia, Pennsylvania

Ziyad M. Hijazi, MD
Professor
Departments of Pediatrics & Internal Medicine
Director, Rush Center for Congenital & Structural
    Heart Disease
Rush University
Chicago, Illinois

Dominique Himbert, MD
Hospital Practitioner
Department of Cardiology
Hôpital Bichat
Paris, France

Eric M. Horlick, MDCM, FRCPC
Assistant Professor
Department of Medicine
University of Toronto
Director, Structural Heart Disease Intervention Service
Department of Medicine
Division of Cardiology
Toronto General Hospital
Toronto, Ontario, Canada

Bernard Iung, MD
Professor of Cardiology
Paris Diderot University
Cardiology Department
Hôpital Bichat
Paris, France

Vladimir Jelnin, MD
Director, 3D Cardiac CT Imaging Laboratory
Department of Interventional Cardiology
Lenox Hill Hospital
New York, New York

Thomas K. Jones, MD
Professor
Department of Pediatrics
University of Washington
Director, Cardiac Catheterization Laboratories
Seattle Children's Hospital
Seattle, Washington

Samir R. Kapadia, MD
Director, Sones Cardiac Catheterization Laboratories
Department of Interventional Cardiology
Cleveland Clinic
Cleveland, Ohio

Morton J. Kern, MD
Professor of Medicine
Associate Chief
Division of Cardiology
University of California, Irvine
Orange, California
Chief Cardiologist
Long Beach Veterans Administration Hospital
Long Beach, California

Michael S. Kim, MD
Assistant Professor
Internal Medicine/Division of Cardiology
University of Washington
Seattle, Washington

Susheel K. Kodali, MD
Co-Director, Transcatheter Aortic Valve Program
Director, Interventional Cardiology Fellowship Program
Columbia University Medical Center
New York-Presbyterian Hospital
New York, New York

Jean-Claude Laborde, MD
Honorary Consultant Cardiologist
Cardiothoracic Unit
St. George's Hospital
London, England

John Lasala, MD, PhD
Professor of Medicine
Department of Internal Medicine (Cardiology)
Washington University School of Medicine
Director, Cardiac Catheterization
Barnes-Jewish Hospital
St. Louis, Missouri

Evan Lau, MD
Fellow, Interventional Cardiology
Department of Cardiology
Cleveland Clinic Foundation
Cleveland, Ohio

Martin B. Leon, MD
Professor of Medicine
Director, Center for Interventional Vascular Therapy
New York Presbyterian Hospital
Columbia University Medical Center
Chairman Emeritus, Cardiovascular Research Foundation
    in New York City
New York, New York

C. Huie Lin, MD, PhD
Fellow, Interventional Cardiology
Department of Medicine
Washington University School of Medicine
Barnes-Jewish Hospital
St. Louis, Missouri

Philipp C. Lurz, MD
Senior Clinical Fellow
Department of Internal Medicine/Cardiology and
    Grown Up Congenital Heart Disease
University of Leipzig – Heart Center
Leipzig, Germany

Michael Mack, MD
Baylor Health Care System
Dallas, Texas

Mark D. Osten, MD, FRCPC
Assistant Professor
Department of Medicine
University of Toronto
Interventional Cardiologist
Division of Cardiology
University Health Network, Toronto General Hospital
Toronto, Ontario, Canada

Paul Poommipanit, MD
Interventional Cardiologist
Advanced Cardiovascular Consultants
Department of Medicine
Trinity Medical Center
Rock Island, Illinois

Robert A. Quaife, MD
Associate Professor of Medicine and Radiology
Director, Advance Cardiac Imaging
University of Colorado Denver
Denver, Colorado

Carlos E. Ruiz, MD, PhD
Director, Division of Cardiac Intervention for Structural Heart Disease
Department of Interventional Cardiology
Lenox Hill Hospital
New York, New York

Ernesto E. Salcedo, MD
Professor of Medicine
University of Colorado Denver
Denver, Colorado
Director, Echocardiography
University of Colorado Hospital
Aurora, Colorado

Joachim Schofer, MD
Professor
Hamburg University Cardiovascular Center
Hamburg University
Medical Director
Cardiovascular Center
Medical Care Center
Hamburg, Germany

Horst Sievert, MD
Associate Professor
Department of Internal Medicine
University of Frankfurt
Director
Cardiovascular Center Frankfurt
Frankfurt, Germany

Daniel H. Steinberg, MD
Assistant Professor of Medicine
Division of Cardiology
Medical University of South Carolina
Charleston, South Carolina

Jonathan Tobis, MD
Professor
Department of Medicine
University of California – Los Angeles
Director, Interventional Cardiology
Department of Medicine
University of California – Los Angeles Medical Center
Los Angeles, California

Stefan Toggweiler, MD
Division of Cardiology
St. Paul's Hospital
The University of British Columbia
Vancouver, British Columbia, Canada

Alejandro J. Torres, MD
Assistant Professor of Pediatrics
Department of Pediatric Cardiology
Columbia University
Children's Hospital of New York-Presbyterian
New York, New York

Christophe Tron, MD
Department of Cardiology
Rouen University Hospital
Rouen, France

E. Murat Tuzcu, MD
Vice Chairman
Robert and Suzanne Tomsich Department of Cardiology
Cleveland Clinic Foundation
Cleveland, Ohio

Alec Vahanian, FESC, FRCP(Edin.)
Head of Service
Cardiology Department
Hôpital Bichat
Paris, France

John G. Webb, MD, FACC
McLeod Professor of Heart Valve Intervention
University of British Columbia
Director, Cardiac Catheterization and Interventional Cardiology
St. Paul's Hospital
Vancouver, British Columbia, Canada

Jens Wiebe, MD
Institute of Applied Physics
Hamburg University
Hamburg, Germany

Alexander B. Willson, MBBS, MPH
Fellow, Interventional Cardiology
Interventional Cardiology Research
St. Paul's Hospital
Vancouver, British Columbia, Canada

Nina Wunderlich, MD
Director of Non-Invasive Cardiology
CardioVascular Center Frankfurt
Frankfurt, Germany

CORE KNOWLEDGE IN STRUCTURAL HEART DISEASE INTERVENTION

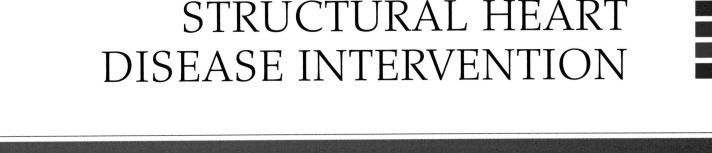
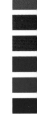

CHAPTER 1

Building a Structural Heart Disease Program

Quang T. Bui and Howard C. Herrmann

The first percutaneous transluminal coronary angioplasty (PTCA) procedure performed by Dr. Andreas Gruentzig in 1977 ushered in a new era of interventional cardiovascular medicine.[1,2] The field of interventional cardiology has subsequently grown to encompass not only coronary interventions but also those outside the confines of the coronary bed including interventions in the peripheral vasculature. The cognitive and technical skills required to perform coronary and noncoronary interventions have evolved, such that the American Board of Internal Medicine (ABIM) in 1999 added an additional Added Qualification Exam for interventional cardiology, thus recognizing it as a distinct subspecialty within the field of cardiovascular medicine.

Over the past 30 years, innovation has driven the field to move outside the confines of the vascular bed to tackle diseases involving cardiac structural and valvular abnormalities. This has created a new field within interventional cardiology: namely that of interventions pertaining to structural heart disease (SHD). Historically, pediatric interventional cardiologists have led the way, employing percutaneous transcatheter technology to successfully treat children with congenital maladies. The adaptation of these early techniques and their continued evolution has fueled the development of new percutaneous SHD procedures to treat both congenital and acquired heart disease involving not only structural but also functional abnormalities that include heart valves, cardiac chambers, and the proximal great vessels.

Recognizing the future growth and the complexities of SHD interventions, the Society for Cardiovascular Angiography and Interventions (SCAI) created a Council on Structural Heart Disease in 2008 to provide future guidance and leadership regarding this emerging field. In 2010, a survey commissioned by the Council was published. Practice patterns from 107 US-based physicians across all regions of the country were sampled. Sixty-eight percent of these physicians personally and currently perform SHD cardiac interventions with a majority of respondents (80%) performing closure of interatrial communication defects (patent foramen ovale, atrial septal defect).[3] Although only 20% of respondents (range 8%–68%) anticipate doing new procedures in the next 3 years, it is likely that the rapid growth and development of transcatheter therapies that now include valve implantation and repair will heighten the interest of clinical programs to establish SHD programs to fill the anticipated need created by this new emerging technology. This chapter provides guiding principles upon which to build a successful adult SHD program that ensures high-quality patient care, supports and contributes to the growing knowledge base of SHD interventions, and allows for monitoring of quality.

SHD PROGRAM GOALS

The goal of building a SHD program is to establish a clinical center that provides a high level of clinical performance in procedures for patients with SHD. It requires an assembly of specialists with the intellectual

3

and technical knowledge base germane to SHD interventions with the appropriate ancillary support staff and facilities. Current centers with established interventional cardiology programs operate on four principles as per the American College of Cardiology (ACC) Training Statement on Recommendations for the Structure of an Optimal Adult Interventional Cardiology Program.[4] These principles can also be adapted for programs performing SHD interventions as follows:

- To understand the effectiveness and limitations of SHD interventional procedures in order to select patients and procedure types appropriately.
- To achieve the appropriate cognitive knowledge and technical skills needed to perform SHD interventional procedures at the level of quality attainable through the present state of the art.
- To foster an attitude of lifelong learning and critical thinking skills needed to gain from experience and incorporate new developments.
- To understand and commit to quality assessment and improvement in procedure performance.

With these tenets serving as a foundation, those seeking to build a successful SHD program should, at a minimum, seek to establish four additional goals:

- To acquire and establish the technical and intellectual knowledge base to perform SHD interventions.
- To establish a multidisciplinary team to facilitate execution of these procedures.
- To create a physical and intellectual environment where SHD procedures will be performed.
- To establish a mechanism to maintain procedural proficiency and allow for adaptation of new technology.

Establishing a Technical and Intellectual Knowledge Base for SHD Interventions

It is assumed that these newly developed SHD programs have a strong preexisting expertise in interventional cardiology at their foundation. However, SHD interventions represent a deviation from conventional coronary and noncoronary vascular procedures, which utilize over-the-wire technology to operate within the walls of the well-defined intravascular space. SHD interventions typically involve navigation of catheters and guidewires in more open three-dimensional (3D) space, where the limitations of fluoroscopy and angiography are most exposed. Taking into account interactions with moving anatomic structures and using existing catheter-based technology, operators may deploy various plugs, valves, clips, or cinching devices to modify existing anatomic structures. A representative list of technical skills and procedures that are

TABLE 1-1 Technical Knowledge Base for Structural Heart Disease Intervention

Core Interventional Skills

- Transseptal catheterization technique
- Catheter-based hemodynamic evaluation for SHD interventions
- Image guidance using intracardiac and transesophageal echocardiography for SHD interventions
- Vascular access and closure techniques for SHD interventions

Closure of Congenital and Acquired Cardiac Defects in Adults

- Closure of patent foramen ovale
- Closure of atrial septal defects
- Closure of ventricular septal defects
- Closure of fistula and patent ductus arteriosus
- Closure of paravalvular leaks
- Closure of left atrial appendage

Transcatheter Therapy for Valvular Disease

- Aortic balloon valvuloplasty
- Percutaneous mitral balloon commissurotomy
- Transcatheter aortic valve implantation
- Transcatheter mitral valve repair
- Pulmonic valve valvuloplasty and implantation in adults

Other Specialized Procedures

- Percutaneous treatment of coarctation of the aorta
- Septal ablation in obstructive hypertrophic cardiomyopathy
- Insertion of percutaneous left ventricular assist devices

currently available under the rubric of SHD interventions can be found in Table 1-1. They range from closure of simple interatrial communications and escalate in technical difficulty to encompass transcatheter valve repair and implantation and transcatheter closure of paravalvular leaks. This list not only reflects the rich diversity of SHD interventions, but also underscores the complexity of performing these procedures.

Several academic centers in the US now offer formal training in advanced SHD interventions in the form of an additional 1-year dedicated fellowship following the conventional Accreditation Council for Graduate Medical Education (ACGME)–approved interventional cardiology training pathway. However, this pathway may not be suitable to all current operators at programs interested in moving forward with establishing a SHD program in the near future, particularly as there is no mechanism for funding these positions within usual training program grants. In addition, there are no formal training guidelines regarding SHD interventions.

TABLE 1-2 Core Knowledge Base in SHD Intervention

- Anatomy of the cardiac valves
- Anatomy of the cardiac chambers
- CTA and MRA in patient assessment and procedural guidance
- TTE, ICE, and TEE in patient assessment and procedural guidance
- Invasive and noninvasive hemodynamic evaluation for SHD interventions
- Practical interventional pharmacologic management for SHD interventions
- Vascular access and closure issues in SHD interventions
- Clinical and natural history of structural, valvular, and adult congenital heart diseases

CTA, computed tomography angiography; ICE, intracardiac echocardiography; MRA, magnetic resonance angiography; TEE, transesophageal echocardiography; TTE, transthoracic echocardiography.

As with the early experiences involving coronary angioplasty, seasoned operators who want to gain expertise in advanced SHD interventions will need to rely on their knowledge as cardiovascular disease experts and their skills with cardiac catheterization and intervention to carry them through with "on-the-job" experience.

The successful operator should possess a core knowledge base (Table 1-2) that centers on a strong conceptual understanding of cardiac anatomy, physiology, and pathophysiology. Understanding the role of adjunctive imaging (e.g., computed tomography angiography [CTA], magnetic resonance angiography [MRA], transthoracic/transesophageal/intracardiac echocardiography) in patient assessment and procedural guidance is critical to preprocedural planning and procedural success. Core technical skills (Table 1-1) at a minimum should include adept skills with general catheterization laboratory techniques and close familiarity with transseptal left heart catheterization, intimate knowledge of catheter-based hemodynamic assessment, and interpretation as well as performance and interpretation of intracardiac ultrasound. Armed with these minimal core cognitive and technical skills, operators may then rely on simulation-based training and proctored procedures to gain proficiency in some SHD interventions. It is likely that, given the diversity of SHD interventions that range in complexity and frequency of occurrence, not all SHD interventional operators and SHD programs will gain sufficient experience to be proficient to perform all possible procedures. The range in complexity with SHD interventions will necessitate regionalization of more complex procedures (e.g., transcatheter valve repair/implantation or transcatheter perivalvular leak repair) to tertiary and quaternary medical centers, where procedural volumes will be higher for low-volume SHD procedures.

Assembling a Multidisciplinary SHD Team

The diversity that is present in SHD provides for varying levels of complexity in regard to potential SHD therapeutic interventions. Having a single disciplinary team led by the interventional cardiologist with an expertise in SHD interventions would be sufficient to complete a transcatheter closure of a noncomplex interatrial communication.

In contrast, a complex patient with symptomatic critical aortic stenosis and severe peripheral vascular disease who is a poor operative candidate and is being considered for transcatheter aortic valve implantation (TAVI) would be best served by a team of specialists across multiple disciplines. Cardiac and peripheral noninvasive imaging provided by an imaging specialist allow for careful planning in determining a transapical procedural approach. Transesophageal echocardiography preprocedure via the cardiac anesthesiologists allows for proper selection of prosthesis size and, when performed during the procedure, provides adjunctive imaging guidance. A collaborative effort between both interventional cardiologist and cardiac surgeon brings together complementary skills sets when performing the TAVI procedure. When performed in conjunction with cardiac anesthesia, an additional buffer of support is provided in the form of preprocedural, periprocedural, and postprocedural monitoring, thereby maximizing the chances of a favorable outcome. This multidisciplinary team approach works well in the procedure room, whether a catheterization laboratory or hybrid operating room (OR), and this relationship should be extended beyond these walls to include interdisciplinary conferences where differing viewpoints regarding clinical management can be voiced so that patients can be properly assessed in a manner that ensures appropriate patient selection for the procedure (Fig. 1-1). A multidisciplinary SHD team working in this fashion should serve as a model for other complex SHD interventions and is an essential component of a successful SHD program.

Creating and Maintaining an Environment for Conducting SHD Procedures

At a minimum, there are two essential components to creating an environment for a SHD program. The first deals with that of the physical environment. Ideally, these procedures should be performed in a space that

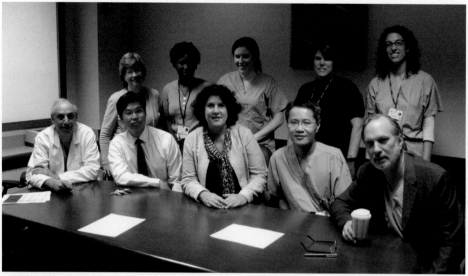

FIGURE 1-1.

The multidisciplinary transcatheter aortic valve implantation (TAVI) team meets weekly to review cases and discuss management of complex patients with aortic stenosis. Members include interventional cardiologists, cardiac surgeons, cardiac anesthesiologists, research nurses, clinical nurses, echocardiographers, and an administrative assistant. Both surgical and cardiology fellows often attend as well.

will accommodate not only the primary operators but also all ancillary support teams including the anesthetists, noninvasive cardiologists, cardiovascular perfusionist, surgical and catheterization ancillary staff, and their requisite equipment. The space should have the characteristics of a sterile OR, but also maintain the minimal X-ray equipment complement consisting of a single plane cine-radiographic unit with high-resolution digital video image processing capability with full hemodynamic monitoring such as can be found in a fully equipped catheterization laboratory; the so-called hybrid OR (Fig. 1-2).

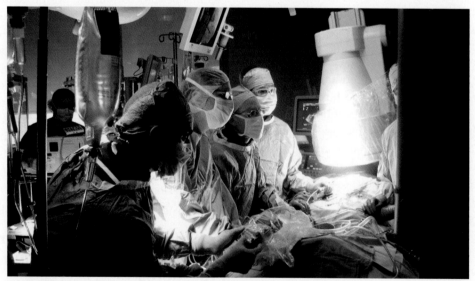

FIGURE 1-2.

Interventional cardiologists (IC) and cardiac surgeons (CS) working side by side in a hybrid operating room at the University of Pennsylvania performing a transcatheter aortic valve implantation. From left: Drs. Amr Bannan (IC), Joseph Bavaria (CS), Howard Herrmann (IC), and Wilson Szeto (CS).

The second essential component to creating an environment for an SHD program involves creating an "intellectual" environment to complement the physical environment. This "intellectual" environment represents academic and scholarly activity that is characteristic of most vibrant medical communities. This should include interdisciplinary clinical conferences, journal clubs, and clinical outcomes research. Interventional cardiologists and cardiac surgeons, adult and pediatric specialists, proceduralists, and noninvasive imaging experts must all acknowledge the need to learn from each other. These activities serve to refine our thinking by continually challenging our understanding of conventional clinical practice, ultimately driving innovation and advancement of the field.

Maintenance of Procedural Proficiency and Adaptation of New Technology

The field of SHD interventions is poised for future expansive growth as innovation continues to push the frontier of technology forward. As the technical knowledge base continues to expand, maintaining proficiency in current SHD procedures while adapting to new emerging techniques will be challenging. The volume-based standards employed to define training standards for coronary interventions are likely not to pertain to SHD interventions, as they tend to be low-volume procedures in general. It is likely necessary that SHD programs adopt practice patterns based on the hub-and-spoke distribution paradigm with smaller SHD programs on the periphery offering expertise in SHD interventions for the more common procedures while referring less common and more complex SHD interventions to the hub or central SHD program. This regionalization of care allows for proficiency to be maintained for low-volume and higher complex SHD procedures at larger SHD programs where larger procedural volume will allow for the development of expertise and likely improved clinical outcomes. As new potential therapeutic procedures become available, they will certainly create new methodological challenges; however, training in SHD interventions is likely to be a lifelong endeavor. A strong foundation rooted in the cognitive and technical core skills discussed in this chapter should allow for the basic skills to adapt to new technologies as they arise with the same "on-the-job" learning paradigm that has served the interventional cardiology community since its inception.

QUALITY MONITORING

The assessment of quality assurance (QA) for structured and valvular interventions is more difficult than for percutaneous coronary intervention (PCI) due to a number of unique aspects of this field. As described in this chapter, the knowledge base is distinct from coronary disease and not as routinely acquired during an adult cardiovascular fellowship. A specialized core curriculum that encompasses both pediatric and adult cardiology, as well as adult congenital heart disease, is required.[5] In addition, the volume for many procedures may be too low to use this as a surrogate for competency.[3]

Nonetheless, some analogies to PCI can be drawn. Operators should be assessed for clinical proficiency. This assessment includes cognitive knowledge, procedural skills, clinical judgment, and procedural outcomes.[6] For some of the most complex and technically demanding procedures that occur least commonly (e.g., ventricular septal defect and paravalvular leak closure), quantitative measure of success or experience are not possible. However, in this case, there may need to be a greater emphasis on basic technical skills, such as intracardiac or transesophageal echo and transseptal puncture, in order to ensure competency in the fundamental technical and knowledge skills necessary for successful completion of this procedure.

For PCI, a minimum number of procedures (e.g., ≥75/year, ≥400/lab) are often used to ensure adequate skills for either an operator or a laboratory. Similar thresholds could be developed for common structural and valvular interventions (e.g., atrial septal defect [ASD] closure and TAVI), or for the laboratory volume of a group of procedures. This may also be important for laboratory inventory issues and access to devices. For example, a facility that does less than 15 to 20 ASD closures per year will have difficulty maintaining both proficiency and adequate device size inventory to ensure adequate quality of procedural outcomes.

QUALITY IMPROVEMENT

The second aspect of quality monitoring requires a component of continuous quality improvement (QI). This is an organized scientific process for evaluating, planning, improving, and controlling quality in order to improve performance.[7] Catheterization laboratory directors need to develop variables to assess the quality of care. For structural and valvular interventions, these may include procedural successes or complications specific to these procedures. Examples might include tamponade during transseptal puncture, severe mitral regurgitation after balloon valvuloplasty, embolization of device during septal defect or leak closure, or need for a permanent pacemaker after alcohol septal ablation.

These variables for success and complications must be systematically collected prospectively. The key to successful QI also entails the provision of feedback to operators (or trainees) on solutions to any issues that are identified. In this regard, participation in registries for structural and valvular interventions will be essential for benchmarking of individual operator or laboratory results. Professional organizations including the ACC and SCAI should be encouraged to take the lead in the organization of such a registry. Hospitals will need to fund an adequate level of staff support to collect and submit outcome data.

In the future, it is conceivable that specific board requirements or certification will be developed for structural and valvular interventions, although there is presently little interest for this among operators or training program directors.[3] Due to the new core knowledge base for this field, the diversity of diseases, and the low frequency of interventions, the cardiovascular community will be challenged to devise new training standards, credentialing approaches, and QA and QI programs.

CONCLUSION

The field of interventional cardiology encompassed by SHD disease interventions is an exciting field that is evolving quickly. Although guidelines establishing standards for training and care are rudimentary, this advancing field offering new therapeutic options will drive the creation of clinical centers offering SHD interventions. We have attempted to provide guiding principles upon which clinical centers may draw in their attempts to build their own clinical SHD programs.

REFERENCES

1. Gruentzig AR. Transluminal dilation of coronary-artery stenosis. *Lancet.* 1978;1:263.
2. Gruentzig AR, Senning A, Siegenthaler WE. Non-operative dilation of coronary-artery stenosis: percutaneous transluminal coronary angioplasty. *N Engl J Med.* 1979;301:61–68.
3. Herrmann HC, Baxter S, Ruiz CE, et al. Results of the SCAI survey of physicians and training directors on procedures for structural and valvular heart disease. *Catheter Cardiovasc Interv.* 2010;76:E106–E110.
4. Hirshfeld JW, Banas JS, Cowley M, et al. American College of Cardiology training statement on recommendations for the structure of an optimal adult interventional cardiology training program. *J Am Coll Cardiol.* 1999;7:2141–2147.
5. Ruiz ER, Feldman TE, Hijazi ZM, et al. Interventional fellowship in structural heart and congenital heart disease for adults. *Catheter Cardiovasc Interv.* 2010;76:E90–E105.
6. Bashore TM, Bates ER, Berger PB, et al. American College of Cardiology/Society for Cardiac Angiography and Interventions clinical expert consensus document on cardiac catheterization laboratory standards. A report of the American College of Cardiology task force on clinical expert consensus documents. *J Am Coll Cardiol.* 2001;37:37:2170–2214.
7. Brindis RG. Quality of care in interventional cardiology. In: Topol EJ, ed. *Textbook of Interventional Cardiology.* 5th ed. Philadelphia: Saunders Publishers; 2008:1221–1240.

CHAPTER 2

Facilities: The Structural Heart Disease Interventional Lab and the Hybrid Operating Room

John D. Carroll* and Michael Mack

T his chapter explores what is needed in a facility to perform structural heart disease (SHD) interventions that include both a specialized cardiac catheterization laboratory (i.e., the SHD interventional lab) and a hybrid operating room (i.e., the hybrid OR). These novel facilities should be optimally designed, equipped, and staffed to perform these unique procedures and operations. Commercial technology is rapidly evolving to meet these new needs.

The SHD interventional lab and the hybrid OR are closely related but have a major difference: whether or not open surgical operations are routine or only rarely performed. In addition, the location of the hybrid facility may be within the operating theater or within the cardiac catheterization suites, and this will determine both the name and other uses of the room. This distinction between a specialized lab and specialized OR is at times clear, but the boundaries have become less distinct between the two worlds of interventional cardiology and cardiac surgery using these facilities. This shift away from past models of specialty focus is especially true with a new spirit of partnership between cardiology and surgery. A major professional evolution is occurring with cardiac surgeons acquiring catheter-based skills, image guidance technology and know-how, and the growth of new procedures, such as transapical valve implantation.[1]

GETTING STARTED

Building a facility to perform SHD interventions starts with a planning process that is much more involved than choosing imaging equipment. Table 2-1 outlines the key factors and steps that must be addressed in building both a hybrid OR and an SHD interventional lab. Furthermore, the reader is referred to Chapter 1 for advice and insights on program development.

The planning process must be site specific and may involve renovation versus building an SHD intervention facility as part of an entirely new hospital or tower. In addition, hospitals are undergoing major transitions in relevant technology such as the information technology infrastructure, expanding availability of multiple modalities of cardiovascular imaging, and co-location of procedure rooms, ORs, preprocedure preparation areas, postprocedure recovery areas, and intensive care units.

Facilities are filled with physicians, allied health professionals, staff, and managers who provide direct patient care and manage these facilities. SHD has seen the merging of old teams and the emergence of new teams of physicians and nurses bringing together a variety of skill sets and interacting in a new fashion in the evaluation of patients and the performance of SHD procedures and operations.[1-3] Table 2-2 presents the likely composition of the committees to plan and operate these facilities in most hospitals.

*Dr. Carroll receives research grant support, royalties, speaking, and consulting honoraria from Philips HealthCare.

TABLE 2-1 Getting Started: Key Factors to Address when Building a Hybrid Operating Room as well as an SHD Interventional Lab

1. Perform a formal needs assessment and strategic vision: Does your hospital really need these dedicated and often very expensive facilities?
   - Make a list of all the possible hybrid procedures and nonhybrid procedures that will be performed in the proposed facility.
   - Where will cases come from?
   - Formalize the business model in parallel to the clinical case for the facility.
2. Build consensus among potential physician users and clinical department heads: Are turf issues addressed?
3. Engage the hospital CEO and board.
   - Build your case, highlighting patient care and marketing advantages to hybrid procedures. Use the example of other successful programs such as vascular aneurysm volumes and revenue.
   - Gain support to diffuse department conflicts surrounding charging, scheduling, and productivity.
4. Motivate the directors and managers of both the OR and the cardiac catheterization laboratory. Their support, knowledge, and ability to adapt are key determinants of success.
5. Assemble hybrid teams utilizing staff from both OR and cath lab.
6. Obtain facility plans and involve the facility VP to understand structural limitation for room layout and design.
7. Understand your local and state certificate of need and other relevant regulatory issues.
8. Assess your infrastructure and support for multidisciplinary clinical trials and other postmarketing studies. What facility and staffing issues are relevant for this data collection?
9. Formulate an RFP to have competitive bids from multiple imaging and other vendors.
10. Plan on at least several site visits to learn the lessons others have discovered, the technologies they use, and see how their solution may or may not fit your needs.

CEO, chief operating officer; OR, operating room; RFP, request for proposal; VP, vice president.

THE PROBLEMS OF USING OLDER FACILITIES

Most interventional procedure rooms were designed and equipped in the coronary and vascular interventional era. As a result, the performance of SHD interventions in the traditional cardiac catheterization

TABLE 2-2 Key People: Members of the Hybrid OR and SHD Facility Planning and Oversight Committees

- An administrative leader, consensus builder, and problem solver
- Cardiologist
- Surgeon
- Anesthesiologist
- OR director
- Cath lab director
- Architect
- Construction project manager
- Facility plant manager
- Infection control manager
- Information systems manager
- Multiple OR vendor teams
- Representative from research group

laboratory has many challenges, as listed in Table 2-3. The nature of SHD interventions is very different from coronary and vascular interventions, and these differences are reflected in the facility needs.[4] Furthermore, the traditional OR does not function as a hybrid room by simply bringing in a portable fluoroscopy unit. The experiences of vascular surgery and interventional radiology in building hybrid rooms for other types of interventions have many parallels to the SHD facility issues.[5-7] Figure 2-1 demonstrates the dramatic changes in image quality and image guidance accuracy in performing transcatheter aortic valve implantation (TAVI) with old technology versus the appropriate newer technology.

WHAT IS UNIQUE ABOUT A FACILITY FOR SHD INTERVENTIONS?

Table 2-4 presents additional design variables and technology needs that should be considered when embarking in the process of building either an SHD interventional lab or a hybrid OR. Combining this list with Table 2-3 provides a checklist for the members of a planning team to consider and modify according to their local needs, strategy, and resources. We have tried to consider the facility needs to perform the

TABLE 2-3 Problems with Existing Facilities: The Challenges in Performing SHD Interventions in the Traditional Cardiac Catheterization Laboratory

- Imaging system
  - FD size too small
  - May lack DSA, rotational acquisition, and many other functions
- No convenient and radiation-safe place for anesthesiology and echocardiography teams
  - Especially with floor-mounted X-ray systems
- Lack of flexibility in room setup
  - Positioning of table, monitors, shields, lighting, and gantry
- No integration of ultrasound technology
  - TTE, TEE, vascular, transcranial Doppler, and ICE
  - Ultrasound not part of room configuration design, the image display monitors, tableside controls, and the archiving system
- Suboptimal image display
  - Small monitors
  - Limited visibility of monitors
    - Not seen well by others in the room including anesthesiology and echocardiography teams
- Room size inadequate
  - Multiple teams
  - Additional equipment including a heart-lung machine
- Storage space limited and inventory incomplete
  - Specialized supplies and equipment needed during SHD interventions
- Conversion to an open surgical operation difficult
  - Suboptimal level of sterility
    - Differing concepts of "sterile technique"
    - Air flow management
    - Personnel attire and access via control room and limited recognition of "red line"
    - Scrub sinks in-room
  - Lack of availability of anesthesia and pump equipment
  - Lack of availability of surgical supplies
  - Unfamiliarity of cath lab personnel with surgical processes and practices
  - Inadequate overhead lighting for surgical procedures

DSA, digital subtraction angiography; FD, flat detector; ICE, intracardiac echocardiography; SHD, structural heart disease; TEE, transesophageal echocardiography; TTE, transthoracic echocardiography.

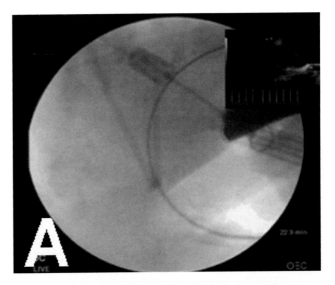

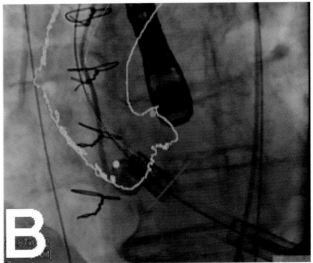

FIGURE 2-1.

The hybrid room needs state-of-the-art imaging systems. Transcatheter aortic valve implantation procedures performed with low-quality portable fluoroscopic imaging **(A)** and with high-quality flat detector fixed X-ray imaging system **(B)** that includes segmented computed tomographic angiography overlay. This comparison demonstrates the marked differences in image quality and the requirement for modern imaging applications.

broad array of procedures that are described in the rest of this book. In the future, the devices, the procedures, and the imaging guidance technologies will evolve, but the basic principles outlined here will hold for the most part.

THE ROOM: HOW TO PUT IT ALL TOGETHER

The Treatment Environment

Hospitals have become more patient-centric in the design of their facilities. Humanizing the treatment environment is not a matter of marketing but has an impact on the patient's experience and potentially their outcome. The SHD facility should likewise be

TABLE 2-4 Building the Best: Additional Unique Design and Other Features of SHD Intervention Room and Hybrid Operating Room

- Room size
  - SHD interventional lab: 600–800 sq ft
  - Hybrid OR: >800 sq ft
    - Rectangular shape
    - 10-ft ceilings
    - In-room storage cabinets for catheters and wires
    - Control room
    - Leaded walls
- Room layout considerations
  - Imaging equipment: C-arm/robotic arm/table movement and relationship with anesthesia location
  - Monitor booms: able to view by both the surgeon and cardiologist
  - Surgical lighting: free from overhead obstruction
  - Medical gases: combination of floor-, wall-, or ceiling-mounted
  - Perfusion equipment
- Room location
  - Proximity to ICU is more important than proximity to ED
- Advanced mechanical and rhythm support on-site
  - Percutaneous ventricular assist devices
  - Pacemaker units capable of high rates
- Invasive hemodynamic physiologic equipment
  - In-room display of results
  - Ability to compare pre- and postintervention data
  - Report generation with waveforms
- Multimodality image integration is the future: plan ahead
  - Robotic catheter control systems integrated into imaging systems
  - Magnetic resonance guidance
- IT infrastructure that addresses current and future needs
  - In-room information management, procedure planning tools, and tableside controls to optimize work flow
  - Interface with hospital EMR
  - Connections to external registries
  - Ability to transmit video of cases for conferences
- Supplies: How will they come into the space?
  - Model 1: The OR model: Per case supply delivery
  - Model 2: The cath lab model: Bulk supply delivery and large inventory stored in room

ED, emergency department; EMR, emergency medical response; ICU, intensive care unit; IT, information technology; OR, operating room; SHD, structural heart disease.

designed to reduce patient anxiety utilizing nonpharmacologic techniques via lightening, music, colors, and access to entertainment video. This is especially true in the interventional lab where most patients will be lightly sedated.

Room Size

Because of the multiple teams and the requirements of imaging, anesthesia, heart-lung bypass, and many other forms of equipment, the hybrid OR and the SHD interventional lab need to be large. Approximately 600 to 800 sq ft of working space is needed in the main room of an SHD interventional lab and over 800 sq ft is needed for a hybrid OR (Fig. 2-2). Both types of facilities need extra room for storage and for device preparation (Fig. 2-3).

The Operating Table

The table must have the flexibility and maneuverability of a traditional OR table for patient positioning yet also have the imaging capabilities of a cath lab table. Most manufacturers now have tables that do serve this purpose, but careful integration with the imaging equipment vendor is critical (Fig. 2-4).

Lighting for the Hybrid OR

The integration of lighting commensurate with typical OR requirements and the tracking systems for the imaging gantry is also a critical design and construction issue (Fig. 2-5).

Control Room

This room needs to have excellent visibility of the main room (Fig. 2-6). Ample room is needed for the recording equipment, workstations, and monitors as well as for the nurse or technician operating them. In addition, the nonsterile control room needs to have adequate space for the frequent internal staff as well as external visitors who are observing cases. The control room or another room immediately adjacent should also have image review stations that will allow the review of all imaging modalities. This is important for not only preprocedure planning but also during the actual procedure itself when there will be occasional need to review previously acquired studies.

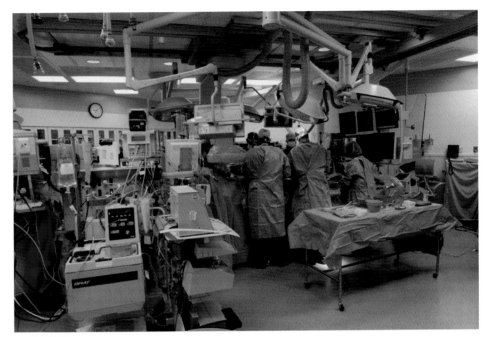

FIGURE 2-2.

This panoramic view of the hybrid operating room captures the complexity of the technology and the multiple people forming the team. Note the room available for all equipment and the rectangular shape; room size is 880 sq ft.

Conference Room

These procedures need careful planning by the entire team to allow execution of the procedure in the safest and most efficient manner. There must be a room where all parties can have a preprocedure review of upcoming cases and a rehearsal of the planned sequence of events and potential major challenges to be overcome. Postintervention debriefing sessions also are critical and the convenience of a room next to the SHD facility will maximize its use. In this conference room, all relevant patient data, including images, must be retrievable and displayed for the group.

IMAGING TECHNOLOGY FOR SHD INTERVENTIONS

Part 1: X-Ray Imaging

The X-ray system remains the workhorse imaging modality for many portions of SHD interventions. It is the most expensive equipment in the room, and

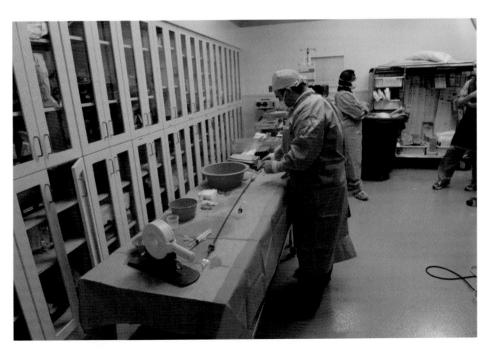

FIGURE 2-3.

The structural heart disease interventional lab and hybrid operating room must have ample in-room storage and space to allow for device preparation.

FIGURE 2-4.

The operating room table must be designed for both traditional open operations as well as image-guided procedures.

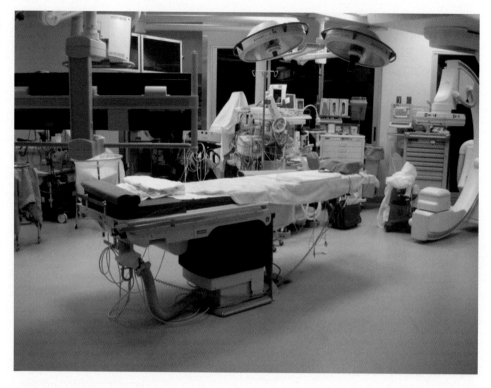

vendor selection is a central step in the planning process. Furthermore, the X-ray system, including the table, monitors, workstation, and tableside controls, is the major foundation around which the rest of the room is organized. Table 2-5 outlines the many considerations that should be considered in choosing an X-ray system.

The X-ray systems to perform percutaneous coronary work were not designed to accommodate anesthesiology and echocardiography teams often needed for SHD interventions. Specifically, the X-ray system commonly used was floor-mounted at the patient's head. This gantry location and its physical motions make it difficult for these teams to gain access to the patient for monitoring

FIGURE 2-5.

The integration of operating room lighting and the tracks for the imaging system is critical in the layout of the hybrid operating room.

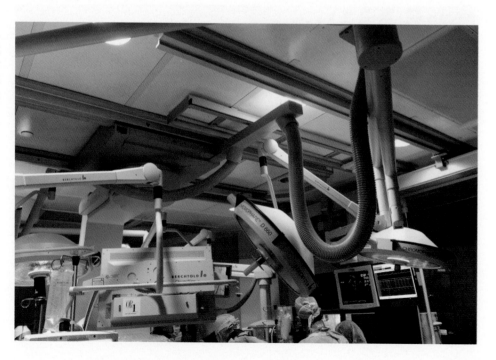

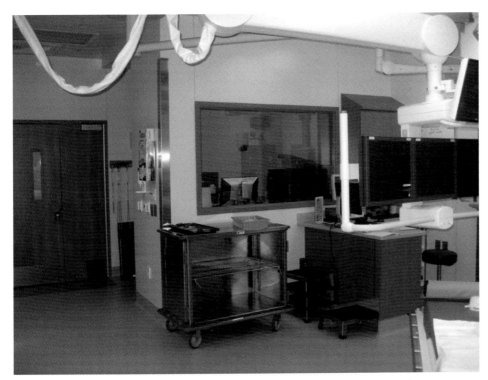

FIGURE 2-6.

The control room in the hybrid operating room is separated from the main room to provide radiation protection to the technologist.

and airway access. The hybrid coronary revascularization strategy and the use of completion angiography after coronary bypass grafting have provided experience in the integration of angiographic X-ray systems into a form of hybrid room specialized for coronary and vascular work.[8] Innovations in optimizing gantry position for coronary interventions provides the concepts and tools that can be adapted to optimizing gantry position for TAVI and other SHD interventions.[9,10]

X-ray systems with more flexibility in location and that can be moved are best for the SHD interventional lab and the hybrid OR (Fig. 2-7). The floor-mounted robotic arm has gained prominence due to this need for flexibility despite its higher cost.[2] These highly flexible systems allow positioning in angular, orbital, lateral, and longitudinal directions. Ceiling-mounted systems help in the ability to reconfigure the space to provide access to the patient. All systems do not totally eliminate the potential for collisions with staff. There have been some concerns that hygienic concerns may be different between floor-mounted and ceiling-mounted systems. The use of biplane X-ray systems is possible but clearly adds to the complexity of the room setup and operation. Biplane imaging has not proved to be particularly useful, rather quite cumbersome in adult SHD procedures. On the other hand, some pediatric centers have incorporated biplane systems into the hybrid OR design. These and other facility issues have been encountered with

the emergence of hybrid interventional strategies in congenital heart disease and are worthy of examination in planning adult SHD facilities for some hospitals.[11–14]

Part 2: Ultrasound Imaging

The most dramatic change that SHD interventions have brought to the therapeutic facility has been a fundamental shift in the imaging guidance modalities. Ultrasound has become a real-time image guidance technology for SHD interventions. Echocardiographic technology, especially real-time three-dimensional (3D), and professional societies are starting to adapt to this major area of growth and development.[15–20] In the traditional OR, there has been frequent use of transesophageal echocardiography immediately presurgery and postsurgery but not for actual image guidance of the operation itself. This is stimulating new interactions between anesthesiology and the cardiology echocardiology professional communities.

Ultrasound, in general, is now equal to X-ray in terms of importance and frequency of use for SHD interventions.[4,16] However, the type of ultrasound and the role of ultrasound vary in its utility based on the specific procedure being performed.[15] The use of ultrasound for different SHD interventions is covered in depth in Chapters 6 and 7, as well in the chapters focused on specific SHD interventions.

TABLE 2-5 The X-Ray System: Imaging Equipment Considerations

Images
- FD with large image formats
- Best image quality that is possible but with ability to easily choose low-dose/lower image quality for many procedures
- DSA and full peripheral interventional tool set
- Ability to image very obese patients
- Strongly consider single very large, programmable monitors for optimal display and, in the future, in-room decision support

Radiation
- Radiation doses relative to image quality
- Monitoring of doses
- Ability to store and archive fluoroscopic images
- Ability to collimate and use shields

Gantry performance
- Ability to achieve steep angles
- Flexibility of gantry position
- Rotational acquisition capabilities
- Ability to pan from head to toes
- Ease of isocentering

Table
- Maximum table weight at least 350–450 lbs with stability during CPR
- Full functionality as a surgical operating table
- Extra length to accommodate supplies and extra personnel at feet end
- Ability to tilt in all directions
- Ease of panning even with obese patients
- Removable arm boards
- Table-mounted contrast injection system

Computer imaging workstation
- Ability to import preprocedure CTA and MRA data, display, and register with fluoroscopy
- Three-dimensional reconstruction software from rotational images
- Software to simulate angiographic image in different gantry positions
- Software to calculate gantry positions for TAVI
- Consider currently EP mapping systems that may be adapted to SHD
- Device radiographic enhancement software: currently only for stents
- C-arm CT software upgrade capability for the future

Tableside controls
- User friendly controls for display monitors, X-ray system, and computer workstation applications
- Consider IVUS and OCT tableside systems

Ultrasound
- X-ray system features described here must have flexibility to accommodate integration of ultrasound into the room infrastructure

CPR, cardiopulmonary resuscitation; CTA, computed tomographic angiography; DSA, digital subtraction angiography; EP, electrophysiology; FD, flat detector; IVUS, intravascular ultrasound; MRA, magnetic resonance angiography; OCT, optical coherence tomography; SHD, structural heart disease; TAVI, transcatheter aortic valve implantation.

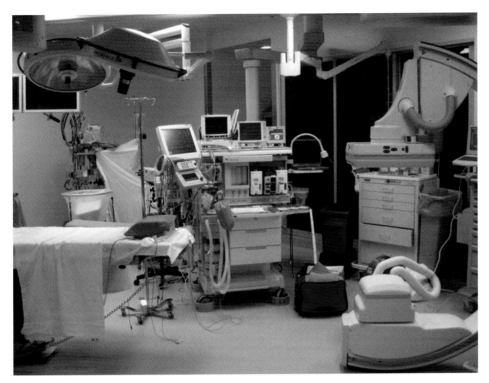

FIGURE 2-7.

Room layout and work flow are critical concerns in the hybrid room. Anesthesiologists bring their equipment to the hybrid room as well as the need for access to the patient. Note the placement of the equipment does not impede the movement of the X-ray gantry, which is shown rotated out of the working field.

From a facility design perspective, it is important to recognize this major shift in image guidance brought about by the SHD revolution in interventions. Multiple lessons have been learned in the recent years, including the following[20,21]:

- Both ultrasound and X-ray are used in most interventions, and the facility must allow simultaneous display for all parties.
- Implantable device and catheter technology have traditionally been designed to optimize image guidance by X-ray and this is changing.
- The target of most SHD interventions is soft tissue, and thus, ultrasound guidance is likely to increase further.
- Many SHD interventions are complex, and there is a need for a new level of precision of guidance and placement that translates to higher image resolution.
- Some SHD interventions require navigating delivery systems in "open" 3D space; that is, cardiac chambers, and using either two-dimensional (2D) X-ray projection or 2D echocardiographic cross-sectional images for completing these tasks is challenging. The field of view for ultrasound, even 3D, is limited such that large field navigation continues to be guided by X-ray.
- Ultrasound carries no inherent risk. In contrast, the risks of fluoroscopy are not insignificant for complex interventions.
- Both technologies continue to evolve and for ultrasound real-time 3D and new intracardiac

echocardiography (ICE) technology are likely to profoundly alter SHD image guidance and future facility, training, and equipment needs.

Transcatheter valve interventions represent the area with the most recent growth; therefore, these are discussed briefly in this chapter. The goal is to use two concrete examples of the determinants of image guidance technology needs that should be understood in designing new facilities.

Example 1: TAVI Guidance: Although transesophageal echocardiography (TEE) has a critical role in TAVI, fluoroscopy is still the predominant mode of imaging used for valve implantation. Numerous reports describe TAVI being performed under ultrasound guidance only to avoid contrast load in patients with impaired renal function, but because the implanted devices still have a significant X-ray signature, the use of ultrasound for deployment is still somewhat hampered. The use of 3D TEE for device placement in TAVI has not proven to be particularly useful for most groups. The current value of TEE for TAVI procedures is in the assessment of valve function and quantification of paravalvular leak immediately after valve implantation.

Example 2: MitraClip Guidance: The role of ultrasound for transcatheter mitral valve procedures, on the other hand, is central to the successful performance of the procedures. The use of not only 3D echo but also multiple plane imaging (i.e., two simultaneously displayed 2D ultrasound perspectives) significantly facilitates placement of the Evalve clip device. From the performance of the transseptal crossing to the perpendicular alignment of the clip to the mitral commissures to the assessment of device deployment and residual regurgitation, 3D echo is now the gold standard for transcatheter mitral valve procedures. The new smaller size TEE probes and 3D ICE catheters now in development will offer the ability for these procedures to be performed under local anesthesia and conscious sedation.

The now routine use of ultrasound guidance has revealed the lack of ultrasound integration in the procedure lab (Fig. 2-8). This is a similar history to the initial use of coronary intravascular ultrasound that required rolling in a specialized machine for each case that has now been replaced by integrated intravascular ultrasound (IVUS) systems using the procedure room monitor, tableside control, and plug-and-play imaging catheters.

The integration of ultrasound into procedure and ORs is a topic that is a key facility issue that is likely to rapidly evolve in the next several years. Integration has several levels and starts with the display of the ultrasound images on the procedure room monitors. This may require cables that are draped across the floor and then plugged into the back of the monitor block. More imbedded ultrasound units and connections are needed.

The second level of ultrasound integration is how the images are displayed in terms of perspective. Traditional ultrasound images could only be displayed from the perspective of the ultrasound array. Thus, transthoracic echocardiography (TTE) images produced images from the perspective of the chest wall and TEE images were from the esophageal perspective (e.g., the "surgeon's view" of the mitral valve). With the advent of 3D ultrasound imaging, the resultant volumetric data set can be reformatted to allow display in any perspective. Thus, despite the esophageal location of the TEE ultrasound probe, the mitral valve can be viewed from the left ventricular perspective. This ability to change the ultrasound perspective is a new feature and its impact on image guidance of SHD interventions is just starting to be appreciated and refined.

The third level of ultrasound integration is the ability to fuse or register ultrasound images with images from another modality. Registration with live fluoroscopy and with preprocedure acquired computed tomographic angiography (CTA) and MRI images are being explored.

The fourth level of ultrasound integration is in the control and manipulation of the images by the interventionalist or the surgeon. Currently, this control is in the hands of the echocardiographer or the anesthesiologist. The advent of catheter-based imaging of cardiac chambers and valves has arrived in the form of ICE. The use of ICE has already transformed the performance of many SHD interventions and further improvements are likely to further expand its use.

FIGURE 2-8.

The integration of ultrasound into the structural heart disease interventional lab is evolving. Shown here is an echocardiographer performing a transesophageal echocardiograph during an intervention. The room setup must be flexible to allow these procedures. Further improvements in ultrasound integration, radiation safety, and image display are needed.

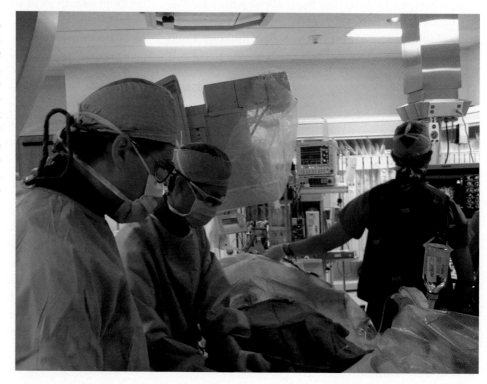

Part 3: Other Forms of Multimodality Imaging

Preprocedure CTA and magnetic resonance angiography (MRA) can now be imported, segmented, and registered in the SHD interventional lab.[20–24] As discussed in Chapter 5, the in-room use of the preprocedurally acquired CTA and MRI images can facilitate the performance of several different SHD interventions. The facility requirements for this advanced multimodality approach are several. First, there must be an image workstation that is part of the procedure room or hybrid OR. This workstation must be capable of accessing images from the CT and MR labs. The applications on the workstation should allow the CT and MR images to be manipulated and segmented to optimize their use for the intervention. The resultant images must be displayed in-room. Finally, the interface of the X-ray system must be such that coregistration of fluoroscopy and the CT and MR images is possible (Fig. 2-9). The resultant hybrid image is displayed in-room and allows the operator an enhanced level of visual guidance for certain interventions. Specific SHD clinical applications using CTA/MRA integration that have some clinical experience include transcatheter paravalvular leak closure, TAVI, pulmonary artery stenting, and septal defect closure.

Part 4: Vascular Access Imaging

Vascular imaging can involve all of the previously described modalities. Several of the new SHD interventions require very large catheters to be inserted, generally from the femoral artery or femoral veins. Some of the major complications in the transcatheter aortic valve implantation procedure using the femoral artery have been related to vascular access.

Vascular imaging capabilities are necessary for both the SHD procedure lab and hybrid OR. The X-ray system must have the ability to visualize down to the legs, must have digital subtraction angiography (DSA) and run-off capabilities, and the necessary image display capabilities like overlay to facilitate vascular interventions. Ultrasound is likely to be increasingly used to facilitate percutaneous access and allow immediate post-vascular closure results. Current vascular ultrasound technologies are separate and freestanding units that must be rolled in and rolled out of procedure rooms. It is expected that vendors will develop and sell more integrated units in the near term.

Part 5: Next Generation Angiography: Rotational Angiography and C-Arm CT Reconstruction

Careful consideration should be given in planning and outfitting an SHD procedure room or a hybrid OR with an X-ray system that has first generation applications or that can be upgraded to more advanced capabilities. The modern gantry system is capable of isocentric rotations during angiographic acquisitions that, by themselves, produce a 3D-like image for the

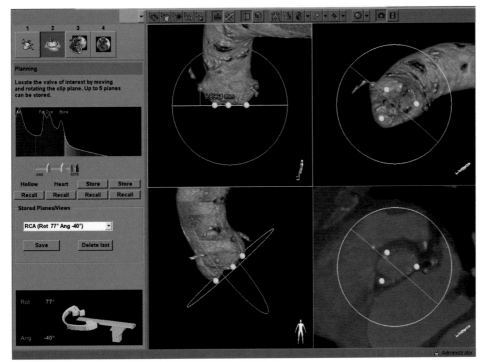

FIGURE 2-9.

Computer imaging workstations bring advanced applications to the hybrid operating room and structural heart disease interventional lab. Shown here is a three-dimensional reconstruction of the aortic root. This in-room application allows identification of landmarks defining the plane of the aortic valve that can be used to determine an optimal gantry position for valve deployment as part of transcatheter aortic valve implantation.

physician. Perhaps more exciting and potentially useful is the ability to take the rotational angiographic images and process them into a volumetric 3D or even four-dimensional (i.e., 3D plus time) reconstruction. The technology has been developed and used in early clinical feasibility studies focused on 3D reconstruction of coronary arteries and intracardiac devices.[25,26] Application of this C-Arm CT concept to cardiac chambers and the entire heart is an exciting next area of development that could profoundly impact SHD interventions as well as electrophysiology procedures.[27–30]

In brief, the flat detector mounted on the C-arm can function as a CT scanner providing imaging of contrast-filled as well as soft tissues (Fig. 2-10). Therefore, the SHD procedure room as well as the hybrid OR should optimally be equipped with systems that can perform rotational acquisitions and have the ability to be upgradable to the necessary software and image processing workstations associated with them. These capabilities are available now from multiple vendors for ungated reconstructions (i.e., XperCT, DynaCT, and InnovaCT), but they are inadequate for intracardiac work unless the heart is transiently arrested during image acquisition, as with rapid ventricular pacing.

In summary, the interventionalist and cardiac surgeon need to understand image guidance technology and the imaging needs in performing SHD interventions. In-depth understanding and clinical experience are necessary in order to optimally design and use the facility today, but also be prepared for major challenges in the next few years.

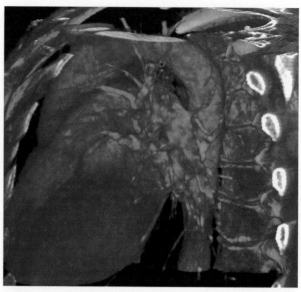

FIGURE 2-10.

The flat detector can be rotated around the patient to produce computed tomography–like images that potentially can be useful for structural heart disease interventions. This is a work-in-progress.

IMAGING DISPLAY

Given the fundamental reality that SHD procedures are image guided, the issue of how images are presented is very important. Monitor location in the crowded hybrid OR needs to be carefully planned (Fig. 2-11).

FIGURE 2-11.

Monitors display images and other important data for in-room use. The hybrid operating room and structural heart disease interventional lab need monitors placed so all members of the team have access to the information. In this photograph, note the multiple monitors and all operators looking in the same direction.

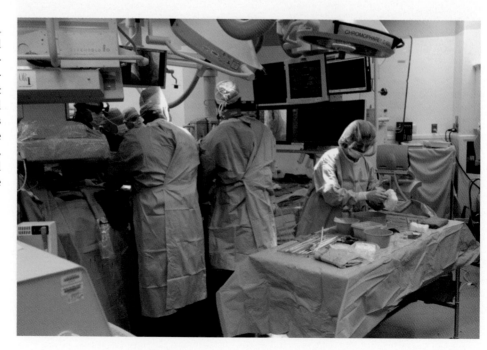

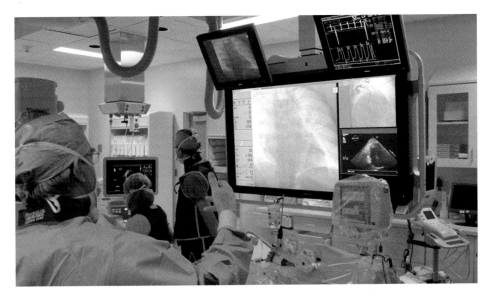

FIGURE 2-12.

Large flat display monitors bring added functionality to the structural heart disease interventional lab and hybrid operating room. They can be programmed to display different images from different sources. They have much higher resolution than home television technology. They also provide the means to display other information such as checklists, flow sheets for protocols, and instructions for use.

Monitor technology is undergoing a transition with very large monitors now available (Fig. 2-12) that produce very high resolution images, approximately 3,840 by 2,160 pixels. The next generation of large displays will have even higher spatial resolution. Monitors also must have flexibility in displaying large numbers of inputs (Fig. 2-13). This is especially important with SHD interventions using different imaging modalities and with the sequence of tasks to be performed requiring a different mix of fluoroscopy and ultrasound.

In addition, the large displays are especially useful when there are multiple teams and numerous individuals who need to see the images, hemodynamic, and other information being displayed. Older and smaller monitors were scaled primarily for the use of the single primary operator and required that operator to be within a few feet of the monitor. In the work of SHD interventions, there is a need for a display system with "no bad seats" for those working as a team. Finally, there are more futuristic image display technologies

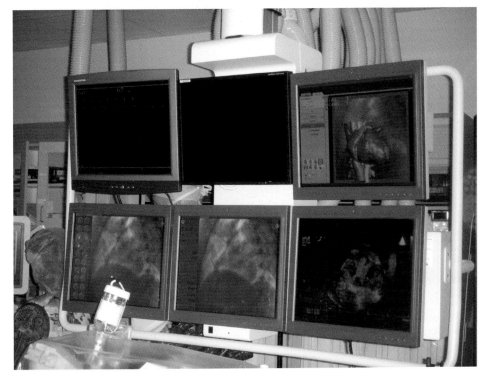

FIGURE 2-13.

Multiple modalities of imaging are needed in these new facilities. Here, a six-monitor bank shows live fluoroscopy, a road map, computed tomographic angiography overlay, three-dimensional transesophageal echocardiography, and hemodynamics.

including 3D holography that are under development and may have some special value to the performance of SHD interventions.

Image Archiving and Systems Integration

Images from the procedure must be archived automatically during and at the end of the case. Modern archiving systems are available from multiple vendors.

Angiographic Injectors and Contrast Management Systems

Integrated automatic contrast and saline injector systems have become common in cardiac catheterization labs and have replaced traditional manifold systems and separate stand-alone large volume, high-rate injectors for chamber visualization. These systems have multiple advantages including their integration to the procedure table, the reduced chance of air embolism, the ability to easily switch from one injection routine to another type (i.e., coronary angiography and left ventricular cineangiography), and the ability to precisely control injection rates, timing, and total volumes.[31] These capabilities of the automatic injectors are especially valuable when performing rotational angiography and peripheral angiography using DSA. They also will be needed in robotic catheter guidance systems.

HEMODYNAMIC ASSESSMENT IN THE SHD PROCEDURE LAB AND HYBRID OR

The traditional cardiac catheterization laboratory was the home of hemodynamic assessment that included the quantification of valvular abnormalities, cardiac function, and shunts (Fig. 2-14). The emergence of noninvasive assessment with echocardiography and Doppler slowly and almost completely transferred this function from the cardiac catheterization laboratory to the noninvasive arena. The performance of SHD interventions is now making an important impact on hemodynamic knowledge and skills in the procedure room. Not only are the noninvasive methods being applied during the intervention, but catheter-based hemodynamics are being brought back to aid in decision making during an intervention.

The facility for performing SHD interventions must therefore have capabilities for hemodynamic assessment. Staff must be thoroughly trained. The hemodynamic data must be displayed and integrated

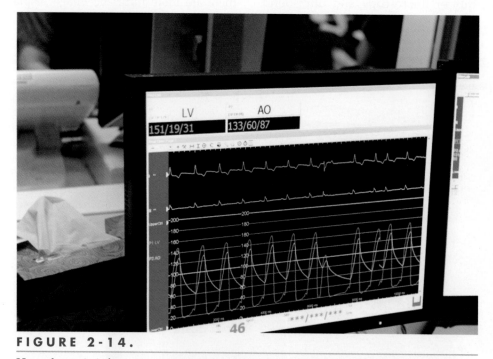

FIGURE 2-14.

Hemodynamic information is central to patient care in the structural heart disease interventional facility. This information needs to be displayed in-room with key measurements shown in a paired fashion before and after intervention.

with echocardiographic and Doppler data. All of these data and its analysis ultimately needed to end up in a report that is generated quickly and is presented in a form that effectively communicates the key findings.

OTHER INFORMATION TECHNOLOGY CONSIDERATIONS

Cardiac catheterization laboratory workflow was dramatically altered with the need to document in detail the procedure log, the inventory used, the medical team present, the radiation doses, contrast volumes, and a variety of specific metrics for monitoring quality. This led to the hemodynamic recorder becoming a computer-based recording of all details and variables of the case. The data are organized for the generation of a final report. Increasingly, certain data fields have become standardized to meet regulatory and quality of care reporting requirements. Cath-PCI is a national registry that requires data to be downloaded from the majority of sites in the US performing percutaneous coronary intervention (PCI). All these data functions will be needed in the SHD procedure room and hybrid OR.

It is expected that many SHD interventions will be monitored carefully for clinical and cost outcomes. It is likely that hospitals performing some of the next generation SHD interventions will be required to report results to national registries—either as part of device surveillances mandates, quality improvement initiatives, or registry design—to enable comparative effectiveness research. Planning and operating an SHD intervention room or hybrid OR must take into consideration these present and future needs in reporting. The SHD facility of the future will immediately and seamlessly download fields of text data, measurements, and images into a hospital emergency management system that connects to these national registries.

Another information technology infrastructure consideration in planning facilities for SHD interventions is the ability to transmit live or recorded cases. Many of these advanced rooms have been developed and continue to be planned for centers that have a regional, national, and international presence. In addition, it may be of interest for all institutions to have the ability to transmit cases internally for educational and training purposes. Therefore, it is key to install the appropriate video and transmission infrastructure. Retrofitting facilities for these capabilities is much more expensive than having infrastructure installed during the original build.

MANAGING RADIATION EXPOSURE

Both the SHD procedure room and hybrid OR have important issues related to radiation exposure to both the patient and also the staff and physicians. In the SHD procedure room, the staff and cardiologists theoretically should be knowledgeable to the basic principles of radiation and be practicing "as low as reasonably achievable" (ALARA). There is mounting concern that there has been inadequate attention to radiation safety during cardiac imaging, that there is an incomplete understanding of the risks, and that new efforts need to be instituted to reduce unnecessary radiation during medical imaging, including during image-guided interventions.[32–35]

Unfortunately, radiation safety awareness has been less than optimal, misconceptions are common (Table 2-6), and it has been shown that cardiologist are often unaware of the doses received by their patients.[36] Anesthesiologists and the echocardiography team are exposed to the highest doses of scatter radiation during many SHD interventions because of their proximity, the imaging systems, and also the frequent lack of movable shields that are standard for the cardiologist's location. In the hybrid OR, the surgeon may be close to the patient and X-ray system, especially during procedures such as transapical aortic valve implantation. Although radiation exposure times are less for transapical compared with transfemoral TAVI, the proximity of the operator to the radiation beam (especially with

TABLE 2-6 Radiation Myths: Radiation Falsehoods and Misconceptions for the SHD Procedure Room and Hybrid OR

- Radiation is not a major issue in the design and management of these new facilities
- High-radiation doses are generally due to old or poorly maintained equipment
- Modern flat detector systems have eliminated radiation concerns
- All patients and all procedures have a similar risk of radiation injury
- There is little the surgeon or cardiologist can do during an SHD intervention to reduce radiation risks

TABLE 2-7 Radiation Solutions: Key Items for Radiation Management in Designing and Operating Structural Heart Disease Procedure Rooms and Hybrid Operating Rooms

System Feature	Justification
Quantify and displaying in the room both real-time but also cumulative radiation doses to the patient. Notifying when high doses reached.	Older systems had no or minimal in-room display capabilities and focused on crude parameters such as fluoroscopy time.
Monitoring of radiation exposure to all medical personnel is essential and is optimal if available in real-time rather than the monthly or yearly report.	Feedback on radiation doses received/delivered in a timely and easy-to-understand format is part of building a team culture of radiation safety.
Shielding must be placed in locations to protect those closest to the patient and receiving the highest doses of scatter radiation.	Multiple new member of the SHD team need protection during procedures.
Patients at higher risk of radiation injury should be identified (i.e., obese and young patients), and those having procedures associated with potentially high radiation doses.	Radiation dose management, as contrast volume management, needs to be especially stressed when the risk of radiation injury is high.
Both cardiologists and surgeons need specific credentialing for the use of fluoroscopy and their practices must be monitored to ensure best practices are employed.	Operator techniques in minimizing radiation are well known but often not performed. Currently, there is no reporting of exposure data or other accountability, but this will change.

hands frequently exposed) leads to greater radiation exposure. In addition, shielding may be both cumbersome and be thought of as a potential compromise to sterility.

These are important issues in radiation safety that need to be recognized and approached for the SHD facility, as outlined in Table 2-7. New technologies to monitor real-time radiation exposure are now available (Fig. 2-15). Education and training in the principles and practices of radiation safety need to be

Fluo	**Normal**
Time	**2:19**
K̇	**100** ← Skin dose rate mGy/min.
	6 ← Safe working time min.
AK	**2096.65** mGy

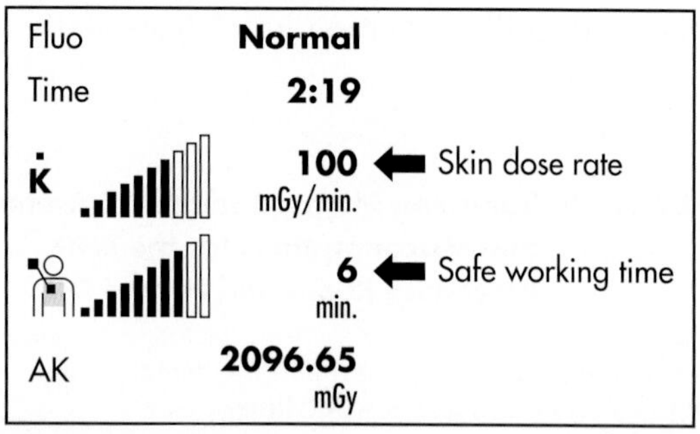

FIGURE 2-15.

Radiation monitoring is important in the hybrid operating room and structural heart disease interventional lab. Real-time display of data using realistic measurements of radiation dose are now available and will more routinely enter into in-room decision making as has occurred with monitoring of contrast volume, blood loss, and other traditional variables.

addressed in the facility planning process because these topics may be new to many on the SHD interventional team. Cardiac surgeons planning on a career including image-guided procedures need to be aware of the reported significant DNA damage in high-volume interventional cardiologists.[37,38]

CONCLUSION

This chapter provides a background on facility issues related to providing SHD interventional services. The facility issues include multiple unique requirements that have become apparent in the first decade of major growth in the type, diversity, and volume of SHD interventions. Two types of facilities have been discussed: the hybrid OR and the SHD interventional lab. A major caveat has been the dynamic nature of this field as new devices, new procedures, and new imaging guidance technologies become available (Fig. 2-16). The hybrid OR and the SHD interventional lab of the future are exciting to consider but major barriers exist and need to be overcome in the development, assessment of impact, approval, distribution, and effective use of new technologies.[39,40] These topics are also highly relevant to planning and building an SHD interventional facility today. These facilities are major investments and careful planning for today's needs is important.

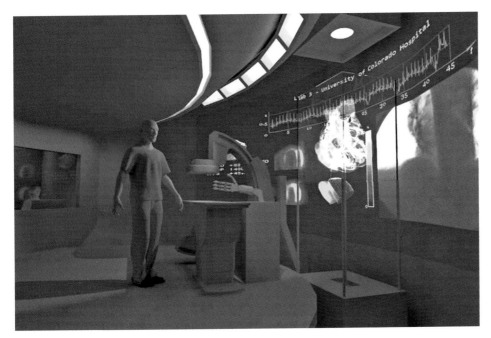

FIGURE 2-16.

The future interventional laboratory as well as hybrid operating room is expected to evolve with advances in image guidance, robotics, image display, decision support, and other technologies. (Futuristic lab rendering created by Adam Hansgen of the 3D Lab at the University of Colorado Denver.)

REFERENCES

1. Carroll JD. The evolving treatment of aortic stenosis: do new procedures provide new treatment options for the highest-risk patients? *Circulation.* 2006;114:533–535.
2. Nollert G, Wich S. Planning a cardiovascular hybrid operating room: the technical point of view. *Heart Surg Forum.* 2009;12(3):E125–E130.
3. Urbanowitz JA, Taylor G. Hybrid OR: is it in your future? *Nurs Manage.* 2010;41:22–26.
4. Carroll JD, Chen SYJ, Kim M, et al. Structural heart disease interventions: rapid clinical growth and challenges in image guidance. *Medica Mundi.* 2008;52:43–50.
5. Sikkink CJ, Reijnen MM, Zeebregts CJ. The creation of the optimal dedicated endovascular suite. *Eur Endovasc Surg.* 2008;35:198–204.
6. Cate G, Fosse E, Hol PK, et al. Integrating surgery and radiology in one suite: a multicenter study. *J Vasc Surg.* 2004;40(3):494–499.
7. Field ML, Sammut J, Kuduvalli M, et al. Hybrid theatres: nicety or necessity? *J R Soc Med.* 2009;102:92–97.
8. Zhao DX, Leachhe M, Balaguer JM, et al. Routine intraoperative completion angiography after coronary artery bypass grafting and 1-stop hybrid revascularization: results from a fully integrated hybrid catheterization laboratory/operating room. *J Am Coll Card.* 2009;53:232–241.
9. Chen SY, Carroll JD. 3-D reconstruction of arterial tree to optimize angiographic visualization. *IEEE Trans Med Imaging.* 2000;19(4):318–336.
10. Garcia J, Movassaghi B, Casserly I, et al. Determination of optimal viewing regions for X-ray coronary angiography based on a quantitative analysis of 3D reconstructed models. *Int J Cardiovasc Imaging.* 2009;25:455–462.
11. Galantowicz M, Cheatham JP. Lesson learned from the development of a new hybrid strategy for the management of hypoplastic left heart syndrome. *Pediatr Cardiol.* 2005;26:190–199.
12. Bacha EA, Daves S, Hardin J, et al. Single-ventricle palliation for high-risk neonates: the emergence of alternative hybrid stage I strategy. *J Thorac Cardiovasc Surg.* 2006;131:163–171.
13. Bacha EA, Marshall AC, McElhinney DB, et al. Expanding the hybrid concept in congenital heart. *Semin Thorac Cardiovasc Surg Pediatr Card Surg Annu.* 2007:146–150.
14. Hirsch R. The hybrid cardiac catheterization laboratory for congenital heart disease: from conception to completion. *Catheter Cardiovasc Interv.* 2008;71:418–428.
15. Hudson PA, Eng MH, Kim MA, et al. A comparison of echocardiographic modalities to guide structural heart disease interventions. *J Interv Cardiol.* 2008;21:535–546.
16. Silvestry FE, Kerber RE, Brook MM, et al. Echocardiography-guided interventions. *J Am Soc Echocardiogr.* 2009;22:213–231.
17. Kim M, Casserly I, Garcia J, et al. Percutaneous transcatheter closure of prosthetic mitral paravalvular leaks: are we there yet? *JACC Cardiovasc Interv.* 2009;2:81–90.
18. Eng M, Salcedo E, Quaife R, et al. Implementation of real time three-dimensional transesophageal echocardiography in percutaneous mitral balloon valvuloplasty and structural heart disease interventions. *Echocardiography.* 2009;26:958–966.
19. Salcedo EE, Quaife RA, Seres T, et al. A framework for systematic characterization of the mitral valve by real-time three-dimensional transesophageal echocardiography. *J Am Soc Echocardiogr.* 2009;10:1087–1099.

20. Carroll JD. The future of image guidance of cardiac interventions. *Catheter Cardiovasc Interv.* 2007;70:783.

21. Carroll JD. Dynamic imaging for structural heart disease interventions. *Cardiac Interventions Today.* 2008;2:65–68.

22. Garcia J, Eng MH, Chen SY, et al. Image guidance of percutaneous coronary and structural heart disease interventions using a computed tomography and fluoroscopic integration. *Vascular Disease Management.* 2007;4:87–89.

23. Garcia J, Bhakta S, Kay J, et al. On-line multi-slice computed tomography interactive overlay with conventional X-ray: a new and advanced imaging fusion concept. *Int J Cardiol.* 2009;133(3):e101–e105.

24. Wink O, Hecht H, Ruiters D. Coronary computed tomographic angiography in the cardiac catheterization laboratory: current applications and future developments. *Cardiol Clin.* 2009;27:513–529.

25. Neubauer A, Garcia JA, Messenger JC, et al. Clinical feasibility of a fully automated 3D reconstruction of rotational coronary X-ray angiograms. *Circ Cardiovasc Interv.* 2010;3:71–79.

26. Schoonenberg G, Florent R, Lelong P, et al. Projection-based motion compensation and reconstruction of coronary segments and cardiac implantable devices using rotational X-ray angiography. *Med Image Anal.* 2009;13:785–792.

27. Orlov MV, Hoffmeister P, Chaudhry GM, et al. Three-dimensional rotational angiography of the left atrium and esophagus—A virtual computed tomography scan in the electrophysiology lab? *Heart Rhythm.* 2007;4:37–43.

28. Thiagalingam A, Manzke R, D'Avila A, et al. Intra-procedural volume imaging of the left atrium and pulmonary veins with rotational X-ray angiography: implications for catheter ablation of atrial fibrillation. *J Cardiovasc Electrophysiol.* 2008;19:293–300.

29. Carroll JD. The death or the rebirth of the left ventriculogram? *Catheter Cardiovasc Interv.* 2009;73:241–242.

30. Glatz AC, Zhu X, Gillespie MJ, et al. Use of angiographic CT imaging in the cardiac catheterization laboratory for congenital heart disease. *JACC Cardiovasc Imaging.* 2010;3:1149–1157.

31. Messenger JC, Casserly I. Advances in contrast media and contrast injectors. *Cardiol Clin.* 2009;27:407–415.

32. U.S. Food and Drug Administration. Initiative to reduce unnecessary radiation exposure from medical imaging. Available at: http://www.fda.gov/radiation-emitting-products/radiationsafety/radiationdosereduction/ucm199904.htm. Accessed December 31, 2010.

33. Chen J, Einstein AJ, Fazel R, et al. Cumulative exposure to ionizing radiation from diagnostic and therapeutic cardiac imaging procedures: a population-based analysis. *J Am Coll Cardiol.* 2010;56:702–711.

34. Budoff MJ, Gupta M. Radiation exposure from cardiac imaging procedures: Do the risks outweigh the benefits? *J Am Coll Cardiol.* 2010;56:712–714.

35. Gerber TC, Carr JJ, Arai AE, et al. Ionizing radiation in cardiac imaging: a science advisory from the American Heart Association Committee on Cardiac Imaging of the Council on Clinical Cardiology and Committee on Cardiovascular Imaging and Intervention of the Council on Cardiovascular Radiology and Intervention. *Circulation.* 2009;119:1056–1065.

36. Gurley JC. Flat detectors and new aspects of radiation safety. *Cardiol Clin.* 2009;27:385–394.

37. Boyaci B, Yalcin R, Cengel A, et al. Evaluation of DNA damage in lymphocytes of cardiologists exposed to radiation during cardiac catheterization by the COMET ASSAY. *Jpn Heart J.* 2004;45:845–853.

38. Andreassi MG, Cioppa A, Botto N, et al. Somatic DNA damage in interventional cardiologists: a case-control study. *FASEB J.* 2005;19:998–999.

39. Chen SYJ, Hansgen A, Carroll JD. The future cardiac catheterization laboratory. *Cardiol Clin.* 2009;27:541–548.

40. Chen SYJ, Carroll JC. Coronary angiography: the need for improvement and the barriers to adoption of new technology. *Cardiol Clin.* 2009;27:373–383.

CHAPTER 3

Anatomy of Cardiac Valves for the Interventionalist

Thomas J. Helton and Samir R. Kapadia

With the expanding feasibility of structural interventions, in-depth understanding of the cardiac valvular anatomy has become an integral part of training. Understanding the gross anatomy and its correlation to the various imaging modalities is critical for successful application of knowledge in the catheterization laboratory. This chapter outlines the gross anatomy with fluoroscopy, computed tomography (CT), and echocardiography correlates to make the anatomy relevant to interventionalists. Some relevant pathologic anatomy findings in clinical context are also discussed.

GENERAL ORIENTATION OF THE VALVES

The heart is normally situated obliquely in the chest such that the interventricular and interatrial septa are approximately 45 degrees to the anteroposterior (AP) projection (Fig. 3-1). Therefore, a 45-degree left anterior oblique (LAO) projection will allow distinction of the left and right structures, whereas a 45-degree right anterior oblique (RAO) projection will discriminate anterior and posterior structures. The planes of the mitral and tricuspid valves are virtually at right angles to the septal plane, with some inferior tilt, and with the mitral plane situated slightly posterior to the tricuspid valve plane. In other words, LAO 45 degrees caudal 15 degrees may visualize the mitral and tricuspid valves en face,

whereas RAO 45 degrees caudal 15 degrees may provide one of the side views for these valves. The inflow and outflow of the left ventricle are aligned closely with an angle of 15 to 20 degrees in a normal heart, whereas the inflow and outflow of right ventricle are aligned almost at 90 degrees.

The aortic valve plane is typically tilted caudally and leftward, with the end on view being either LAO 60 degrees caudal 35 degrees or RAO 30 degrees cranial 45 degrees. Side views can be obtained with either RAO 20 degrees caudal 20 degrees to LAO 40 degrees cranial 30 degrees projections. The pulmonary valve is tilted quite posteriorly and to the right, such that the end on view can be obtained with LAO and steep (>45 degrees) caudal angulation and the pulmonary valve plane ranges from RAO cranial to lateral projections. The right ventricle wraps around the outflow of the left ventricle, being mostly anterior to the left ventricle, with only the inferior margin to the right of the left ventricle; the outflow tract of the right ventricle is superior and to the left of the aortic valve. The left atrium forms most of the posterior aspect of the heart as appreciated on lateral fluoroscopic views.

FIBROUS SKELETON OF THE HEART

Fibrous skeleton of the heart forms the base on which the valve leaflets are attached and, therefore, accurate anatomical understanding of this is critical for valvular

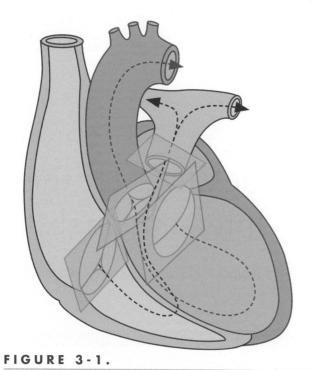

FIGURE 3-1.

Orientation of cardiac valve planes.

interventions. The mitral, tricuspid, and aortic orifices are intimately connected at a central fibrous body which is also referred to as right fibrous trigone. The annuli of the valves are not simple fibrous rings but are made up of fibrocollagenous elements of varying consistency from which the fibrous core of the cusps take origin. The aortic annulus is formed by semilunar attachments of the cusps in a crownlike fashion and lacks a true circular ring. The left fibrous trigone is the area closer to the anterolateral commissure of the mitral valve, and the right fibrous trigone is a central fibrous mass that is the confluence of the aortic, mitral, and tricuspid valves. Away from the central body, the fibrous skeleton becomes less robust with less discrete organization.

The pulmonary valve annulus is anterior and to the left of the aortic annulus and is connected to the same by another fibrous band referred to as the conus ligament. The anterior mitral leaflet is contiguous with the adjacent left and noncoronary cusps (NCCs) of the aortic valve, commonly referred to as the aortomitral curtain. Calcifications of the fibrous networks of the mitral and aortic annuli (mitral annular calcification [MAC]) are of critical importance to the outcome of transcatheter aortic valve implantation (TAVI) with respect to symmetric deployment of the valve and resultant perivalvular leak.

AORTIC VALVE

Gross Anatomy

Aortic Annulus

The aortic root is a complex and dynamic structure involving the interface of the aortic annulus, sinotubular (ST) junction, sinuses of Valsalva, the commissures of the aortic valve leaflets, and the leaflets themselves. Anatomically, the annulus is typically considered as the semilunar lines of attachment of the aortic valve leaflets to the aortic sinuses. However, when measurements of the aortic annular diameter are made, the aortic annulus is measured often times at the hinge points of the valves. These two definitions obviously have important differences and implications in clinical practice. As the aortic leaflets are attached to the aortic root in crown-shaped manner, three triangular areas (trigones) are created in between three cusps in the part of the aorta that extends below the aortic valve.[1] The trigone between the left and noncoronary sinus is contiguous with the anterior leaflet of the mitral valve. The trigone between the noncoronary and the right cusp is contiguous with the membranous septum. The remaining trigone between the two coronary cusps attaches to the muscular septum.

The aortic root is often described as resembling a crown that is transected by three horizontal planes.[1] The top of the crown, represented by an imaginary plane that transects the ring-shaped ST junction in a horizontal fashion, is formed by the peripheral attachments of the aortic valve leaflets near the commissures. The base of the crown is a virtual plane, formed by horizontal transection of the basal attachments of the aortic valve leaflets.[1] Between these two planes exists the true anatomic aortoventricular junction forming the third imaginary horizontal plane of the aortic root (Fig. 3-2). It is important to note that these planes are not necessarily parallel to each other due to the fact that there is reflection of left and right coronary cusp (RCC) over the muscular septum.

Traditionally, the aortic annulus is measured along the virtual basal plane of the crown, in the left ventricular outflow tract (LVOT) at the inferior most aspect of the aortic valve leaflet hinge points (Fig. 3-2), in the parasternal long axis or apical five-chamber views by two-dimensional (2D) transthoracic echocardiography (TTE).[1] The aortic annulus can also be measured by transesophageal echocardiography (TEE) in the 125- to 140-degree long-axis view of the left ventricle. This measurement is taken from the inner edge of the septal endocardium to the inner edge of the anterior leaflet of

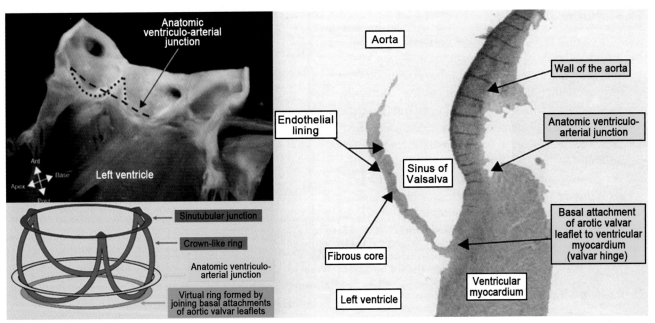

FIGURE 3-2.

Aortic annulus, ventriculo-arterial junction, and "virtual crown." (Modified from Piazza N, de Jaegere P, Schultz C, et al. Anatomy of the aortic valvar complex and its implications for transcatheter implantation of the aortic valve. *Circ Cardiovasc Interv.* 2008;1[1]:74–81.)

the mitral valve at the hinge point of the aortic valve leaflets in midsystole.[2] There are several important points about the measurement of the annulus. The annulus is not circular and, therefore, different modalities that measure different planes of the annulus do not necessarily yield same results.[3] When the largest diameter of annulus is measured by 2D methods (typical for TEE or TTE), special care has to be taken to get the maximal diameter because symmetric opening of the leaflets (where typically the views are obtained) does not necessarily provide the largest diameter (Fig. 3-3).[4] In addition to measuring the aortic annulus or LVOT dimensions, measurements of the ST junction and the ascending aorta are also important.

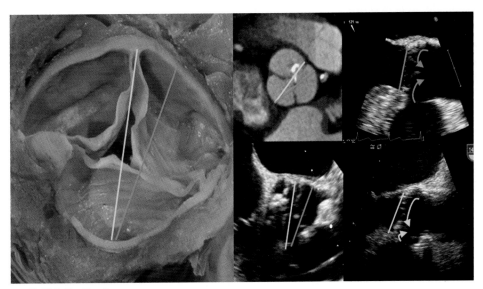

FIGURE 3-3.

Correlative pathologic, cardiac computed tomography, and echocardiographic measurements of the aortic annulus. The *yellow line* represents the correct measurement, whereas the *green line* represents common erroneous ■ measurements.

Sinotubular Junction

The ST junction is a circular ridge of fibroelastic tissue that provides an anchoring mechanism for the aortic valve by serving as a peripheral attachment zone for the fibrous connections of the leaflets. Anatomically, the ST junction marks the transition point from the aortic root to the ascending aorta. Severe calcification of the ST junction can be problematic for balloon-expandable TAVI. If the calcification is circumferential and the ST junction diameter is smaller or comparable to the diameter of the annulus, there is some risk of "watermelon seeding" of the balloon in the ventricular direction at the time of valve deployment. Precariously, this can lead to severe aortic insufficiency or even valve embolization into the left ventricle.

Sinuses of Valsalva

Bound distally by the ST ridge and proximally by the attachment of the aortic valve leaflets, the sinuses of Valsalva are expanded portions of the aortic root that are interconnected by a network of fibrous triangles and function to provide support to the aortic valve. There are three sinuses of Valsalva, each named for the coronary artery to which it is associated: right coronary, left coronary, and noncoronary. A unique aspect of the noncoronary sinus is that it rests on the interatrial septum. This relationship has several implications for the interventionalist. When doing a transeptal puncture, visualization of this sinus by contrast injection or catheter placement in the sinus is critical to avoid puncturing the aorta. The fossa ovalis and patent foramen ovale (PFO) are located directly posterior to the noncoronary sinus. If the aorta is dilated, and there is a large Eustachian valve, this can result in torsion of the intra-atrial septum effectively tenting open the PFO, leading to platypnea-orthodeoxia. Another important aspect of this relationship is that the pericardial reflection does not extend to the bottom of the noncoronary sinus; however, the upper region between the NCC and intra-atrial septum can be intrapericardial. Therefore, accidental puncture in the aorta in this region can lead to tamponade, whereas a puncture of the aorta in the lower aspect of the sinus can often be treated conservatively, if only the needle entered the aorta and the hole has not been dilated.

Leaflets

The aortic valve is normally comprised of three semilunar leaflets or cusps of nonuniform size that are attached peripherally to the aortic root at the level of the ST junction by crescent-shaped fibrous bands of tissue. Functionally, these leaflets separate the aorta from the left ventricle during ventricular diastole. Each leaflet derives its name from the associated coronary artery that arises near the cusp: RCC, left coronary cusp (LCC), and NCC. The leaflets are attached to each other for a very short segment at their bases and these areas of attachment form apposition lines referred to as commissures.

Anatomic Relationships

The anatomic relationships of aortic valve to the vascular and conduction system have become even more important to the interventionalist in the current era of TAVI. The aortic valve is the fundamental centerpiece of the heart with respect to the other valves. Positioned behind the pulmonic trunk and infundibulum, the aortic valve lies anteriorly between the tricuspid and mitral valves (Fig. 3-4). Because of this rather unique juxtaposition, deployment of a percutaneous aortic valve in a suboptimal location (more ventricular) can have untoward effects on the neighboring valves, especially the mitral valve.

The relationship with coronary ostia is also crucial; the ostia of the coronary arteries typically arise in the superior margin of the sinuses of Valsalva immediately below the ST junction. Some variation in the origin of the ostia of the coronary arteries is well described; the most common variance is that the ostia arise more than 2 mm below the ST junction in 10% of the population.[5] This can be problematic for percutaneous valve deployment if the skirt of the percutaneous valve or, more commonly, the native leaflet of the aortic valve covers the ostia of the coronary artery.[6] The native leaflet is more likely to close the lower origin of the left main coronary artery when it arises from the center of the cusp rather than its typical location, which is from the posterior aspect of the left sinus at variable distance from the noncoronary leaflet attachment. As the left coronary artery courses anteriorly behind the pulmonary artery, the ostium of the left main may assume a funnel-like configuration in the aorta with the superior and posterior aspects being more proximal and the posterior inferior aspects being more distal.

Careful consideration should be given prior to stenting the left main trunk in patients intended to have a TAVI. In the absence of beveled stents, the inferior aspect of left main stent often extrudes into the aortic lumen. It is conceivable that a percutaneously placed valve may crush the native valve leaflets against a protruding left main stent. If left main percutaneous

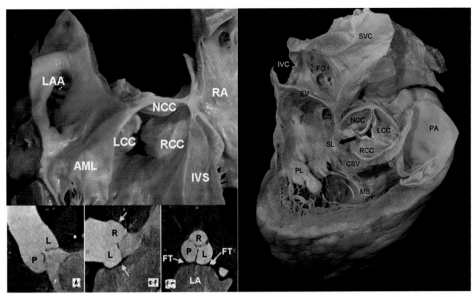

FIGURE 3-4.

Top: Human heart specimens looking from the posterior aspect with right-side oriented to the right of the picture. Note the septal leaflet of the tricuspid valve and its relation to the membranous septum (*black arrow*) and the aortic valve is continuous with the anterior leaflet of the mitral valve.

Bottom left: Computed tomography scan image demonstrating the aortoventricular continuation. The right leaflet as it rests on the interventricular septum has an "attachment" to the aortic tissue (*yellow arrow*) that is distinct from the "hinge point" of the leaflet (*red arrow*). Conversely, the left and noncoronary leaflets have these points in close proximity (*yellow* and *red arrow*). To the right, the heart opened by removing the right ventricle, which shows anterior relations of the aorta. AML, anterior mitral leaflet; CS, coronary sinus; CSV, coronary sinus vein; EV, Eustachian valve; FO, fossa ovalis; FT, fibrous trigone; IVC, inferior vena cava; IVS, interventricular septum; L, left coronary cusp; LA, left atrium; LAA, left atrial appendage; LCC, left coronary cusp; MB, moderator band; NCC, noncoronary cusp; P, posterior or non-coronary cusp; PA, pulmonary artery; PL, posterior leaflet; R, right coronary cusp; RA, right atrium; RCC, right coronary cusp; SL, septal leaflet; SVC, superior vena cava. (Modified from Agarwal S, Tuzcu EM, Rodriguez ER, et al. Interventional cardiology perspective of functional tricuspid regurgitation. *Circ Cardiovasc Interv.* 2009;2[6]:565–573.)

intervention is undertaken in such patients, precise stent placement to avoid "hanging out" into the aorta is paramount. Shallow LAO or AP cranial projections (instead of the typical LAO caudal or AP caudal views) may be useful to allow conservative stent positioning.

In addition to a low origination of the coronary ostia in the aortic sinus, other characteristics that increase the risk of left main occlusion during percutaneous valve implantation are related to size and calcification of the native valve. Large native valve leaflets near the origin of the left main and bulky calcification of those leaflets increase the likelihood of left main compromise during these procedures as result of the leaflets being plastered over the ostium of the left main. Aortomitral continuity via the intervalvular fibrous skeleton allows complete straightening of the left coronary leaflet, hence, potentially placing the left coronary ostium at a higher risk. The right coronary artery does not have these same exposures, because the interventricular septum anchors the right

coronary leaflet, thereby limiting the upward movement of the leaflet. On the contrary, surgical aortic valve replacement more commonly compromises the right coronary artery. This may be related to the fact that, during surgical implantation, the prosthetic valve is placed on top of the interventricular septum and, therefore, comes in close proximity to the right coronary artery, particularly if the septum is hypertrophied and angulated.

Conduction system disturbances are also common during percutaneous valve implantations especially with the self-expanding longer valves—with some series reporting a 20% to 30% incidence of permanent pacemaker implantation as a result.[7] Anatomically, this reflects the close proximity of the atrioventricular (AV) node to the interventricular septum. The AV node lies in the apex of Koch's triangle in the right atrium near the membranous septum and gives rise to the bundle of His, which traverses the membranous septum in the subaortic region to become the fascicles of the left bundle. Fascicles of the left bundle course between the right and NCC cusp of the aortic valve in the interval-vular fibrous triangle making it particularly vulnerable to disruption with placement of a percutaneous aortic valve, especially when a self-expanding valve is placed lower in the LVOT.[8]

Pathologic Anatomy

Three basic types of aortic stenosis (AS) are recognized: (1) degenerative calcific aortic stenosis, (2) congenitally bicuspid aortic stenosis, and (3) rheumatic aortic stenosis. Degenerative calcific aortic stenosis is present in approximately 2% to 3% population over the age of 65 and approximately 4% of patients over the age of 85.[9] Nearly one-third (29%) of patients have calcific aortic sclerosis without stenosis.[9] Degenerative calcific aortic stenosis represents the majority of patients over the age of 70 undergoing traditional aortic valve replacement. Congenitally bicuspid aortic stenosis is the most common etiology of aortic stenosis in younger patients and has been reported to occur in 1% to 2% of the population. The hemodynamic perturbations associated with the bicuspid fusion of leaflets in combination with fibrillin-1 deficient microfibrils are responsible for the premature loss of the structural integrity of the valve as well as premature degeneration of the aortic media.[10] As such, bicuspid aortic stenosis is often associated with dilatation of the aortic root and aneurysm formation. These patients typically present in their fifth and sixth decade of life with symptomatic aortic stenosis, with or without a dilated aortic root, and present a unique challenge for percutaneous valve therapy. Large annular diameter, dilated aortic sinuses, and eccentric leaflet calcification often translate into suboptimal candidacy for TAVI. Even crossing the bicuspid valve can be difficult in these patients, an AL-1 catheter and a straight 0.35-inch wire can be used to accomplish this occasionally arduous task. If the left coronary leaflet is involved in the fusion (left-right or left-non) an RAO projection is often helpful in crossing these valves, whereas a traditional LAO projection is most useful for crossing valves with fusion of the right and noncoronary leaflets.

Fluoroscopic Anatomy

Pivotal to performing TAVI and other structural heart interventions is a fundamental understanding of fluoroscopic anatomy. Two basic views commonly used for fluoroscopic imaging of the aortic valve are RAO 30 degrees and LAO 60 degrees. In the RAO view,

the RCC is the most anterior located cusp (closest to the anterior wall of the left ventricle); conversely, the NCC is the most posterior located cusp (closest to the inferior wall of the left ventricle) (Fig. 3-5). The LCC lies between the NCC and RCC in the RAO projection. Conversely, in the LAO projection, the LCC is well visualized (closest to the lateral wall of the ventricle), whereas the NCC and RCC are superimposed on one another with NCC lying slightly below RCC (Fig. 3-5).

Achieving a uniform alignment of the coronary cusps for TAVI typically requires slight caudal angulation for the RAO view and slight cranial angulation for the LAO view (Fig. 3-5). Fluoroscopy is also important for recognizing other important anatomic

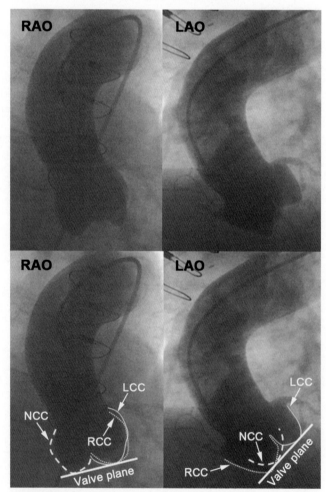

FIGURE 3-5.

Aortic root angiography and alignment of the aortic valve plane for transcatheter aortic valve implantation. Views are LAO 40 degrees with 20 degrees cranial and RAO 20 degrees with 20 degrees caudal. LAO, left anterior oblique; LCC, left coronary cusp; NCC, noncoronary cusp; RAO, right anterior oblique; RCC, right coronary cusp.

considerations for TAVI such as curvature of the aortic arch, aortic valve calcification (AVC), calcification of the ST junction, as well as aortoiliac calcification and diameter, and movement of equipment through the aortoiliac system.

CT Anatomy

CT conventions for interrogating aortic valve have not been formalized; however, the anatomic assessment of the aortic valve has become a standard practice prior to TAVI. Several anatomic issues can be addressed by CT scanning, including severity and location of calcification, anatomy of the aortic valve (bicuspid, etc.), annulus diameter with accurate minimal and maximal diameter measurements,[11] ST junction assessment, plane of aortic annulus,[12] location of coronary ostia (as previously described), and aortic valve area.

Age-related degenerative changes in the aortic valve are those of progressive calcification and fibrosis (intrinsic and extrinsic cusp calcification).[13] Two patterns of calcification have been described: (1) coaptation pattern calcification occurs along the line of cusp coaptation; and (2) radial pattern calcification occurs as spokes of a wheel, spreading from the peripheral cusp attachments toward the center. However, in advanced stages, the calcification pattern becomes unidentifiable.[14]

AVC can be scored by cardiac CT. In studies quantifying AVC by electron beam CT (EBT), it has been determined that a high calcium score correlates with severity of aortic valve stenosis.[15–18] Contrast enhanced electrocardiography (ECG)-gated multidetector row CT (MDCT) decreases motion artifacts, resulting in better characterization of aortic valve morphology.

Bicuspid aortic valves are present in 1% to 2% of the population and are the second most common etiology of aortic stenosis. Fusion of the left and right cusp is the most frequent morphologic change resulting in a bicuspid valve; fusion of right and NCCs is the second most common pattern of fusion. These structural changes in the bicuspid aortic valve straighten the line of lateral attachment, thereby limiting the mobility of the valve and subjecting the valve to hemodynamic perturbations that facilitate premature degeneration and calcification of the valve.

In addition to evaluation of the aortic valve, many other parameters are ascertained during the acquisition of cardiac CT that are routinely used in planning a TAVI: aortic dimensions, diameter of the aortic annulus, and ST junction. Likewise, ECG-gated MDCT allows accurate evaluation of aortic valve leaflet motion and measurement of aortic valve area (AVA) with good correlation with TEE.[19,20]

AVA assessment by TEE and MDCT is primarily that of planimetry of the aortic, whereas the continuity equation is used for assessment by TTE. TEE and MDCT evaluate anatomic valve area instead of effective area, which is instead evaluated by TTE. Therefore, AVA measured by TEE and MDCT is larger than that measured by TTE.[21–24] Although there is no dearth of data supporting the validity of MDCT in evaluating aortic stenosis, it is not used routinely, except in those being evaluated for TAVI, because of limitations such as radiation exposure, heart rate variability, chronic kidney disease, and contrast dye allergy.

Echocardiographic Anatomy

Echocardiography provides excellent temporal and spatial resolution for investigating not only the anatomy but also the function of the aortic valve. Identification of various anatomic relationships in different transthoracic and transesophageal views is critical for planning and image guidance of structural interventions. Two-dimensional TTE is the most commonly used tool for assessing the severity of aortic valve stenosis. This can be accomplished by planimetry of the valve, measuring the peak transvalvular velocity and the peak and mean pressure gradients across the valve.[25] Peak pressure gradient can be calculated from the peak velocity by the Bernoulli equation ($\Delta P = 4V^2$ [ΔP is pressure gradient, V is flow velocity in m/s at the site of obstruction]). AVA can also be estimated by use of the continuity equation and Doppler-derived transvalvular velocities in conjunction with anatomic measurements of the LVOT (AV area is cross-sectional area of LVOT*LVOT VTI [velocity time integral]/aortic valve VTI).[2]

In the presence of aortic valve regurgitation (AR) or significant left ventricular (LV) dysfunction, measuring aortic valve gradient alone is inadequate to determine the severity of aortic stenosis. In these situations, AVA should also be measured because the continuity equation is reliable even in presence of aortic and mitral insufficiency and independent from transaortic flow.[26]

Many indices have been investigated for determining the severity of AS, namely, dimensionless index, jet width at the aortic valve level, valve resistance, percent LV stroke work loss, and modified ventricular-vascular coupling. However, none of these adjunctive measures have proven to be more reliable than transvalvular gradient, AVA, and jet velocity. As such, current guidelines define the severity of aortic stenosis based on these parameters[2]:

1. Mild AS: AVA >1.5 cm^2; mean gradient <20 mm Hg; jet velocity <3.0 m/sec
2. Moderate AS: AVA 1.0–1.5 cm^2; mean gradient 20–40 mm Hg; jet velocity 3.0–4.0 m/sec
3. Severe AS: AVA ≤1.0 cm^2; mean gradient >40 mm Hg; jet velocity >4.0 m/sec

The dimensionless index is the ratio of the systolic velocity flow in the LVOT to the systolic velocity integral in the aortic jet and may be useful in the setting of severe LV dysfunction. Dimensionless index <0.3 is consistent with severe AS and has a high sensitivity and specificity for diagnosis severe AS.[27] Not surprisingly, TTE has limitations; poor acoustic windows and severe calcification of mitral and aortic annulus may lead to inaccurate measurement of LVOT diameter and AV gradients translating to erroneous calculations of aortic valve area.[28] Nonparallel interrogations of jet velocity may lead to underestimation of the severity of stenosis[29] because of the higher central velocity of aortic flow through the valve. In the presence of mitral regurgitation (MR), irregular heart rhythms, or subvalvular or supravalvular stenosis, transvalvular velocities can be overestimated.[30] Low cardiac output or significant LV dysfunction may lead to underestimation of AS severity.[2]

MITRAL VALVE

Gross Anatomy

The mitral valve apparatus is a very complex structure with the annulus, leaflets, chordae, and papillary muscles being the integral parts for proper functioning (Fig. 3-6).

Annulus

The annulus of the valve is more than a simple fibrous ring, but is made up of fibrocollagenous elements of varying consistency from which the fibrous core of the cusps take origin. These variations allow major changes in the shape and dimension of the annulus at different stages of the cardiac cycle. The annulus is strongest near the commissures at the left and right fibrous trigones. Extending from the fibrous trigones, the anterior and posterior coronary prongs (which are tapering fibrous subendocardial tendons) partly encircle the orifice at the AV junction. Between the tips of the prongs in the posterolateral aspect there is a thinner sheet of deformable fibroelastic connective tissue. Spanning anteriorly between the trigones is a fibrous subaortic curtain that descends from the adjacent halves of the left and NCCs of the aortic valve to the anterior mitral leaflet.

The mitral annulus is saddle shaped with the part near both commissures being more ventricular and the part supporting middle parts of the leaflets being more atrial,

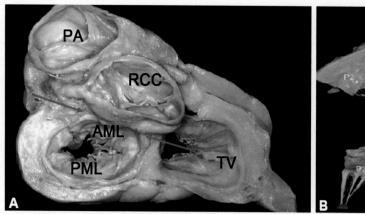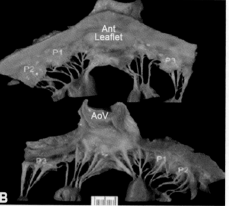

FIGURE 3-6.

Anatomy of the mitral valve. **A:** The cephalad view of the base of heart after removal of the atria. The aortic valve is central in location. The anterior leaflet of the mitral valve is a direct continuation of the part of left and noncoronary cusp of the aortic valve. The *red arrows* indicate the right and left fibrous trigone. **B:** The leaflets are dissected out to show the span of anterior and posterior mitral leaflets. The attachments of the chordae and the relation of papillary muscles to the commissural area are also well delineated. AML, anterior mitral leaflet; AoV, aortic valve; P1, first scallop of posterior mitral leaflet; P2, second scallop of posterior mitral leaflet; PA, pulmonary artery; PML, posterior mitral leaflet; RCC, right coronary cusp; TV, tricuspid valve. (Reprinted from Kapadia SR, Schoenhagen P, Stewart W, et al. Imaging for transcatheter valve procedures. *Curr Probl Cardiol.* 2010;35:228–276, with permission from Elsevier.)

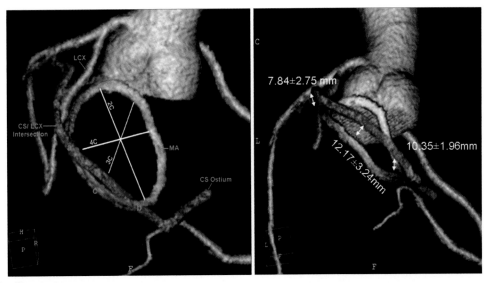

FIGURE 3-7.

Reconstructed 3-dimensional image of mitral annulus (MA), coronary sinus (CS), coronary arteries, and aorta. (*a*) Mitral annulus diameter in four-chamber view (4C), (*b*) Mitral annulus diameter in two-chamber view (2C), and (*c*) mitral annulus diameter in three-chamber view (3C). All MA to CS measurements obtained in two-dimensional images. LCX, left circumflex coronary artery. (Reprinted from Choure AJ, Garcia MJ, Hesse B, et al. In vivo analysis of the anatomic relationship of coronary sinus to mitral annulus and left circumflex coronary artery using cardiac multidetector computed tomography: implications for percutaneous coronary sinus mitral annuloplasty. *J Am Coll Cardiol.* 2006;48[10]:1938–1945, with permission from Elsevier.)

giving it a saddle-shaped appearance (Fig. 3-7). The relationship of the annulus to coronary sinus is of particular importance due to potential devices that can modify annular shape and size. The coronary sinus opens in the right atrium just behind and to the right of the posteromedial commissure of the mitral valve. If one traces the coronary sinus more proximally, it runs on the atrial side of the mitral annulus with 0.5 to 1 cm of distance between the two. As the mitral annulus flattens in patients with severe MR, this distance increases. Anterolateral commissure of the mitral valve is close to where the anterior cardiac vein becomes the coronary sinus.

The annulus area of the mitral valve is approximately 8 cm^2 in men and 6.5 cm^2 in women. The circumference is 10 cm and 9 cm, respectively. The AP diameter is about 4 cm and the commissural diameter is about 5 cm. The annulus can be divided in the anterior and posterior part by the commissures. The anterior part of the annulus is related to the left ventricle, left fibrous trigone, left coronary sinus, noncoronary sinus, right fibrous trigone, and the interventricular septum, from the lateral to medial direction. The posterior commissure is related to the interventricular septum and then the free wall of the left ventricle going from medial to lateral direction. The intertrigonal part of the annulus is relatively fixed, whereas the lateral part of the annulus is the most mobile. The annulus supports the attachments of LV myocardial fibers that arrange from a

right-hand helix in the subendocardium to a left-hand helix in the subepicardium creating a wringing effect on the ventricle, essentially pulling down the annulus with each ventricular systole.

Leaflets

The anterior leaflet is a larger leaflet encompassing a third of the circumference of the annulus with few or no marginal indentations. The leaflet is attached to the left and right fibrous trigone on either side and continues up to the aortic valve and aortomitral curtain. Near the tip of the leaflet there is a deep, crescentic, rough zone on the ventricular side where chordae tendineae are attached. The ridge demarcating the proximal margin of the rough zone indicates the maximal extent of surface coaptation zone. The anterior leaflet does not have basal zone because it forms the smooth boundaries for the ventricular outlet. Segmentation of the anterior leaflet is artificial with different parts of the leaflet demarcated as A1, A2, and A3 from lateral to medial corresponding to similar segments of the posterior leaflet (Fig. 3-6).

The posterior leaflet, although shorter, encompasses larger circumference (two-thirds) of the annulus. The posterior leaflet has two indentations delineating three scallops: a relatively large middle scallop and smaller anterolateral and posteromedial commissural scallops. Each scallop has a crescentic, opaque, rough zone, and receives the attachments of the chordae on its ventricular aspect. This rough area, which is larger than the comparable area on the anterior leaflet, identifies the area of apposition of the leaflets. From the rough zone to within 2–3 mm of its annular attachment, there is a membranous clear zone devoid of chordae. Contrary to the anterior leaflet, the basal 2–3 mm of the posterior leaflet is thick and vascular and receives basal chordae.

Chordae Tendineae

True chordae of the mitral valve may be divided into commissural chordae, rough zone chordae, and basal chordae. Most true chordae divide into branches from a single stem soon after their origin from the apical one-third of a papillary muscle, or proceed as single chordae that divide into several branches near their attachment. Basal chordae are solitary bands passing from the ventricular wall to the base of the posterior leaflet. In the majority of hearts, the chordae support the entire free edges of the valvular cusps. As the chordae originate in a fanlike shape from the papillary muscles, their density is higher in the subcommissural area. This is important to recognize because the percutaneous clip can get tangled in the chordae more easily in the commissural area than in the middle of the valve. Further, the lack of basal chordae on the anterior leaflet allows one to pass catheters in the ventricular side of leaflets in the subannular space, which is important for percutaneous direct annuloplasty. False chordae, chordae that are not inserted into the valve leaflet, occur in about 50% of left ventricles and often cross the subaortic outflow. Their role, if any, is yet to be determined.

Papillary Muscles

There are two papillary muscles with large variation in the size, shape, and location. The anterolateral muscle arises from the anterolateral free wall of the myocardium and the posteromedial from the inferior wall. The posteromedial muscle is frequently U-shaped or with multiple heads. The anterior papillary muscle usually has one head. Chordae tendineae arise mostly from the tip and apical one-third of each muscle, but sometimes take origin near their base. The chordae from each papillary muscle diverge and are attached to corresponding rough zone on both leaflets. The anteroapical displacement of the papillary muscle can lead to systolic anterior motion of the mitral valve, thereby leading to LV outflow obstruction. The anterolateral muscle has dual blood supply, whereas the posteromedial muscle gets single blood supply from the right coronary artery making it more vulnerable to rupture, leading to severe MR postmyocardial infarction. Global LV dilatation as seen in dilated cardiomyopathy displaces the papillary

muscles apically, causing symmetric tethering of the mitral leaflets leading to central malapposition and central MR. On the other hand, inferior myocardial infarction can cause increased tension in the chordae arising from the posteromedial commissure leading to posteriorly directed MR that can originate more medially, sometimes approaching the posteromedial commissure. Posterior annuloplasty may work better for this type of situation than with apical tethering. Further, clipping may be difficult if the funnel-shaped regurgitant orifice extends up to the posteromedial commissure.

Pathological Anatomy

Mitral Stenosis

Anatomy of mitral valve in rheumatic mitral stenosis is very important to distinguish from that calcified mitral stenosis from extension of annular calcification in the leaflets. Rheumatic process affects the tips and commissures causing thickening and restriction of the tips. Further, there is fibrosis and shortening of the chordae. Balloon mitral valvuloplasty works well in patients with severe symmetric commissural fusion with minimal calcification and relatively well-preserved subvalvular apparatus. In patients with nonrheumatic mitral stenosis, balloon valvuloplasty does not work because balloon dilatation cannot mobilize the leaflets. Similarly, when the subvalvular fibrosis is severe with significantly shortened chordae (anterior chordae with less than 8 mm length from the tip of the mitral valve to the papillary muscle), commissural separation with balloon valvuloplasty will not be able to release the leaflet enough for good long-term success. These observations have led to the description of several anatomic scores to predict balloon mitral valvuloplasty outcomes.[31–33]

Mitral Regurgitation

Anatomic or functional abnormalities of any of the structures in the mitral valve apparatus may lead to MR.[34–36] The disease process leading to MR may be a primary mitral valve disease, secondary regurgitation resulting from another cardiac disease, or mitral valve involvement in a systemic inflammatory disease.

Various terminologies are used to characterize the mechanisms of MR. The morphologic description, proposed by Carpentier, classifies the mechanism of regurgitation according to leaflet pathophysiology.[37,38] Type I regurgitation occurs in the presence of normal leaflet motion and is usually caused by annular dilatation or leaflet perforation. Type II is caused by leaflet prolapse, which is commonly the result of degenerative (myxomatous) disease, chordal elongation or rupture, or papillary muscle elongation or rupture. Type III is due to restricted leaflet motion, which may be due to posterior wall motion abnormality or papillary muscle dysfunction from ischemic cardiac disease, or commissural fusion and/or leaflet or chordal thickening from rheumatic heart disease. This simplification has utility in terms of both the surgical and percutaneous approaches because the goal of therapy is to restore normal leaflet function, but not necessarily normal valve anatomy.

Another common method of categorizing MR is based on the etiology and mechanism of MR. This classification is commonly used in literature to study the clinical outcomes of patients. In this classification scheme, MR is divided loosely based on an abnormal ("primary") or normal ("secondary") MR: degenerative or rheumatic disease (primary MR), and functional or ischemic disease (secondary MR). Of note, the terms functional, ischemic, and secondary MR are often used interchangeably and may represent many different mechanisms and morphologic variants. Degenerative disease includes Barlow's disease (myxomatous degeneration) and fibroelastic deficiency, both of which can result in MR leaflet prolapse and MR. Fibroelastic deficiency is the most common etiology to present for surgical mitral valve repair, representing approximately 70% of the US surgical population. MR in rheumatic disease is a result of leaflet deformity due to severe calcification and apical leaflet doming. Although this is a common cause of MR worldwide, it is less frequently encountered in the United States.

Functional MR occurs in the setting of LV dysfunction and is seen in patients with coronary artery disease (ischemic MR) or in patients with dilated cardiomyopathy from other causes. Ischemic MR results from decreased closing force and increased tethering force on the leaflets.[39] Various factors can decrease closing force including diminished LV ejection fraction, LV dyssynchrony, and diminished annular motion and, similarly, many factors increase tethering forces like papillary muscle displacement, LV remodeling, annular dilatation, and so forth. It is becoming increasingly clear that there is tremendous interaction of ventricular, valvular, and annular factors in generation, perpetuation, and progression of "functional" MR.

Fluoroscopic Anatomy

Orientation of the leaflets of mitral valve is best imagined by knowing the commissures in every projection. The anterolateral commissure is near the left anterior descending artery ostium and the posteromedial commissure is close to the origin of the posterior descending artery. The RAO view shows the anterolateral commissure on the

top and the posteromedial commissure on the bottom; both the anterior and posterior leaflets are superimposed and lie in the middle (Fig. 3-8). The relation of anterior mitral leaflet to the NCC of the aortic valve is also appreciated in this view. Anterior and posterior papillary muscles are well visualized in systole during ventriculogram.

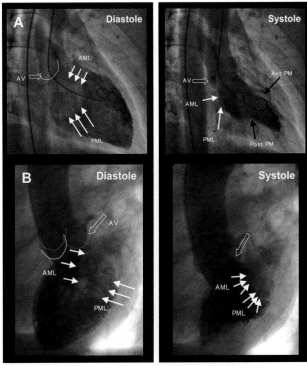

FIGURE 3-8.

A: Right anterior oblique (RAO) 30-degree view of the left ventricle in diastole and systole. The aortic valve (*open arrow*) with three leaflets (right coronary cusp [RCC], blue lines; noncoronary cusp [NCC], white lines; and left coronary cusp [LCC], red lines), mitral valve (*solid white arrow*), and the papillary muscles (*solid black arrows*) are shown. In diastole, mitral valve is open and there is clearance of contrast as the blood enters the left ventricle from left atrium. Anterior and posterior leaflets are seen separate in diastole (*left panel*). In systole, mitral valve is closed and aortic valve is open (*right panel*). In this view anterior, apex, and the inferior walls can be assessed. **B:** Left anterior oblique (LAO) 60-degree view of the left ventricle in diastole and systole. *Open arrow* shows the aortic valve with three leaflets (RCC, blue lines; NCC, white lines; and LCC, red lines), *solid white arrow* shows the mitral valve, and the *black arrows* point to the papillary muscles. In diastole, mitral valve is open and there is clearance of contrast as the blood without contrast enters the left ventricle from left atrium. Anterior and posterior leaflets are seen separate in diastole. In this view, the lateral and the septal walls can be assessed. AML, anterior mitral leaflet; Ant PM, anterolateral papillary muscle; AV, aortic valve; PML, posterior mitral leaflet; Post PM, posterolateral papillary muscle. (Reprinted from Kapadia SR, Schoenhagen P, Stewart W, et al. Imaging for transcatheter valve procedures. *Curr Probl Cardiol.* 2010;35:228–276, with permission from Elsevier.)

The LAO view gives appreciation of the mitral annulus and the circumference of anterior and posterior leaflets. Different segments (A1, A2, A3 and P1, P2, P3) of the leaflets are well appreciated in this view. The relation of the papillary muscle to the leaflets is also well delineated. The LVOT is well seen in this orientation, although some cranial angulation may help to eliminate foreshortening of the outflow tract. Relation of the mitral annulus to the different structures is well appreciated in this view.

Echocardiographic Anatomy

For imaging of the mitral valve, two important planes can be visualized at 0 degree, one in the mid esophagus and the other in the transgastric location.

The correlation of these views to the fluoroscopic anatomy is shown in Figure 3-9. The mid esophageal 0-degree view provides a four-chamber view of the mitral and tricuspid valves. The relation of interatrial septal puncture site or septal devices to the mitral valve can be best assessed in this view. When the TEE probe is advanced to the transgastric location with flexion, a short-axis view of the left ventricle at the mitral valve level can be obtained. This view is critical for evaluating the mitral valve in short axis, which can be very helpful in several mitral interventions (e.g., commissure evaluation during mitral valvuloplasty, assessing the orientation of clip in relation to valve coaptation line during MitraClip procedure). The

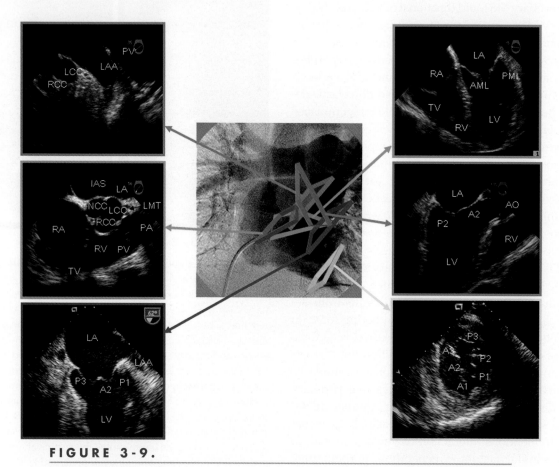

FIGURE 3-9.

Fluoroscopic image of the heart and corresponding transesophageal electrocardiography images are shown. Mitral and aortic valve details are outlined. A1, first scallop of the anterior mitral leaflet; A2, second scallop of the anterior mitral leaflet; A3, third scallop of the anterior mitral leaflet; AML, anterior mitral leaflet; AO, aorta; IAS, intra-atrial septum; LA, left atrium; LAA, left atrial appendage; LCC, left coronary cusp; LMT, left main trunk; LV, left ventricle; NCC, noncoronary cusp; P1, first scallop of the posterior mitral leaflet, ; P2, second scallop of the posterior mitral leaflet; P3, third scallop of the posterior mitral leaflet ; PA, pulmonary artery; PML, posterior mitral leaflet; PV, pulmonic valve; RA, right atrium; RCC, right coronary cusp; RV, right ventricle; TV, tricuspid valve. (Reprinted from Kapadia SR, Schoenhagen P, Stewart W, et al. Imaging for transcatheter valve procedures. *Curr Probl Cardiol.* 2010;35:228–276, with permission from Elsevier.)

orientation of different segments of mitral leaflets is shown in Figure 3-9. When the transducer is rotated at 40 to 60 degrees, and the probe is advanced to the mid esophageal level, mitral valve commissural views can be obtained. In this view, A2 is typically located in the middle of the LV inflow with P1 and P3 on each side. Figure 3-9 shows the aortic long-axis view that is typically obtained at the mid esophageal level with 120-degree rotation. As the probe is pulled up, the interatrial septum can also be visualized. Anterior and posterior leaflets (typically A2 and P2) are seen in this view, although rotating the probe from side to side can allow interrogation of the entire mitral valve apparatus.

Biplane TEE is at times very helpful when devices are being advanced into the left atrium. Three-dimensional (3D) TEE has significantly improved the ability to visualize the valve from the "surgeon's view." This reconstruction, as one looks at the short-axis view of the mitral valve from the esophagus, is very helpful to visualize the exact segment of the mitral valve that is prolapsing and the orientation of the device in relation to pathology.

CT Anatomy

Because of limited temporal resolution of CT, TEE is certainly superior in identifying the mechanism of MR and defining anatomic details of the leaflets with motion; however, CT can provide very useful information. Radiation doses increase when high-resolution images are obtained. It is easier to measure annular size with CT because of the possibility to reconstruct mitral annular plane from a 3D data set. Further, one can assess restriction and tenting of each part of the mitral apparatus, which may be very critical to determine precise mechanism of MR in patients with functional MR.

CT provides a unique opportunity to study the mitral annulus and its relation to the surrounding structures (Fig. 3-7). The relation of the mitral annulus to the coronary sinus can be easily investigated by MDCT. However, due to limited temporal resolution, the relation of mitral annulus to coronary sinus in different phases of cardiac cycle can be difficult to determine. There is no standard method to measure this distance; however, two-, three-, or four-chamber views can be used to determine this distance. It may be important to measure the angle between coronary sinus plane and the mitral annulus. This angle may provide some insight into the direction of pull of the device in the coronary sinus to the mitral annulus. Despite these measurements, the success of a device can still be difficult to predict from CT prior to procedure.[40] Qualitative assessment to judge the calcification of the mitral annulus is also very

important if placement of coronary sinus (CS) devices is planned. Typically, significant calcification can be considered a relative contraindication for this approach.

TRICUSPID VALVE

Annulus

Not unlike the mitral valve, the tricuspid annulus derives its support from the fibrous skeleton of the heart (right AV ring as opposed to the left AV ring). The tricuspid valve is made up of a fibrous core that attaches to the base of the heart via the supportive network of fibrocollagenous tissue of the right AV ring. In healthy population, the tricuspid annulus has an ellipsoid and nonplanar morphology appearing somewhat saddle-shaped in configuration. The highest point of the annulus is in the anteroseptal segment in close proximity to the right ventricular outflow tract (RVOT) and the aortic valve. The lowest point of the annulus is the posteroseptal segment, which is closer to the right ventricular apex. Interestingly, this geometry changes in patients with severe functional tricuspid regurgitation. As the severity of tricuspid regurgitation increases, the annulus takes on a more planar and circular configuration as the anteroposterior distance increases disproportionately to the septal-lateral distance and the vertical axis decreases.[41,42] Unlike the mitral annulus, the tricuspid annulus does not contract independently, thus making it potentially more susceptible to the function of the periannular myocardium.[43] Additionally, the fibrous skeleton supporting the annulus is not as extensively anchored in the periphery as the mitral annulus, which in turn allows it to be more malleable in regard to remodeling.

Leaflets

As implied by the name, the tricuspid valve consists of three cusps (leaflets), each named in accordance to its location with reference to the right ventricle (anterior, posterior, and septal) (Fig. 3-10). Typically, the anterior cusp is the largest, extending from the septum medially along the anterior margin of the AV groove terminating at the commissure of the posterior leaflet. Originating at the posteroseptal commissure of the posterior wall of the right ventricle, the septal leaflet traverses both the muscular and membranous septum to terminate at the anteroseptal commissure. Spanning the distance between the anterior and septal leaflets is the posterior cusp.[43] Together, these cusps are anchored to the ventricular myocardium through chordal attachments to the papillary muscles (trabeculae carneae). Although the posterior

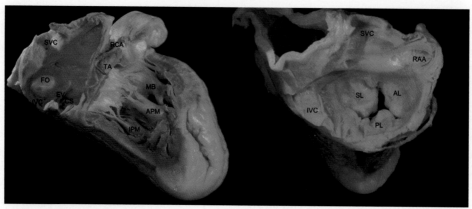

FIGURE 3-10.

Anatomy of the tricuspid valve and the valvular apparatus. The anterolateral wall of right ventricle and right atrium is removed to demonstrate tricuspid valve attachment to the ventricle. The relation of tricuspid annulus to the right coronary artery is visualized. Interatrial septal relations with superior vena cava (SVC), inferior vena cava (IVC), and the coronary sinus (CS) are clearly visualized. AL, anterior leaflet of tricuspid valve; APM, anterior papillary muscle; EV, Eustachian valve; FO, fossa ovalis; IPM, inferior papillary muscle; MB, moderator band; PL, posterior leaflet of the tricuspid valve; RAA, right atrial appendage; RCA, right coronary artery; SL, septal leaflet of the tricuspid valve; TA, tricuspid annulus. (Modified from Agarwal S, Tuzcu EM, Rodriguez ER, et al. Interventional cardiology perspective of functional tricuspid regurgitation. *Circ Cardiovasc Interv.* 2009;2[6]:565–573.)

and septal walls of the right ventricle occasionally have chordae tendineae that arise directly from the myocardium to anchor their respective cusp.[44]

Chordae Tendineae

The right ventricle has three papillary muscles, named according to their location of origin in the right ventricle. Arising from the lateral aspect of the anterior wall of the right ventricle, beneath the anteroposterior commissure, the anterior papillary muscle is the largest and most consistent in origin. Conversely, the posterior papillary muscle arises from the posterior aspect of the right ventricle inferior to the posteroseptal commissure and morphologically is often bifid or trifid. Typically, the septal papillary muscle is the most inconsistent in origin and often has associated chordae that arise directly from the myocardium. Another unique aspect of the right ventricle is the presence of the septomarginal trabeculae (moderator band); the moderator band is a muscular ridge that connects the anterior wall of the right ventricle to the interventricular septum carrying with it the right bundle branch fibers of the conduction system.

Pathological Anatomy

Tricuspid Regurgitation

Tricuspid regurgitation is typically referred to as functional (not related to a primary valvular pathology) or valvular. Valvular tricuspid regurgitation is less

common as the etiology for tricuspid regurgitation (when it is considered the mechanism), many etiologies exist, and the two broad descriptive categories are rheumatic or nonrheumatic. Nonrheumatic involves a host of disease processes that affect the tricuspid valve, including infective endocarditis, Ebstein's anomaly, carcinoid syndrome, connective tissue diseases such as Marfan's, papillary muscle dysfunction, valvular prolapse, or other structural problems in the valve complex either congenital or trauma related.

Functional tricuspid regurgitation is the most frequent etiology of tricuspid regurgitation and, although oversimplified, typically results from dilation of the right ventricle and tricuspid annulus. The clinical context in which this occurs is generally related mitral valve disease. The complex interplay between the tricuspid annulus, chordae, leaflets, and papillary muscles is ultimately responsible for development of functional tricuspid regurgitation. Many factors correlate with functional tricuspid regurgitation including annular size and shape, papillary and tricuspid valve tethering, right ventricular shape and function, severity of pulmonary hypertension, atria size, and LV systolic function.[43] The majority of current surgical and percutaneous techniques incorporate reduction in tricuspid valve annular size to correct functional tricuspid regurgitation. Current techniques, primarily reserved for mild to moderate tricuspid regurgitation, include plication of the annulus of the posterior (bicuspidization with obliteration of the posterior leaflet) and purse-string–like reduction of the anterior and posterior annular diameter (De Vega style technique). More severe regurgitation is often treated with the use of flexible bands or rings (rigid or flexible), again with the goal of reduction of annular diameter to achieve congruent leaflet coaptation. Tricuspid valve replacement is typically reserved for nonrepairable primary leaflet pathology. Percutaneous approaches to both repair and replacement have been described,[45,46] but are not yet ready for human use.

Fluoroscopic Anatomy

Two projections that are useful to gain a fluoroscopic understanding of the anatomy of the right-sided cardiac structures are the posteroanterior view and lateral view. During ventricular systole, the posteroanterior view provides excellent visualization of the right atrium, right ventricle, tricuspid valve, and the pulmonary artery (Fig. 3-11). Conversely, in ventricular diastole, the lateral view nicely delineates the relationships of the superior and inferior vena cava to the right atrium and ventricle. Additionally, the lateral view also provides another vantage point of the pulmonary artery, RVOT, and the pulmonic valve (Fig. 3-11).

Echocardiographic Anatomy

The 0-degree mid esophageal four-chamber view is often a good starting point for imaging of the tricuspid valve. Often, the etiology of the tricuspid

regurgitation can be identified in this view, although supplemental views are helpful. In this view, the septal leaflet and nonseptal leaflet (anterior or posterior) are well seen as is the degree of tricuspid regurgitation. The nonseptal leaflet can be either anterior or posterior depending on the positioning of the probe and degree of flexion or anteflexion.[47] The 60-degree mid esophageal right ventricular inflow-outflow view is well suited for visualization of the anterior and posterior leaflets of the tricuspid valve as well as the right ventricular inflow and pulmonic valve.[47] Better visualization of the chordae tendineae and papillary muscles can be accomplished with rotation of the probe to 120 degrees for a long-axis view of the right ventricular inflow. The single best view to visualize all three leaflets together is the transgastric short axis (~30 degrees).

CT Anatomy

The role of cardiac CT for tricuspid valve procedures is paramount in patients with congenital heart disease as the etiology for their tricuspid valve disease, but the utility otherwise remains to be proven. As previously described, the tricuspid valve separates the right atrium from the morphologic right ventricle and consists of the same components as the mitral valve (leaflets/cusps, commissures, chordae tendineae, and papillary muscles). Distinguishing the morphologic left and right ventricles can be difficult in patients with complex congenital heart disease. Fortunately, there

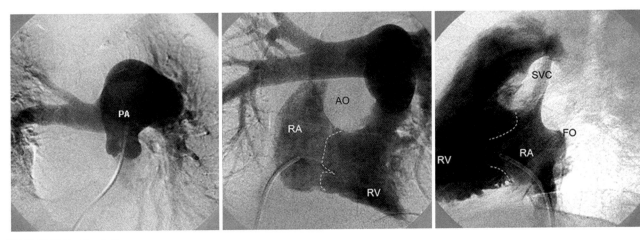

FIGURE 3-11.

Pulmonary angiography on the left to assess pulmonic valve using the NIH catheter. Note the presence of mild pulmonary insufficiency and poststenotic pulmonary artery dilatation. Digital subtraction was used for better visualization. The middle and right panel show injection of the dye in right atrium (RA). AO, aorta; FO, foramen ovale ; PA, pulmonary artery; RA, right atrium; RV, right ventricle; SVC, superior vena cava. (Modified from Agarwal S, Tuzcu EM, Rodriguez ER, et al. Interventional cardiology perspective of functional tricuspid regurgitation. *Circ Cardiovasc Interv.* 2009;2[6]:565–573.)

are several unique characteristics that make this possible by CT: the moderator band, a heavily trabeculated apex, well-developed infundibulum, septal papillary muscles, and the lack of fibrous continuity of the aortic valve and outflow.

Cardiac CT is also very useful for evaluating leaflet morphology and thickening as well as leaflet apposition but may not add much to TEE in this regard. Leaflet nonapposition is best determined at the end of ventricular systole in an ECG-gated CT. Other indirect markers of tricuspid valve disease are the presence of contrast in the hepatic veins or inferior vena cava during the first pass phase of CT (very sensitive marker for tricuspid regurgitation), bowing of the interventricular septum into the left ventricle during systole (indicative of elevated right-sided filling pressures), and lastly, right atrial and ventricular dilatation may alert one to the presence of tricuspid regurgitant disease. Constrictive pericarditis and pulmonary hypertension are important etiologies to consider when evaluating the tricuspid valve by cardiac CT. In patients with tricuspid stenosis, CT imaging is good at identifying fusion of the leaflet edges and shortening of the chordae tendineae.

PULMONIC VALVE

Positioned in the outflow tract of the right ventricle at the apex of the infundibulum, the pulmonary valve functions to partition the right ventricle from the pulmonary trunk. Not unlike the aortic valve, the pulmonary valve is a trileaflet valve made up of three semilunar cusps (anterior, left, and right; named according to their anatomic position prior to embryologic rotation of the great vessels to their respective ventricles). Similar to the aortic annulus, the annulus of the pulmonary valve consists of three "rings," which are described by their anatomic relationship to the pulmonary valve. Superiorly, commissural apposition occurs at the ST junction of the pulmonary trunk, signifying the location of the first ring. The ventriculo-arterial junction marks the location of the second ring; the third ring is the basal-most ring, occurring within the ventricle at the level of the base of the sinuses.

Pathologic Anatomy

Pulmonic Stenosis

Pulmonic stenosis (PS) produces RVOT obstruction and the resultant pressure overload increase in the right ventricular systolic pressure and hypertrophy. Progressively, PS leads to right ventricular failure and dilatation and, ultimately, tricuspid regurgitation. Four types of PS are often described: valvular PS, supravalvular PS (stenosis of the main pulmonary artery), subvalvular PS, and peripheral PS (branch pulmonary artery stenosis). True valvular PS usually occurs as an isolated congenital defect and is rarely the result of rheumatic fever, endocarditis, or carcinoid syndrome.

Valvular PS characteristically gives rise to a fibrotic dome-shaped valve that is rarely calcified and, as a result, is usually amenable to percutaneous balloon valvuloplasty. Conversely, subvalvular PS (outflow tract hypertrophy) and dysplastic valves are not particularly pliable or responsive to balloon valvuloplasty. The normal pulmonic valve orifice area is 2 cm^2 per square meter of body surface area. The other units can be expressed as 0.5 cm^2/m^2 and 1 to 2 cm^2/m^2 for clarity. Current guidelines would suggest that balloon valvotomy of the pulmonic valve is indicated for asymptomatic patients with a mean transvalvular gradient >40 mm Hg or peak instantaneous gradient of >60 mm Hg. For symptomatic patients, the threshold for intervention is somewhat lower, with mean gradient >30 mm Hg or peak instantaneous gradient >50 mm Hg.[49] Since the inception of percutaneous balloon valvotomy, it has now become the standard of care for patients with isolated severe valvular PS.[49]

Percutaneous treatment is recommended as the treatment modality of choice for focal branch and/or peripheral PS with more than a 50% stenosis and an elevated right ventricular systolic pressure greater than 50 mm Hg, with or without symptoms. In general, surgery is recommended for patients with severe PS and associated hypoplastic pulmonary annulus, severe pulmonary regurgitation, subvalvular PS, or supravalvular PS. Surgery is also preferred when there is other concomitant valve disease, such as severe tricuspid regurgitation, or if the pulmonary valve is heavily calcified or dysplastic.[49]

Pulmonary Regurgitation

Pulmonary regurgitation is principally the result of long-standing pulmonary hypertension and patients usually remain asymptomatic for many decades, although it can contribute to right-sided volume overload and dysfunction. Percutaneous therapies for pulmonary regurgitation are limited, although percutaneous pulmonary valve implantation has been successfully performed in patients with congenital heart disease and conduit dysfunction (stenosis or regurgitation).[50,51]

Fluoroscopic Anatomy

Right ventricular angiography is performed as a routine part of pulmonic valvuloplasty in both anteroposterior and lateral projections to precisely locate the pulmonic valve and measure the annulus. The lateral projection is particularly helpful in delineating the anatomy of the RVOT, infundibular obstruction, right ventricular function, and mobility of the pulmonic valve. Pulmonary angiography is also very useful to determine the degree of pulmonary regurgitation and evaluate for other lesions such as supravalvular or peripheral PS.

Complete or near complete outflow tract obstruction by ventricular angiography should alert the operator to the likelihood of "suicide ventricle" physiology that may occur immediately after balloon valvuloplasty as the result of a sudden reduction in ventricular afterload and hypertrophic obstructive cardiomyopathy-like physiology with increased outflow tract obstruction in the setting of afterload reduction. Patients exhibiting "suicide ventricle" physiology should be treated with beta-blockers and intravenous fluids and not inotropic agents because these may exacerbate the outflow tract obstruction and hypotension. In the ensuing days to weeks, the outflow hypertrophy will regress in size and the subvalvular gradient will diminish. With a pigtail in the right ventricle, the markers on the pigtail may be used to assess the diameter of the annulus to aid in balloon sizing; typically, the goal is balloon-to-annulus ratio of 1.2:1.4. A successful procedure is defined as one in which the final transvalvular gradient is <20 mm Hg.

Echocardiographic Anatomy

Transesophageal echocardiographic imaging of the pulmonary valve is often of limited utility and not routinely used in pulmonic valvuloplasty. Success is largely defined on the basis of transvalvular gradient reduction as determined by use of dual lumen pigtail catheter. However, if TEE imaging is needed, the pulmonic valve is best visualized in 60-degree mid esophageal inflow-outflow view. In this view, doming of the leaflets, calcification, mobility, and leaflet thickening can be assessed. Supplemental mid and upper esophageal short-axis views may also be beneficial when assessing degree of mobility, valve morphology, and procedural success.

CT Anatomy

Cardiac CT is very useful in planning pulmonary valve procedures because these patients commonly have congenital heart disease and complex anatomy. RVOT obstruction has many potential etiologies as previously outlined and therein lies the utility of cardiac CT in planning the appropriate treatment approach. Appropriate preprocedural imaging with cardiac CT or MRI may also tip off the operator to potential poor candidates for percutaneous valvuloplasty—that is, those with bicuspid or unicuspid valves (<20% incidence) or myxomatous dysplastic valves.

Because of the ordinarily slender and delicate appearance of the pulmonic valve it may not always be readily seen. If it easily visible by CT it is likely to be thickened. Like the tricuspid valve, the morphology of the pulmonic valve can be directly assessed by CT. In contradistinction to the tricuspid valve, the pulmonic leaflet apposition is best appreciated at the end-diastole and the extent of leaflet excursion is better viewed in end-systole.[48] Moderate to severe PS is typically associated with poststenotic dilatation of the pulmonary artery and right ventricular hypertrophy. Pulmonary regurgitation occurs as the result of dilatation of the pulmonic annulus, usually in the presence of pulmonary hypertension or dilatation of the pulmonary artery, either idiopathic or secondary to another disease process as mentioned previously.

Similar to CT evaluation of the tricuspid valve, examination of the chamber size and thickness of the right heart should be performed when pulmonic valve pathology is suspected. Right atrial and ventricular dilation/hypertrophy may be present and pulmonary trunk dimensions should also be scrutinized. Bowing of the interventricular septum into the LV cavity in systole is consistent with pressure overload; however, if septal bowing is present in both systole and diastole, this is most consistent with right-sided volume and pressure overload.[48]

CONCLUSION

In-depth understanding of anatomy and its implications in different interventions is increasingly important with expanding structural interventions and revolution in imaging capabilities.

REFERENCES

1. Serruys PW. *Transcatheter Aortic Valve Implantation: Tips and Tricks to Avoid Failure.* New York: Informa Healthcare; 2010.

2. Baumgartner H, Hung J, Bermejo J, et al. Echocardiographic assessment of valve stenosis: EAE/ASE recommendations for clinical practice. *J Am Soc Echocardiogr.* 2009;22(1):1–23; quiz 101–102.

3. Schoenhagen P, Tuzcu EM, Kapadia SR, et al. Three-dimensional imaging of the aortic valve and aortic root with computed tomography: new standards in an era of transcatheter valve repair/implantation. *Eur Heart J.* 2009;30(17):2079–2086.

4. Piazza N, de Jaegere P, Schultz C, et al. Anatomy of the aortic valvar complex and its implications for transcatheter implantation of the aortic valve. *Circ Cardiovasc Interv.* 2008;1(1):74–81.

5. Turner K, Navaratnam V. The positions of coronary arterial ostia. *Clin Anat.* 1996;9(6):376–380.

6. Kapadia SR, Svensson L, Tuzcu EM. Successful percutaneous management of left main trunk occlusion during percutaneous aortic valve replacement. *Catheter Cardiovasc Interv.* 2009;73(7):966–972.

7. Bleiziffer S, Ruge H, Horer J, et al. Predictors for new-onset complete heart block after transcatheter aortic valve implantation. *JACC Cardiovasc Interv.* 2010;3(5):524–530.

8. Piazza N, Grube E, Gerckens U, et al. Procedural and 30-day outcomes following transcatheter aortic valve implantation using the third generation (18 Fr) corevalve revalving system: results from the multicentre, expanded evaluation registry 1-year following CE mark approval. *EuroIntervention.* 2008;4(2):242–249.

9. Otto CM, Lind BK, Kitzman DW, et al. Association of aortic-valve sclerosis with cardiovascular mortality and morbidity in the elderly. *N Engl J Med.* 1999;341(3):142–147.

10. Fedak PW, Verma S, David TE, et al. Clinical and pathophysiological implications of a bicuspid aortic valve. *Circulation.* 2002;106(8):900–904.

11. Delgado V, Tops LF, Schuijf JD, et al. Successful deployment of a transcatheter aortic valve in bicuspid aortic stenosis: role of imaging with multislice computed tomography. *Circ Cardiovasc Imaging.* 2009;2(2):e12–e13.

12. Kurra V, Kapadia SR, Tuzcu EM, et al. Pre-procedural imaging of aortic root orientation and dimensions: comparison between X-ray angiographic planar imaging and 3-dimensional multidetector row computed tomography. *JACC Cardiovasc Interv.* 2010;3(1):105–113.

13. Butany J, Collins MJ, Demellawy DE, et al. Morphological and clinical findings in 247 surgically excised native aortic valves. *Can J Cardiol.* 2005;21(9):747–755.

14. Thubrikar MJ, Aouad J, Nolan SP. Patterns of calcific deposits in operatively excised stenotic or purely regurgitant aortic valves and their relation to mechanical stress. *Am J Cardiol.* 1986;58(3):304–308.

15. Kaden JJ, Freyer S, Weisser G, et al. Correlation of degree of aortic valve stenosis by Doppler echocardiogram to quantity of calcium in the valve by electron beam tomography. *Am J Cardiol.* 2002;90(5):554–557.

16. Shavelle DM, Budoff MJ, Buljubasic N, et al. Usefulness of aortic valve calcium scores by electron beam computed tomography as a marker for aortic stenosis. *Am J Cardiol.* 2003;92(3):349–353.

17. Messika-Zeitoun D, Aubry MC, Detaint D, et al. Evaluation and clinical implications of aortic valve calcification measured by electron-beam computed tomography. *Circulation.* 2004;110(3):356–362.

18. Walsh CR, Larson MG, Kupka MJ, et al. Association of aortic valve calcium detected by electron beam computed tomography with echocardiographic aortic valve disease and with calcium deposits in the coronary arteries and thoracic aorta. *Am J Cardiol.* 2004;93(4):421–425.

19. Baumert B, Plass A, Bettex D, et al. Dynamic cine mode imaging of the normal aortic valve using 16-channel multidetector row computed tomography. *Invest Radiol.* 2005;40(10):637–647.

20. Feuchtner GM, Dichtl W, Friedrich GJ, et al. Multislice computed tomography for detection of patients with aortic valve stenosis and quantification of severity. *J Am Coll Cardiol.* 2006;47(7):1410–1417.

21. Alkadhi H, Wildermuth S, Plass A, et al. Aortic stenosis: comparative evaluation of 16-detector row CT and echocardiography. *Radiology.* 2006;240(1):47–55.

22. Bouvier E, Logeart D, Sablayrolles JL, et al. Diagnosis of aortic valvular stenosis by multislice cardiac computed tomography. *Eur Heart J.* 2006;27(24):3033–3038.

23. Pouleur AC, le Polain de Waroux JB, Pasquet A, et al. Aortic valve area assessment: multidetector CT compared with cine MR imaging and transthoracic and transesophageal echocardiography. *Radiology.* 2007;244(3):745–754.

24. Habis M, Daoud B, Roger VL, et al. Comparison of 64-slice computed tomography planimetry and Doppler echocardiography in the assessment of aortic valve stenosis. *J Heart Valve Dis.* 2007;16(3):216–224.

25. Rispler S, Rinkevich D, Markiewicz W, et al. Missed diagnosis of severe symptomatic aortic stenosis. *Am J Cardiol.* 1995;76(10):728–730.

26. Skjaerpe T, Hegrenaes L, Hatle L. Noninvasive estimation of valve area in patients with aortic stenosis by Doppler ultrasound and two-dimensional echocardiography. *Circulation.* 1985;72(4):810–818.

27. Oh JK, Taliercio CP, Holmes DR Jr, et al. Prediction of the severity of aortic stenosis by Doppler aortic valve area determination: prospective Doppler-catheterization correlation in 100 patients. *J Am Coll Cardiol.* 1988;11(6):1227–1234.

28. Vengala S, Nanda NC, Dod HS, et al. Images in geriatric cardiology. Usefulness of live three-dimensional transthoracic echocardiography in aortic valve stenosis evaluation. *Am J Geriatr Cardiol.* 2004;13(5):279–284.

29. Yeager M, Yock PG, Popp RL. Comparison of Doppler-derived pressure gradient to that determined

at cardiac catheterization in adults with aortic valve stenosis: implications for management. *Am J Cardiol.* 1986;57(8):644–648.

30. Mallavarapu RK, Nanda NC. Three-dimensional transthoracic echocardiographic assessment of aortic stenosis and regurgitation. *Cardiol Clin.* 2007;25(2): 327–334.

31. Shaw TR, Sutaria N, Prendergast B. Clinical and haemodynamic profiles of young, middle aged, and elderly patients with mitral stenosis undergoing mitral balloon valvotomy. *Heart.* 2003;89(12):1430–1436.

32. Wilkins GT, Weyman AE, Abascal VM, et al. Percutaneous balloon dilatation of the mitral valve: an analysis of echocardiographic variables related to outcome and the mechanism of dilatation. *Br Heart J.* 1988;60(4):299–308.

33. Iung B, Cormier B, Ducimetiere P, et al. Immediate results of percutaneous mitral commissurotomy. A predictive model on a series of 1514 patients. *Circulation.* 1996;94(9):2124–2130.

34. Roberts WC, Perloff JK. Mitral valvular disease. A clinicopathologic survey of the conditions causing the mitral valve to function abnormally. *Ann Intern Med.* 1972;77(6):939–975.

35. Braunwald E. Valvular heart disease. In: Zipes DP, Braunwald E, eds. *Braunwald's Heart Disease: A Textbook of Cardiovascular Medicine.* Vol 2. 7th ed. Philadelphia: W.B. Saunders; 2005.

36. Braunwald E. *Braunwald's Heart Disease: A Textbook of Cardiovascular Medicine.* 7th ed. Philadelphia: W.B. Saunders; 2005.

37. Ribeiro EJ, Carvalho RG, Brofman PR, et al. [Conservative surgery of the mitral valve]. *Arq Bras Cardiol.* 1983;41(4):341–343.

38. Carpentier A. Cardiac valve surgery—the "French correction." *J Thorac Cardiovasc Surg.* 1983;86(3):323–337.

39. Levine RA, Schwammenthal E. Ischemic mitral regurgitation on the threshold of a solution: from paradoxes to unifying concepts. *Circulation.* 2005;112(5): 745–758.

40. Choure AJ, Garcia MJ, Hesse B, et al. In vivo analysis of the anatomical relationship of coronary sinus to mitral annulus and left circumflex coronary artery using cardiac multidetector computed tomography: implications for percutaneous coronary sinus mitral annuloplasty. *J Am Coll Cardiol.* 2006;48(10):1938–1945.

41. Fukuda S, Saracino G, Matsumura Y, et al. Three-dimensional geometry of the tricuspid annulus in healthy subjects and in patients with functional tricuspid regurgitation: a real-time, 3-dimensional echocardiographic study. *Circulation.* 2006;114(1 Suppl):I492–498.

42. Ton-Nu TT, Levine RA, Handschumacher MD, et al. Geometric determinants of functional tricuspid regurgitation: insights from 3-dimensional echocardiography. *Circulation.* 2006;114(2):143–149.

43. Agarwal S, Tuzcu EM, Rodriguez ER, et al. Interventional cardiology perspective of functional tricuspid regurgitation. *Circ Cardiovasc Interv.* 2009;2(6): 565–573.

44. Drake RL, Vogl W, Mitchell AWM, et al. *Gray's Anatomy for Students.* 2nd ed. Philadelphia: Churchill Livingstone/Elsevier; 2010.

45. Boudjemline Y, Agnoletti G, Bonnet D, et al. Steps toward the percutaneous replacement of atrioventricular valves an experimental study. *J Am Coll Cardiol.* 2005;46(2):360–365.

46. Zegdi R, Khabbaz Z, Borenstein N, et al. A repositionable valved stent for endovascular treatment of deteriorated bioprostheses. *J Am Coll Cardiol.* 2006; 48(7):1365–1368.

47. Mathew JP, Ayoub CM. *Clinical Manual and Review of Transesophageal Echocardiography.* New York: McGraw-Hill; 2005.

48. Manghat NE, Rachapalli V, Van Lingen R, et al. Imaging the heart valves using ECG-gated 64-detector row cardiac CT. *Br J Radiol.* 2008;81(964):275–290.

49. Warnes CA, Williams RG, Bashore TM, et al. ACC/AHA 2008 Guidelines for the Management of Adults with Congenital Heart Disease: a report of the American College of Cardiology/American Heart Association Task Force on Practice Guidelines (writing committee to develop guidelines on the management of adults with congenital heart disease). *Circulation.* 2008;118(23):e714–e833.

50. Lurz P, Bonhoeffer P, Taylor AM. Percutaneous pulmonary valve implantation: an update. *Expert Rev Cardiovasc Ther.* 2009;7(7):823–833.

51. Bonhoeffer P, Boudjemline Y, Qureshi SA, et al. Percutaneous insertion of the pulmonary valve. *J Am Coll Cardiol.* 2002;39(10):1664–1669.

CHAPTER 4

Anatomy of the Cardiac Chambers for the Interventionalist

Michael S. Kim and Adam R. Hansgen

The treatment of patients with congenital and acquired structural heart disease (SHD) through transcatheter techniques represents a major area of growth in interventional cardiology. The advent of novel devices (occluders and plugs, transcatheter valves and clips, etc.) and unique delivery catheters, coupled with advances in noninvasive imaging that enhance visualization of cardiovascular anatomy in three-dimensions (3D), have provided interventionalists the opportunity to treat a diverse range of structural heart defects that traditionally were only approached surgically. As a result, interventionalists now face the challenge of expanding their knowledge of cardiovascular anatomy to include a detailed understanding of the cardiac chambers and the spatial relationships of surrounding valvular and vascular structures.

This chapter includes an overview of the general anatomic structure with subsequent highlighting of major anatomic characteristics and landmarks of the right and left atria, left atrial (LA) appendage, atrial septum, and right and left ventricular (LV) chambers. A detailed description of gross anatomic imaging correlations is beyond the scope of this chapter and is reviewed elsewhere in this book.

ATTITUDINALLY APPROPRIATE NOMENCLATURE

Conventional nomenclature dictates that structures within the body are best described relative to the subject's anatomic position: standing upright and facing the observer (Fig. 4-1). Spatial descriptions are subsequently derived according to three orthogonal planes: sagittal, coronal, and axial. In the sagittal plane, structures are described as being anterior (closer to the sternum) or posterior (closer to the spine). Within the coronal (frontal) plane, structures are described as being medial or lateral relative to a center line/central plane, which itself is described as having superior (closer to the head) and inferior (closer to the feet) ends.

Although the rationale underlying such "attitudinally appropriate nomenclature" appears obvious, examining the heart in isolation (as many anatomists and pathologists do) typically results in such attitudinal orientation being forgotten. Instead, it is common to adopt the attitudinally incorrect "Valentine" approach to cardiac anatomy where the heart is described as if standing on its apex with its long axes positioned in the sagittal and coronal planes. Thus, in the Valentine heart, the right atrium (RA) and right ventricle (RV) are located rightward, whereas the LA and LV are located leftward (Fig. 4-2). In situ, however, all interventionalists know this Valentine orientation to be fundamentally inaccurate. Rather, the human heart is both rotated and oriented at an angle with the apex pointing to the left. Consequently, when viewed in the frontal plane (i.e., anterior to posterior), the right heart chambers overlap the left heart chambers with the atrial chambers situated posteriorly and rightward relative to the ventricular chambers (Fig. 4-3). In this review of cardiac anatomy, we strive to describe and exhibit cardiac structures in true attitudinal fashion[1] whenever possible, while continuing to use certain terms that are not strictly attitudinal (e.g., right, left) in the spirit of convention.

RIGHT AND LEFT ATRIA

In attitudinally appropriate terms, the names of the two atria are far from accurate. When viewed from the front, the "right" atrium in situ is positioned rightward and anterior to its "left" counterpart (Fig. 4-4), such that very little of the LA is seen in this view. The two atria share the same basic anatomic components: a venous component, an appendage, and a vestibule leading into the atrioventricular (AV) valves (i.e., tricuspid and mitral valves). Although they share these basic anatomic elements, the atria themselves differ dramatically in both structure and morphology.

Right Atrium

The venous component of the RA is composed of the superior vena cava (SVC) and inferior vena cava (IVC),

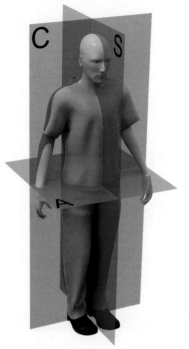

FIGURE 4-1.

Conventional anatomic and spatial nomenclature. A, axial plane; C, coronal plane; S, sagittal plane.

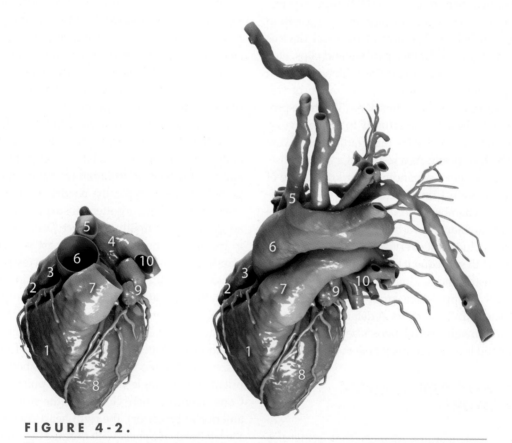

FIGURE 4-2.

The "Valentine" heart orientation. 1, right ventricle; 2, right atrium; 3, right atrial appendage; 4, left atrium; 5, superior vena cava; 6, aorta; 7, pulmonary artery; 8, left ventricle; 9, left atrial appendage; 10, left upper pulmonary vein.

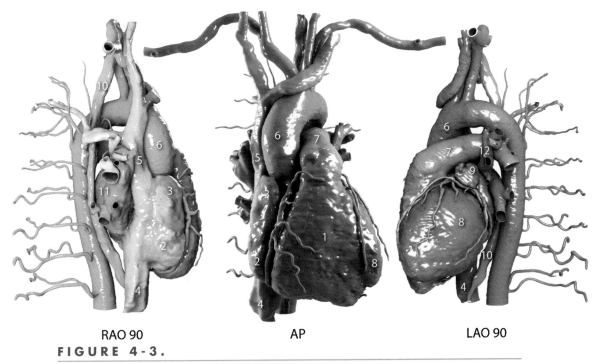

RAO 90   AP   LAO 90

FIGURE 4-3.

The heart's orientation in situ. **A:** Right anterior oblique 90 degrees. **B:** Anteroposterior. **C:** Left anterior oblique 90 degrees. 1, right ventricle; 2, right atrium; 3, right atrial appendage; 4, inferior vena cava; 5, superior vena cava; 6, aorta; 7, pulmonary artery; 8, left ventricle; 9, left atrial appendage; 10, esophagus; 11, left atrium; 12, left upper pulmonary vein.

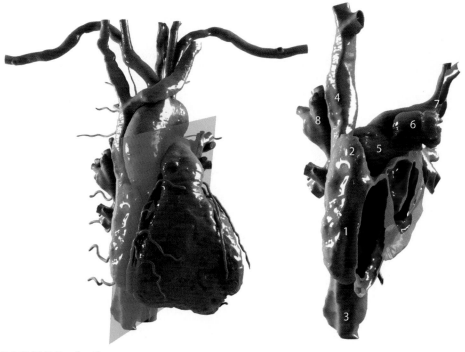

FIGURE 4-4.

Orientation of the atria in situ. The right atrium is oriented both rightward **(A)** and anterior **(B)** to the left atrium. 1, right atrium; 2, right atrial appendage; 3, inferior vena cava; 4, superior vena cava; 5, left atrium; 6, left atrial appendage; 7, left upper pulmonary vein; 8, right upper pulmonary vein.

which enter the RA at obtuse angles and with the SVC oriented slightly anterior to the IVC. The entrance to the IVC is guarded by the Eustachian valve, a triangular flap of fibrous or fibromuscular tissue extending from the lateral aspect of the IVC orifice over to the ridge of atrial tissue separating the IVC and coronary sinus (i.e., the sinus septum or "Eustachian ridge"). The Eustachian valve may vary dramatically in humans, from being very large to virtually absent, muscular to membrane-like, or well-defined to a lace-like Chiari network.[2] Similar to the IVC orifice, the RA entrance of the coronary sinus is guarded by the Thebesian valve. Although the Thebesian valve is typically described as a small crescentric flap (oftentimes with fenestrations), like the Eustachian valve, it, too, may exhibit wide variation in its morphology.[3] In some patients, the Thebesian valve may be quite extensive, potentially inhibiting the placement of a catheter or pacing wire into the coronary sinus. Together, the Eustachian and Thebesian valves converge into the tendon of Todaro, which itself is the anatomic "continuation" of the

Eustachian ridge as it courses along the posterior wall of the RA (Fig. 4-5).

The dominant feature of the RA is the large atrial appendage, which forms the entire anterior wall of the RA. The RA appendage is triangular in shape and projects anteriorly with a superiorly directed apex (Fig. 4-6). On the endocardial surface, the RA appendage is easily distinguished from the remainder of the RA by its characteristics ridges (i.e., pectinate muscles). The pectinate muscles arise and extend from yet another major anatomic feature of the RA, the terminal crest.

The terminal crest (i.e., crista terminalis) is a muscle bundle delineating the border between the ridge-lined atrial appendage and the smooth venous component. It sweeps around the RA in the shape of a twisted C, originating from the septal wall, passing anterior to the entrance of the SVC, descending posteriorly and laterally, and finally turning anterior again to pass rightward to the orifice of the IVC (Fig. 4-7). At this point, the terminal crest extends as an array

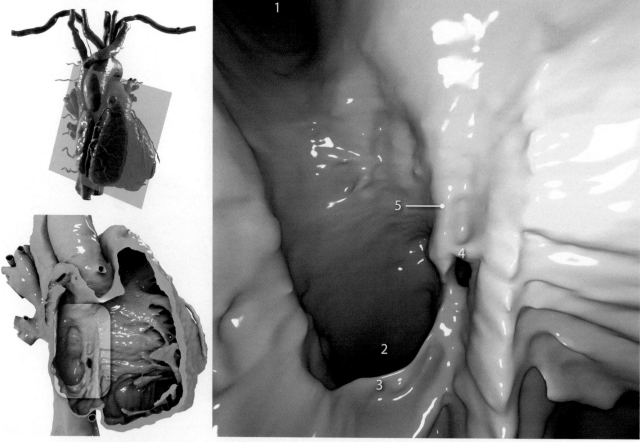

FIGURE 4-5.

Endocardial landmarks of the right atrium. 1, superior vena cava; 2, inferior vena cava; 3, Eustachian ridge; 4, Thebesian valve; 5, tendon of Todaro.

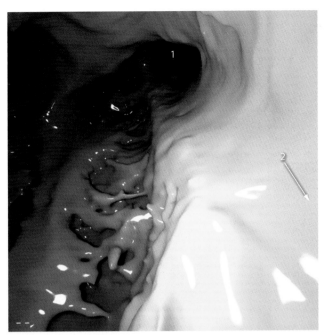

FIGURE 4-6.

Right atrial appendage. 1, superior vena cava; 2, inferior vena cava.

of fine bundles known as the cavotricuspid isthmus, which itself is a critical component in common atrial flutter circuits.

All of the muscle ridges terminate in the vestibule, the inlet to the tricuspid valve, thus marking the termination of the atrial myocardium. The major anatomic landmark of the RA vestibular component is the triangle of Koch, whose borders are formed by the tendon of Todaro posteriorly, the hinge line of the septal leaflet of the tricuspid valve anteriorly, and the orifice of the coronary sinus at the base (Fig. 4-8). Within the angle enclosed by the anterior and posterior borders of the triangle of Koch lie the AV node and its fiber bundles.

Left Atrium

Whereas the RA has several important anatomic landmarks and is dominated by its large appendage, the LA is relatively featureless with the majority of its size composed of a smooth walled body. Although a detailed review of the LA myoarchitecture is beyond the scope of a review of gross chamber anatomy, it is important to note that whereas the endocardial surface of the LA is smooth, the transmural architecture of the LA is remarkably complex and is composed of multiple overlapping myofibers in an array of orientations/bundles (e.g., Bachmann's bundle, septopulmonary bundle, septoatrial bundle) initially described by Papez in 1920.[3]

The posteriorly oriented venous component of the LA receives the pulmonary veins. The venoatrial transition is smooth and often indistinct with atrial musculature extending over and into the walls of the pulmonary veins to varying degrees. Traditionally, the venous component is described as being composed of four pulmonary veins (two veins from each lung) entering the LA, although modern imaging techniques have demonstrated considerably greater variation in both the number and arrangement of pulmonary venous origins.[4] The venous component lies immediately anterior to the esophagus, with the walls of the two structures separated only by the fibrous pericardium.[5]

The vestibular component marks the LA outlet and forms the mitral isthmus, which lies between the orifice of the left inferior pulmonary vein and the annular attachment of the mitral valve.[6] Along the inferior quadrant of the vestibule is the coronary sinus, which occupies the left AV groove.

Left Atrial Appendage

Although not as significant in size relative to its right-sided counterpart, the LA appendage far surpasses the RA appendage as a focus of clinical interest. As close to 90% of clinical embolic events in patients with atrial arrhythmias and/or mitral valve disease result from intracardiac thrombi originating in the LA appendage, exploring mechanisms to prevent thrombus

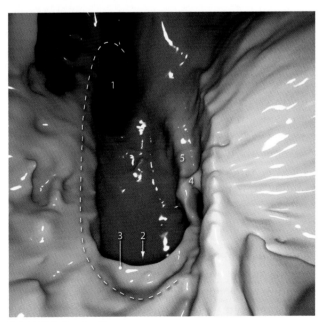

FIGURE 4-7.

Terminal crest. Borders of the terminal crest, (dashed line); 1, superior vena cava; 2, inferior vena cava; 3, Eustachian ridge; 4, Thebesian valve; 5, tendon of Todaro.

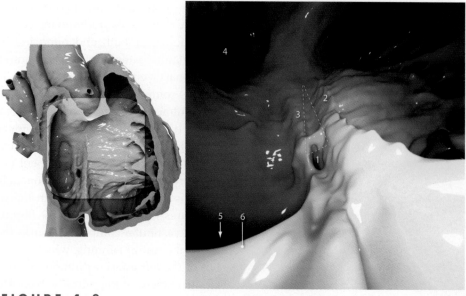

FIGURE 4-8.

Triangle of Koch. 1, coronary sinus os; 2, septal leaflet of the tricuspid valve; 3, tendon of Todaro; 4, superior vena cava; 5, inferior vena cava; 6, Eustachian ridge.

formation within the LA appendage has remained an area of active investigation for several decades. Although long-term anticoagulation has been shown to dramatically reduce the risk of thromboembolic events in patients with atrial arrhythmias and mitral valve disease, such treatment is often either burdened by challenges or outright contraindicated in many patients.[7] With the advent of transcatheter LA appendage occlusion devices (Fig. 4-9), interventionalists have yet another reason to better understand and appreciate LA appendage anatomy and morphology beyond its propensity for thrombus formation.

Unlike the true LA, which is formed from the outgrowth of the pulmonary veins (thereby accounting for its smooth-walled endocardial surface), the LA appendage is the remnant of the original embryonic LA. Anatomically, the LA appendage has a narrow base or os and is long and hook-like in shape with the apex pointing downward (Fig. 4-10). Unlike the smooth-walled LA, the LA appendage inner wall resembles its right-sided counterpart, with trabeculations and pectinate muscles. Several notable autopsy studies have confirmed a wide variation in LA appendage anatomy with regard to volume, length, and os diameter.[8–10] In addition, LA appendages from patients with atrial fibrillation were noted to be larger in volume with broader os diameters when compared to LA appendages from patients with known sinus rhythm.[9,11]

Beyond the inherent LA appendage anatomic variations that exist among all patients, and especially

in those with underlying atrial or valvular pathologies, several aspects of LA appendage gross and spatial anatomy are worth addressing in today's era of transcatheter LA appendage occlusion. First, the shape of the LA appendage os has been shown to be consistently elliptical, and not circular, in shape[12]; thus, a circular occlusion device may in fact leave crevices around the device resulting in an incomplete seal of the os, which raises debate as to the potential residual risk of thromboembolic events in patients with incomplete occlusion of the LA appendage os.[13,14] Second, autopsy studies have demonstrated that close to 70% of LA appendages follow a principle axis that is either markedly bent or spiral (Fig. 4-11) in orientation.[9] Although it has been suggested that the relationship between the overall length of the LA appendage and the diameter of the os is critical in successful and complete deployment of an occlusion device into the LA appendage,[15] some experts suggest that the distance between the LA appendage os and the point at first significant path deviation may in fact be the crucial measurement when considering device occlusion of the LA appendage.[10] Third, autopsy studies have demonstrated that over half of LA appendage specimens studied had evidence of "pits and troughs" that either occur in isolation or in clusters.[10] Perhaps more importantly, the atrial wall thickness within these depressions is often paper-thin, potentially increasing the risk of perforation during wire or catheter navigation within the LA appendage. Finally, a thoughtful understanding of

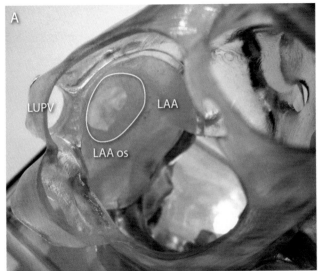

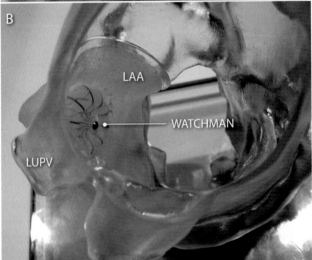

FIGURE 4-9.

Left atrial appendage (LAA) occlusion device. **A:** Model of the LAA. **B:** Model of the LAA with a WATCHMAN LAA Closure Device (Atritech Inc., Plymouth, MN) in place. LUPV, left upper pulmonary vein.

the spatial relationship of the LA appendage to surrounding structures is of supreme importance when considering options for transcatheter occlusion. For example, although clinical studies have demonstrated no evidence of pulmonary vein inflow or mitral valve disruption following implantation of various LA appendage occlusion devices,[16–18] other surrounding structures such as the left anterior descending coronary artery, circumflex coronary artery, and great cardiac vein may be vulnerable to trauma following LA appendage occlusion device implantation, particularly in cases where devices are sized to be 20% to 40% larger than the os (Fig. 4-11).[10] Moreover, with LA appendage occlusion devices delivered via an epicardial approach, there exists the potential risk to disrupt the left phrenic nerve that may run along the pericardium directly overlying the LA appendage.[19]

ATRIAL SEPTUM

The atrial septum remains an intracardiac structure at the "heart" of both intense investigation and, oftentimes, equally intense controversy.[20–26] Surface features of the atrial septum are best appreciated on the RA side, whereas the LA aspect of the septum demonstrates rather featureless topography. The "true" atrial septum (i.e., septum primum) remains limited to the "flap valve" component, which is composed of the floor of the fossa ovalis and the muscular rim at the anteroinferior border, and is confluent with the floor of the triangle of Koch (Fig. 4-12).[3,27] The majority of the atrial septum as well as the entirety of the superior, posterior, and much of the anterior rims of the fossa ovalis (including the major muscular rim, the limbus) are composed of in-foldings of the atrial walls and

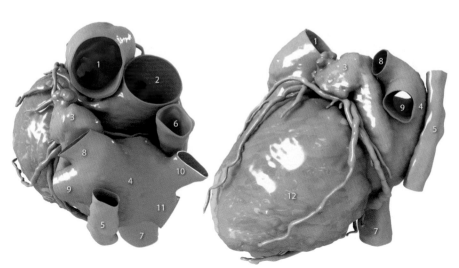

FIGURE 4-10.

Orientation and shape of the left atrial appendage. 1, pulmonary artery; 2, aorta; 3, left atrial appendage; 4, left atrium; 5, esophagus; 6, superior vena cava; 7, inferior vena cava; 8, left upper pulmonary vein; 9, left lower pulmonary vein; 10, right upper pulmonary vein; 11, right lower pulmonary vein; 12, left ventricle.

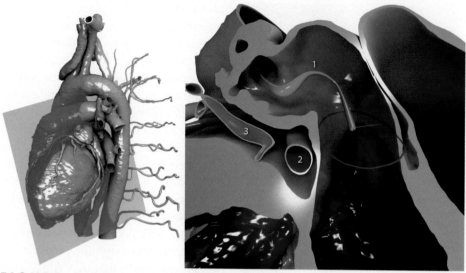

FIGURE 4-11.

Left atrial appendage. 1, bent/spiral principle axis (centerline color and thickness exaggerated as the line moves closer to/farther from the camera viewpoint), spatial orientation of the left atrial appendage to the circumflex coronary artery and great cardiac vein; 2, left circumflex artery; 3, great cardiac vein.

comprise the embryonic septum secundum (Fig. 4-12). The area of the fossa ovalis that extends from its superior border to the ostium of the SVC is formed by an in-folding of the RA wall and is filled with extracardiac adipose tissue. The superior margin of the fossa ovalis is formed by a slightly protruding rim (i.e., limbus). The segment of the septal wall located superiorly and

anteriorly to the fossa ovalis directly overlies the aorta (and not the LA) and is known as the aortic mound (Fig. 4-12).[28]

The floor of the fossa ovalis, flap valve of the septum primum, septum secundum, and limbus may all vary widely in their respective degrees of thickness. The limbus may be quite prominent and can often be felt

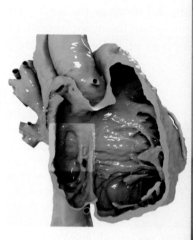

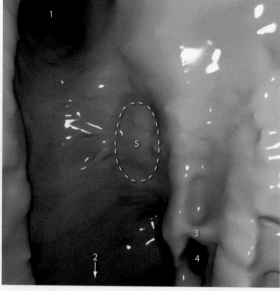

FIGURE 4-12.

Atrial septum. 1, superior vena cava; 2, inferior vena cava; 3, Thebesian valve; 4, coronary sinus os; 5, fossa ovalis.

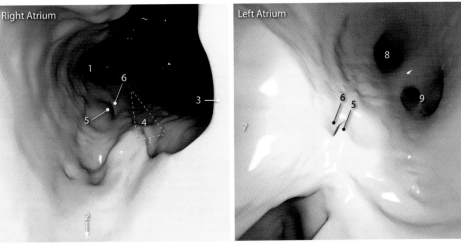

FIGURE 4-13.

Patent foramen ovale. 1, superior vena cava; 2, inferior vena cava; 3, Eustachian ridge; 4, triangle of Koch; 5, septum primum; 6, septum secundum; 7, mitral valve; 8, right upper pulmonary vein; 9, right lower pulmonary vein.

and observed by interventionalists as a "jump" as the tip of a catheter drops into the flap valve component of the fossa ovalis. The flap valve itself is generally thin (i.e., approximately 2 mm), and, in some cases, may be so thin and redundant as to become aneurysmal in appearance throughout the cardiac cycle.[28]

The flap valve of septum primum closes shut so long as LA pressure exceeds RA pressure, and closure of the fossa is complete when the flap is completely adhered to the rim. In approximately 25% to 30% of the population, the seal between the septum primum and septum secundum is incomplete, resulting in a probe patent fossa (i.e., patent foramen ovale), which is thought to be a route for paradoxical emboli (Fig. 4-13).[22]

RIGHT VENTRICLE

For many years, the RV was often overlooked in lieu of its left-sided counterpart. Thus, although LV function and the correlation to clinical outcomes have been the focus of extensive investigation, interest in the RV has traditionally failed to garner similar interest. The recent interest in structural heart interventions, especially in patients with congenital heart disease where the RV is often the "center of attention,"[29] however, has fostered a renewed appreciation for RV anatomy and morphology.

In the normal heart, the RV is the anterior-most structure with a retrosternal location. The RV is triangular in shape when viewed laterally (Fig. 4-14A)

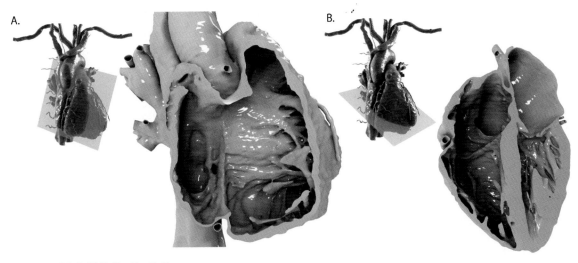

FIGURE 4-14.

The right ventricle. **A:** Lateral section. **B:** Cross-section.

FIGURE 4-15.

Components of the right ventricle. **A:** Bipartate concept. **B:** Tripartate concept. 1, inflow; 2, infundibulum/outflow; 3, apical trabecular.

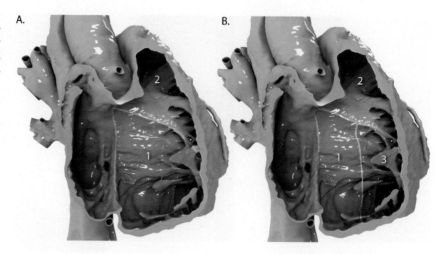

and crescent shape when viewed in cross-section (Fig. 4-14B).[30] Morphologically, the RV is distinguished from the LV by its more prominent trabeculae, thinner myocardial wall, presence of a moderator band, and absence of fibrous continuity between the tricuspid and pulmonic valves.[31]

Traditionally, the RV is described in terms of two components (Fig. 4-15A): the sinus (inflow) and the conus (infundibulum/outflow).[30] A tripartite concept (Fig. 4-15B) has also been proposed to describe the RV, dividing it into inflow, apical trabecular, and outlet components,[32] which may be of potential benefit in describing and analyzing congenitally malformed hearts. The apical trabecular component allows direct distinction between the morphologic RV and LV (irrespective of the chamber location within the entirety of cardiac mass), a critical tool in defining anatomy in patients with congenital malformations. In the two-component description, the RV inflow includes the trabeculated apical portion of the RV. As previously mentioned, the muscular trabeculations in the apical morphologic RV are significantly coarser than the fine, criss-cross patterned trabeculations seen in the LV.[33]

The inflow portion of the RV extends over the length of the AV junction and tricuspid valve (i.e., from the hingeline of the tricuspid valve to the insertions of the papillary muscles) (Fig. 4-15). Although a detailed description of tricuspid valve anatomy is beyond the scope of this chapter, it is important to note that the three leaflets (i.e., septal, anterosuperior, and posterior) of the tricuspid valve are supported by a varied array of papillary muscles, whose inconsistent number and arrangement helps to distinguish it from the mitral valve apparatus.

The tricuspid and pulmonic valves are oriented perpendicular to one another and, thus, the inflow

and outflow portions of the RV are oriented at 90 degrees to each other (Fig. 4-16).[34] The pulmonary valve is separated from the tricuspid valve by the ventriculo-infundibular fold of the crista supraventricularis, which courses superiorly into the subpulmonary infundibulum of the RV outflow tract. The anterosuperior wall of the RV completes the subpulmonary infundibulum, which itself courses into the pulmonic valve (Fig. 4-17).[33] The relationship between the pulmonic valve and subpulmonary infundibulum is an important one in that, because the infundibulum serves to lift the pulmonic valve clear of the interventricular septum, the entire pulmonary valve can be successfully excised for use as an autograft in the Ross procedure without incursion into the LV cavity.[35]

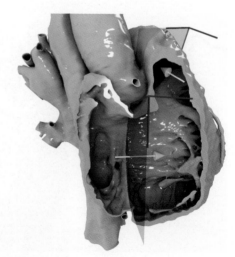

FIGURE 4-16.

Orientation of right ventricular inflow and outflow demonstrating unidirectional flow of blood.

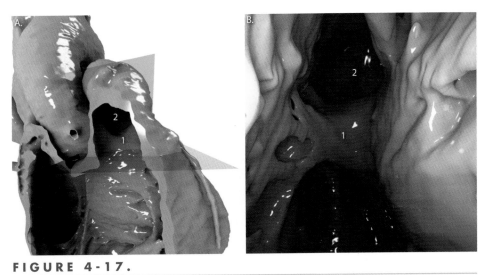

FIGURE 4-17.

Subpulmonary infundibulum of the right ventricular outflow tract. 1, subpulmonary infundibulum; 2, pulmonary valve.

LEFT VENTRICLE

The normal LV shape is a truncated ellipsoid with its long axis oriented from its base to apex.[34] In simplistic terms, the LV is cone-shaped, is thickest at its base and thinnest at its apex, and is effectively "hugged" by the RV.[36] From the anterior view, the vast majority of the LV is hidden "beneath" the RV. The LV endocardial surface is characterized by a network of thin muscle bundles (trabeculations) that encompass the apical third of the chamber. Finally, the left ventricular outflow tract (LVOT) is composed of thick muscle bundles lining the anterosuperior, posteroinferior, and posterior walls, whereas the septal wall of the LVOT is relatively smooth.

Similar to the RV, the LV has both an inlet (mitral valve) and outlet (aortic valve) that are in continuity. Unlike the RV whose inlet and outlet are oriented at 90 degrees to one another and are separated by a muscular fold that ultimately courses into the subpulmonary infundibulum, the LV inlet and outlet are oriented only 30 degrees to each other, are separated only by a thin membrane (the anterior mitral valve leaflet), and essentially overlap one another (Fig. 4-18). Thus, whereas blood flow in the RV is essentially unidirectional, blood flow in the LV is truly bidirectional with blood entering and leaving the LV through essentially the same orifice (i.e., blood flows vertically into the LV chamber through the mitral valve and then flows out through the aortic valve in the same vertical axis through the opposite vector) (Fig. 4-19). It is this bidirectional flow of blood that is required to generate systolic blood pressures in excess of 120 mm Hg.[34]

RAPID PROTOTYPING

Historically, preserved hearts obtained at autopsy were used to teach cardiac anatomy to students and physicians. Even today, gross pathologic specimens are used to provide insight to physicians exploring new operative procedures. Practically speaking, however, neither autopsy specimens nor cardiac pathologists are readily available to most clinicians. In addition, these specimens may not accurately reflect the true 3D spatial relationships present in situ because they are often collapsed. Interventionalists have struggled for years to find

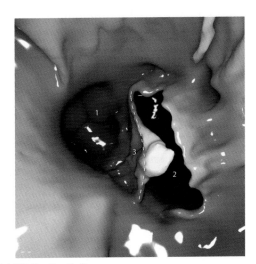

FIGURE 4-18.

Orientation of the left ventricular inflow (mitral valve) and outflow (aortic valve) separated by the anterior mitral valve leaflet. 1, aortic valve; 2, mitral valve; 3, anterior mitral valve leaflet.

Bidirectional blood flow through the left ventricle. 1, aortic valve; 2, mitral valve.

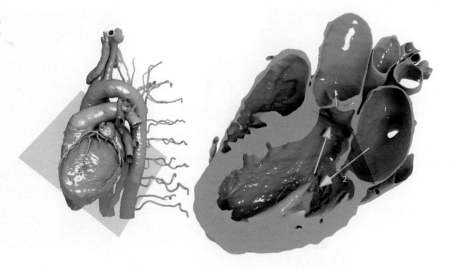

mechanisms to appreciate 3D cardiac anatomy in a manner similar to the way cardiac surgeons have directly visualized 3D anatomy for years. Standard two-dimensional (2D) imaging modalities (e.g., echocardiography, fluoroscopy, computed tomography [CT], and magnetic resonance imaging [MRI]) are widespread and demonstrate undeniable clinical value, yet remain limited in their ability to clearly represent the complex 3D spatial relationships present in SHD. Rather, physicians are forced to integrate the representative 2D images in his or her mind and conceptually extract the relevant 3D relationships. Computer graphics have allowed for "3D volume reconstructions" to be generated to provide an improved overview of 3D anatomy, but even this advance is limited by its lack of realism and inability to be tangibly manipulated.

The application of rapid prototyping, a method by which 2D images are processed into 3D physical models, in SHD education and management represents a major step forward in providing interventionalists the opportunity to more clearly understand the complex anatomic and spatial relationships present in the heart (Fig. 4-20).[37] In addition, physical models may potentially serve as an effective bridge between traditional medical imaging and actual patient anatomy. In providing an ex vivo representation of the complex anatomy present in congenital and acquired SHD, physical models may help to clarify the potential procedural challenges, likelihood of success or failure, and ideal equipment/devices needed in order to maximize patient safety and procedural success.[38]

CONCLUSION

The care and management of patients with congenital and acquired SHD represents a major area of growth in cardiology. Given the dramatic increase in the number of both approved and investigative catheter-based therapies that involve both structural modification and device implantation, interventionalists are compelled, now more than ever, to possess a solid foundational

Physical model of the heart created through rapid prototyping.

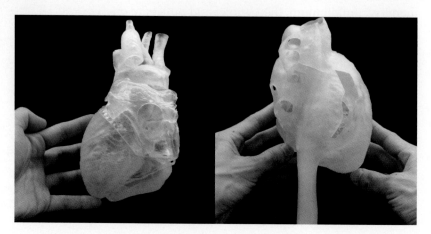

knowledge of cardiac anatomy and anatomic spatial relationships. The application of novel technologies to create patient-specific 3D physical models of hearts may serve as an effective bridge between noninvasive imaging and in vivo cardiac anatomy, thereby providing an available modality, beyond rare autopsy specimens, to acquire this necessary knowledge. Such a knowledge base not only assists in safe catheter navigation of the 3D space of cardiac chambers, but also may aid in interventionalists' appreciation of both the benefits and limitations of novel catheter-based therapies and implantable devices.

REFERENCES

1. Cosio FG, Anderson RH, Kuck KH, et al. Living anatomy of the atrioventricular junctions. A guide to electrophysiologic mapping. A Consensus Statement from the Cardiac Nomenclature Study Group, Working Group of Arrhythmias, European Society of Cardiology, and the Task Force on Cardiac Nomenclature from NASPE. *Circulation.* 1999;100:e31–e37.

2. Ho SY, Anderson RH, Sanchez-Quintana D. Gross structure of the atriums: more than an anatomic curiosity? *Pacing Clin Electrophysiol.* 2002;25:342–350.

3. Ho SY, Sanchez-Quintana D. The importance of atrial structure and fibers. *Clin Anat.* 2009;22:52–63.

4. Kato R, Lickfett L, Meininger G, et al. Pulmonary vein anatomy in patients undergoing catheter ablation of atrial fibrillation: lessons learned by use of magnetic resonance imaging. *Circulation.* 2003;107:2004–2010.

5. Sanchez-Quintana D, Cabrera JA, Climent V, et al. Anatomic relations between the esophagus and left atrium and relevance for ablation of atrial fibrillation. *Circulation.* 2005;112:1400–1405.

6. Wittkampf FH, van Oosterhout MF, Loh P, et al. Where to draw the mitral isthmus line in catheter ablation of atrial fibrillation: histological analysis. *Eur Heart J.* 2005;26:689–695.

7. Al-Saady NM, Obel OA, Camm AJ. Left atrial appendage: structure, function, and role in thromboembolism. *Heart.* 1999;82:547–554.

8. Sharma S, Devine W, Anderson RH, et al. The determination of atrial arrangement by examination of appendage morphology in 1842 heart specimens. *Br Heart J.* 1988;60:227–231.

9. Ernst G, Stollberger C, Abzieher F, et al. Morphology of the left atrial appendage. *Anat Rec.* 1995;242:553–561.

10. Su P, McCarthy KP, Ho SY. Occluding the left atrial appendage: anatomical considerations. *Heart.* 2008; 94:1166–1170.

11. Hara H, Virmani R, Holmes DR, Jr, et al. Is the left atrial appendage more than a simple appendage? *Catheter Cardiovasc Interv.* 2009;74:234–242.

12. Veinot JP, Harrity PJ, Gentile F, et al. Anatomy of the normal left atrial appendage: a quantitative study of age-related changes in 500 autopsy hearts: implications for echocardiographic examination. *Circulation.* 1997;96:3112–3115.

13. Zabalgoitia M, Halperin JL, Pearce LA, et al. Transesophageal echocardiographic correlates of clinical risk of thromboembolism in nonvalvular atrial fibrillation. Stroke Prevention in Atrial Fibrillation III Investigators. *J Am Coll Cardiol.* 1998;31:1622–1626.

14. Schneider B, Finsterer J, Stollberger C. Effects of percutaneous left atrial appendage transcatheter occlusion (PLAATO) on left atrial structure and function. *J Am Coll Cardiol.* 2005;45:634–635; author reply 635.

15. Ramondo A, Maiolino G, Napodano M, et al. Interventional approach to reduce thromboembolic risk in patients with atrial fibrillation ineligible for oral anticoagulation. *Ital Heart J.* 2005;6:414–417.

16. Ostermayer SH, Reisman M, Kramer PH, et al. Percutaneous left atrial appendage transcatheter occlusion (PLAATO system) to prevent stroke in high-risk patients with non-rheumatic atrial fibrillation: results from the international multi-center feasibility trials. *J Am Coll Cardiol.* 2005;46:9–14.

17. Sievert H, Lesh MD, Trepels T, et al. Percutaneous left atrial appendage transcatheter occlusion to prevent stroke in high-risk patients with atrial fibrillation: early clinical experience. *Circulation.* 2002;105:1887–1889.

18. Hanna IR, Kolm P, Martin R, et al. Left atrial structure and function after percutaneous left atrial appendage transcatheter occlusion (PLAATO): six-month echocardiographic follow-up. *J Am Coll Cardiol.* 2004;43:1868–1872.

19. Sanchez-Quintana D, Cabrera JA, Climent V, et al. How close are the phrenic nerves to cardiac structures? Implications for cardiac interventionalists. *J Cardiovasc Electrophysiol.* 2005;16:309–313.

20. Butera G, Biondi-Zoccai GG, Carminati M, et al. Systematic review and meta-analysis of currently available clinical evidence on migraine and patent foramen ovale percutaneous closure: much ado about nothing? *Catheter Cardiovasc Interv.* 2010;75:494–504.

21. Butera G, Agostoni E, Biondi-Zoccai G, et al. Migraine, stroke and patent foramen ovale: a dangerous trio? *J Cardiovasc Med (Hagerstown)* 2008;9:233–238.

22. Kim MS, Klein AJ, Carroll JD. Transcatheter closure of intracardiac defects in adults. *J Interv Cardiol.* 2007;20:524–545.

23. Rao PS. FOCUS: Atrial septal defects. Structural heart disease in adults. *J Invasive Cardiol.* 2009;21:A6, A9–A10.

24. Rao PS. When and how should atrial septal defects be closed in adults? *J Invasive Cardiol.* 2009;21:76–82.

25. Carroll JD. Migraine Intervention With STARFlex Technology trial: a controversial trial of migraine and patent foramen ovale closure. *Circulation.* 2008;117: 1358–1360.

26. Carroll JD. Double standards in the world of ASD and PFO management: closure for paradoxical embolism. *Catheter Cardiovasc Interv.* 2009;74:1070–1071.

27. Anderson RH, Cook AC. The structure and components of the atrial chambers. *Europace.* 2007;9 (suppl 6):vi3–vi9.

28. Tzeis S, Andrikopoulos G, Deisenhofer I, et al. Transseptal catheterization: considerations and caveats. *Pacing Clin Electrophysiol.* 2010;33:231–242.

29. Davlouros PA, Niwa K, Webb G, et al. The right ventricle in congenital heart disease. *Heart.* 2006; 92 (suppl 1):i27–i38.

30. Haddad F, Couture P, Tousignant C, et al. The right ventricle in cardiac surgery, a perioperative perspective: I. Anatomy, physiology, and assessment. *Anesth Analg.* 2009;108:407–421.

31. Sheehan F, Redington A. The right ventricle: anatomy, physiology and clinical imaging. *Heart.* 2008;94: 1510–1515.

32. Goor DA, Lillehei CW. *Congenital Malformations of the Heart.* 1st ed. New York: Grune and Stratton; 1975.

33. Ho SY, Nihoyannopoulos P. Anatomy, echocardiography, and normal right ventricular dimensions. *Heart.* 2006;92(suppl 1):i2–i13.

34. Adhyapak SM, Parachuri VR. Architecture of the left ventricle: insights for optimal surgical ventricular restoration. *Heart Fail Rev.* 2010;15:73–83.

35. Gonzalez-Lavin L, Geens M, Ross DN. Pulmonary valve autograft for aortic valve replacement. *J Thorac Cardiovasc Surg.* 1970;60:322–330.

36. Ho SY. Anatomy and myoarchitecture of the left ventricular wall in normal and in disease. *Eur J Echocardiogr.* 2009;10:iii3–iii7.

37. Kim MS, Hansgen AR, Wink O, et al. Rapid prototyping: a new tool in understanding and treating structural heart disease. *Circulation.* 2008;117: 2388–2394.

38. Kim MS, Hansgen AR, Carroll JD. Use of rapid prototyping in the care of patients with structural heart disease. *Trends Cardiovasc Med.* 2008;18: 210–216.

CHAPTER 5

Cardiac CT and MRI in Patient Assessment and Procedural Guidance in Structural Heart Disease Interventions

Robert A. Quaife and John D. Carroll

T he breadth of structural heart disease interventions (SHDIs) has recently expanded, the result of ongoing improvements in percutaneous devices and patient outcomes. This success is related to the combination of new devices coupled with accurate preprocedure planning using advanced cardiac imaging and new intraprocedural guidance techniques. A cooperative multispecialty effort is essential for such complex procedures that integrate a team of interventionalists, advanced imaging specialists, and echocardiographers. A specific and major component of these results reflects improvements in three-dimensional (3D) imaging using advanced imaging techniques and the experience of the cardiac imagers in combination with a technically skilled interventional cardiologist. Selection of the correct and appropriate patients for SHDIs is perhaps the most important part of procedure. Technical improvements in noninvasive cardiac imaging now enhance standard information gained from routine echocardiography.[1-3]

In this chapter, we discuss the advantages and issues associated with cardiac MRI and cardiac computed tomography (CT) imaging of structural heart disease (SHD). Description of the relative value of these technologies applied to common SHD problems will be discussed for preprocedure planning, intraprocedural guidance, and postprocedural evaluation of results.

ADVANCED CARDIAC IMAGING METHODS

The goal of advanced cardiac imaging is to supplement data routinely available from echocardiography and to reduce the necessity of diagnostic cardiac angiography. Echocardiography still is the most widely available and safe modality to screen for SHD issues. This technology has high temporal and spatial resolution with an accurate assessment of cardiac velocities using Doppler methods. Physicians also have a general familiarity with the information acquired from echocardiography. However, the specific imaging plane and the relationship to other cardiovascular structures are less well defined with routine echocardiography. Despite significant improvements in echocardiography with the advent of 3D echocardiographic imaging using a transesophageal approach, tomographic and volumetric imaging provides a more comprehensive evaluation of the target volume and the structural relationships of adjacent anatomy.[4]

Comprehensive fine resolution of cardiac structures and display of 3D relationships to adjacent structures in combination with a full field of view (FOV) are the strengths of tomographic imaging techniques such as CT and MRI. An interventional structural disease program demands a state-of-the-art advanced cardiac imaging program. This includes high-end MRI and CT scanners to address the variety of unique problems posed by SHDI. The MRI system required is a 1.5- or 3-Tesla MRI scanner equipped with a high-speed gradient system of at least 40 mT/m gradient strength and 150 mT/m/ms slew rate, multichannel phase-array coils suitable for children to adults. Similarly, a CT required has, at a minimum, a 64-slice multidetector rows computed tomography (MDCT) system with a fast gantry rotation (i.e., 400 msec or less per rotation) and multisegment multiphasic retrospective or prospective cardiac gating methods.[5] The need for multiple two-dimensional (2D) and 3D reconstructions necessitates substantial memory and computing power in workstations to rapidly process and display this complex data. Because evaluation of moving formats is necessary to accurately define fine structures, postsurgical relationships, and position of defects, the workstation requires significant computing power. Dedicated four-dimensional (4D) workstations are necessary to process these data-intensive studies in a timely manner.[5]

Cardiac MRI

Cardiac MRI (CMR) is a valuable technique employed to fully evaluate patients with SHD. CMR routinely includes four major pulse sequence types used in the routine assessment of cardiovascular patients.[5,6] Basic technical characteristics simply define T1-weighted imaging as the response of the organ or blood to the primary magnetic field (i.e., the magnet strength), whereas T2-weighted images rely on the local tissue individual magnetic effects (i.e., tissue protons; fat, water, or specific tissues), all resulting in different image intensity signals. Specific imaging sequences focus on these different characteristic to obtain cardiac images. The sequences can be categorized as (1) bright-blood cine sequence, (2) dark-blood T2-weighted sequence, (3) phase-contrast sequence, and (4) MR angiography. Cardiac gating is required to stop cardiac motion and reduce imaging blurring that would normally result from cardiac motion. Commercially available sequences usually employ breath holding to remove respiratory motion. Adults usually breath-hold voluntarily but this is more difficult in adolescents and children. Thus, alternative navigator methods have been developed to average respiratory cycles over multiple breaths allowing acquisition at either inspiration or expiration that provide high-quality nonblurred images.[7]

CMR imaging is usually performed in modules, which include (1) scout/axial localizers, (2) long-axis localizer (orthogonal axis), (3) cardiac function, (4) tissue characterization, (5) phase contrast shunt or flow determinations, (6) myocardial flow/perfusion, (7) MR angiography, and (8) delayed contrast enhancement.

Cardiac function and quantification of volumes and ejection fraction are performed using a bright-blood cine sequence that produces a series of images that are played as a composite movie loop averaged over multiple cardiac cycles (cinematic display). Signal within the ventricles and vessel lumens are encoded bright by implementing a steady-state free precession (SSFP) sequence (Fig. 5-1). Images produced by this sequence are T2 weighted, which is in contradistinction to older gradient-recall echo (GRE) cine sequences. The SSFP sequences provide higher contrast and are resistant to inflow effects. Cine images are acquired in standard cardiac axes. Structural anatomy and physiologic motion of the heart can be evaluated.

Dark-blood sequence produces images at a single cardiac phase with bright soft tissue structures (myocardium and vessel walls) but dark-blood signals inside ventricles and vessel lumen. Employing a breath-hold technique, a double-inversion recovery sequence is used to acquire the images with an improved contrast to noise with fewer artifacts. Dark-blood images are useful for evaluating morphology, tissue characteristic, and

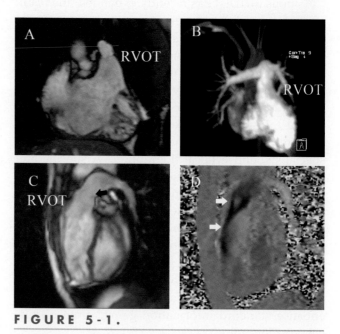

FIGURE 5-1.

Cardiac magnetic resonance (CMR) images shown of the right ventricle in **(A)** steady-state free precession (SSFP), **(B)** MR angiography, and **(C)** magnitude and **(D)** phase-contrast images. These sequences SSFP, MRA dynamic, and phase-contrast define functional characteristics of the right ventricle, which are important for percutaneous valve replacement of the pulmonic valve. Note the *white arrows* indicate a regurgitant jet from pulmonary valve regurgitation. RVOT, right ventricular outflow tract.

connections of the cardiovascular structures. Limited temporal information is a limitation of this technique. Adding a third inversion pulse provides enhanced fluid signal characteristics that help distinguish fluid or edema from fat or tissue. This is important for defining recent inflammation or infarction.

MR angiography (MRA) can be divided into contrast-enhanced technique and non–contrast-enhanced technique. Contrast-enhanced MRA produces high-resolution images, but, due to the inherent noncubical (nonisotropic voxels) resolution, the resolution is slightly more limited than that of CT angiography for evaluating thin structures or fine fistulous tract often present in SHD. MRA is a volumetric technique that allows multiplanar reformatting of the bright, contrast-filled blood vessel, 3D data (Fig. 5-1B).[7] Typically, this technique is not cardiac gated and is used for evaluating noncardiac structures, such as the aorta and the pulmonary arteries. Administration of gadolinium-based contrast agent is required at a concentration of between 0.1 and 0.2 mmol/kg (around 20 to 30 mL) for this technique. Gadolinium contrast is safe under most conditions but is contraindicated in patients with acute or severe chronic renal failure. The concern in adults is a rare condition known as nephrogenic systemic fibrosis (NSF), which is associated with gadolinium contrast use in patients with renal failure. Thus, prudence dictates that gadolinium contrast should not be used in patients with glomerular filtration rate (creatinine clearance less than 30 mL/min).[8] Noncontrast MRA studies are performed using cardiac gated, 3D, navigated echo, SSFP sequences.

Phase-contrast sequences generate quantitative velocity mapping similar to Doppler echocardiography. This method is very useful in quantifying regurgitant volumes and Qp/Qs calculations present in paravalvular leaks and shunt pathology lesions. Phase-contrast sequences for congenital heart disease (CHD) are used to quantify flow and pressure gradient estimated from velocity by the Bernoulli equation. To measure flow, an imaging plane is placed perpendicular to the vessel lumen such that both the cross-section of the vessel and the through-plane velocity of blood are imaged. Total flow is calculated by summing velocity across the luminal cross-section with a known slice thickness providing absolute flow and volume. Therefore, cardiac output, shunt ratio, and valvular regurgitation (Fig. 5-1C,D) can be quantified.[9]

Cardiac CT

Ultrafast CT was one of the first CT imaging systems to be able to detect interatrial shunt employing temporal resolution of approximately 50 ms per frame,

thereby stopping cardiac motion. The advent of faster gantry rotation speeds, increased numbers of detectors, and dual sources improved spatial and temporal resolution, thereby allowing application of multislice CT scanners in SHDI. Imaging of delicate structures present in SHD requires at a minimum a 40- to 64-row detector system and may be enhanced by new 256- or 320-row CT systems that allow information acquisition in one to four heart beats. Utilizing the 64-row or greater CT scanner with a gantry rotation time of 420 ms or faster, tube voltages of 80-100-120 kV, and tube current upward of 800 mA are all required.

Implementation of multiphase contrast injectors and high-concentration contrast agents (Isovue 370 mg/mL) has also dramatically improved the image quality, a necessary requirement for delineation of fine structures (i.e., atrial baffles, paravalvular leaks, and origin of the great vessels). High flow rate and multiphase contrast injectors have allowed minimization of contrast artifacts and the ability to produce differential chamber contrast concentrations. Delivery of an adequately dense contrast bolus to opacify the cardiac chambers while at the same time reducing beam-hardening artifact emanating from the superior vena cava requires fast power injection of the contrast bolus with washout by saline chaser injection. Importantly, reducing the concentration or creating a gradient of the contrast level compared to other structures or chambers is important for the accurate evaluation of SHD.[10–13] To achieve the desired opacification of chambers, the rate of injection and percentage of contrast needs to be varied. It is possible to change the concentration by either diluting the contrast or reducing the rate of injection. These methods provide differential chamber contrast concentration necessary for identification of the shunts, delineation of fine structures, and 3D special relationships often required for preprocedural planning in SHD.[5,10] Thus, clear communication between the interventionalist to the imaging specialist is needed so that the injection protocol optimizes the visualization of the target.

In a typical cardiac exam using a 64-slice scanner, approximately 75 mL of iodinated contrast (Iopamidol–Isovue; 370 mg/mL) is injected in the right anticubital vein at 5 mL/s followed by a 30 to 50 mL saline chase also delivered at 3 to 4 mL/s. However, the site of injection (e.g., right or left anticubital veins or possibly the leg) may be important for the identification of different intracardiac shunts. Information regarding the potential right-to-left direction of atrial septal defect (ASD) shunting can be determined by performing a dynamic contrast-enhanced cardiac exam. Funabashi and colleagues were able to demonstrate shunt directionality in ventricular septal

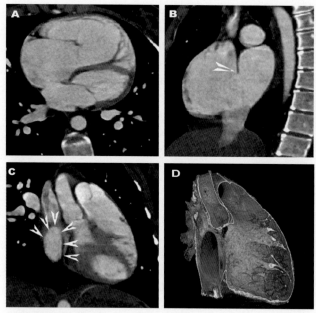

FIGURE 5-2.

Cardiac computed tomographic angiography images of a large atrial septal defect. Orthogonal views of the atrial septal defect (ASD) are shown from the long axes **(A,B)** and short axis **(C)**. The *arrows* delineate the large ASD, also shown as a "hole" in **(D)**. **(D)** A three-dimensional volumetric display of the large ASD with an absent inferior rim. (Reprinted from Quaife RA, Chen MY, Jehle A, et al. Pre-procedural planning for percutaneous atrial septal defect closure: using cardiac computed tomographic angiography. *J Cardiovasc Comput Tomogr.* 2010;4:330–338, with permission from Elsevier.)

defect (VSD), ASD, and patent ductus arteriosus (PDA) by comparing the density of right and left chamber at 5 and 30 seconds after contrast injection.[14] Shunt directionality utilizing a triple phase contrast protocol using 60 mL of iodixanol followed by 40 mL of dilute iodixanol (50:50 with saline), then followed by a 50 mL saline flush demonstrated similar feasibility. Furthermore, the orientation of a contrast jet on dynamic contrasted cardiac CT can be helpful in the differentiation of secundum ASD from patent foramen and, in shunt visualization, from ischemic VSD, perivalvular leak, or other complex CHD (Fig. 5-2).[15]

Optimal acquisition protocols are critical for SHD evaluations using CT and must balance the radiation dose being delivered. Most current systems have radiation dose reduction methods that should be applied whenever possible. These include electrocardiography (ECG) phase dose modulation or "step and shoot" sequential axial imaging technologies. Yet, the dynamic nature of cardiac structures often requires assessment throughout the cardiac cycle. Consideration of patient size is also required to properly tailor tube current and voltage to deliver the minimum radiation

dose to the patient that answers the important question. This is especially important in young individuals who, because of their disease, have often been subjected to multiple procedures using ionizing radiation.[16]

Elimination of motion artifacts is of the utmost importance in obtaining high-quality cardiac images. Cardiac motion is least significant during end systole and mid-to-late diastole making electrocardiogram (ECG) gating a requirement of any cardiac CT exam. The use of oral or intravenous beta-blockers to slow heart rate also helps to limit cardiac motion and improve image acquisition. However, care must be used in patients with pulmonary hypertension, reduced ventricular function, and cardiac conduction abnormalities.

Modality Selection

Advanced cardiac imaging techniques are usually performed after a screening echocardiogram. Selection of the appropriate imaging modality is probably related most to the type of SHD problem to be addressed, but may also be determined by availability and local expertise. Therefore, consideration of the absolute spatial resolution, temporal resolution, FOV, and characterization of different tissue types needs to be identified and addressed. Either CT or cardiovascular magnetic resonance (CMR) provide extended FOV compared to echocardiography; however, they differ significantly in spatial versus temporal resolution (Table 5-1). CT angiography (CTA) possesses inherently greater absolute resolution between 0.4 and 0.6 mm, but is at a cost of lower temporal resolution even when large doses of beta-blockers are used to lower the heart rate and improve nonmotion imaging. CMR in general can be performed at most physiologic heart rate without heart rate-lowering medications, but suffers from a nonuniform voxel size with lower resolution in the z axis of 1.5 to 2 mm. This creates voxels of $1 \times 1 \times 2$ mm, which limits assessment of structures that course out of normal planes. Characterization of tissue edema or scar in addition to flow or shunts is the strength of CMR. Another key question is the potential effect of ionizing radiation on a patient. This relates to patient age, sex, and the region of interest because some tissues are more sensitive than other to effects of radiation. Breast tissue in women is a more sensitive tissue and is directly in the FOV for most cardiac imaging.[16,17] Therefore, careful consideration is required to determine both the short-term benefits (i.e., procedural success) and long-term risks (i.e., future cancer) associated with CTA. In general, CTA is better for fine resolution as long as the heart rate can be lowered

TABLE 5-1 **Value of Different Cardiac Magnetic Resonance and Computed Tomographic Angiography Methods Used in Structural Heart Disease Interventions**

Method	Role	Preprocedure	Intraprocedure	Postprocedure
CTA	Structural characterization	+++	++	+++
CTA	Advanced structural characterization	+++	+	+++
CMR	Advanced structural characterization	++	(++ future)	+
Quant CMR	Shunt characterization	++++	(++ future)	++++
Quant CMR	Shunt and regurgitant lesions evaluation	++++	(++ future)	++++
Quant CMR	Hemodynamic characterization	++++	(++ future)	++++

CMR, cardiac magnetic resonance; CTA, computed tomographic angiography. Utility scale is shown from (+) modestly useful to significantly useful (+++).

without contraindications, whereas CMR is better for larger structures at higher heart rate, or quantification of volumes or shunts is required.

PREPROCEDURE ADVANCED IMAGE PROCESSING FOR OPTIMAL PATIENT SELECTION

The successful percutaneous correction of SHD problems requires not only a thorough clinical evaluation but also comprehensive preprocedure imaging, detailing the SHD abnormality. In most cases, transthoracic echocardiography (TTE) and transesophageal echocardiography (TEE) provide the initial evaluation. However, in the case of large ASDs, for example, the presence or, more importantly, the absence of an inferior rim may not be completely assessed on a TEE.[18,19] Therefore, high-resolution multiplanar CTA or MRA may be required to help identify this problematic anatomy.[20]

Obviously, spatial resolution is critically important, but also important is definition of the structure throughout the cardiac cycle displayed at the correct orientation to identify the correct structure. This is accomplished using multiplanar reconstruction (MPR) and myocardial perfusion imaging (MPI) image display techniques. The 3D nature of both CMR angiography and CTA allows reorientation in thin planes of off-axis data to resolve detailed anatomy not usually visualized in standard cardiac plane. The need for nonstandard planes is especially true for pathologic states such as aortic pseudoaneurysm. However, to understand the true adjacency of structures, 3D volumetric reconstructions are required. Although not as quantitative, they provide the SHD interventionalist with a visual model of the size and orientation of the abnormality (Fig. 5-3). This type of eye–hand visualization can be extended in a technique called rapid prototyping or 3D modeling

printed from a 3D graphic printer.[21] To attain this level of image processing and reconstruction, proper initial processing of CTA and MRA basic data is required, but it also requires fine tuning of image segmentation by a clinically knowledgeable individual.

Postprocessing of the CTA data set is important to select those images that will yield the least cardiac motion. Typically, axial data sets are reconstructed retrospectively from 0% to 90% of the R-R interval at between 0.8 and 1.0-mm slice thickness with 50% slice overlap (0.8/0.4, 1/0.5, or for more noisy data, 2/1 mm). Depending on the presence of metal and the attenuation artifacts from metal, the smoothing image data kernel may be set at a smooth or sharp characteristic. Often the sharpest kernel (for CTA images) is required for assessment of paravalvular leaks where the adjacent prosthetic valve with sewing ring creates significant artifacts that, if not addressed, can obscure the target paravalvular leak. The concepts of targeting and interventional path planning identification are crucial for successful interventions (Fig. 5-4).

Data may then be evaluated using MPR images or maximum intensity projection (MIP) image sets in orthogonal views of the target, which provide the basis for assessment of SHD (Fig. 5-4). Use of 3D display methods is less well standardized and often requires imager interface to display the structure in a meaningful way.[22] Intensity inversion threshold methods are often required to view structures within the chambers. This method codes the contrast dark, allowing tissue (gray structures) to stand out from the contrast in the chambers. Addition of cinematic motion of these images often allows significantly improved visualization of such abnormal structures.

MRA, on the other hand, is acquired with the image data parameters obtained at the time of imaging. Only MRA images can be postprocessed similar to those

FIGURE 5-3.

Rapid prototype models provide insight into the three-dimensional (3D) orientation of the target, in this case, an atrial septal defect (ASD). Images on the left depict the standard Amplatzer delivery system **(A)** and, on the right, the Hausdorf-Lock delivery catheter **(B)** with orientation of device in relationship to the defect. Top images simulate fluoroscopy and the middle four images are multiplanar reconstruction images from a computed tomography image of an ASD cardiac model in the anterior and left anterior oblique projections. Volumetric 3D images are shown on the bottom. (From Quaife RA & Carroll JD. In: Hijazi ZM, Feldman T, Abdullah Al-Qbandi MH, Sievert H, eds. *Transcatheter Closure of Atrial Septal Defects & Patent Foramen Ovale: A Comprehensive Assessment.* 2010. Used with permission from Cardiotext Publishing.)

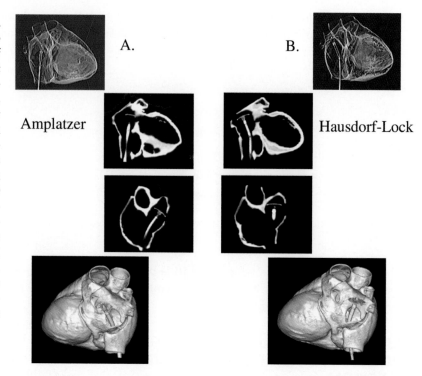

of CTA. MPR and MIP image orientation and display are the hallmarks of image analysis for SHD. Selection of the timed segments of the dynamic gadolinium contrast injection is most critical to identify cardiac structure such as the right atrium (RA), right ventricle (RV), pulmonary outflow tract and pulmonary artery (PA) versus pulmonary veins, left atrium (LA), left ventricle (LV), and aorta. Once the segment is selected,

MR vendors often have preset image "galleries" or color-coded volumetric 3D display packages to render the 2D image into a 3D format. Because CMR has less signal to noise than CTA, these presets are often too stringent for these images and require individual manipulation. Despite this minor limitation of MRA images, similar image quality is provided to those of CTA once adjusted correctly.

FIGURE 5-4.

The key preprocedural imaging characteristics are outlined for a paravalvular leak case. Planning begins with orientation of the interatrial septum and the probable location of the transseptal puncture. This is followed by identification of the target, and the pathway or trajectory to the target and the relationship to important factors, such as the sewing ring of the valve, leaflets, and orientation, in order to successfully deploy a leak closing device. AV, atrioventricular valve; IAS, interatrial septa; IVC, inferior vena cava; LA, left atrium; LAA, left atrium appendage; LV, left ventricle; MV, mitral valve; RA, right atrium; RV, right ventricle; SVC, superior vena cava; TV, tricuspid valve.

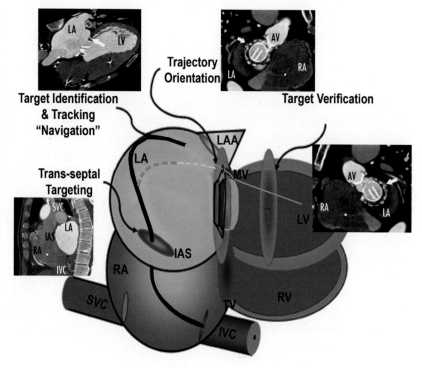

Identifying the critical structures involved in a nonsurgical approach to SHD is problem specific. The characteristics of SHDI are determined by the anatomic variations and technologic limitations of the proposed procedure. Advanced cardiac imaging provides a valuable resource of heart- and vessel-specific information to evaluate exclusionary characteristics, presizing, procedural risk assessment, and subsequent complication assessment. This requires a cooperative effort between the imager who understands the major issues of a specific procedure and interventionalist who can visualize the procedure and then evaluate the image data. It is the responsibility of the imager to display the data in a meaningful method to allow the proceduralist to assess the anatomy and characteristics of the intervention, from which both contribute data about the procedural risks and the potential for long-term complications.[5] In more complex cases, this may be enhanced by creation of a physical model of a defect or aneurysm. Although only a single cardiac phase depiction, the model sheds light about the size, orientation, and adjacencies around the target point. Additionally, these models may also be used to model positioning of catheters or devices prior to actual implantation (Fig. 5-3). Simplified identification of complex anatomic angulations and potential stress points can be simulated prior to actual device implantation. Use of these preprocedural imaging methods hopefully improve the safety and possibly shorten the time of SHDI.[21,22]

Atrial Septal Defects

CTA is a high-resolution and wide FOV technique that allows detailed anatomy resolution, assessment, and spatial orientation of the pulmonary veins, coronary sinus, and of specific ASD morphologic characteristics (i.e., rim dimensions and tissue quality) (Fig. 5-2).

Similarly, CMR is an accurate method of determining ASD size defect size, spatial orientation of the pulmonary veins, and coronary sinus while providing more quantitative determinations of the magnitude of shunting and the degree of RV volume overload. RV enlargement and a significant left-to-right shunt are factors defining the necessity of closure for ASDs (Fig. 5-5). This information is invaluable in clarifying the feasibility of percutaneous defect closure with occluder devices.[20,23,24]

In a feasibility study, we studied CTA for evaluation of patients with a secundum ASD prior to possible transcatheter closure and found that CTA was better than echocardiography in determining the size and tissue quality of the inferior rim in large septal defects.[20] Single-plane imaging modalities such as TEE are limited in their capacity to thoroughly evaluate ASDs with deficient inferior rims.[25,26] The angulation of TEE planes, despite multiplane technology, is still limited by the esophageal location. Furthermore, oblong defects may be cut tangentially, thereby resulting in a misinterpretation of the size of the defect and/or the presence or absence of rims, which are key factors for procedural success. Our investigation of the utility of CTA was performed before the availability of 3D TEE echocardiography methods, and such technology may also provide similar information.[20,23] CTA and the full FOV with CTA may better define percutaneous versus surgical candidates when compared to standard 2D TEE. Measurements obtained by CTA in either the axial or sagittal projections appeared to correlate with the maximum diameter determined by invasive balloon sizing by intracardiac echocardiography (ICE). Comparable results between balloon sizing of ASD size by CMR and CTA are reported, but CTA offers the advantage of providing superior multiplanar resolution and, when coupled with 3D image display, allows operators an insight into potential procedural success.[23,27]

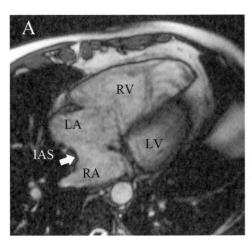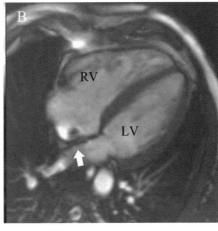

FIGURE 5-5.

A,B: Cardiac magnetic resonance evaluation of a large secundum atrial septal defect (ASD) is shown. Note the absent posterior interatrial rim and the associated right ventricle enlargement and hypertrophy. **B:** An ASD closure device is in place (*arrow*) in the interatrial septum from a different patient. IAS, interatrial septa; LA, left atrium; LV, left ventricle; RA, right atrium; RV, right ventricle.

During viewing of CTA data, it is critical to define orthogonal planes to accurately assess the size, location, and rim components. CTA also provides the ability to assess the dynamic nature of interatrial septal defects necessary for accurate sizing of the hole. Key measurements that are important for successful closure include the superoinferior and anteroposterior defect measurements, distance between defect edge to the right superior pulmonary vein, and distance from the edge of the defect to the anterior mitral valve leaflets. Also, atrial dilation in the chronic volume overload from a large ASD can distort the axis of the interatrial septum and lead to a more difficult 2D echocardiographic assessment of rim tissue. Absence of inferior rim tissue in one report was the most predictive of an unsuccessful percutaneous closure attempt.[28] Thus, preprocedure identification of such anatomy by CTA in selected cases (i.e., in large ASDs [over 20 mm] or inferiorly positioned ASDs) potentially could eliminate attempts at percutaneous closure with a low chance of success and triage them to surgical closure. Volumetric 3D display of CTA data may also help clarify important relationships to pulmonary veins, coronary sinus, and of mitral valve leaflet (Fig. 5-2). Further studies are needed to see if these patient-specific 3D anatomic features, which are easily determined by CTA, can be used to improve device closure procedures and avoid device–anatomy size mismatch or misalignment that lead to complications such as ASD device embolization and erosion. Animal studies using CTA are being used to enhance our understanding of ASD device–anatomy interactions and the risk of erosion.[29]

Congenital and Ischemic Ventricular Septal Defects

VSD is a common form of CHD in children and is rarely identified and diagnosed in adulthood. Most are membranous VSD with less frequent muscular VSDs detected. However, many VSDs that are identified are an unexpected finding during the evaluation of shortness of breath and pulmonary hypertension. SHDI using devices aimed at closing muscular VSDs is now common. Closure of these VSDs relatively late in adulthood still appears to generate improvement in LV systolic function and modulation of pulmonary arterial hypertension. Retrospective evaluations of surgical VSD closures demonstrate an 18% residual shunt and higher risk of atrioventricular (AV) conduction problems and arrhythmias. Percutaneous closure methods appear to have lower complication rates than those experienced with surgical closure.[30] Characterization of the size and location

of these defects is important for planning percutaneous interventions.[31,32] CMR provides quantification of the severity of shunt and the magnitude of pulmonary hypertension using phase contrast sequences. Generally, identification of the defect is comparable to that of CTA, although in small VSDs (which are associated with hypertrophy and trabeculation) this may be more difficult. CTA allows MPR characterization of the entire tract through the trabeculation of these VSDs.

Unlike congenital VSD patients who are often clinically stable, postinfarct VSD patients are often unstable with cardiogenic shock requiring intra-aortic balloon pump or other support devices. Postinfarction VSD is a highly lethal complication of ischemic heart disease with mortalities of 20% to 50% soon after recognition and 90% mortality if untreated. Sizing of these defects is difficult due to the underlying process resulting in essentially a tearing of tissue with necrotic tissue borders (Fig. 5-6). As a result, postinfarction VSDs have a major deviation from the idealized circular geometry of congenital defects and, in addition, defect size may dramatically change during the cardiac cycle and with alterations in loading conditions.[33,34] In many cases, cardiogenic shock limits CMR evaluation. CTA provides an alternative method of 3D assessment of the defect, but there are numerous challenges. Renal insufficiency and often tachycardia are potential limitations for using CTA, although they are not absolute contraindications. Echocardiography still remains the initial imaging modality most transportable and widely available. However, the exact characterization is limited by both transthoracic with limited spatial resolution and transesophageal echocardiography, which often requires difficult transgastric views.

Specific characterization of the defects is complicated by the complex shape of these tears in the myocardium. These perforations may have multiple orifices and extensive tunnels that make it difficult to identify the LV entrance and RV exit sites. CTA with adequate heart rate control resulting in suspension of cardiac motion provides the multiplanar method to reorient the septal muscle fiber necessary to identify the defect tracts. This appears to be similar to that obtained by real-time 3D TEE. When planning percutaneous closure of these defects, not only is the size important for the adequacy of available device sizes, but the tract length and deployment orientation are also key to defining potential success and recommendations for procedure performance. Perforations adjacent to the moderator band common in apical–septal VSDs may limit deployment of the device successfully or adequate closure of the defect. Simulation measurements of the planned device in the defect to surrounding structures from the CTA images may help define an initial starting

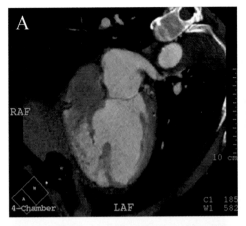

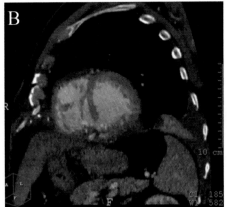

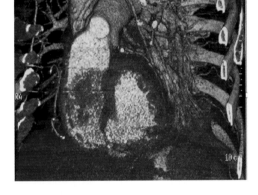

FIGURE 5-6.

A large ischemic postinfarct ventricular septal defect is shown in orthogonal views **(A,B)** and in three-dimensional volumetric format **(C)**. Note the inferior-septal location with limited free wall rim and complex nature of the defect. LAF, left arcuate fasciculus; RAF, right arcuate fasciculus.

point. Figure 5-7 shows a device in place in an apical VSD. These examples exemplify some of the major issues of associated SHDI in postinfarct VSDs.

Aortic Pseudoaneurysms

Recent technical advances in transcatheter device development have allowed transcatheter therapies for aortic pseudoaneurysms in what has been primarily a surgical treatment world. Both CMR and CTA have similar value in the clinical evaluation of this entity. Because object motion does not pose a significant problem, these studies can be performed without beta-blocker administration. Most SHDIs in aortic pseudoaneurysms are in nonsurgical candidates with potential life-threatening problems. Much like ASD, definition of the size, presence

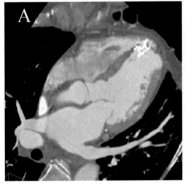

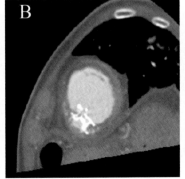

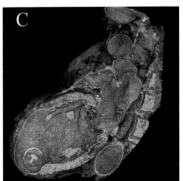

FIGURE 5-7.

A-C: Postischemic ventricular septal defect (VSD) device placement is shown depicting the difficulty in defining the orientation of the defect, tissue, and the device. This apical–septal VSD was successfully closed but did not completely stop left-to-right flow. Thirty months later, the patient is physically active despite the small residual leak.

FIGURE 5-8.

A: The dilemma over the best method to guide this procedure, transesophageal echocardiography (TEE) versus transthoracic echocardiography (TTE), is depicted. TTE was selected based on the cardiac magnetic resonance imaging. TEE would involve a greater distance from the esophagus to the target and ultrasound signal transmission limitation through the left bronchus. The echocardiogram images show the aortic pseudoaneurysm before **(B)** and after **(C)** device deployment using biplane echocardiography.

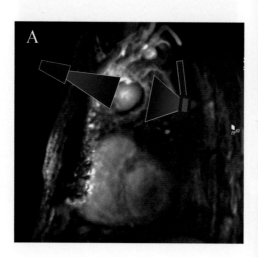

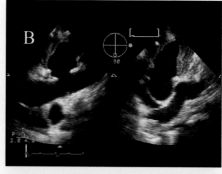

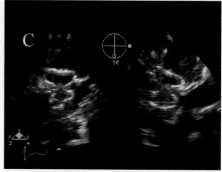

of rims of tissue defining a neck, and adjacency to other structure are critical preplanning characteristics.[35] Most interventions not involving "stent grafts" are in the ascending aorta. Technical challenges for these interventions include tortuosity of the ascending and arch aorta and catheter choices to provide stability for deployment of a device (Fig. 5-8). Many of these issues can be defined either by 3D image displays or physical models. An example of CMR preintervention and postintervention is shown in Figure 5-9.

Transcatheter Aortic Valve Implantation

Recent advances in valve technologies have led to catheter-mounted valves that may be deployed percutaneously.[36] This technology is becoming a major therapy for patients with severe aortic stenosis.[37] CTA has become a significant part of the management of transcatheter aortic valve implantation (TAVI) patients. Its ability to characterize extensive calcification in addition to defining relationships between the aorta and the origins of the coronary vessels provides key pieces of data necessary for patient selection for this procedure.[38] CMR and echocardiography are limited in the assessment in calcification within or around the aortic valve. Outcomes related to this procedure are importantly related to how to select the most appropriate candidates for these interventions.

In a CTA study that evaluated patients undergoing TAVI by del Valle-Fernandez and coauthors,[38] they characterized several key items that help define procedural success. These parameters included diameters of the annulus, cusp, and sinotubular junction of the aorta; the angulation between the aorta and the LV; and the distance between the AV leaflet insertion and the origins of both the right and left coronary ostia.[38–42] These parameters determine sizing and positioning and are critical because malpositioning of the device/valve stent can result in significant regurgitation and impairment of the mitral valve apparatus. Therefore, selection of the correct patients is as important as selection of the size of the valve. Shown in Figure 5-10 are measurements made prior to TAVI with a follow-up study defining the positioning of the device. Assessment of the ascending, thoracic, and abdominal aorta is a critical factor in the decision whether percutaneous versus transapical approach is selected (Fig. 5-11).[43,44] Additionally, preprocedural planning of the trajectory of the placement of wires and balloon catheters are shown using a physical model of the aorta and aortic valve from the CTA of this patient. The position may exert disproportionate stress of one leaflet compared to another (Fig. 5-12). Development of such imaging-based techniques or tools will assist in the successful deployment of these valves. Shown in Figure 5-13 is the preprocedural and postprocedural CTA, in which one can understand the alignment and placement of

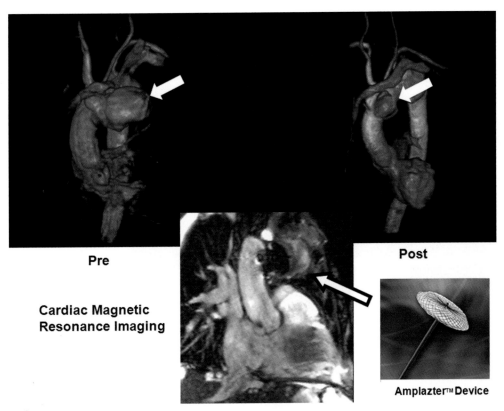

FIGURE 5-9.

Precardiac and postcardiac magnetic resonance angiography (MRA) and steady-state free precision images are shown for an aortic pseudoaneurysm. The susceptibility artifact in the postprocedural image is shown (white arrow) in the shape similar to the device (*lower right*). The defect from the device postprocedure is on the right of the image. There was complete closure of the pseudoaneurysm.

the valve. An example of TAVI is shown in Figure 5-14. Similar methods can be applied to the pulmonary valve and percutaneous placement of the Melody or SAPIEN prosthesis in CHD patients.

Paravalvular Leaks

The percutaneous treatment of paravalvular leaks may be a tedious and difficult proposition. Most often, like aortic pseudoaneurysm, transcatheter paravalvular leak closure is performed in individuals with a high risk of cardiac surgery reoperation. It is frequently characterized by episode of decompensated heart failure and often accompanied by hemolysis.[45] These leaks are often identified by color flow Doppler but the size and shape are not well defined by echocardiography because of the adjacency of significant metal reverberation artifacts. Again, CMR is limited in defining the origin of the leak but is able to quantify the severity of regurgitation.

CTA is the best method to characterize these somewhat illusive perforations but still has limitations. The extensive metal and often calcification may limit evaluation of the size of the defect. Multiphase CTA acquisitions and reconstructions are often required to determine the size and shape of the hole (Fig. 5-15). In some cases, these may be multiple. The size from the sewing ring to the edge and the arc length are important for determining the type and size of devices to be attempted. Maximal size often is noted during one part of the cardiac cycle and is not consistently diastole or systole. Thus, this then requires the higher radiation dose multisegment/phase acquisition method. Next attention must turn to the relationship to the leaflet for orientation under fluoroscopy and to other structures. This is very important because, in the aortic position, they are often adjacent to the left main coronary ostium. The position of the valve leaflets to the perforation, especially if they are a tilting disk or a bileaflet valve, is critical for assessing the risk of entrapment of the leaflet with the device. Also, planning for use of antegrade, retrograde, or transapical approaches is aided by this prior assessment of the likelihood of entrapment. Even catheter base angulations and approach

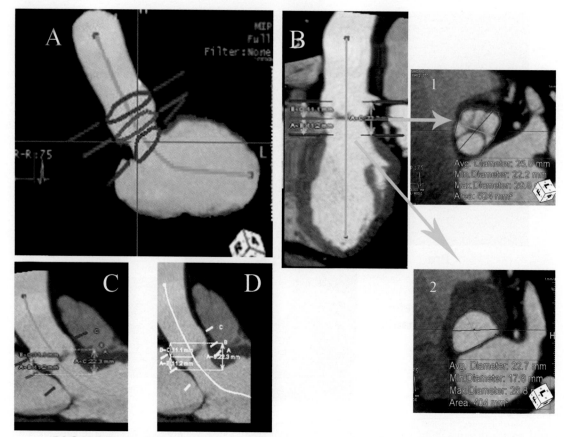

FIGURE 5-10.

Computed tomographic angiography–simulated measurements necessary for transcatheter aortic valve implantation (TAVI) are shown in initial orientation **(A)** and curved multiplanar reconstruction used to obtain measurements **(B)**. The distance from the outflow tract to the aortic valve annulus and the distance from the annulus to the left coronary ostium are measured prior to TAVI **(C,D)**. Note the more oval shape of both the left ventricular outflow tract and the aortic valve annulus **(B1,B2)**.

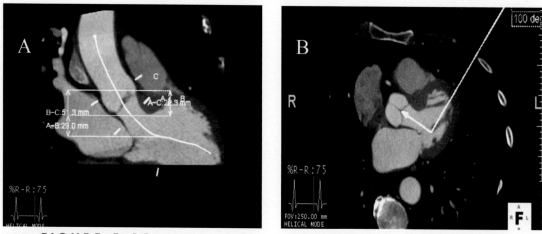

FIGURE 5-11.

A percutaneous pathway for transcatheter aortic valve implantation is shown **(A)** along with a transapical planning map **(B)**.

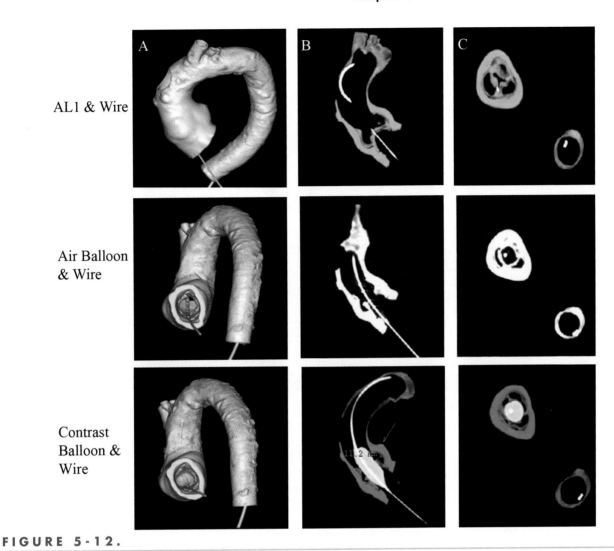

FIGURE 5-12.

A–C: Planning of catheter and wire placement prior to the procedure can be modeled, which allows selection of the most specific combination to engage the target and minimize potential complications. Note the wire position and the stress placed on the inferior leaflet when the balloon is expanded (either air or contrast).

may be modeled, as shown in Figure 5-16. It is these factors that help guide the interventionalist toward the type of devices likely to be successful.

Pulmonary Arterial and Valvular Interventions

Patients living with repaired CHD are a growing segment of the cardiovascular disease population. Approximately 85% of these people reach adulthood and the most common CHD syndromes in this population are tetralogy of Fallot (TOF) followed by pulmonary stenosis and atresia and transposition of the great vessels. Many of these individuals require pulmonary valve replacements during their lives and often this may be required multiple times throughout lives. Pulmonary arterial and branch stenoses are also associated with

the RV outflow tract (RVOT) obstruction. The advent of percutaneous interventions for these two specific problems is part of modern SHDI not available previously. Advanced imaging with either CMR or CTA is well suited to provide critical noninvasive measurements of the pulmonary annulus, RVOT angulations and orientations, and severity of stenoses in the pulmonary vessels. This is in addition to quantization of the velocities in the RVOT and also the quantified regurgitant volume. Strict criteria are mandated for percutaneous valve implantation in the pulmonary position such that the diameter of the outflow tract needs to be between 16 and 22 mm for valves such as the Melody valve (Medtronic, Inc., Minneapolis, MN) or 18 to 25 mm for the SAPIEN valve (Edwards Lifesciences, Irvine, CA). Not only is the size important but also the angulation prior to and after the valve annular region.[46]

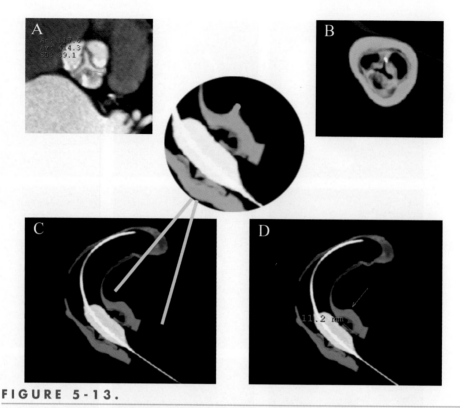

FIGURE 5-13.

A: Orientation of computed tomographic angiography image and aortic valve with severe stenosis. **B:** The computed tomography image of the model of the valve. This allows preplanning of the orientation as well as anticipating possible complications of initial balloon valvuloplasty due to angulation of the balloon in the tortuous aorta as modeled by the physical model reimaged with the balloon in place **(A,C)**. Note the difference in angulation of the superior leaflet compared to the bottom. This simulation may define greater stress on the bottom leaflet compared to the top leaflet. **D:** The distance between the aortic valve annulus and the left main coronary ostium.

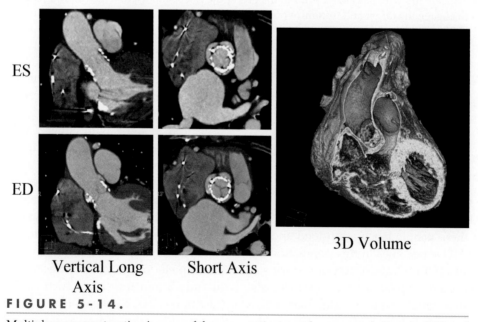

FIGURE 5-14.

Multiplanar reconstruction images of the same patient are shown at end-diastole (*ED*) and end-systole (*ES*) following transcatheter aortic valve implantation. The three-dimensional volume image shows the stent structure suspending the valve.

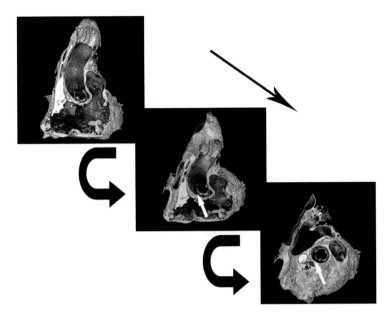

Volumetric three-dimensional (3D) display of the computed tomographic angiography image is used to rotate into the perpendicular view to identify the target (paravalvular leak in this case; *white arrows*). This requires rotation of the data in 3D to visualize the tract in order to help plan approach and best view angulation.

Pulmonary vascular intervention can be challenging in the identification of the exact sites of stenosis and the orientation when performed under fluoroscopy. CTA more than CMR can provide high-quality images even when prior hardware is present. Planning of the orientations and best angiographic view may now be identified following the CTA and prior to the interventional procedure. This preprocedural planning can be taken a step further to segment the arteries in the target vessel to provide centerlines that, on a 3D workstation, can be rotated into the orientation used in the angiographic suite. Using software such as TrueView (Philips Medical, Best, The Netherlands), the best projections with the least overlap of adjacent structures are selected and incorporated into the angiographic procedure (Fig. 5-17).

CTA   Fluoroscopy

FIGURE 5-16.

Complex procedural guidance is shown with preprocedural computed tomographic (CT) angiography planning on the left and periprocedural image on the right. The plane of the interatrial septum and the orientation to the target paravalvular leak are identified. A centerline is drawn as a pathway through the defect into the left ventricle to follow during the procedure (lower left). These data with CT are imported into the angiographic suite and registered with fluoroscopy (upper right). As a result, the CT image rotates with the C-arm during the case. The fluoroscopic image on the lower right shows the identical path to that of the centerline defined before the procedure. IAS, interatrial septa; LA, left atrium; LAA, left atrial appendage; LV, left ventricle.

FIGURE 5-17.

A,B: Computed tomographic angiography identification of a right branch pulmonary artery stenosis in orthogonal views. **C,D:** Precontrast and postcontrast angiogram and angioplasty. The *green line* is the centerline to help guide the interventionalist when the data are imported into the angiographic suite.

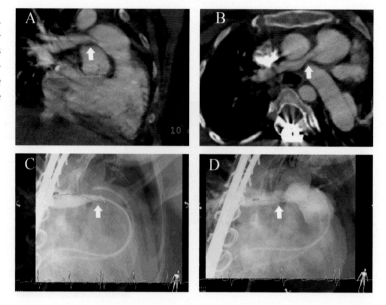

This methodology appears to reduce contrast total usage and may shorten the procedure time.

INTRAPROCEDURE GUIDANCE

One of the major limitations of fluoroscopic guidance of SHDI is the lack of tissue/structure identification. Therefore, marriage of CT tissue characterization overlay with the X-ray method provides the advantage of visualization of the cardiac soft tissue during guidance of SHDIs. This also allows preplanning of pathways for an approach identified by the prior imaging techniques, often providing a road map guidance tool using centerline methods. Rotation of the 3D data set into orientations achievable with fluoroscopic has the advantage of determining the optimal views or projections to lessen structure overlap and provide orthogonal views for guidance. This prior planning allows familiarity of the anatomic structures and relationships prior to the actual procedure. An additional advantage is the limitation of radiation dose when trial and error projection simulations are defined in advance of the SHDI. Shown in Figure 5-16 is a paravalvular leak in which the "guidance centerline" was constructed from the CTA data set. This predicted the crossing point of the interatrial transseptal puncture, the course through the atrial targeting, and identified the leak under the left atrial appendage. This centerline method provides a path for placement of guidewires through the paravalvular leak. This was verified both fluoroscopically and using CTA image overlay. More investigation is warranted, but this methodology may shorten procedure time and result in lower procedural radiation dose.[47,48]

Simulation of structure and function relationship may also be enhanced when disease-specific 3D models are generated. Orientation of catheters or devices can be tried in order to experience the complexities of angulations and constraints prior to actual procedures. Such models could provide key information about anatomic idiosyncrasies on a patient by patient basis to improve outcomes in percutaneous valve repair subjects or other types of SHDIs.[22]

Combination of tissue visualization and contrast angiography at the time of the procedure may provide guidance advantages. C-arm cone beam CT represents a technology that has been commercialized for noncardiac applications and involves rotational angiography with subsequent 3D reconstruction. The resultant CT-like 3D representations of vascular structures for neurologic interventions and soft tissue objects for abdominal interventions represent current uses. Adaptation of this technology and technique to the cardiac environment is challenging and will require both ungated and gated approaches to reconstructions. Cardiac and breathing motion, more complex injection protocols, and the need for cardiologists to gain experience in using CT applications in the procedure room are some of the challenges to be overcome. In Figure 5-18, the 3D reconstruction of the heart is seen in different projections.

CONCLUSION

Advanced cardiac imaging provides important tissue characteristics and spacial relationships necessary and key to successful SHDI. Merging of these technologies may help improve the safety, reduce procedural duration, and enhance the durability of such interventions.

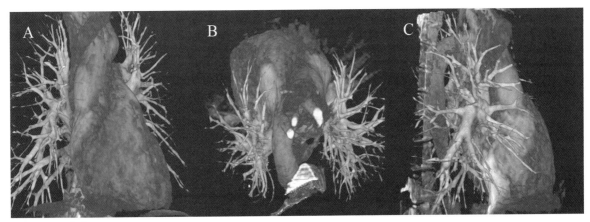

FIGURE 5-18.

An example of whole-heart flat-panel angiography is shown in anterior **(A)**, superior (head, **B**), and right lateral **(C)** projections.

REFERENCES

1. Hilliard AA, Nishimura RA. The interventional cardiologist and structural heart disease: the need for a team approach. *JACC Cardiovasc Imaging.* 2009;2:8–10.
2. Hudson PA, Eng MH, Kim MS, et al. A comparison of echocardiographic modalities to guide structural heart disease interventions. *J Interv Cardiol.* 2008;21: 535–546.
3. Silvestry FE, Kerber RE, Brook MM, et al. Echocardiography-guided interventions. *J Am Soc Echocardiogr.* 2009;22:213–231; quiz 316–317.
4. Eng MH, Salcedo EE, Quaife RA, et al. Implementation of real time three-dimensional transesophageal echocardiography in percutaneous mitral balloon valvuloplasty and structural heart disease interventions. *Echocardiography.* 2009;26(8):958–966.
5. Chan FP. MR and CT imaging of the pediatric patient with structural heart disease. *Semin Thorac Cardiovasc Surg Ped Card Surg Ann.* 2009;12:99–105.
6. Valente AM, Powell AJ. Clinical applications of cardiovascular magnetic resonance in congenital heart disease. *Cardiol Clin.* 2007;25:97–110.
7. Gutierrez FR, Ho ML, Siegel MJ. Practical applications of magnetic resonance in congenital heart disease. *Magn Reson Imaging Clin N Am.* 2008;16:403–435.
8. Thomsen HS, Marckmann P, Logager VB. Update on nephrogenic systemic fibrosis. *Magn Reson Imaging Clin N Am.* 2008;16:551–560.
9. Gatehouse PD, Keegan J, Crowe LA, et al. Applications of phase-contrast flow and velocity imaging in cardiovascular MRI. *Eur Radiol.* 2005;15:2172–2184.
10. Chan FP. Cardiac MDCT. In: Fishman EK, Jeffrey RB, eds. *Multidetector CT.* Philadelphia, PA: Lippincott Williams and Wilkins; 2004:129–158.
11. Steiner RM, Reddy GP, Flicker S. Congenital cardiovascular disease in the adult patient: imaging update. *J Thorac Imaging.* 2002;17(1):1–17.
12. Lipton MJ, Higgins CB, Farmer D, et al. Cardiac imaging with a high-speed Cine-CT Scanner: preliminary results. *Radiology.* 1984;152(3):579–582.
13. Skotnicki R, MacMillan RM, Rees MR, et al. Detection of atrial septal defect by contrast-enhanced ultrafast computed tomography. *Cathet Cardiovasc Diagn.* 1986;12(2):103–106.
14. Funabashi N, Asano M, Sekine T, et al. Direction, location, and size of shunt flow in congenital heart disease evaluated by ECG-gated multislice computed tomography. *Int J Cardiol.* 2006;112(3):399–404.
15. Quaife RA, Carroll JD. CT evaluation of the interatrial septum in atrial septal defects. In: Hijazi ZM, Feldman T, Abdullah Al-Qbandi MH, Sievert H, eds. *Transcatheter Closure of Atrial Septal Defects & Patent Foramen Ovale: A Comprehensive Assessment.* Minneapolis, MN: Cardiotext; 2010.
16. Einstein AJ, Moser KW, Thompson RC, et al. Radiation dose to patients from cardiac diagnostic imaging. *Circulation.* 2007;116:1290–1305.
17. Einstein AJ, Henzlova MJ, Rajagopalan S. Estimating risk of cancer associated with radiation exposure from 64-slice computed tomography coronary angiography. *JAMA.* 2007;298:317–323.
18. Khan AA, Tan JL, Li W, et al. The impact of transcatheter atrial septal defect closure in the older population: a prospective study. *JACC Cardiovasc Interv.* 2010;3(3):276–281.
19. Huang X, Shen J, Huang Y, et al. En face view of atrial septal defect by two-dimensional transthoracic echocardiography: comparison to real-time three-dimensional transesophageal echocardiography. *J Am Soc Echocardiogr.* 2010;23:714–721.
20. Quaife RA, Chen MY, Jehle A, et al. Pre-procedural planning for percutaneous atrial septal defect closure: using cardiac computed tomographic angiography. *J Cardiovasc Comput Tomogr.* 2010;4:330–338.
21. Kim MS, Hansgen AR, Carroll JD. Use of rapid prototyping in the care of patients with structural heart disease. *Trends Cardiovasc Med.* 2008;18(6):210–216.
22. Carroll JD. The future of image guidance of cardiac interventions. *Catheter Cardiovasc Interven* 2007;70:783.

23. Gade CL, Bergman G, Naidu S, et al. Comprehensive evaluation of atrial septal defects in individuals undergoing percutaneous repair by 64-detector row computed tomography. *Int J Cardiovasc Imaging*. 2007; 23(3):397–404.

24. Kim YJ, Hur J, Choe KO, et al. Interatrial shunt detected in coronary computed tomography angiography: differential features of a patent foramen ovale and an atrial septal defect. *J Comput Assist Tomogr*. 2008;32(5):663–667.

25. Berger F, Ewert P, Abdul-Khaliq H, et al. Percutaneous closure of large atrial septal defects with the Amplatzer septal occluder: technical overkill or recommendable alternative treatment? *J Interv Cardiol*. 2001;14(1):63–67.

26. Schwinger ME, Gindea AJ, Freedberg RS, et al. The anatomy of the interatrial septum: a transesophageal echocardiographic study. *Am Heart J*. 1990;119(6): 1401–1405.

27. Piaw CS, Kiam OT, Rapaee A, et al. Use of non-invasive phase contrast magnetic resonance imaging for estimation of atrial septal defect size and morphology: a comparison with transesophageal echo. *Cardiovasc Intervent Radiol*. 2006;29(2):230–234.

28. Durongpisitkul K, Tang NL, Soongswang J, et al. Predictors of successful transcatheter closure of atrial septal defect by cardiac magnetic resonance imaging. *Pediatr Cardiol*. 2004;25(2):124–130.

29. Ivekari AA, Haynes SE, Amelon R, et al. Analysis of real time in-vivo Amplatzer septal occluder deformation. Presentation at: Computer Methods for Cardiovascular Device Design and Evaluation. NIH, NSF, FDA Workshop; June 1–2, 2010. Bethesda, MD.

30. Al-Kashkari W, Balan P, Kavinsky CJ, et al. Percutaneous device closure of congenital & iatrogenic ventricular septal defects in adult patients. *Catheter Cardiovasc Interv*. 2011;77(2):260–267.

31. Hein R, Buscheck F, Fischer E, et al. Atrial and ventricular septal defects can safely be closed by percutaneous intervention. *J Interv Cardiol*. 2005;18(6): 515–522.

32. Hijazi ZM. Catheter closure of atrial septal and ventricular septal defects using the Amplatzer devices. *Heart Lung Circ*. 2003;12(suppl 2):S63–S72.

33. Holzer R, Balzer D, Amin Z, et al. Transcatheter closure of post-infarction ventricular septal defects using the Amplatzer muscular VSD occluder: results of a US registry. *Catheter Cardiovasc Interv*. 2004;61:196–201.

34. Halpren DG, Perk G, Ruiz C, et al. Percutaneous closure of a post infarction ventricular septal defect guided by real-time three-dimensional echocardiography. *Eur J Echocardiogr*. 2009;10:569–571.

35. Bashir F, Quaife R, Carroll JD. Percutaneous closure of ascending aortic pseudoaneurysm using Amplatzer septal occluder device: the first clinical case report and literature review. *Catheter Cardiovasc Interv*. 2005;65(4):547–551.

36. Webb JG, Altwegg L, Boone RH, et al. Transcatheter aortic valve implantation: impact on clinical and valve-related outcomes. *Circulation*. 2009;119:3009–3016.

37. Masson JB, Kovac J, Schuler G, et al. Transcatheter aortic valve implantation: review of the nature, management, and avoidance of procedural complications. *J Am Coll Cardiol Intv*. 2009;2:811–820.

38. del Valle-Fernandez R, Jelnin V, Panagopoulos G, et al. A method for standardization computed tomography angiography-based measurement of aortic valular stuctures. *Eur Hrt J*. 2010;31:2170–2178.

39. Wong DR, Ye J, Cheung A, et al. Technical considerations to avoid pitfalls during transapical aortic valve implantation. *J Thorac Cardiovasc Surg*. 2010;140: 196–202.

40. Leipsic J, Wood D, Manders D, et al. The evolving role of MDCT in transcatheter aortic valve replacement: a radiologists' perspective. *Am J Roentgenol*. 2009; 193:W214–W233.

41. Ng AC, Delgado V, Van der Kley F, et al. Comparison of aortic root dimensions and geometries before and after transcatheter aortic valve implantation by 2- and 3-dimensional transesophageal echocardiography and multislice computed tomography. *Circ Cardiovasc Imaging*. 2010;3:94–102.

42. Tops LF, Wood DA, Delgado V, et al. Noninvasive evaluation of the aortic root with multislice computed tomography implications for transcatheter aortic valve replacement. *J Am Coll Cardiol Img*. 2008;1:321–330.

43. Wood DA, Tops LF, Mayo JR, et al. Role of multislice computed tomography in transcatheter aortic valve replacement. *Am J Cardiol*. 2009;103:1295–1301.

44. Gurvitch R, Wood DA, Leipsic J, et al. Multislice computed tomography for prediction of optimal angiographic deployment projections during transcatheter aortic valve implantation. *J Am Coll Cardiol Intv*. 2010;3:1157–1165.

45. Pate GE, Al Zubaidi A, Chandavimol M, et al. Percutaneous closure of prosthetic peri-valvular leaks: case series and review. *Catheter Cardiovasc Interv*. 2006;68:528–533.

46. Demkow M, Biernacka EK, Spiewak M, et al. Percutaneous pulmonary valve implantation preceded by routine prestenting with bare metal stent. *Catheter Cardiovasc Interv*. 2011;77(3):381–389.

47. Garcia JA, Eng MH, Chen SY, et al. Image guidance of percutaneous coronary and structural heart disease interventions using a computed tomography and fluoroscopic integration. *Vas Dis Manag*. 2007;4:89–97.

49. Wallace MJ, Kuo MD, Glaiberman C, et al. Three-dimensional C-arm cone-beam CT: applications in interventional suite. *J Vasc Interv Radiol*. 2008;19: 799–813.

CHAPTER 6

Echocardiography in Patient Assessment and Procedural Guidance in Structural Heart Disease Interventions

Ernesto E. Salcedo and John D. Carroll

S tructural heart disease interventions (SHDIs) rely on a well-integrated team of interventionalists, advanced imaging specialists, and echocardiographers. Optimal results demand an experienced cardiac imager as well as a highly experienced interventionalists.[1] In this chapter, we highlight the central role that echocardiography plays in the management of patients with structural heart disease (SHD). We review the use of transthoracic and transesophageal echocardiography (TEE) for patient selection and preprocedure planning, intraprocedure guidance, and postprocedure evaluation of results.

The SHD interventionalist needs to be familiar with the different echocardiographic modalities available and needs to clearly understand the strengths and limitations of each echocardiographic technique. A brief description of current echocardiographic methods, of value in the management of patients with SHD, is presented on the opening section of this chapter. We recognize that there are different imaging modalities to assist in SHDIs, as described in other chapters of this manual. Different groups may prefer one imaging technique over another,[2] but echocardiography, because of its availability and diagnostic strengths, is the most commonly used imaging tool for the management of patients with SHD and to guide their interventions.[3]

ECHOCARDIOGRAPHIC METHODS

Table 6-1 and Figure 6-1 summarize the current echocardiographic tools for the assistance of SHDIs. Transthoracic echocardiography (TTE) is of great value for the morphologic characterization of most of the SHD abnormalities that are considered for percutaneous interventions.[3–6] TTE is routinely used for obtaining standard cardiac chamber dimensions and parameters of right and left ventricular function.[7] TTE is most commonly used for patient selection and preprocedural planning. TEE provides superior image resolution and, when the TTE is technically difficult, TEE is frequently used to better define and qualify an SHD diagnosis prior to the intervention. In addition, TEE has become the standard imaging technique to assist on catheter guidance and device deployment in many SHDIs.[3] Color Doppler and spectral Doppler can be used with both TTE and TEE. Doppler methods assist in the evaluation of cardiac shunts, regurgitant and stenotic lesions, and hemodynamic assessment.[4] Injection of agitated saline is used primarily to evaluate for the presence and degree of intracardiac shunting. It is of particular help in the detection of interatrial shunts secondary to either atrial septal defects (ASDs) or patent foramen ovale (PFO). Real-time three-dimensional (3D) echocardiography is fast becoming the standard

TABLE 6-1 Value of Different Echocardiographic Methods Used in Structural Heart Disease Interventions

Method	Role	Preprocedure (in Echo Lab)	Intraprocedure (in Cath Lab)	Postprocedure (in Cath Lab)
2D TTE	Structural characterization	++	++	++
3D TTE	Advanced structural characterization	++		++
2D TEE	Advanced structural characterization	+++	+++	+++
3D TEE	Advanced structural characterization	++++	++++	++++
Contrast echo	Shunt characterization	++++		++++
Color Doppler	Shunt and regurgitant lesions evaluation	++++		++++
Spectral Doppler	Hemodynamic characterization	++++	++++	++++

++, adequate value; +++, good value; ++++, preferred technique.
2D, two-dimensional; 3D, three-dimensional; TEE, transesophageal echocardiography; TTE, transthoracic echocardiography.

for echocardiography. Many SHDIs benefit from the exquisite anatomic detail that real-time 3D TEE provides.[8]

Patient Selection and Preprocedure Planning

The successful percutaneous correction of SHD problems requires not only a thorough clinical evaluation but also comprehensive imaging to precisely characterize the SHD abnormality. In most cases, TTE and TEE provide this information. For example, in patients with mitral stenosis being considered for mitral valve balloon valvuloplasty or percutaneous mitral commissurotomy (PMC), TTE provides the diagnosis, estimation of stenosis severity, and the feasibility of a successful intervention through the assessment of leaflet thickness, calcification mobility, and presence of subvalvular stenosis.[9] Some patients with mitral stenosis will not be suitable candidates for PMC because of mitral insufficiency, left atrial thrombus, or asymmetric degree of commissural fusion and calcification.

Echocardiography is ideally suited to provide precise quantification of the SHD abnormality being considered for intervention. Echo Doppler estimation of stenotic and regurgitant lesions is well established and is considered the gold standard in many situations. Recognizing associated pathology, such as tricuspid

regurgitation, pulmonary hypertension, and pericardial effusion, will be of added value in the preprocedure planning for an intervention.

Intraprocedure Guidance

Both TTE and TEE can be used for intraprocedure guidance of SHDIs. If the patient is going to be intubated and receive general anesthesia, we use TEE because of better image resolution. If the patient is awake and conscious sedation is planned, we will evaluate the quality of the TTE on the supine position, or with a small degree of left lateral rotation. If the images are adequate, we will proceed with TTE guidance; if not, we will use a TEE probe and conscious sedation.

After deciding what echocardiographic method will be used for guidance (TTE vs. TEE), the diagnosis is confirmed, the need for intervention is reviewed, and the desirable goals for the intervention are discussed. A preintervention echocardiogram detailing the area of interest is recorded to use for comparison with a postprocedure echocardiogram.

Transseptal puncture for delivery of catheters and devices in the left heart is frequently the first intraprocedure step where echo plays a pivotal role. This is explained in detail in the section of echocardiographic guidance for specific SHDIs.

Recognizing guidewires, catheters, and devices with echocardiography may be difficult and requires

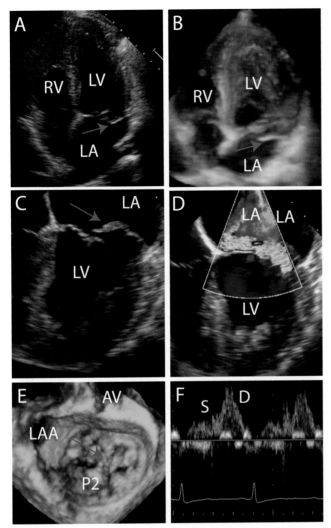

FIGURE 6-1.

Echo modalities used to assist structural heart disease interventions. Patient with flail mitral valve (P2) segment and severe eccentric mitral regurgitation being evaluated for percutaneous mitral valve repair. **A:** Two-dimensional transthoracic echocardiography (TTE): apical four-chamber view demonstrating the flail posterior leaflet. **B:** Three-dimensional TTE: Note the improved depiction of the flail segment rendered by the added dimension. **C:** Two-dimensional transesophageal echocardiography (TEE): The flail segment is clearly depicted with this approach. **D:** Two-dimensional TEE with color Doppler: Illustrating an eccentric mitral regurgitation jet of moderate to severe degree. **E:** Three-dimensional TEE: "Surgeon's view" of the mitral valve from the left atrium clearly illustrating the P2 segment flail and the ruptured chordae. **F:** Pulsed Doppler demonstrating systolic blunting of pulmonary flow consistent with moderate/severe mitral regurgitation. The *red arrows* point to the flail mitral valve segment. AV, aortic valve; LA, left atrium; LAA, left atrial appendage; LV, left ventricle; RV, right ventricle; S and D, systolic and diastolic phases of pulmonary venous flow.

experience and practice. The catheter, guidewire, or device may not be readily apparent on the echocardiogram because they are off the anatomic echocardiographic plane. This problem is minimized by using 3D echocardiography or by enlarging the angle of view. Another problem is the inability of echo to distinguish between the tip of the catheter and parts of the body of the catheter. Moving the catheter in and out of the imaging plane helps in recognizing the actual catheter tip. Small wires are not very echogenic and can only be seen when they are moved. An additional point to keep in mind is the presence of "shadowing" from the catheters that can create the appearance of a catheter when there is none or, in 3D, the appearance of a tear (shadowing) in cardiac tissue.

The main advantage of using echocardiography over X-ray methods to assist in the guidance of SHDIs resides in the ability of ultrasound to visualize soft tissue. This is of great value in avoiding complications. By knowing the exact position of a catheter tip or device, in relation to the surrounding anatomic structures, the interventionalist can advance or retrieve a catheter or device, thereby minimizing the chances of perforation.

EVALUATION OF RESULTS

The achievement of expected goals of an SHDI can be immediately assessed with echocardiography. The baseline echocardiogram is used for direct comparison to evaluate the beneficial effects of the intervention. Morphologic information is obtained with two-dimensional (2D) or 3D echocardiography and functional information through the use of spectral and color Doppler. If the expected goal is not achieved, the intervention can be repeated as long as no major complications are recognized. When the expected goal is achieved, a diligent search for potential complications is done. Of particular interest are the presence and size of pericardial effusions, the presence and size of catheter-induced ASDs postseptal puncture, and the presence of thrombus in any cardiac chamber or structure. The search and avoidance of specific complications will be detailed under each intervention.

In the following section, we describe the role of echocardiography in assisting the most common SHDIs. Table 6-2 outlines the preferred echocardiographic tool to aid in the different types of SHDIs. In Table 6-2, we also provide references for the interventions which, because of lack of space, we do not cover in the text of this chapter.

TABLE 6-2 **Preferred Echocardiographic Methods to Assist Structural Heart Disease Interventions**

Intervention	Preprocedure (in Echo Lab)	Intraprocedure (in Cath Lab)	Postprocedure (in Cath Lab)
Shunt Interventions			
PFO closure	TTE color and contrast	ICE color and contrast	TTE color and contrast
	TEE color and contrast		TEE color and contrast
ASD closure	TTE color and contrast	2D and 3D TEE	TEE color and contrast
	TEE color and contrast		3D TEE
VSD closure	TTE color	2D and 3D TEE	2D and 3D TEE
Fistula closure[10]	TTE contrast and color	2D and 3D TEE	2D and 3D TEE
PDA closure[11]	TTE contrast and color	TTE contrast and color	TTE contrast and color
Closure of baffle leaks[12]	2D TEE, color Doppler	2D and 3D TEE	2D and 3D TEE
	Doppler hemodynamics	Color Doppler	Color Doppler
Valve Interventions			
Aortic balloon valvuloplasty	TTE	TTE	TTE
	Doppler hemodynamics	Doppler hemodynamics	Doppler hemodynamics
Transcatheter aortic valve implantation[13–19]	TTE	Doppler hemodynamics	Doppler hemodynamics
	Doppler hemodynamics	2D and 3D TEE	2D and 3D TEE
	2D and 3D TEE		
Mitral balloon commissurotomy	TTE	Doppler hemodynamics	Doppler hemodynamics
	Doppler hemodynamics	2D and 3D TEE	2D and 3D TEE
Edge-to-edge MV repair	2D TEE, color Doppler	2D and 3D TEE	2D and 3D TEE
	Doppler hemodynamics	Color Doppler	Color Doppler
Pulmonic balloon valvuloplasty[20]	TTE	TTE	TTE
	Doppler hemodynamics	Doppler hemodynamics	Doppler hemodynamics
Transcatheter pulmonic valve implantation[21]	TTE	Doppler hemodynamics	Doppler hemodynamics
	Doppler hemodynamics	2D and 3D TEE	2D and 3D TEE
	2D and 3D TEE		
Paravalvular leaks closure	2D TEE	2D and 3D TEE	2D and 3D TEE
	Color Doppler	Color Doppler	Color Doppler
	Doppler hemodynamics		
Other Interventions			
Alcohol septal ablation	TTE	TTE	TTE
	Color Doppler	Color Doppler	Color Doppler
	Doppler hemodynamics	Doppler hemodynamics	Doppler hemodynamics
LAA closure[22,23]	2D TEE	2D and 3D TEE	2D and 3D TEE
Pseudoaneurysm of aorta closure[24]	2D and 3D TTE, TEE	2D and 3D TTE, TEE	2D and 3D TTE, TEE
	Color Doppler	Color Doppler	Color Doppler

ASD, atrial septal defect; ICE, intracardiac echocardiography; LAA, left atrial appendage; MV, mitral valve; PDA, patent ductus arteriosus; PFO, patent foramen ovale; TEE, transesophageal echocardiography; TTE, transthoracic echocardiography; VSD, ventricular septal defect.

Echocardiographic Guidance for Specific Structural Heart Disease Interventions

Transseptal Puncture

Many SHDIs require transseptal puncture.[25] In this section, we describe the role of 2D and 3D TEE in assisting with this procedure.

PREPROCEDURE CHARACTERIZATION OF INTERATRIAL SEPTUM AND ATRIA

Key echocardiographic points include:

1. Morphologic characterization: A TEE is performed to assess left and right atrial size and to ensure that the left atrium (LA) and left atrial appendage are free of thrombus. The anatomy of the intra-atrial septum is clearly defined. The presence of a PFO or ASD is also noted. In addition, presence and size of a Eustachian valve or ridge and presence and size of a Chiari network is noted. Septal thickness and presence of interatrial septal aneurysm are noted. The fossa ovalis rims are carefully delineated: The posterior rim is made of a fold of atrial tissue, fat, and pericardial space between the left and right atria; the superior rim is bounded by the superior vena cava (SVC); the anterosuperior rim is bounded by the noncoronary sinus of Valsalva of the aortic valve; the anterior rim is demarcated by the septal tricuspid annulus; the anteroinferior rim is next to the coronary sinus os; and the inferior rim is next to the inferior vena cava (IVC) (Fig. 6-2).

2. Avoiding complications: The most important structures to avoid puncturing, during transseptal puncture, are the aortic valve and root as well as the posterior pericardial fold between both atria.

Understanding the anatomy of the interatrial septum as depicted in Figure 6-3 and, as described next, will help immensely on avoiding complications related to inappropriate puncture sites.

INTRAPROCEDURE GUIDANCE

1. TEE catheter guidance to the fossa ovalis: The transseptal assembly consisting of the needle, dilator, and sheath are first placed in the SVC near its entrance to the right atrium (RA); under fluoroscopy and 2D or 3D TEE guidance, the assembly is moved toward the center of the fossa ovalis. By putting pressure with the guiding catheter over the membrane of the fossa ovalis, "tenting" of this structure occurs (Fig. 6-4).

2. Determining point of septal puncture: The point of maximal tenting will be the area where the puncture will take place, so it is important to recognize that this point is away from the aorta and that is not situated too posterior. The bicaval view is used to choose the anterosuperior point of puncture; the aortic short-axis view is used to choose the anteroposterior point of puncture. After the septal puncture has taken place, it is customary to inject agitated saline into the LA to make sure the guiding catheter is in the left atrial cavity.

EVALUATION OF RESULTS

1. Once the intervention is completed, a 2D TEE image of the interatrial septum with color Doppler is performed to assess the size of the residual septal puncture-induced ASD (Fig. 6-4). Only rarely do these defects have any clinical significance as to require percutaneous closure.

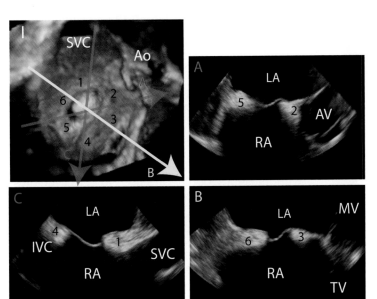

FIGURE 6-2.

Interatrial septum rims. Real-time three-dimensional transesophageal echocardiography views of the interatrial septum as seen from the right atrium (*I*). **A–C:** Multiplane reconstructions following the direction of the arrows. The *red arrow* (*A*) follows a short-axis view of the aortic valve and transects the posterior (*5*) and anterior (*2*) rims. The *yellow arrow* (*B*) follows a four-chamber view and transects the posterosuperior rim (*6*) and anteroinferior (*3*) rim. The *green arrow* (*C*) follows a bicaval orientation and transects the superior (*1*) and inferior (*4*) rim. Ao, aorta; AV, aortic valve; IVC, inferior vena cava; LA, left atrium; MV, mitral valve; RA, right atrium; SVC, superior vena cava; TV, tricuspid valve.

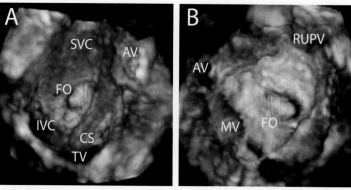

FIGURE 6-3.

Anatomy of the interatrial septum. Real-time three-dimensional transesophageal echocardiography views of the interatrial septum as seen from the right atrium **(A)** and from the left atrium **(B)**. The view from the right atrium is presented with the correct anatomic orientation: the superior vena cava *(SVC)* on top, the inferior vena cava *(IVC)* on the bottom, and the aortic valve *(AV)* anteriorly. The fossa ovalis *(FO)* is seen in the center of the image. In the view from the left atrium, the fossa ovalis is again seen in the center. The mitral valve *(MV)* and the aortic valve *(AV)* are to the left of the picture and the right upper pulmonary vein *(RUPV)* is seen in the top right of the image. CS, coronary sinus; TV, tricuspid valve.

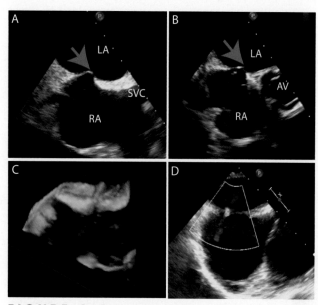

FIGURE 6-4.

Transseptal puncture. Two-dimensional and three-dimensional (3D) transesophageal echocardiography (TEE) images obtained during and after transseptal puncture. **A:** Bicaval view shows the typical "tenting" of the interatrial septum during septal puncture. This view permits selecting the appropriate superoinferior point of puncture. **B:** Short-axis aortic valve *(AV)* view shows similar "tenting" but allows selecting the appropriate anteroposterior point of puncture and avoidance of puncturing the aorta. **C:** A real-time 3D TEE image of the catheter entering the left atrium *(LA)*. **D:** The small residual atrial septal defect after septal puncture, with color Doppler. RA, right atrium; SVC, superior vena cava.

2. Ruling out complications: Presence or absence of pericardial effusion is determined immediately after septal puncture and at the end of the intervention. Presence of intracardiac thrombus is searched for. New valvular regurgitant lesions are ruled out.

Shunt Lesions

Patent Foramen Ovale Closure

Percutaneous closure of PFOs is one of the most common SHDIs performed today.[26–28] TTE and TEE play a central role in the diagnosis, quantification of shunt size, and suitability for percutaneous closure. PFO device closure is frequently guided by intracardiac echo (ICE) unless the PFO is complex in appearance or there are congenital remnants in the RA that can be better discerned with TEE.

PREPROCEDURE CHARACTERIZATION OF PATENT
FORAMEN OVALE

Key echocardiographic points include (PFO protocol):

1. TTE apical four and subcostal views (with and without color Doppler) are used to detect the presence and location of a PFO. These views also permit the detection of interatrial septum aneurysm and presence and size of Eustachian valve and Chiari network.

2. Right-to-left shunting at the atrial level is demonstrated by injecting agitated saline (10 mL of saline, 1 mL of air, a few drops of blood) in an antecubital

vein. This is done on the supine position at rest, after Valsalva (release phase), with cough, and in the upright position. Arrival of microbubbles in the LA before five cardiac cycles is considered positive for intracardiac shunt. After five beats, it is considered positive for intrapulmonary shunt.

3. Injection of agitated saline during supine bike exercise or immediately following treadmill exercise is done in patients suspected to have exercise-induced shunting at the PFO level. In these patients, O_2 saturation during exercise is obtained to search for hypoxemia.

4. A semiquantitative assessment of the degree of shunting is recommended. We use the following scale: grade 0, none; grade 1, mild, one to five bubbles; grade 2, moderate, 6 to 20 bubbles; grade 3, severe, >20 bubbles.

5. Transcranial Doppler can also be used to demonstrate the presence of venous to arterial shunting.[29] We have found this to be of particular use during exercise.

6. TEE is performed when TTE fails to demonstrate a shunt and the suspicion of a PFO remains high. TEE is performed in patients with a PFO being considered for percutaneous PFO closure (Fig. 6-5). TEE facilitates characterizing a PFO by determining its exact location, size, presence, and length of a "tunnel" and associated findings. High-stroke risk TEE findings in patients with PFO include presence of atrial septal aneurysm and prominent Eustachian valve. TEE can assist in device selection for percutaneous PFO closure. Patients with a long "tunnel" or a very thick septum secundum near the PFO are perhaps better candidates for a Helex-type device.

INTRAPROCEDURE GUIDANCE

At our institution, most percutaneous PFO closures are guided by ICE. Occasionally, when the PFO morphology is complex or there are prominent right atrial remnants, we use TEE for intraprocedure guidance. This guidance is very similar to the one described for ASD closure in following text.

EVALUATION OF RESULTS

1. We also use ICE for the immediate evaluation of PFO device closure results in the cath lab.

2. A TTE is performed before discharge to document appropriate device location; absence of significant residual shunt (injection of agitated saline at rest and with cough and Valsalva); absence of postprocedure complications such as pericardial effusion, mitral aortic, and tricuspid insufficiency; and absence of peridevice thrombus formation.

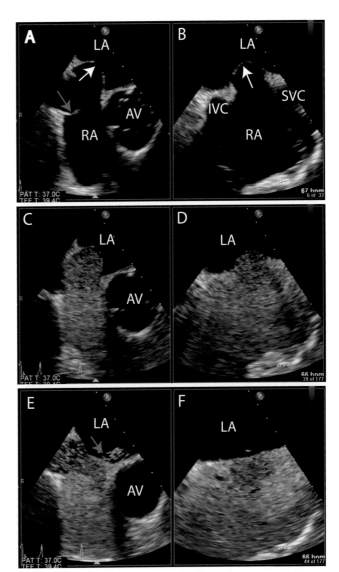

FIGURE 6-5.

High-risk patent foramen ovale (PFO). Contrast transesophageal echocardiography in a patient being considered for PFO device closure. In addition to having right to left shunt (**E**, *green arrow*) as demonstrated by microbubbles passing from the right atrium (*RA*) to the left atrium (*LA*), there is a prominent Eustachian valve (**A**, *red arrow*) and a large interatrial septal aneurysm (**A,B**, *white arrows*). **A,C,E:** Views of the interatrial septum in the plane of the aortic valve short axis. **B,D,F:** Views of the interatrial septum from the bicaval view. AV, aortic valve; IVC, inferior vena cava; SVC, superior vena cava.

Atrial Septal Defect Closure

Ostium secundum ASDs are nowadays almost exclusively closed percutaneously.[30,31] TTE and TEE are the premier imaging tools to diagnose and typify ASDs as well as to quantify the size of the shunt and the degree of the resulting right ventricular volume overload.

Preprocedure Characterization

Key echocardiographic points include:

1. Diagnosis of ASD by echo: With TTE, the apical four-chamber and subcostal views provide the best windows to visualize an ASD. Color Doppler demonstrates the presence and location of interatrial left-to-right shunting and the injection of agitated saline demonstrates the presence of left-to-right shunting by the washout of contrast in the RA from blood coming from the LA. It is also common to see microbubbles passing from the RA to the LA during parts of the cardiac cycle demonstrating the presence of some degree of right-to-left shunting. ASDs with significant shunts have evidence of right ventricular volume overload or shunt-related pulmonary hypertension. An attempt is made to characterize all pulmonary veins.

2. ASD type: At present, the only ASDs that are amenable to percutaneous closure are ostium secundum type. It is therefore critical to make the correct diagnosis of the ASD type. TTE and TEE are quite useful in distinguishing ostium secundum from ostium primum and sinus venosus defects.

3. ASD size: Having an accurate size of an ASD is of critical importance on determining feasibility of percutaneous closure and for device sizing. TEE is the preferred echo tool to adequately size an ASD. Multiple imaging planes are register to obtain the maximal dimensions. It should be noted that an ASD frequently is oval in shape and different dimensions can be obtained depending on the plane of view. 3D TEE permits a more accurate depiction of the size and shape of the defect by presenting the interatrial septum en face (Fig. 6-6).

4. ASD rims: When all the rims are present and well developed, one can think of the interatrial septum with a secundum ASD as a small bagel. In some patients, a bite is taken from this bagel, thereby creating an ASD with an inadequate rim. Patients with deficient rims (<5 mm) may not be good candidates for percutaneous ASD closure. In the preprocedure TEE, an effort is made to characterize and measure all of the rims, but particular attention is paid to the inferior rim, which, when deficient, can be the source of device embolization.

5. Multiple ASDs and fenestrations: Not infrequently, fenestrations and/or multiple ASDs are present. TEE can characterize the presence of fenestrations and, with color Doppler, it is possible to determine the number of ASDs if more than one is present. It is also important to determine if there is an associated PFO.

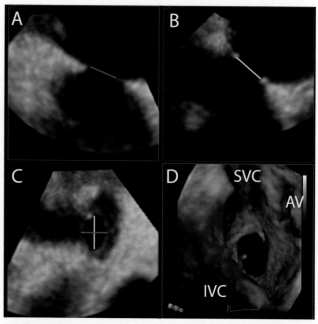

FIGURE 6-6.

Atrial septal defect (ASD) sizing. **A,B:** The multiplane reconstruction views from which the vertical and horizontal dimensions are obtained. **C:** Obtained from an en face multiplane reconstruction view depicting an oval-shaped defect with the vertical diameter (*yellow*) larger than the horizontal diameter (*red*). **D:** A real-time three-dimensional transesophageal echocardiographic view of a large secundum ASD in a patient being considered for percutaneous ASD closure. AV, aortic valve; IVC, inferior vena cava; SVC, superior vena cava.

Intraprocedure Guidance

1. Choosing device size: TEE is used to measure the length of the interatrial septum in three planes. This will confirm that there is enough interatrial septal tissue to support the device discs without impinging in surrounding cardiac structures. In addition, the discs have to be large enough to have adequate support from the ASD rims. Determining device size requires knowledge of ASD diameters and orifice area as described in the previous section. Balloon sizing is also used to choose device size. Under TEE guidance, a balloon is inflated in the ASD until flow through the defect ceases; at this point, the diameter of the waist of the balloon as seen longitudinally is measured on TEE (Fig. 6-7). This diameter is used to determine device size.

2. Device deployment: Under fluoroscopy and 2D or 3D TEE guidance, the guidewire, delivery sheath, and the occluder device are advanced into the LA. The left atrial disc is deployed and pulled back to abut the interatrial septum. Echo is particularly helpful

in maintaining a parallel orientation of the disc with the interatrial septum so as to have the best device/interatrial septum apposition. After the left hemi-disc is deployed, the waist and right hemi-disc are deployed again, thereby maintaining the best possible parallel orientation between the device and the interatrial septum. We find this can be best accomplished by the use of a biplane TEE depiction of the interatrial septum from a bicaval view and a short-axis view of the interatrial septum at the level of the aortic valve or with 3D TEE guidance (Fig. 6-8). After the device is deployed, absence of ASD flow is demonstrated with color Doppler after the "push and pull" maneuver to also ensure device stability. Before releasing the device, a surveillance TEE is done

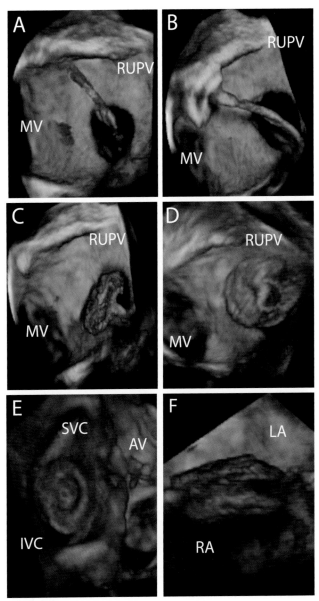

FIGURE 6-8.

Amplatzer atrial septal defect (ASD) closure device deployment. Real-time three-dimensional transesophageal echocardiography images obtained during percutaneous ASD closure. **A:** The guide catheter entering the left atrium through the ASD. **B:** The left atrial hemi-disc has been deployed. **C:** The device is pulled back toward the ASD. **D:** The device is abutted against the ASD rims. **E:** The device as seen from the right atrium (*RA*) after the right atrial hemi-disc is deployed. **F:** Both hemi-discs deployed with good support from the surrounding rims. AV, aortic valve; IVC, inferior vena cava; LA, left atrium; MV, mitral valve; RUPV, right upper pulmonary vein; SVC, superior vena cava.

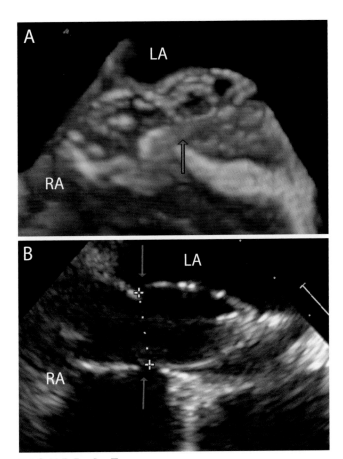

FIGURE 6-7.

Atrial septal defect (ASD) balloon sizing. **A:** A three-dimensional transesophageal echocardiography (TEE) image of an inflated ASD balloon sizing device. The *red arrow* points to the waist that is formed by the ASD rims as they constrict the inflated balloon. **B:** A two-dimensional TEE image of the same balloon. The *red arrows* point to the waist of the balloon, the diameter of which is measured by the *dotted line* and serves as reference to choose the ASD closure device size. LA, left atrium; RA, right atrium.

to make sure the mitral and tricuspid leaflets are not impinged by the device and that the hemi-discs are not compressing any adjacent cardiac structures. At this point, the device is released, commonly shifting the plane of the device to some degree. TEE is used again to document any residual transoccluder flow and or peridevice residual flow.

Evaluation of Results

1. Device stability: After completing the deployment, device stability is checked with TEE for several minutes to ensure there is no immediate embolization.
2. Residual shunt assessment: TEE color Doppler is used to assess for any residual peridevice shunt. It is not uncommon to see low-velocity transdevice shunting of mild degree.
3. Search for complications: Presence of pericardial effusion is ruled out. Tears in interatrial septal tissue are searched for. Presence of peridevice thrombus is excluded. Mitral and tricuspid valve impingement and regurgitation is noted.
4. Predischarge echo: We usually perform a limited TTE the next morning prior to discharge. Device stability is noted. Presence and degree of residual shunt is noted with color Doppler and agitated saline. Pericardial effusion is searched for.

Ventricular Septal Defect Closure

Congenital ventricular septal defects (VSDs) in children are commonly closed percutaneously. In adults, acquired VSDs, usually resulting from complication of myocardial infarction, are now with increasing frequency being closed percutaneously by interventionalists.[32,33] Percutaneous closure of VSDs has been described in adults with congenital muscular or perimembranous defects, VSD postmyocardial infarction, residual or recurrent VSD postsurgical repair, and VSD postseptal reduction for hypertrophic cardiomyopathy. TTE with color Doppler usually provides the initial confirmation of the presence of a VSD complicating a myocardial infarction and helps in characterizing its location, size, and suitability for percutaneous closure.

Preprocedure Characterization

Key echocardiographic points include:

1. Characterizing VSD size and location: TTE can characterize location and size of the VSD as well as left and right ventricular global and segmental function. In addition, associated valvular abnormalities and the presence and severity of pulmonary hypertension can be assessed.

2. Color Doppler and spectral Doppler aid in the detection of shunt flow through the defect when the presence of the anatomic defect is not well seen on 2D echocardiography.
3. TEE better characterizes the size, location, and shape of the VSD and frequently clarifies the suitability of a given patient for percutaneous closure.

Intraprocedure Guidance

1. Creation of arteriovenous loop: The deployment of a VSD closure device requires the creation of an arteriovenous wire loop. A guidewire is introduced in a femoral artery; it is advanced through the aorta and aortic valve into the left ventricle. Through the VSD, the wire is advanced into the right ventricle and RA and it is finally sneered with a gooseneck snare into the SVC and pulled out through the internal jugular vein.
2. TEE complements fluoroscopy in guiding the wire to create the arteriovenous loop and then advancing the delivery catheter and deploying the closure device. TEE is particularly helpful in aligning the closing device hemi-discs parallel to the long axis of the interventricular septum and outside of the VSD tract.
3. We have found that 3D TEE helps clarifying the complex morphologic findings associated with postmyocardial infarct VSD and currently is our preferred imaging tool to guide percutaneous VSD closures.

Evaluation of Results

1. Immediately after deploying a VSD closure device, echocardiography is used to determine stability of the closure device and the presence and degree of residual shunt.
2. In addition, impingement of surrounding cardiac structures is noted if present.

Valve Lesions

Balloon Aortic Valvuloplasty

Balloon aortic valvuloplasty (BAV) is a well-established procedure in patients with severe aortic stenosis who are not candidates for surgical aortic valve replacement[34,35]; it can also be used as a bridge to improve and stabilize the general clinical status of patients with critical aortic stenosis in preparation for percutaneous or surgical aortic valve replacement. Although an antegrade approach through an interatrial septal puncture is possible, a retrograde femoral approach is more commonly done.

PREPROCEDURE CHARACTERIZATION

Key echocardiographic points include:

1. In patients with aortic stenosis TTE and Doppler methods are the main techniques to characterize the aortic valve morphology its severity and suitability for BAV.

2. Morphologic characterization: Evaluation of the number of cusps and location of a raphe if present; assessment of cusp mobility and degree of commissural fusion; assessment of valve calcification; assessment of left ventricular outflow tract (LVOT) size; assessment of aortic root size and presence and degree of calcification and complex plaques in aortic root; and assessment of presence and severity of aortic insufficiency.

3. Aortic stenosis severity: Patients being considered for BAV will usually have critical aortic stenosis (<0.7 cm^2) as determined by echocardiographic 2D planimetry, or preferably by Doppler-derived gradients and continuity equation. In patients with severely compromised left ventricular function, the Doppler-derived velocity ratio of the LVOT and the aortic valve is used.

4. Suitability for BAV: Potential candidates for BAV will have critical aortic stenosis, absence of severe aortic insufficiency, and absence of severe calcification of the aortic root or presence of complex aortic root plaques.

INTRAPROCEDURE GUIDANCE

1. Echocardiography can be used to complement fluoroscopy in guiding the guidewire and balloon through the stenotic aortic valve and to follow the gradients and degree of aortic insufficiency after each balloon inflation.

2. If the retrograde approach is used, echocardiography will be particularly useful in guiding the septal puncture and navigating the guidewires and catheters through the LA, mitral valve, and left ventricle.

EVALUATION OF RESULTS

1. Reduction of aortic stenosis severity: In most patients undergoing BAV, only a modest improvement of aortic stenosis severity is expected. Significant hemodynamic improvement is frequently gained by going from critical to severe aortic stenosis. Measuring gradients and valve area by echocardiography after each balloon inflation will facilitate reaching this goal and avoid the presence of severe aortic insufficiency and other potential complications.

2. Search for complications: Complications common to all SHDIs, such as pericardial effusion and tamponade as well as thrombus formation, are searched for. In BAV, the relevant complications include aortic leaflet disruption with concomitant severe aortic insufficiency.

Percutaneous Mitral Commissurotomy

Percutaneous mitral valve balloon commissurotomy (PMC) has replaced surgery as the preferred initial intervention in most patients with severe mitral stenosis.[9,36–39] TTE is recognized as the best imaging tool to characterize the presence and severity of mitral stenosis and, with the aid of Doppler methods, it allows for an accurate hemodynamic assessment of the mitral stenosis burden. TTE is also recognized as the gold standard to select suitable candidates for PMC. TEE is best suited to provide guidance during PMC.

PREPROCEDURE CHARACTERIZATION

Key echocardiographic points include (Fig. 6-9):

1. Mitral valve area is obtained by planimetry from the parasternal short-axis view.
2. Mean mitral valve gradient.
3. Mitral valve area by pressure half time.
4. Measurement of systolic pulmonary pressure.
5. Presence and severity of mitral regurgitation (MR).
6. Wilkins score[9]: A mitral valve with a Wilkins score of 8 to 9 with no more than moderate MR is deemed suited for PMC.
7. Degree of commissural fusion.
8. Measurement of mitral valve annular diameter (to determine balloon size selection).

INTRAPROCEDURE GUIDANCE (FIG. 6-10)

1. Septal puncture (see section of transseptal puncture)
2. Catheter and balloon guidance: After the septal puncture, under fluoroscopy and 2D or 3D TEE guidance, a coiled-tip guidewire is placed into the LA through the Brockenbrough sheath. Next, the Inoue balloon catheter is advanced over the coiled-tip wire. Once the balloon catheter has crossed the interatrial septum, the catheter is placed in the LA, thereby forming a loop with the tip facing the mitral valve orifice, and the balloon catheter is moved toward and through the mitral valve orifice. We find these maneuvers are best guided by a wide sector real-time 3D TEE view.
3. Balloon positioning and inflation: After the balloon catheter has passed into the left ventricle, a real-time 3D TEE four-chamber view is used to best align the depth and central orientation of the balloon catheter. This same view is used to follow the distal, proximal, and medial inflation of the balloon.

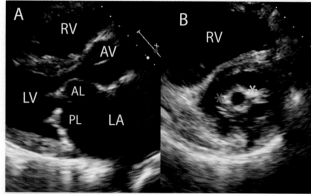

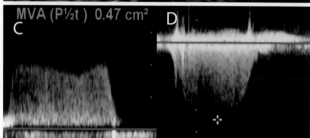

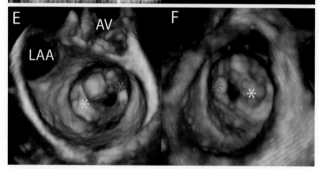

FIGURE 6-9.

Mitral stenosis: preprocedure assessment. **A,B:** Transthoracic long- and short-axis views of the mitral valve in a patient being considered for percutaneous mitral valve commissurotomy. The typical hockey stick deformity of the anterior leaflet (*AL*) is present. The posterior leaflet (*PL*) is thickened and has a fixed and vertical orientation. The left atrium (*LA*) is markedly enlarged. **B:** The narrowed mitral valve orifice is noted. Both commissures are fused (*red asterisk*, medial commissure; *yellow asterisk*, lateral commissure). **C:** The spectral Doppler signal through the mitral valve with an estimated mitral valve area by the pressure half method (MVA/P 1/2t) of 0.5 cm², consistent with severe mitral stenosis. **D:** The tricuspid regurgitant velocity from which estimation of systolic pulmonary arterial pressure is estimated. **E,F:** Three-dimensional transesophageal echocardiographic renditions of the stenotic mitral valve as seen from the left atrium (**E**) and from the left ventricle (**F**). The *yellow asterisk* demarks the lateral commissure; the *red asterisk* demarks the medial. AV, aortic valve; LAA, left atrial appendage; LV, left ventricle; RV, right ventricle.

4. Determining need for reinflation: Immediately after the balloon is inflated, color Doppler is used to assess for the presence and severity of MR. A short-axis view of the mitral valve is imaged to assess for the degree of commissural splitting and to measure mitral valve area by planimetry. The mean transmitral valve pressure gradient is noted. Reinflation is done if there is incomplete commissure splitting

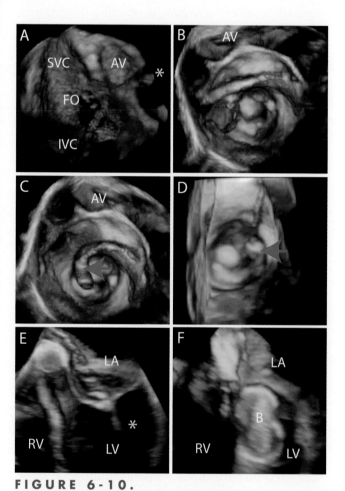

FIGURE 6-10.

Mitral stenosis: intraprocedure guidance. **A:** The guiding catheter entering from the inferior vena cava (*IVC*) into the right atrium (*red asterisk*) passing through the fossa ovalis (*FO*) and ending in the left atrium (*yellow asterisk*). **B:** The guiding wire and the delivery catheter have been advanced into the left atrium. **C:** The deflated balloon (*red arrow*) is being directed toward the narrow mitral valve orifice. **D:** The deflated balloon has entered the mitral valve orifice. **E:** The delivery catheter and the deflated balloon are seen from a four-chamber perspective through the mitral orifice and into the inflow of the left ventricle (*LV*). This view permits orientation of the balloon along the center of the long-axis plane of the LV. **F:** The inflated balloon (*B*) overriding the mitral annulus; a waist is formed by the stenotic mitral valve. AV, aortic valve; LA, left atrium; RA, right atrium; SVC, superior vena cava.

and the valve area is less than 1.5 cm² by planimetry. No further inflations are done when adequate commissure splitting is obtained or if there is significant mitral insufficiency.

EVALUATION OF RESULTS (FIG. 6-11)

1. Immediate procedural success is recognized by having a valve area of ≥1.5 cm², splitting of both commissures, and absence of significant mitral insufficiency.
2. Recognition and avoidance of complications: Most complications of this procedure occur during the manipulation of catheters and balloon. Echocardiography plays a major role in minimizing these

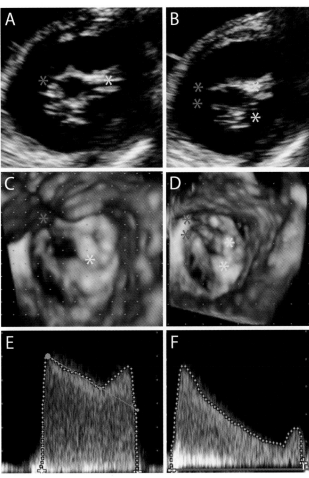

FIGURE 6-11.

Mitral stenosis: pre- and post–percutaneous mitral commissurotomy (PMC). **A,B:** Transthoracic short-axis views of the mitral valve before and after PMC. Note the splitting of the commissures in B. **C,D:** Similar findings on three-dimensional transesophageal echocardiography. **E,F:** The drop in transmitral pressure gradient post-PMC as registered by spectral Doppler. *Red asterisks* demark the medial commissure; *yellow asterisks* demark the lateral commissure. *Single asterisks* demark the commissures prior to PMC; *double asterisks* demark the splitted commissures after PMC.

problems by providing soft tissue definition of the interface between the catheters and cardiac structures. During the process of interatrial septum puncture, manipulation of the Inoue balloon catheter in the LA and commissurotomy of the mitral valve by Inoue balloon catheter TEE guidance assist the interventionalist in avoiding puncturing inappropriate sites by recognizing malpositioning of the catheters.

Edge-to-Edge Mitral Valve Repair

Currently, there are several approaches to percutaneously correct either functional or structural severe mitral insufficency.[40–44] In this section, we discuss the use of echocardiography in assisting the guidance of the most common form of percutaneous mitral valve repair with the e-Valve device (Fig. 6-12).

Preprocedure Characterization

Key echocardiographic points include:

1. Demonstration of structural or functional moderate (3+) or severe (4+) MR.
2. TTE characterization of left ventricle size and function (M mode left ventricular end-systolic diameter and 2D end diastolic and end-systolic volumes and ejection fraction).
3. Assessment of pulmonary pressure by tricuspid regurgitant jet velocity and right atrial pressure estimate derived from IVC diameter.
4. MR grading: Moderate or severe MR is defined echocardiographically by the presence of at least three of the following criteria: (1) color flow MR jet area (>6 cm² or >30% left atrial area); (2) systolic blunting or reversal of pulmonary vein flow; (3) vena contracta width >0.5 cm in parasternal long-axis view; (4) regurgitant volume of >45 mL/beat; (5) regurgitant fraction >40%; and/or (6) regurgitant orifice area >30 cm².
5. Basic TEE views to obtain (0-degree omniplane): (1) superior, mid esophageal five-chamber equivalent with views of A1 and P1 mitral valve segments; (2) central, the probe is advanced 1 to 3 cm to visualize A2 and P2 segments; and (3) inferior, the probe is advanced further by 1 to 3 cm to visualize the A3 and P3 segments.
6. Additional TEE views to obtain: 60- to 90-degree omniplane with anterior angulation to visualize A1, A2, and A3 scallops; at midline to obtain the bi-commissural view; and with posterior angulation to visualize the P1, P2, and P3 scallops. In addition, right superior and left superior pulmonary

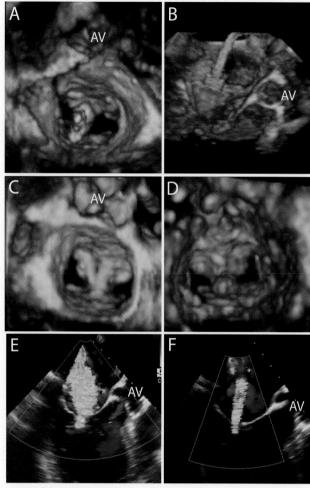

FIGURE 6-12.

Edge-to-edge percutaneous mitral valve repair. **A,B:** Three-dimensional transesophageal echocardiography images obtained during the Evalve clip guidance to the mitral leaflet edges. **A:** A view of the mitral valve from the left atrium; note that the clip is at the center of mitral valve orifice and is oriented perpendicular to the mitral leaflets line of coaptation. **C,D:** The clip in place with the double orifice mitral valve as seen from the left atrium **(C)** and from the left ventricle **(D)**. **E:** The presence of severe mitral insufficiency as seen prior to the clip repair and **(F)** the presence of only mild mitral regurgitation postrepair. AV, aortic valve.

veins and flow are registered. A transgastric short-axis view of the mitral valve is done to measure flail width if present. A basal short-axis view at 15 to 45 degrees is obtained to visualize the inter-atrial septum, the aortic valve in short axis, and RA and LA. Finally, a LVOT view is recorded at 110 to 130 degrees to demonstrate mal-coaptation of A2 and P2 if present.

7. TEE anatomic measurements: (1) flail gap, vertical separation between anterior and posterior leaflets where the flail gap is the largest; (2) coaptation depth, vertical distance from the mitral annulus to the leaflet coaptation point where the coaptation depth is greatest; (3) coaptation length, vertical distance at the line of leaflet coaptation where the coaptation length is the shortest.

Intraprocedure Guidance

1. Transseptal puncture: Please see section on transseptal puncture for general guidelines. For the edge-to-edge mitral repair, a septal puncture site is selected to optimize the trajectory of the steerable sleeve to permit directing the clip at the center of the mitral valve orifice and perpendicular to the coaptation line of the mitral valve leaflets. Frequently, this requires puncturing the fossa ovalis posterosuperiorly.

2. Deployment of clip delivery system: After the transseptal puncture and under fluoroscopic and TEE guidance, the steerable guide and steerable sleeve are advanced into the LA and positioned near the center of the mitral valve orifice. The clip is then steered over the mitral regurgitant jet. The clip is rotated until its arms become perpendicular to the coaptation line of the mitral valve leaflets and advanced through the mitral orifice into the left ventricle. We use 3D TEE guidance for this maneuver because it provides visualization of a large segment of the catheters and detailed anatomic information of the mitral leaflet scallops and surrounding structures.

3. Clip deployment: For the actual deployment of the clip, we use orthogonal biplane TEE echocardiographic views to optimize visualization of the flail segments. By having orthogonal views minor adjustments on the anterior and posterior axis as well as the medial and lateral axis are possible, thereby enhancing the ability to grasp the leaflets in the best possible place.

Evaluation of Results

1. Immediately after the leaflets have been grasped, the presence and degree of residual MR is assessed, the stability and correct positioning of the clip is investigated, and in the absence of problems, the clip is released.

2. A successful edge-to-edge repair is considered if there is a decrease of MR severity to 2+ or less.

3. Presence and size of postseptal puncture ASD is documented.

4. Any other complications such as device embolus, worsening of MR, and pericardial effusion are searched for.

Paravalvular Leaks Closure

Percutaneous closure of prosthetic paravalvular leaks is being reported with increasing frequency.[45–48] Many of these patients are not candidates for a reoperation, and a percutaneous alternative is a welcomed alternative by these patients' surgeons and cardiologists.

Preprocedure Characterization

Key echocardiographic points include:

1. Diagnosis of periprosthetic leaks. Transthoracic echo can suggest the presence of a periprosthetic leak by demonstrating a regurgitant jet between the prosthetic suture ring and the tissue surrounding it. TEE is usually required to confirm the exact location and determine the magnitude of the prosthetic suture ring dehiscence and the severity of the leak.
2. Candidacy for percutaneous approach. In patients with hemodynamically significant periprosthetic leaks or with significant hemolytic anemia, TEE can aid in determining what patients are potential candidates for percutaneous closure. The location, size, and number of leaks need to be clearly delineated with TEE to assess their potential for percutaneous closure. Large dehiscences are unlikely to be closed with the percutaneous approach. Although it is possible to percutaneously close multiple perivalvular leaks, TEE can provide detail information regarding the suitability of having adjacent closure devices or plugs.

Intraprocedure Guidance

1. Mitral prosthesis perivalvular leaks: Percutaneous closure, at our institution, is usually done antegradely via interatrial septal puncture. Depending on the location of the leak, it may be possible to puncture the septum, under TEE guidance, in a point that will favor directing the guidewire and closure device through the most appropriate trajectory. We have found color Doppler, saline injection, and 3D TEE facilitate in directing the guidewire to the area of ring dehiscence. It is also critical to monitor with TEE prosthetic leaflet motion (particularly mechanical prosthesis) when the occluder device is being deployed.
2. Aortic prosthesis perivalvular leaks: Percutaneous closure is usually done retrogradely via a femoral approach. The preferred TEE views to assist include the mid esophageal short-axis view of the aorta and the mid esophageal long-axis view of the aorta. Using these two orthogonal planes, it is possible to direct the guidewire and closure device to the area of dehiscence. It is important to visualize the left main trunk and right coronary ostium to avoid device impingement. Closure device prosthetic leaflet dysfunction should be repeatedly searched for during the procedure.

Evaluation of Results

1. Leak closure: Color Doppler and TEE are used to determine the absence or, if present, the size and residual regurgitant volume of the leak. Although ideally one would like to see no residual periprosthetic shunt at the end of device deployment, it is not uncommon to see some degree of shunt through the device.
2. Search for complications: If the transseptal approach is used, there should be only a small catheter-induced ASD. Pericardial effusion, if not present at the start of the procedure, should alert for the possibility of perforation and potential tamponade. Prosthetic dysfunction in the form of stenosis or insufficiency, if present, is documented and quantified. Detailed inspection of the cardiac chambers and prosthetic valves in search of thrombus is performed.

Alcohol Septal Ablation

Alcohol septal ablation has become a reasonable alternative to surgical myectomy for the treatment of patients with severely symptomatic hypertrophic obstructive cardiomyopathy (HOCM) not responding to medical therapy.[49] Echocardiography plays an important role in patient selection and procedure guidance (Fig. 6-13).

Preprocedure Characterization

Patients with HOCM and New York Heart Association class III/IV despite maximal medical therapy are considered candidates for septal ablation when the following echocardiographic criteria are met:

1. Septal hypertrophy with septal thickness of ≥1.5 cm.
2. LVOT gradient of ≥30 mm Hg at rest or ≥50 mm Hg with Valsalva, amyl nitrite, or exercise. To define latent pressure gradients, exercise testing with Doppler echocardiography is the most physiologic and preferred method to establish the diagnosis of HOCM with a provocable gradient.
3. Additional preprocedure echocardiographic characterization includes determining the presence and severity of systolic anterior motion (SAM) of the mitral valve and presence, severity, and direction (usually posterior) of MR. Additional valvular abnormalities need to be characterized because this may preclude percutaneous treatment of HOCM.

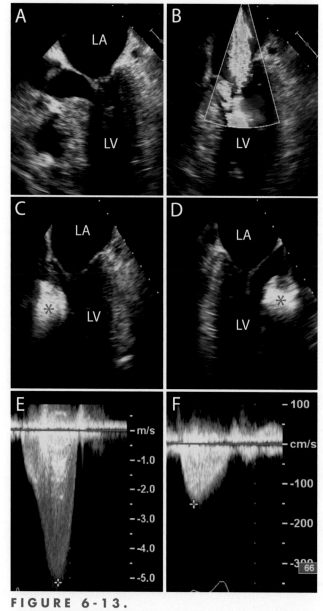

FIGURE 6-13.

Alcohol septal ablation in hypertrophic obstructive cardiomyopathy (HOCM). **A,B:** The typical findings of HOCM on transesophageal echocardiography: septal hypertrophy, systolic anterior motion of the mitral valve, and mitral insufficiency. **C,D:** Four- and three-chamber views of the left ventricle after contrast has been injected in the first septal perforator. The basal septum is opacified (*red asterisk*), thereby confirming an appropriate target zone for alcohol septal ablation. **E,F:** The significant drop in left ventricular outflow tract gradient obtained with alcohol septal ablation. LA, left atrium; LV, left ventricle; red asterisk, xxx.

Intraprocedure Guidance

1. Baseline echocardiographic parameters obtained in the catheterization lab: TTE apical 4, apical 5, and long-axis left ventricular views are obtained with and without color Doppler. Location of maximal

septal thickness, presence and degree of SAM of the mitral valve, and presence and degree of MR is noted. TEE is performed if inadequate transthoracic windows are present.

2. LVOT gradients at rest and, if necessary, after amyl nitrite and after catheter-induced premature ventricular contraction (PVC) are recorded.

3. Myocardial contrast echocardiography[50]: To determine if the selected septal perforator irrigates the septal bulge responsible for the LVOT obstruction, 1 mL of a mixture of radiographic contrast, agitated saline, and blood is injected into the angiographically most promising septal perforator. Ideally, the septal opacification will occur in the proximal septum; in the area of septum/SAM contact, it will be transmural and will not affect the inferior septum, right ventricle, moderator band, the papillary muscles, and anterior or lateral walls. Additional views such as parasternal short- and long-axis views of the left and right ventricle are frequently required to exclude opacification of undesirable locations.

4. Monitoring alcohol injection: After selecting the most appropriate septal perforator for septal ablation, echocardiography is used to monitor the progression of the alcohol injection. We monitor the progression of the alcohol injection by obtaining orthogonal views (usually apical 5 and long-axis left ventricle views) after each milliliter of alcohol injected. We monitor for continued enhancement of the appropriate septal area, for the presence of microbubbles in the left or right ventricle (if present, the rate of alcohol injection is decreased), for changes in the contractility of the basal septum (and hypokinesia in undesirable left or right ventricle segments—in which case the alcohol injection is stopped), and changes in the degree of SAM and LVOT gradients.

Evaluation of Results

After the target amount of alcohol (3–5 mL) has been injected, the following echocardiographic parameters are recorded:

1. Transthoracic apical 4, apical 5, and long-axis left ventricle views are obtained with and without color Doppler. Maximal septal thickness is measured, presence and degree of SAM of the mitral valve, and presence and degree of MR is noted.

2. LVOT gradients at rest and post–catheter-induced PVC are recorded.

3. Search for potential procedure complications: pericardial effusion, segmental wall motion abnormalities other than in the basal septum, and VSD.

CONCLUSION

SHDIs represent a major advance in the treatment of patients with a multitude of cardiovascular problems. This is a fast-moving field with advances occurring constantly. A successful program of SHDIs mandates a well-integrated team of SHD interventionalists working hand in hand with a team of cardiovascular imagers. In this chapter, we emphasize the central role that echocardiography plays in managing SHDIs by (1) diagnosing the SHD abnormality, (2) determining patient candidacy for an intervention, (3) assisting in guiding the intervention, (4) assisting in device selection and size, (5) evaluating immediate results, (6) recognizing and helping in the management of complications, and (7) in the long-term follow up of patients with SHD.

We present the role of TTE and TEE in the most common SHDIs and provide references for the conditions we did not have space to cover. We describe the protocols we currently use in our program and present illustrations for the most salient features of echocardiographic guidance of SHDIs.

REFERENCES

1. Hilliard AA, Nishimura RA. The interventional cardiologist and structural heart disease: the need for a team approach. *JACC Cardiovasc Imaging*. 2009;2(1):8–10.
2. Hudson PA, Eng MH, Kim MS, et al. A comparison of echocardiographic modalities to guide structural heart disease interventions. *J Interv Cardiol*. 2008;21(6):535–546.
3. Silvestry FE, Kerber RE, Brook MM, et al. Echocardiography-guided interventions. *J Am Soc Echocardiogr*. 2009;22(3):213–231; quiz 316–317.
4. Zoghbi WA, Enriquez-Sarano M, Foster E, et al. Recommendations for evaluation of the severity of native valvular regurgitation with two-dimensional and Doppler echocardiography. *J Am Soc Echocardiogr*. 2003;16(7):777–802.
5. Baumgartner H, Hung J, Bermejo J, et al. Echocardiographic assessment of valve stenosis: EAE/ASE recommendations for clinical practice. *Eur J Echocardiogr*. 2009;10(1):1–25.
6. Flachskampf FA, Badano L, Daniel WG, et al. Recommendations for transoesophageal echocardiography: update 2010. *Eur J Echocardiogr*. 2010;11(7):557–576.
7. Lang RM, Bierig M, Devereux RB, et al. Recommendations for chamber quantification: a report from the American Society of Echocardiography's Guidelines and Standards Committee and the Chamber Quantification Writing Group, developed in conjunction with the European Association of Echocardiography, a branch of the European Society of Cardiology. *J Am Soc Echocardiogr*. 2005;18(12):1440–1463.
8. Salcedo EE, Quaife RA, Seres T, et al. A framework for systematic characterization of the mitral valve by real-time three-dimensional transesophageal echocardiography. *J Am Soc Echocardiogr*. 2009;22(10):1087–1099.
9. Wilkins GT, Weyman AE, Abascal VM, et al. Percutaneous balloon dilatation of the mitral valve: an analysis of echocardiographic variables related to outcome and the mechanism of dilatation. *Br Heart J*. 1988;60(4):299–308.
10. Feldman T, Salinger MH, Das S, et al. Percutaneous closure of an aorta to left atrium fistula with an Amplatzer duct occluder. *Catheter Cardiovasc Interv*. 2006;67(1):132–138.
11. Brunetti M, Ringel R, Owada C, et al. Percutaneous closure of patent ductus arteriosus: a multi-institutional registry comparing multiple devices. *Catheter Cardiovasc Interv*. 2010;76(5):696–702.
12. Klein AJ, Kim MS, Salcedo E, et al. The missing leak: a case report of a baffle-leak closure using real-time 3D transoesophageal guidance. *Eur J Echocardiogr*. 2009;10(3):464–467.
13. Grube E, Buellesfeld L, Mueller R, et al. Progress and current status of percutaneous aortic valve replacement: results of three device generations of the CoreValve Revalving system. *Circ Cardiovasc Interv*. 2008;1(3):167–175.
14. Piazza N, de Jaegere P, Schultz C, et al. Anatomy of the aortic valvar complex and its implications for transcatheter implantation of the aortic valve. *Circ Cardiovasc Interv*. 2008;1(1):74–81.
15. Carroll JD. Optimizing technique and outcomes in structural heart disease interventions: rapid pacing during aortic valvuloplasty? *Catheter Cardiovasc Interv*. 2010;75(3):453–454.
16. Moss RR, Ivens E, Pasupati S, et al. Role of echocardiography in percutaneous aortic valve implantation. *JACC Cardiovasc Imaging*. 2008;1(1):15–24.
17. Masson JB, Kovac J, Schuler G, et al. Transcatheter aortic valve implantation: review of the nature, management, and avoidance of procedural complications. *JACC Cardiovasc Interv*. 2009;2(9):811–820.
18. Dumonteil N, Marcheix B, Berthoumieu P, et al. Transfemoral aortic valve implantation with pre-existent mechanical mitral prosthesis: evidence of feasibility. *JACC Cardiovasc Interv*. 2009;2(9):897–898.
19. Lerakis S, Babaliaros VC, Block PC, et al. Transesophageal echocardiography to help position and deploy a transcatheter heart valve. *JACC Cardiovasc Imaging*. 2010;3(2):219–221.
20. Jassal DS, Thakrar A, Schaffer SA, et al. Percutaneous balloon valvuloplasty for pulmonic stenosis: the role of multimodality imaging. *Echocardiography*. 2008;25(2):231–235.
21. Marianeschi SM, Santoro F, Ribera E, et al. Pulmonary valve implantation with the new Shelhigh

Injectable Stented Pulmonic Valve. *Ann Thorac Surg.* 2008;86(5):1466–1471; discussion 1472.

22. Ussia GP, Mule M, Cammalleri V, et al. Percutaneous closure of left atrial appendage to prevent embolic events in high-risk patients with chronic atrial fibrillation. *Catheter Cardiovasc Interv.* 2009;74(2):217–222.

23. Singh IM, Holmes DR Jr. Left atrial appendage closure. *Curr Cardiol Rep.* 2010;12(5):413–421.

24. Stasek J, Polansky P, Bis J, et al. The percutaneous closure of a large pseudoaneurysm of the ascending aorta with an atrial septal defect Amplatzer occluder: two-year follow-up. *Can J Cardiol.* 2008;24(12): e99–e101.

25. Earley MJ. How to perform a transseptal puncture. *Heart.* 2009;95(1):85–92.

26. Fazio G, Ferro G, Carita P, et al. The PFO anatomy evaluation as possible tool to stratify the associated risks and the benefits arising from the closure. *Eur J Echocardiogr.* 2010;11(6):488–491.

27. Rana BS, Thomas MR, Calvert PA, et al. Echocardiographic evaluation of patent foramen ovale prior to device closure. *JACC Cardiovasc Imaging.* 2010;3(7):749–760.

28. Rigatelli G, Dell'Avvocata F, Ronco F, et al. Primary transcatheter patent foramen ovale closure is effective in improving migraine in patients with high-risk anatomic and functional characteristics for paradoxical embolism. *JACC Cardiovasc Interv.* 2010;3(3):282–287.

29. Kampen J, Koch A, Struck N. Methodological remarks on transcranial Doppler ultrasonography for PFO detection. *Anesthesiology.* 2001;95(3):808–809.

30. Jategaonkar S, Scholtz W, Schmidt H, et al. Percutaneous closure of atrial septal defects: echocardiographic and functional results in patients older than 60 years. *Circ Cardiovasc Interv.* 2009;2(2):85–89.

31. Huang X, Shen J, Huang Y, et al. En face view of atrial septal defect by two-dimensional transthoracic echocardiography: comparison to real-time three-dimensional transesophageal echocardiography. *J Am Soc Echocardiogr.* 2010;23(7):714–721.

32. Halpern DG, Perk G, Ruiz C, et al. Percutaneous closure of a post-myocardial infarction ventricular septal defect guided by real-time three-dimensional echocardiography. *Eur J Echocardiogr.* 2009;10(4): 569–571.

33. De Wolf D, Taeymans Y, Suys B, et al. Percutaneous closure of a ventricular septal defect after surgical treatment of hypertrophic cardiomyopathy. *J Thorac Cardiovasc Surg.* 2006;132(1):173–174.

34. Bourgault C, Rodes-Cabau J, Cote JM, et al. Usefulness of Doppler echocardiography guidance during balloon aortic valvuloplasty for the treatment of congenital aortic stenosis. *Int J Cardiol.* 2008;128(1):30–37.

35. Shareghi S, Rasouli L, Shavelle DM, et al. Current results of balloon aortic valvuloplasty in high-risk patients. *J Invasive Cardiol.* 2007;19(1):1–5.

36. Carabello BA. Modern management of mitral stenosis. *Circulation.* 2005;112(3):432–437.

37. Eng MH, Salcedo EE, Quaife RA, et al. Implementation of real time three-dimensional transesophageal echocardiography in percutaneous mitral balloon valvuloplasty and structural heart disease interventions. *Echocardiography.* 2009;26(8):958–966.

38. Van Mieghem NM, Piazza N, Anderson RH, et al. Anatomy of the mitral valvular complex and its implications for transcatheter interventions for mitral regurgitation. *J Am Coll Cardiol.* 2010;56(8):617–626.

39. Abascal VM, Wilkins GT, Choong CY, et al. Echocardiographic evaluation of mitral valve structure and function in patients followed for at least 6 months after percutaneous balloon mitral valvuloplasty. *J Am Coll Cardiol.* 1988;12(3):606–615.

40. Swaans MJ, Van den Branden BJ, Van der Heyden JA, et al. Three-dimensional transoesophageal echocardiography in a patient undergoing percutaneous mitral valve repair using the edge-to-edge clip technique. *Eur J Echocardiogr.* 2009;10(8):982–983.

41. Bader SO, Lattouf OM, Sniecinski RM. Transesophageal echocardiography of the edge-to-edge technique of mitral valve repair. *Anesth Analg.* 2007;105(5): 1231–1232.

42. Kuduvalli M, Ghotkar SV, Grayson AD, et al. Edge-to-edge technique for mitral valve repair: medium-term results with echocardiographic follow-up. *Ann Thorac Surg.* 2006;82(4):1356–1361.

43. Herrmann HC, Rohatgi S, Wasserman HS, et al. Mitral valve hemodynamic effects of percutaneous edge-to-edge repair with the MitraClip device for mitral regurgitation. *Catheter Cardiovasc Interv.* 2006;68(6):821–828.

44. Feldman T, Wasserman HS, Herrmann HC, et al. Percutaneous mitral valve repair using the edge-to-edge technique: six-month results of the EVEREST Phase I Clinical Trial. *J Am Coll Cardiol.* 2005;46(11):2134–2140.

45. Hagler DJ, Cabalka AK, Sorajja P, et al. Assessment of percutaneous catheter treatment of paravalvular prosthetic regurgitation. *JACC Cardiovasc Imaging.* 2010;3(1):88–91.

46. Hamilton-Craig C, Boga T, Platts D, et al. The role of 3D transesophageal echocardiography during percutaneous closure of paravalvular mitral regurgitation. *JACC Cardiovasc Imaging.* 2009;2(6):771–773.

47. Horton KD, Whisenant B, Horton S. Percutaneous closure of a mitral perivalvular leak using three dimensional real time and color flow imaging. *J Am Soc Echocardiogr.* 2010;23(8):e905–e907.

48. Kim MS, Casserly IP, Garcia JA, et al. Percutaneous transcatheter closure of prosthetic mitral paravalvular leaks: are we there yet? *JACC Cardiovasc Interv.* 2009;2(2):81–90.

49. Agarwal S, Tuzcu EM, Desai MY, et al. Updated meta-analysis of septal alcohol ablation versus myectomy for hypertrophic cardiomyopathy. *J Am Coll Cardiol.* 2010;55(8):823–834.

50. Himbert D, Brochet E, Ducrocq G, et al. Contrast echocardiography guidance for alcohol septal ablation of hypertrophic obstructive cardiomyopathy. *Eur Heart J.* 2010;31(9):1148.

SPECIALIZED SKILLS FOR THE INTERVENTIONALIST

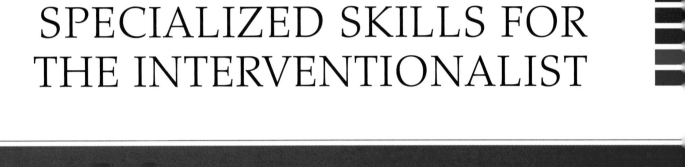

CHAPTER 7

Intracardiac Echocardiography for Structural Heart Disease Interventions

C. Huie Lin and John Lasala

A lthough intracardiac echocardiography (ICE) may have been conceptualized as early as the 1950s,[1] practical widespread application has only been recently possible because of advancements in ultrasound technology that have allowed the production of a phased-array ultrasound transducer the size of an 8 French catheter. At present, ICE catheters are capable of producing frequencies between 5 and 10 MHz, resulting in adequate imaging up to 10 cm from the transducer (Table 7-1).[2] Combined with color, continuous, and pulsed-wave Doppler and four-way steering, contemporary ICE has become a powerful and indispensable component in the toolbox of the structural interventionalist, with virtually infinite applications yet to be described.

SELECTION OF AN INTRACARDIAC ECHOCARDIOGRAPHY SYSTEM

The present generation of ICE probes are generally similar in size; however, a number of differences in design should be taken into consideration when selecting a system for use. The probes range from 8 to 10 French in diameter, and generally, the 8 French probes do not sacrifice imaging or technical quality. Steering capability of the probes is dependent on the model and is a crucial component in imaging of structural heart disease (SHD; see Practical Guide later in this chapter). Although some models are only able to perform anteroposterior tilt, others are able to also perform left/right tilt, allowing additional degrees of freedom in imaging. The conformation of the imaging array may be a consideration for some applications. Our preference has been to use the side-firing array systems exclusively; these systems give a 90-degree arc of view in the plane of the transducer, similar to traditional two-dimensional transthoracic and transesophageal echocardiography (TTE and TEE, respectively). Such images are likely more intuitive for most cardiologists. In contrast, radial array systems are available that yield a circular 360-degree image in a plane orthogonal to the probe, similar to the current generation of intravascular ultrasound probes. The Doppler capability of each system is dependent on both the probe and the generator; however, current applications of ICE for SHD generally require only color Doppler. As with all echocardiographic modalities, the position of the ICE probe allows for unique views and interrogation of structures that are otherwise challenging, if not impossible, from outside the heart. Therefore, as applications of ICE imaging expand, pulsed-wave, continuous wave, and tissue Doppler will likely become more useful. Finally, refurbished and resterilized ICE probes are available, as are services to recycle used probes. Such services should be investigated before committing to a single system.

TABLE 7-1 Commercially Available Intracardiac Echocardiography Catheters

Catheter Name	Company	Catheter Size (French)	Steering	Doppler	Additional Features
ViewFlex Plus	St. Jude Medical	9	Anterior/posterior	Yes	Tissue Doppler capable
AcuNav	Biosense-Webster	8 or 10	Anterior/posterior Left/right	Yes	
ClearICE	St. Jude Medical		Anterior/posterior Left/right	Yes	Tissue Doppler, speckle tracking, integration with NavX
SoundStar	Biosense-Webster	10			Integration with CARTO system

CONCEPTUAL ISSUES AND ORIENTATION

Although the ICE catheter may be introduced from above (internal jugular or subclavian approach), this guide is written from the perspective of a femoral venous approach with the operator at the patient's right side, and the patient's head to the left of the operator. Most commonly, the probe is positioned in the right atrium (RA), from which an atrial septal defect (ASD) closure can be guided and completed. The on-screen orientation marker (Fig. 7-1) describes the position of

the handle such that, in the example given, inferior structures are on the left of the screen, whereas superior structures are on the right of the screen. The range of views for a full survey of the cardiac structures involved can be completed by a combination of the following: (1) clockwise/counterclockwise rotation, (2) anteroposterior tilt, (3) left/right tilt, and (4) advancement/withdrawal of the probe. Clockwise rotation of the probe allows a sweep toward posterior structures, whereas counterclockwise rotation sweeps the view toward anterior structures. Anteroposterior tilt allows a sweep toward superior and inferior structures, respectively,

FIGURE 7-1.

Home view. Catheter is advanced to mid-right atrium. Probe is neutral, without rotation or bend. RA, right atrium; RV, right ventricle; TV, tricuspid valve.

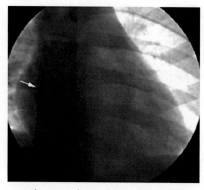

• Catheter is advanced to mid Right Atrium
• Probe is neutral, without rotation or bend

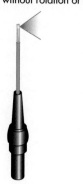

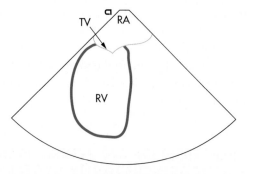

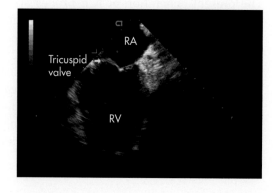

but also allows steering of the catheter if repositioning in other cardiac structures (e.g., across the tricuspid valve into the right ventricle) is necessary. Similarly, left and right tilt allow steering of the catheter but, more importantly, the tilt of the probe allows visualization of structures out of plane to the orientation of the rest of the catheter. This can be conceptualized as similar to TEE multiplanar rotation. Finally, advancement and withdrawal of the probe allows centering in view structures that are superior and inferior to the field of view of the catheter. In combination, these maneuvers allow for excellent visualization of structures that may not be well seen from other echocardiographic modalities, but also may lead to confusing views. When such disorientation occurs, ICE instructors universally recommend returning the probe to neutral position and reacquiring the "home view," described in later text.

PRACTICAL GUIDE TO USE OF INTRACARDIAC ECHOCARDIOGRAPHY: ATRIAL SEPTAL DEFECT CLOSURE

Although the use of ICE in electrophysiologic study/ catheter-based ablation procedures has become near universal, the most common application in SHD intervention is in the assistance of device closure of ASDs/ patent foramen ovale. In this context, the remainder of this chapter focuses on the use of ICE in device closure of the ASD/patent foramen ovale as an introduction to the basic echocardiographic views and practical use of the catheter.

Access

Femoral venous access is obtained bilaterally using the standard modified Seldinger technique. From the left femoral vein, our practice is to advance a 0.038-in 145-cm J-tip wire under fluoroscopic guidance. This is done to confirm continuity from the left femoral vein to the inferior vena cava, and prevent injury to any left-sided residual inferior vena cava. An 8 French 25-cm Terumo Pinnacle sheath (Terumo Medical Corporation, Somerset, NJ) is then placed in the left femoral vein through which the ICE catheter is then advanced. The right femoral venous access is reserved for the right heart catheterization and subsequent device closure procedure.

Placement of the Intracardiac Echocardiography Catheter/ Home View

Under fluoroscopic guidance, the ICE catheter is advanced to the mid-RA. Because the catheter is relatively firm at the tip, care is taken not to enter any other venous structures, and gentle anteroposterior tilt can be used to negotiate vascular tortuosity if needed. From the mid-RA, the probe is placed in neutral position. With subtle clockwise/counterclockwise, the probe can be oriented to bring into view the tricuspid valve and right ventricle: the home view (Fig. 7-1). From here, a complete survey (described later) of the atrial septum and relevant cardiac structures can be conducted. Such a survey is recommended prior to initiating device closure, following placement of closure device, and after release of the device. Frequently, multiple steering manipulations will result in unfamiliar views, at which point it may be useful to return the probe to neutral position in the mid-RA and reidentify the home view.

Right Ventricular Outflow Tract

From the home view, clockwise rotation brings right ventricular outflow tract (RVOT), pulmonary artery, and aortic valve into view (Fig. 7-2).

Coronary Sinus Ostium, Atrial Septum View

Additional clockwise rotation of the catheter allows visualization of the coronary sinus ostium as well as the left atrium (Fig. 7-3).

Left Atrial Appendage, Mitral Valve

Further clockwise rotation of the catheter brings the mitral valve into view. With some leftward tilt, the atrial appendage and atrial septum can be brought into plane (Fig. 7-4).

Left Pulmonary Veins

Clockwise rotation brings into view the left pulmonary veins (Fig. 7-5).

Fossa Ovalis

From left pulmonary vein view, fossa ovalis can be seen with some posterior tilt (Fig. 7-6). Image can be centered by advancing or withdrawing the catheter and subtle clockwise/counterclockwise rotation.

Right Pulmonary Veins

After the catheter steer controls are returned to neutral, the right pulmonary veins can be brought into view with additional clockwise rotation (Fig. 7-7).

Interatrial Septum, Short Axis Aorta

The catheter is withdrawn to the inferior RA, and posterior tilt is engaged. Right tilt may need to be applied

FIGURE 7-2.

Right ventricular outflow tract. Catheter is rotated further clockwise (away from the operator). Right ventricle (*RV*) and outflow tract, pulmonary artery (*PA*), and aortic root (*AO*) brought into view. RA, right atrium.

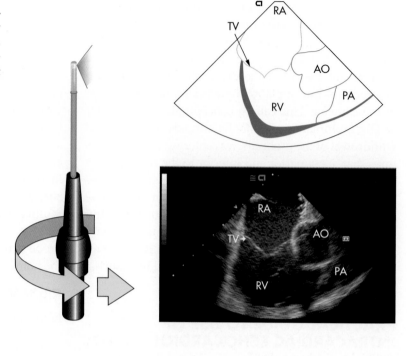

FIGURE 7-3.

Coronary sinus, left atrium. Catheter is rotated further clockwise, directing the ultrasound field slightly posterior. Coronary sinus ostium (*CS*) and left atrium (*LA*) are brought into view. RA, right atrium.

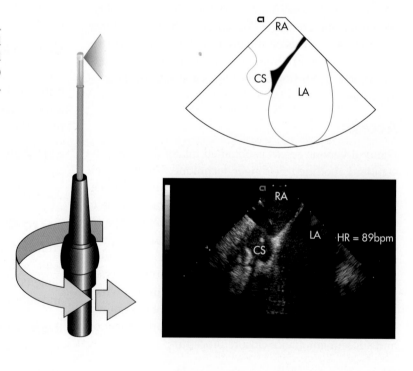

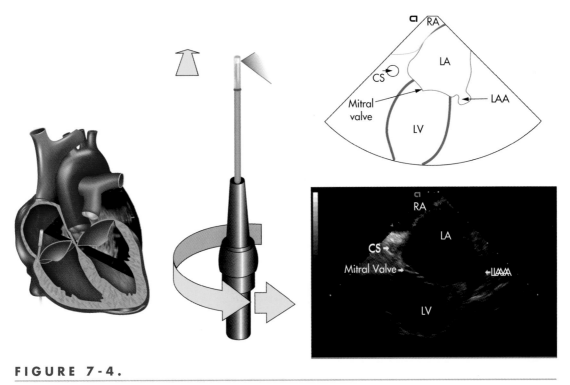

FIGURE 7-4.

Left atrial appendage, mitral valve. Catheter is rotated further clockwise, may need leftward tilt. Left atrium (*LA*), left ventricle (*LV*), mitral valve (*MV*), and left atrial appendage (*LAA*) are brought into view. The interatrial septum is typically seen in the same plane. CS, coronary sinus; RA, right atrium.

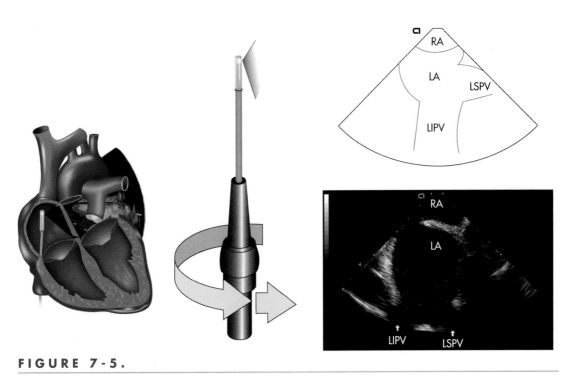

FIGURE 7-5.

Left pulmonary veins. Catheter is again rotated further clockwise. Left atrium (*LA*), left superior pulmonary vein (*LSPV*), and left inferior pulmonary vein (*LIPV*) are brought into view. RA, right atrium.

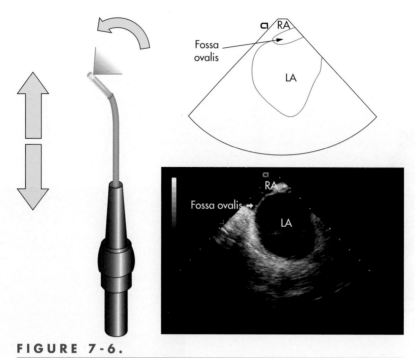

FIGURE 7-6.

Fossa ovalis. From left pulmonary vein view, fossa ovalis can be seen with some posterior tilt. Image can be centered by advancing or withdrawing the catheter and subtle clockwise/counterclockwise rotation. LA, left atrium; RA, right atrium.

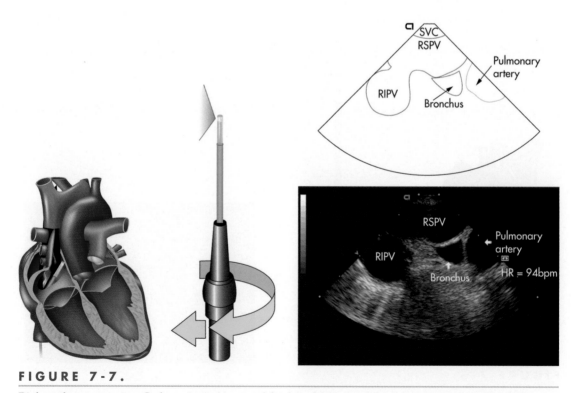

FIGURE 7-7.

Right pulmonary veins. Catheter is again rotated further clockwise. Superior vena cava (*SVC*), right superior pulmonary vein (*RSPV*), and right inferior pulmonary vein (*RIPV*) are brought into view.

as well to bring the interatrial septum and the aorta in short axis in view (Fig. 7-8). Evaluation of device closure is important in this view as both the interatrial septum and part of the aortic rim can be visualized.

Short Axis of the Aortic Valve

The catheter is returned to neutral and advanced to the tricuspid annulus with posterior tilt. From this view, the left atrium, atrial septum, and the aortic valve can be seen (Fig. 7-9). This is another important view for evaluation of device position after deployment. This view completes an initial survey of the atrial septum and associated structures. The left ventricular views are generally reserved for postprocedure assessment.

Left Ventricle Long Axis

The catheter is then advanced with posterior tilt engaged through the tricuspid valve into the right ventricle. The left ventricle can be seen in long axis from this view (Fig. 7-10). Evaluation of the leaflets of the mitral valve, left ventricular function, and assessment for pericardial effusion suggesting perforation can be performed.

Left Ventricle Short Axis

Clockwise rotation, additional posterior tilt, and leftward tilt are engaged to bring the left ventricle into short axis, allowing additional assessment of function (Fig. 7-11).

Balloon Sizing

After crossing the ASD, the sizing balloon catheter is advanced under fluoroscopy. The balloon is then inflated until flow through the defect ceases based on color Doppler on ICE (Fig. 7-12). The width of the balloon on fluoroscopy at the point of "stop–flow" is used to choose the size of the closure device.

Device Placement

Device closure can then be performed according to protocol.[3] The ICE catheter can be placed in the inferior or mid-RA with posterior tilt to guide positioning of the device (Fig. 7-13). Alternatively, the catheter can be placed at the tricuspid annulus with posterior tilt to guide device placement. Once the device has been placed, a thorough survey of the aortic root, valve, mitral and tricuspid valves, pulmonary veins, and coronary sinus should be performed prior to and after device release, including Doppler evaluation of the defect with device in place as described. Finally, the catheter can be advanced to the right ventricle to visualize the left ventricle in long axis and assess for pericardial effusion as a result of occult perforation.

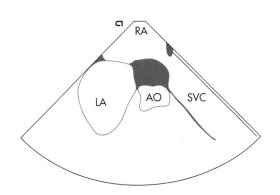

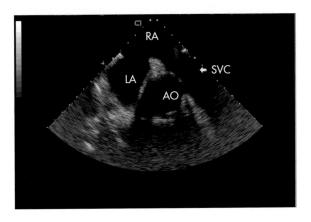

FIGURE 7-8.

Intraatrial septum, superior vena cava. Catheter is withdrawn to inferior right atrium (*RA*), subtle posterior tilt is engaged. Left atrium (*LA*), aorta (*AO*), and superior vena cava (*SVC*) are brought into view. Ideal view for evaluating aortic rim of atrial septum both before and after device placement.

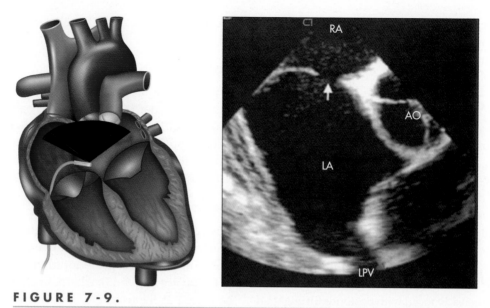

FIGURE 7-9.

Short axis of aortic valve. Catheter is advanced to the tricuspid annulus and posterior tilt is applied. Left atrium (*LA*) and atrial septum, as well as aortic valve (*AO*) in short axis, are brought into view. RA, right atrium.

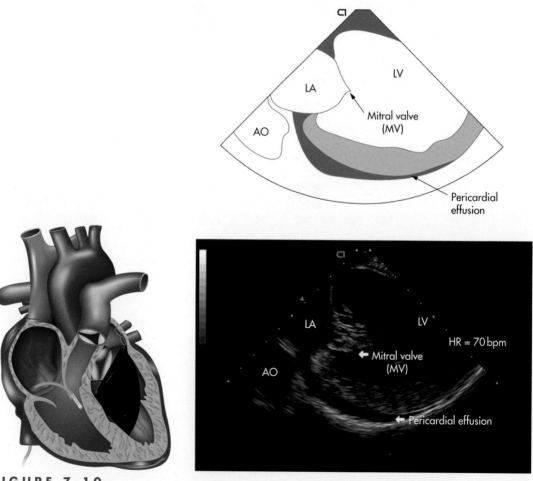

FIGURE 7-10.

Left ventricle long axis. Catheter is then advanced to the right ventricle. Clockwise or counterclockwise rotation may be necessary to direct field toward the left ventricle (*LV*). Ideal view for visualizing mitral valve leaflets and surveying for pericardial effusion. LA, left atrium.

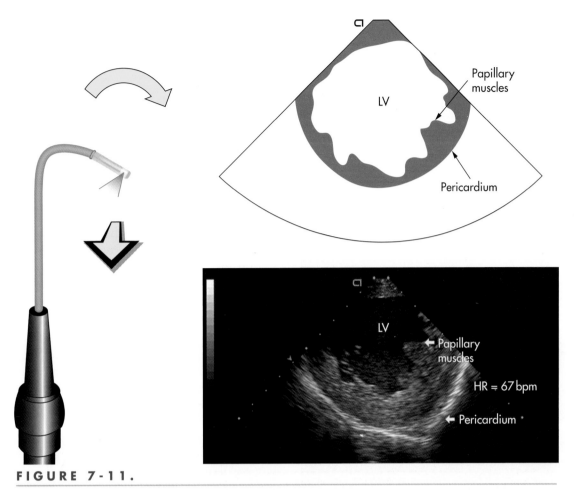

FIGURE 7-11.

Left ventricle short axis. Catheter is rotated further clockwise while positioned in the right ventricle. Left/right tilt may be required to bring left ventricle (*LV*) in short axis into view. Ideal view for examining LV function, papillary muscles, and pericardium.

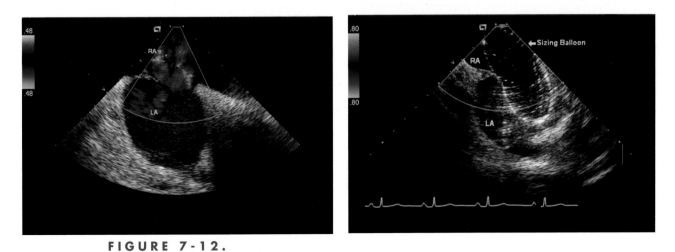

FIGURE 7-12.

Balloon sizing. **Left:** Color Doppler of atrial septal defect. **Right:** Balloon-sizing with "stop–flow." LA, left atrium; RA, right atrium.

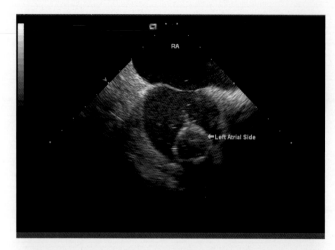

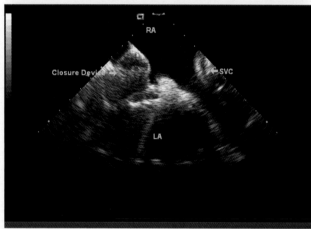

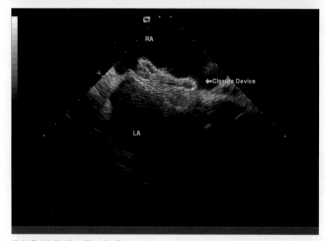

FIGURE 7-13.

Device placement. LA, left atrium; RA, right atrium; SVC, superior vena cava.

ADDITIONAL INTRACARDIAC ECHOCARDIOGRAPHY APPLICATIONS

Device closure of perimembranous ventricular septal defects using ICE guidance has been described.[4] The ventricular septum can generally be visualized from the mid-RA; however, imaging from the left atrium has also provided additional helpful views. Although not required for pulmonary valvuloplasty or transcatheter pulmonary valve replacement, ICE offers excellent views of the RVOT and en face examination of the pulmonary valve or homograft.[5] The RVOT can be seen with the ICE catheter positioned in the RA, although subtle deflections may be necessary depending on the anatomy of the patient (e.g., RVOT conduit). An en face view of the pulmonary valve can be captured if the ICE catheter is advanced through the tricuspid valve into the right ventricle, and subtle anteroposterior tilt is used. Use of ICE for transseptal access during electrophysiologic procedures is common practice and certainly conveys the same added safety and precision to any SHD intervention requiring transseptal access. As discussed previously, ICE can be used to identify the fossa ovalis and guide placement of the transseptal puncture set at the limbus. Following transseptal puncture, ICE can be used to guide balloon atrial septostomy for conditions such as end-stage pulmonary hypertension. In addition to guidance for transseptal puncture, a full survey by ICE prior to intervention can supplant the use of TEE. The left atrial appendage can be assessed for thrombus, and the mitral valve can be fully evaluated prior to valvuloplasty. In addition, the mitral valvuloplasty can be guided by ICE.[6]

CONCLUSION

Percutaneous intrapericardial echocardiography is currently under development and may be helpful in visualizing structures that otherwise may be poorly imaged due to near-field artifact. Similarly, intracoronary sinus ICE has allowed stable positioning of the catheter with improved imaging of structures such as the coronary arterial tree and mitral valve apparatus. In addition, forward-looking as well as real-time three-dimensional and four-dimensional ICE catheters are currently in development. The field of ICE has exploded along with SHD interventions in recent years, and the ongoing expansion of applications and methods will continue to drive the synergistic development of ICE and SHD interventions.

REFERENCES

1. Cieszynski T. Intracardiac method for the investigation of structure of the heart with the aid of ultrasonics. *Arch Immunol Ther Exp (Warsz).* 1960;8:551–557.
2. Kim SS, Hijazi ZM, Lang RM, et al. The use of intracardiac echocardiography and other intracardiac imaging tools to guide noncoronary cardiac interventions. *J Am Coll Cardiol.* 2009;53(23):2117–2128.
3. Amin Z. Transcatheter closure of secundum atrial septal defects. *Catheter Cardiovasc Interv.* 2006;68(5):778–787.
4. Cao QL, Zabal C, Koenig P, et al. Initial clinical experience with intracardiac echocardiography in guiding transcatheter closure of perimembranous ventricular septal defects: feasibility and comparison with transesophageal echocardiography. *Catheter Cardiovasc Interv.* 2005;66(2):258–267.
5. Hijazi ZM, Shivkumar K, Sahn DJ. Intracardiac echocardiography during interventional and electrophysiological cardiac catheterization. *Circulation.* 2009;119(4): 587–596.
6. Green NE, Hansgen AR, Carroll JD. Initial clinical experience with intracardiac echocardiography in guiding balloon mitral valvuloplasty: technique, safety, utility, and limitations. *Catheter Cardiovasc Interv.* 2004;63(3): 385–394.

CHAPTER 8

Catheter-based Hemodynamic Evaluation for Structural Heart Disease Interventions

Morton J. Kern

The widespread use of percutaneous interventional techniques for patients with ischemic and structural heart disease (SHD) (e.g., valvular or atrial septal defects [ASDs]) is now commonplace. This chapter reviews the fundamentals of the hemodynamics of SHD and demonstrates hemodynamic indications, intraprocedural changes, and common findings of complications of common SHD interventions. Complete reviews of hemodynamics in general and those specifically applicable to complex conditions can be found elsewhere.[1-4]

BASIC HEMODYNAMICS

Dr. Carl J. Wiggers (1883–1963) was an eminent cardiovascular physiologist and was the 21st president of the American Physiological Society. He is responsible for a diagram that is most commonly used in the teaching of cardiovascular physiology. All pressure waves of the cardiac cycle can be understood by reviewing the electrical and mechanical activity of the heart as shown on Dr. Wigger's diagram (Fig. 8-1).

The timing of mechanical events, such as contraction and relaxation and the generation of transvalvular and ventricular pressure gradients, can be obtained from the electrocardiogram (ECG) matched to the corresponding pressure waveform. Each electrical event

(e.g., P wave, QRS, T wave) is followed normally by a mechanical function (either contraction or relaxation) resulting in a specific pressure wave.

Although the ECG P wave is responsible for atrial contraction, the QRS for ventricular activation, and the T wave for ventricular relaxation, the normal sequence of contraction and relaxation of the heart muscle is disturbed by arrhythmias and conduction defects. Normal cardiac function may become inefficient or ineffective and can be demonstrated on the associated hemodynamic alterations.

Normal Pressure Wave Forms

Beginning the cardiac cycle, the P wave signals and initiates atrial contraction. Atrial systole and diastole are denoted as the A wave (Fig. 8-1, *point 1*) followed by the x descent, respectively. The P wave (and the A/x pressures) are followed by the QRS signaling depolarization of the ventricles (Fig. 8-1, *point b*). The left ventricle (LV) pressure after the A wave is the left ventricular end diastolic (LVED) pressure that corresponds to the R wave (Fig. 8-1, *vertical line*) intersection with the LV pressure (Fig. 8-1, *point b*). About 15 to 30 msec after the QRS, the ventricles contract, the LV (and right ventricle [RV]) pressure increases rapidly during the isovolumetric contraction period (Fig. 8-1, *interval b-c*). When LV pressure rises above aortic pressure, the aortic valve opens

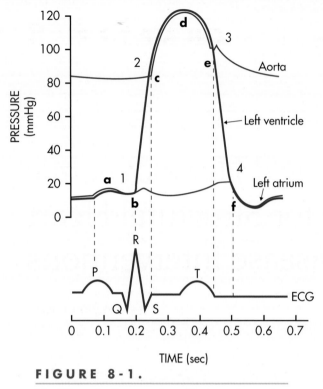

FIGURE 8-1.

The Wigger's diagram of cardiac hemodynamics.

obstruction to outflow, a systolic transvalvular pressure gradient, and correspondingly high transvalvular flow velocity producing characteristic echocardiographic Doppler signals and systolic murmurs. The mitral and tricuspid (atrioventricular [AV]) valves are closed in systole when ventricular pressure is greater than atrial pressure. A regurgitant AV valve that fails to close is characterized hemodynamically by a large regurgitant V wave and long but low flow velocity signals with rumbling systolic murmurs.

In diastole, incompetent semilunar valves fail to seal permitting a continuous backward blood flow into the ventricles with associated echocardiographic flow velocity findings and diastolic murmurs. For the regurgitant AV valve hemodynamics, atrial pressure and volume are highest early in diastole. The stenotic mitral valve has an early LA–LV pressure gradient with high flow velocity into the LV and a decrescendo diastolic rumbling murmur. The more severe the stenosis, the higher the LA pressure and diastolic gradient, persisting across the entire diastolic period.

HEMODYNAMIC ACCURACY

To accurately assess SHD hemodynamics, the operators must eliminate pressure artifacts and use optimal recording methods and best fidelity catheter systems. The most common pressure wave artifact of a fluid-filled system is exaggerated resonance or "ringing" of an underdamped pressure system (Fig. 8-2, *right side*). Be sure to use short stiff tubing, properly debubbled lines, and calibrated recordings. Correct interpretation of hemodynamic waveforms requires review of individual pressure waves and their timing to the ECG. It would not be unusual to have distorted pressure waveforms on the hemodynamic tracing due to an unappreciated electrocardiographic arrhythmia or conduction defect because often only one ECG lead is displayed for the operator.

Accuracy of the pulmonary capillary wedge (PCW) pressure, frequently used to measure mitral valve gradient, is critically important for decisions regarding starting and ending SHD interventions. There should be little hesitation to proceed early to transseptal LA catheterization if there is any doubt about the quality of the PCW. There are two common methods to confirm an accurate PCW pressure that closely agrees with LA pressure. The operator should confirm that PCW pressure wave is not a damped pulmonary artery (PA) pressure by identifying clear A and V waveforms timed against ECG or LV pressure. An end-hole catheter measurement should be used for better PCW fidelity that is connected

(Fig. 8-1, *point c*). Systolic ejection continues until repolarization, signaled by the T wave (Fig. 8-1, *point d*). After the T wave, the LV relaxation produces a fall in the LV and aortic pressure. When the LV pressure falls below the aortic pressure, the aortic valve closes (Fig. 8-1, *point e*). The ventricular pressure continues to fall and when it falls below the left atrial (LA) pressure, the mitral valve opens and the LA empties into the LV (Fig. 8-1, *point f*).

Returning to the atrial pressure wave across the cycle: After the A wave, atrial pressure slowly rises with atrial filling during systole, continuing to increase until the end of systole when the pressure and volume of the LA are nearly maximal, producing a ventricular filling wave, V wave. The V wave peak (Fig. 8-1, *point 4*) is followed by a rapid fall, labeled Y descent, when the mitral valve opens. The peaks and descents of the atrial pressure waves are changed by pathologic conditions such as acute valvular regurgitation, heart failure, and infarction—all potential complications of cardiac interventions.

HEMODYNAMICS OF VALVULAR STENOSIS AND REGURGITATION

To appreciate the hemodynamics of valve dysfunction, recall that the aortic and pulmonary (semilunar) valves open in systole, with LV pressure normally matching aortic pressure. Stenosis of these valves produces

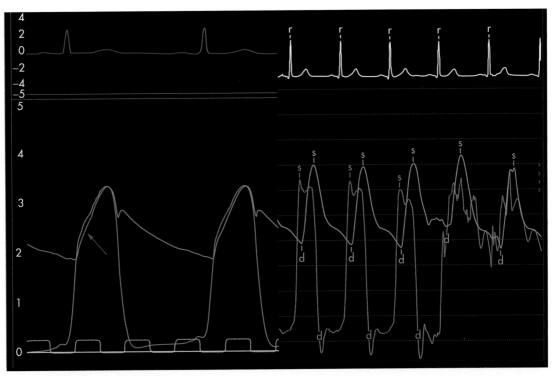

FIGURE 8-2.

Normal left ventricle (LV) and aortic hemodynamics. **Left:** High fidelity LV and simultaneous aortic pressures measured with dual micromanometer catheter. **Right:** Fluid-filled LV and femoral artery pressure waveforms showing underdamped signals. The typical delay in pressure transmission to the femoral artery and its systolic pressure amplification above the LV systolic pressure is evident.

to the pressure transducer with stiff, short pressure tubing thoroughly flushed and bubble free. The operator should note the time delay (i.e., phase shift the PCW pressure V wave to match the LV down stroke). The PCW position (end-hole wedge with balloon deflated) is confirmed by an oxygen saturation >95%. Common hemodynamic problems related to proper pressure recording techniques are reviewed in detail elsewhere.[2,5]

Accurate Left Ventricle–Aortic Pressure Measurements

The hemodynamic assessment of aortic stenosis and its relief after balloon valvuloplasty begins with accurate transvalvular gradient and cardiac output measurements.[6] In most routine measurements, the femoral artery (FA) is used to represent aortic pressure. Due to resonance and peripheral pressure amplification, the FA systolic pressure is higher than central aortic pressure. It is also delayed in time relative to central pressure. The delay and pressure amplification of the FA artificially increases the mean gradient.[7] Figure 8-2 shows the LV–aortic (LV–Ao) pressure measured from a high fidelity catheter with micromanometer pressure

transducers above and below the aortic valve compared to a fluid-filled LV catheter with the fluid-filled FA sheath pressure. Note the delay and overshoot of the femoral pressure. When using femoral pressure, accurate gradients cannot be obtained in patients with peripheral vascular disease at the level of the aortic bifurcation or lower. For better accuracy, a double lumen catheter or two arterial catheters are required.

Techniques to measure LV–Ao pressure gradients from least to most accurate are shown in Table 8-1.

TABLE 8-1 Catheter Techniques to Measure Left Ventricle–Aortic Pressure Gradients

1. Single catheter LV–aorta pullback
2. LV and femoral sheath
3. LV and long aortic sheath
4. Bilateral femoral access
5. Double-lumen pigtail catheter
6. Transseptal LV access with ascending aorta
7. Pressure guidewire with ascending aorta
8. Multitransducer micromanometer catheters

LV, left ventricle.

HEMODYNAMICS OF AORTIC STENOSIS AND VALVULOPLASTY

Balloon valvuloplasty is now frequently used to relieve selected congenital and acquired valvular disorders.[8] In adults, percutaneous balloon aortic valvuloplasty (BAV) has two indications: (1) as a palliative procedure in patients who are not surgical candidates and (2) as an essential prelude to transcatheter aortic valve implantation.

Aortic stenosis is characterized by the delayed upslope of aortic pressure and an LV–Ao pressure gradient (Fig. 8-3).[9] Relief of aortic stenosis will radically alter these two measures. The mean pressure gradient is the area of the superimposed LV–Ao pressure tracings. Operators frequently use the LV and aortic peak-to-peak pressure difference to represent the mean transvalvular pressure gradient.[10] The peak-to-peak gradient is not equivalent to the mean gradient for mild and moderate stenosis but is often close to mean gradient for severe stenosis.

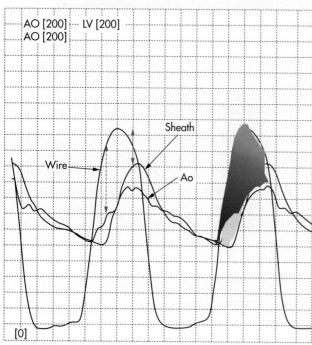

FIGURE 8-3.

Comparison of left ventricular–aortic valve (*Ao*) gradients using central aortic and femoral artery pressure. The femoral artery produces a smaller gradient sheath than the central aortic due to the overshoot of systolic pressure amplification not compensated for by delay in the upstroke. The *dashed red arrow* shows the peak instantaneous pressure gradient and the *solid arrow* shows the peak-to-peak pressure gradient. The *shaded areas* show the difference between gradient of the central and femoral artery pressures. (Redrawn from Fusberg B, Faxon D, Feldman T. Hemodynamic rounds: Transvalvular pressure gradient measurement. *Catheter Cardiovasc Interv.* 2001;53:553–561.)

When using the FA pressure, more accurate valve areas were obtained with unshifted LV–Ao pressure tracings (Fig. 8-3). If the FA pressure is shifted back to match the upstroke of the LV, femoral pressure overshoot (amplification) reduces the true gradient. For highest accuracy, pressures measured immediately above and below the aortic valve should be used, especially for patients with low cardiac output and low transvalvular gradient.[11]

Valve Area Calculations

Stenotic valve areas are calculated from pressure tracings and cardiac output.[12] Cardiac outputs are measured by thermodilution or from the Fick calculation. The Fick calculation uses either assumed oxygen consumption (3 mL/kg O_2) or, for best accuracy, direct oxygen consumption with a metabolic oximeter.

The following Gorlin formula[12] can be applied to both aortic and mitral valves:

$$\text{Area } (\text{cm}^2) = \frac{\text{value flow (mL/s)}}{K \times C \times \sqrt{\text{MVG}}},$$

where MVG is mean valvular gradient (mm Hg), K (44.3) is a derived constant by Gorlin and Gorlin, C is an empirical constant that is 1 for semilunar valves and tricuspid valve and 0.85 for mitral valve, and valve flow is measured in milliliters per second during the diastolic or systolic flow period. For mitral valve flow, the diastolic filling period is used:

$$\frac{\text{CO (mL/min)}}{(\text{diastolic filling period})(\text{HR})}.$$

For aortic valve flow, the systolic ejection period is used:

$$\frac{\text{CO (mL/min)}}{(\text{systolic ejection period})(\text{HR})}$$

where systolic ejection period (sec/min) = systolic period (sec/beat) * HR.

A simplified formula (also known as the Hakke formula[10]) can provide a quick in-laboratory determination of aortic valve area accurately estimated as:

$$\text{Quick valve area} = \text{CO}/ \sqrt{\text{LV–Aortic peak-to-peak}}$$
pressure difference.

For example, peak-to-peak gradient = 65 mm Hg, CO = 5 L/min

$$\text{Quick valve area} = \frac{5 \text{ L/min}}{\sqrt{65}} = \frac{5 \text{ L/min}}{8} = 0.63 \text{ cm}^2$$

The quick formula differs from the Gorlin formula by 18 ± 13% in patients with bradycardia (<65 beats/min) or tachycardia (>100 beats/min). The Gorlin equation overestimates the severity of valve stenosis in low-flow states.[10]

The hemodynamics before and after BAV are compared to assess the results of the procedure. Hemodynamic recording techniques should be identical—that is, the same catheters, tubing, and transducers. An example of a patient's hemodynamics before and after BAV is shown on Figure 8-4. Features denoting success are the reduction of the peak-to-peak gradient (80 to 20 mm Hg) and increase in aortic pressure and decrease in LV peak pressure. The operator should observe the slope of aortic pressure upstroke to avoid mistakenly accepting an erroneous pressure whose zero offset resulted in an increased aortic pressure appearing as a reduced peak-to-peak gradient. A stepwise use of larger balloon inflations can produce gradually enlarged valve area which can be documented by the hemodynamics (Fig. 8-5). The hemodynamic end point of the procedure is a reduction in LV–Ao gradient (<30 mm Hg) and increase in valve area (≥25% of baseline).

An interesting observation is the hemodynamic events during the procedure, which are dramatic but

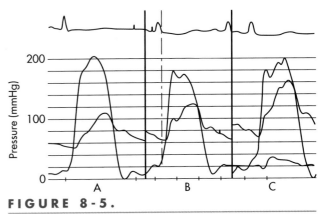

FIGURE 8-5.

Hemodynamics from balloon aortic valvuloplasty procedure using increasing balloon diameters. **A:** Baseline aortic stenosis with left ventricular (LV) pressure of 205 mm Hg, and aortic pressure of 110 mm Hg. **B:** Pressures after initial balloon inflation with fall in LV pressure and increase in aortic pressure. Note change in aortic upslope. **C:** After second larger balloon inflation. LV pressure is not changed but aortic pressure and slope are higher. (Redrawn from Kern MJ, Lim MJ, Goldstein J. *Hemodynamic Rounds: Interpretation of Cardiac Pathophysiology from Pressure Waveform Analysis.* 3rd ed. Hoboken, NJ: Wiley-Blackwell; 2009:178.)

short lived (Fig. 8-6). Rapid ventricular pacing with a transvenous pacemaker is performed to prevent the balloon from "slipping" during inflation. The patient should be observed carefully for syncope and seizures during brief but severe hypotension. Before each BAV balloon inflation, the arterial pressure and PA oxygen saturation (monitored with an oximetric pulmonary catheter) reflecting cardiac output should return to baseline.

AORTIC REGURGITATION AS COMPLICATION OF BALLOON AORTIC VALVULOPLASTY

Aortic regurgitation occurs when there is inadequate closure or malcoaptation of the aortic valve leaflets, allowing blood to enter the LV cavity from the aorta during diastole. It is one of the most common valvular complications of BAV. Depending on the extent of valve leaflet and/or aortic root disruption, some patients may require emergency valve replacement. Figure 8-7 shows a patient with mixed aortic stenosis and regurgitation. Note the wide pulse pressure and rapid LV diastolic filling slope up to the LVED pressure. This patient may not be suitable for BAV.

Figure 8-8 shows the hemodynamic results of BAV that produced acute aortic regurgitation. Measurements

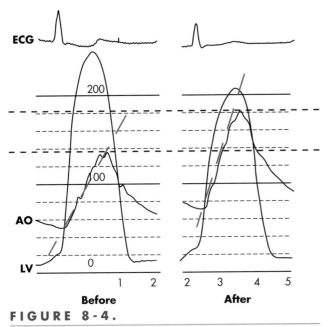

FIGURE 8-4.

Hemodynamics before and after balloon aortic valvuloplasty (BAV). **Left:** Before BAV, there is a large left ventricular (*LV*)–aortic (*Ao*) gradient (100 mm Hg) with delayed upslope of aortic pressure (*red line*). Aortic peak pressure is 138 mm Hg, peak LV pressure is 230 mm Hg. **Right:** After successful BAV, aortic pressure increased to 180 mm Hg and LV pressure decreased to 205 mm Hg, an 80 mm Hg decreased in LV–Ao gradient. Aortic valve area increased from 0.6 to 1.1 cm². Note also the dramatic improvement in the upslope of aortic pressure representing a significant reduction of LV outflow resistance of the previously stenotic valve.

Aortic valvuloplasty

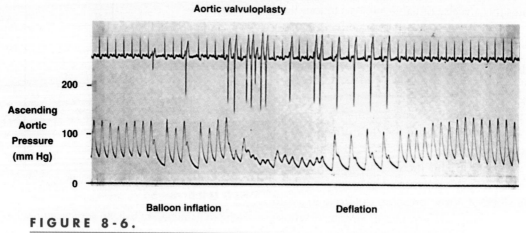

Ascending Aortic Pressure (mm Hg)

Balloon inflation   Deflation

FIGURE 8-6.

Aortic pressure during balloon aortic valvuloplasty balloon inflation. Note transient severe hypotension with recovery. Operators should permit perfusion to be restored before proceeding with subsequent balloon occlusions. (Courtesy of Ted Feldman, MD)

FIGURE 8-7.

Hemodynamics of mixed aortic stenosis and regurgitation. The aortic regurgitation is hemodynamically severe as noted by the wide pulse pressure, the narrow difference between left ventricular end diastolic pressure (*double headed arrow*) and aortic diastolic pressure and the rapid left ventricle filling during diastole (*solid red line* along diastolic pressure).

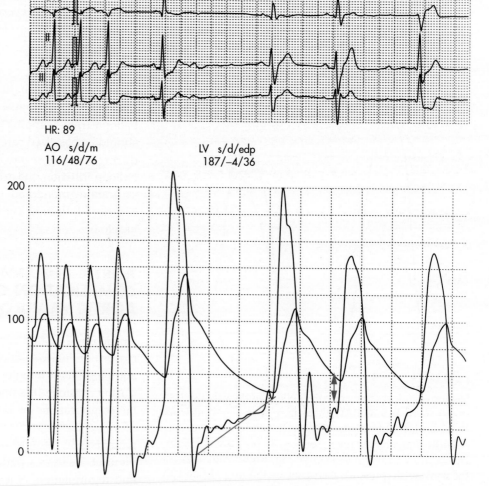

HR: 89

AO s/d/m
116/48/76

LV s/d/edp
187/–4/36

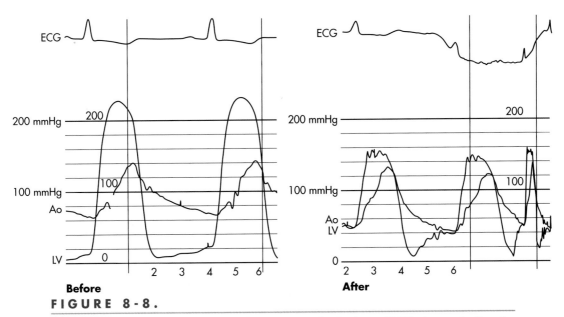

Before

After

FIGURE 8-8.

Hemodynamics before and after balloon aortic valvuloplasty (BAV) demonstrating the marked reduction of systolic gradient and the development of acute aortic insufficiency. Note that after BAV, the aortic (*Ao*) pressure is unchanged but the left ventricular (*LV*) pressure has fallen from 220 to 150 mm Hg and the aortic pressure slope has improved. However, the pulse pressure widened, the LV diastolic filling slope increased rapidly with left ventricular end diastolic pressure rising from 20 to 40 mm Hg. There is equilibration of aortic and LV pressure at end diastole.

made with the stiff exchange wire across a calcific stenotic valve may prop the leaflet open and produce an identical hemodynamic picture.

PULMONARY VALVULOPLASTY

Pulmonary stenosis (pulmonary valve gradient >50 mm Hg) can be easily treated with percutaneous balloon valvuloplasty. The technique is similar to aortic valvuloplasty with a right heart approach. Success is determined by the reduction of pulmonary gradient and reduced right ventricular pressure (Fig. 8-9). A potential complication of pulmonary valvuloplasty is "suicide right ventricle" (severe right ventricular contractility failure). Right ventricular outflow tract obstruction secondary to muscular hypertrophy of the right ventricular outflow tract can be treated with intravenous beta-blockers.[13]

Pre-PTVA

Post-PTVA

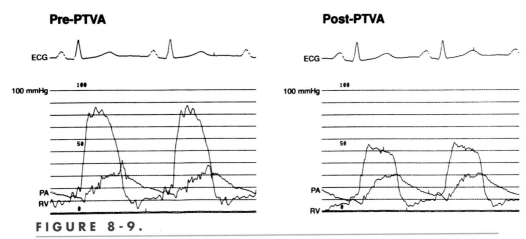

FIGURE 8-9.

Pulmonary balloon valuloplasty hemodynamics. Similar to balloon aortic valvuloplasty, the transvalvular gradient is reduced and the upslope of pulmonary artery (*PA*) pressure improved. PTVA, percutaneous transseptal ventricular assist; RV, right ventricle.

FIGURE 8-10.

Normal left ventricle–pulmonary capillary wedge pressure wave forms. LA, left atrium; LV, left ventricle.

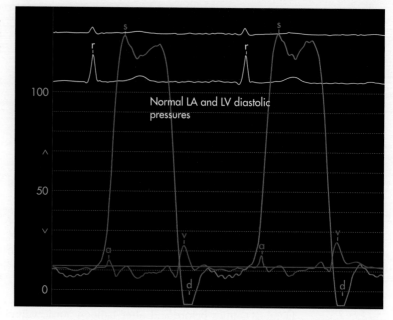

MITRAL VALVE STENOSIS AND VALVULOPLASTY

Percutaneous mitral commissurotomy (PMC) for mitral stenosis has emerged as an excellent alternative to surgical commissurotomy or valve replacement and, in selected patients, is considered as the initial mechanical treatment of choice. PMC has been studied extensively, and when successful, produces marked immediate hemodynamic improvement and sustained clinical benefit. However, not all patients are optimal candidates for PMC. Echocardiography is essential to evaluate mitral valve structure and to exclude LA thrombus.

Hemodynamic assessment of the stenotic mitral valve is performed initially with combined left and right heart hemodynamics comparing PCW pressure to simultaneous LV pressure at rest. Figure 8-10 shows a normal PCW compared to LV pressure. In patients with borderline hemodynamic results, measurements should be made during exercise (e.g., arm lifting with weights). The PCW pressure often overestimates LA pressure in patients with mitral stenosis or prosthetic mitral valves caused in part by the phase delay and poor pressure transmission, making correction and alignment of pressure tracings difficult. Figure 8-11 shows a PCW pressure (*red*) and LA pressure (*orange*),

FIGURE 8-11.

In a patient with suspected mitral stenosis, simultaneous superimposed pulmonary capillary wedge (PCW; *red*) and left atrium (*orange*) pressures demonstrate delayed timing of PCW V waves and higher mean PCW pressure. PCW would falsely increase mitral valve gradient measurement and reduce mitral valve area calculation.

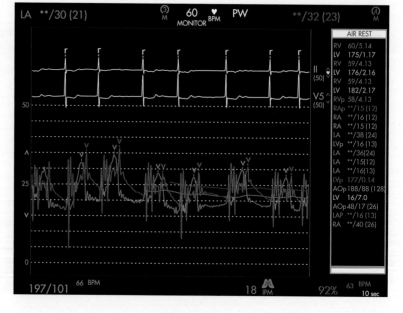

demonstrating different timing of V waves and higher mean for PCW, which would falsely increase mitral valve gradient measurement. LA pressure from transseptal measurement is the most accurate method and should confirm mitral valve gradients prior to mitral valvuloplasty. However, if the PCW/LV pressure tracings show no significant gradients, transseptal catheterization for diagnosis is often unnecessary.[14,15]

The transmitral pressure gradient, calculation of mitral valve area (see previous), and presence of mitral regurgitation (MR) by V wave of LA pressure are used to judge success and need to proceed with or stop the procedure. The echocardiographic assessment of the degree of stenosis and regurgitation as well as commissural separation is also useful both before and immediately after PMC. Figure 8-12 shows a case

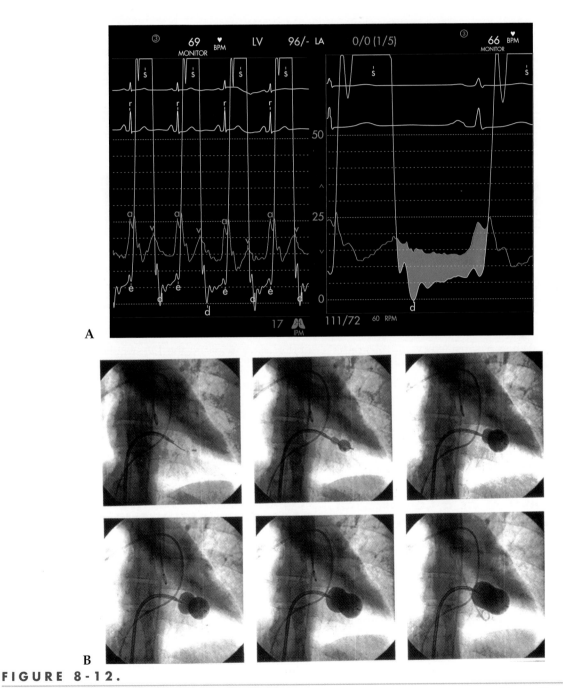

FIGURE 8-12.

A: Mitral stenosis hemodynamics before balloon valvuloplasty. Mean left atrial (*LA*) pressure is 20 mm Hg and mitral valve gradient (MVG) is 12 mm Hg. LA pressure in *orange*, left ventricular (*LV*) pressure is *yellow*. Zero to 50 mm Hg scale. **B:** Cineangiographic frames of Inoue balloon mitral valvuloplasty with serial inflations of the distal then proximal parts of the balloon producing commissural splitting. (Images A,B courtesy of Ted Feldman, MD) *(Continued)*

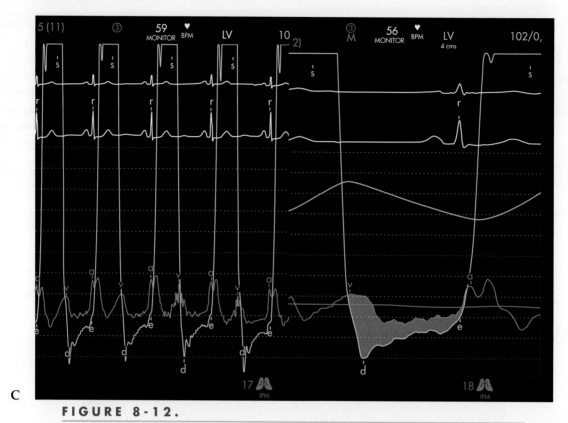

C

FIGURE 8-12.

(Continued) **C:** Mitral stenosis hemodynamics after balloon valuloplasty. There is a modest reduction of LA pressure and MVG to 12 mm Hg and 5 mm Hg, respectively. Mitral valve area improved from 1.1 to 1.8 cm².

example of PMC. When a satisfactory mitral gradient reduction has been achieved, a right-sided oxygen saturation run is obtained to detect residual left-to-right shunting from septal perforation. Successful procedures produce an average decrease in mitral valve gradient of approximately 50% to 75% of the baseline gradient, and a doubling of the mitral valve area, on average about 2 cm².

Mitral Regurgitation as a Complication of Percutaneous Mitral Commissurotomy

The most common complication of PMC is MR because of the unpredictable response to commissural stretching and splitting. Hemodynamically, acute MR is characterized by a new and large V wave (Fig. 8-13). However, as with all hemodynamic wave forms, the compliance changes of pressure and flow also produce changes in V waves in the absence of MR (Fig. 8-14). Nonetheless, a new large V wave after PMC is MR until proven otherwise.

Because the V wave, when obtained from the PCW, and its characteristics are of limited value in the prediction of MR, Freihage et al.[16] reported that the area ratio

under the V wave to the LV systolic area, that is Va/LVa, best correlated with the degree of MR (Fig. 8-15). The ratio was significantly lower in patients with 0 to 1+ MR compared to those with greater than or equal to 2+ MR; 0.14 versus 0.23, (p = .002). The ratio Va:LVa is useful in determining the severity of MR over that of ventriculography.

HYPERTROPHIC OBSTRUCTIVE CARDIOMYOPATHY AND ALCOHOL SEPTAL ABLATION

The hemodynamic evaluation of hypertrophic obstructive cardiomyopathy (HOCM) is crucial for the indications and results of alcohol septal ablation or surgical myomectomy.[17,18] Characteristically, left ventricular outflow tract (LVOT) obstruction in HOCM is dynamic and exquisitely sensitive to ventricular loading conditions and contractility, which can lead to disparities of measurements at different times and under different conditions, thereby explaining some of the discrepancies between echocardiographic findings and invasive catheterization.[18] The LVOT gradient at rest should be compared to dynamic and provocable gradients (e.g., variation with respiration, post–premature ventricular contraction [PVC] accentuation) before, during, and after alcohol septal ablation. The most common methods to assess the LVOT gradient are those used for the assessment of aortic valve stenosis. Although these are acceptable in most circumstances, a pigtail catheter with shaft side holes should not be used because some or all of the holes may be positioned above the intracavitary obstruction, producing an erroneously low LVOT gradient. A Halo catheter with no shaft side holes is preferred. The most accurate hemodynamic assessment of LVOT obstruction uses a transseptal approach with a balloon-tipped catheter placed at the left ventricular inflow region and a pigtail catheter in the ascending aorta for simultaneous measurement of the LVOT gradient. The transseptal approach helps to avoid catheter entrapment, which can be confused for left ventricular pressure of LVOT obstruction. Use of an 8 French Mullins sheath for transseptal access also enables the

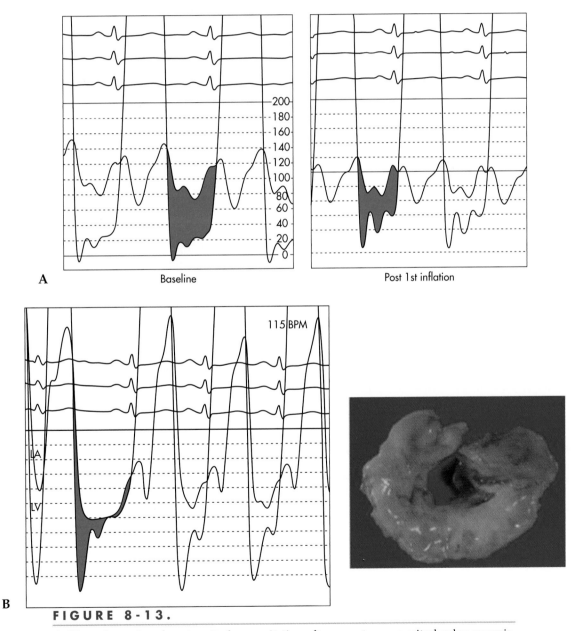

FIGURE 8-13.

A: Hemodynamics of acute mitral regurgitation after percutaneous mitral valve commissurotomy. **Left:** Mitral gradient of 20 mm Hg is reduced to 10 mm Hg after initial balloon inflation. (Courtesy of Dr. Ted Feldman.) **B.** After larger balloon inflation, mitral gradient markedly reduced but large V wave now present indicating acute mitral regurgitation. **Right:** Mitral valve with torn posterior leaflet. *(Continued)*

FIGURE 8-13.

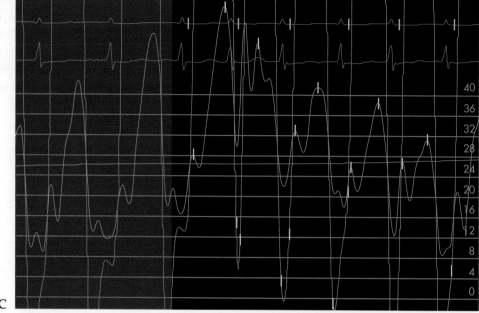

(Continued) **C.** Giant V wave of severe mitral regurgitation. Left atrium pressure is *blue* and left ventricular pressure is *red* (a 0 to 40 mm Hg scale is used).

recording of LA pressure via the sidearm for assessment for concomitant diastolic dysfunction.

Although a temporary pacemaker is used during the procedure, all hemodynamics should be collected with the pacemaker turned off.

A typical HOCM pressure wave from at rest is shown on Figure 8-16. The demonstration of LVOT obstruction is made by pullback of the LV catheter from apex to base (Fig. 8-17). A large LV–aortic gradient

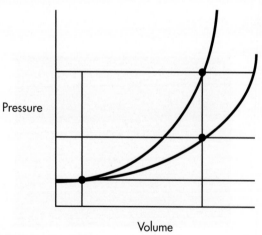

FIGURE 8-14.

Cardiac pressure–volume relationship produces different compliance curves. This graph illustrates the effect of high and lower compliance on a V wave. A highly compliant system (*lower curve*) produces little pressure change as volume increases, whereas a low compliant or stiff chamber (*upper curve*) system produces large pressure increase during similar volume infusion.

disappears when the catheter is positioned just above the mid-cavity obstruction. Left side of the tracing shows large gradient and the right side shows no LVOT gradient while catheter remains in the LV. Note that there is no change of the LV diastolic pressure wave.

The HOCM post-PVC pressure (Fig. 8-16) is associated with three distinct features: (1) the rapid upstroke of aortic pressure, (2) a narrow aortic pulse pressure, and (3) a spike and dome configuration of early vigorous LV ejection followed by delay in ejection of the remaining LV volume, with the resulting the outflow gradient. Another method to demonstrate LVOT in HOCM patients is to perform a Valsalva maneuver. Figure 8-18 shows the hemodynamic changes observed during Valsalva maneuver in a patient with HOCM. The top panel shows the beginning of Valsalva strain phase. Note the increase in LVED and reduced arterial pulse pressure. The LVOT gradient begins to appear and is most pronounced during the plateau phase (bottom panel) during a PVC (middle beat).

The larger post-PVC gradient is present with both aortic stenosis and HOCM. A comparison to the post-PVC hemodynamic responses between HOCM and atrial stenosis is shown on Figure 8-19. Aortic stenosis post-PVC hemodynamics shows a larger pulse pressure, persistently slow aortic upstroke of fixed valve obstruction, and no change in the aortic waveform–all in contrast to the HOCM hemodynamics.

The indications for alcohol septal ablation include cardiac symptoms or syncope refractory to medical therapy, a rest 40 mm Hg LVOT gradient or provocable

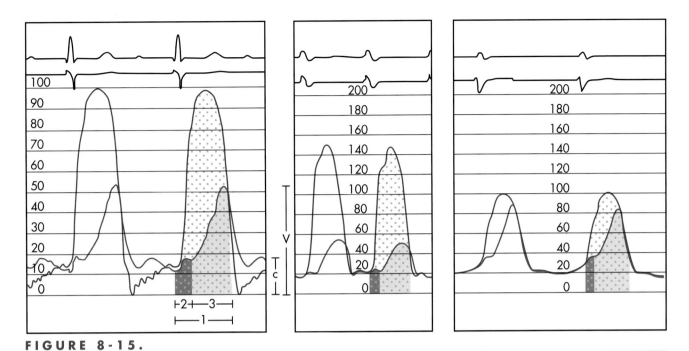

FIGURE 8-15.

Assessment of mitral regurgitation from V waves. **Top:** Simultaneous left ventricle and left atrium (LA) recordings with shaded areas. Small very dark area is C wave area. Gray shaded area is V wave area, and light shaded area is total LA area over systole. **Bottom:** Progression of mitral regurgitation corresponded to enlargement of V wave area relative to total LA area increasing from +2 to +4. (Reproduced from Freihage JH, Joyal D, Arab D, et al. Invasive assessment of mitral regurgitation: Comparison of hemodynamic parameters. *Catheter Cardiovasc Interv.* 2007;69:303–312, with permission.)

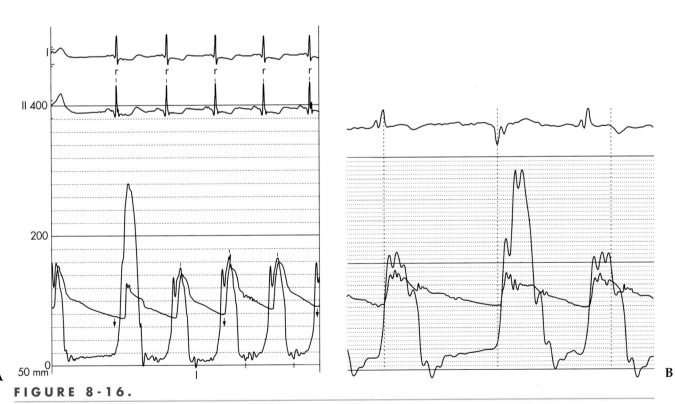

FIGURE 8-16.

A: Patient with hypertrophic obstructive cardiomyopathy (HOCM) with no resting left ventricular outflow tract (LVOT) gradient. **B:** Hemodynamic response to premature ventricular contraction (PVC) shows typical findings of larger LVOT gradient, narrower pulse pressure, and spike and dome aortic waveform with a preserved rapid initial upstroke with left ventricular ejection.

FIGURE 8-17.

Hemodynamics of left ventricular out-flow tract (LVOT) obstruction. Pull-back of left ventricular (LV) catheter from apex to base shows large gradient disappearing just above the mid-cavity obstruction. **Left side** shows large gradient and **right side** shows no LVOT gradient while catheter remains in the LV. Note that there is no change of the LV diastolic pressure wave.

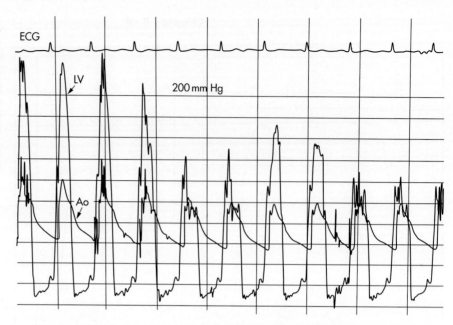

FIGURE 8-18.

Hypertrophic obstructive cardiomyopathy during Valsalva maneuver. Left ventricle (LV) and femoral artery pressures are shown on 0 to 200 mm Hg scale. **Top:** At start of Valsalva maneuver, all pressures increase. As strain progresses, LV filling falls, aortic pulse pressure decreases. **Bottom:** As LV filling continues to be reduced during strain phase of Valsalva, a resting left ventricular outflow tract gradient appears and is exaggerated with a premature ventricular contraction.

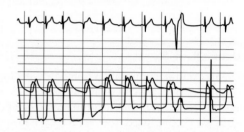

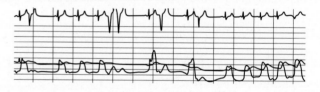

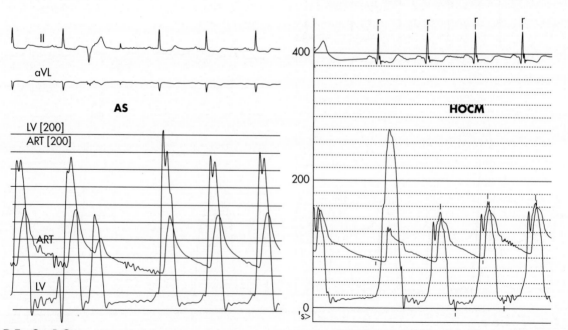

FIGURE 8-19.

The characteristics of post−premature ventricular contraction (PVC) hemodynamics of patients with aortic stenosis **(left)** and hypertrophic obstructive cardiomyopathy (HOCM; **right**) are shown. Aortic stenosis (AS) retains the delayed aortic pressure upstroke and waveform with larger pulse pressure on post-PVC beat. HOCM has dramatic rapid early upslope of aortic pressure with change to spike and dome configuration and narrower pulse pressure.

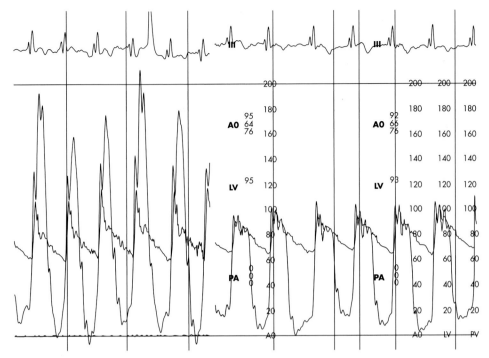

FIGURE 8-20.

Pretransluminal **(left)** and posttransluminal **(right)** alcohol septal ablation procedure hemodynamics. Note the abolition of the left ventricular outflow tract gradient and normalization of the aortic pressure waveform. AO, aorta; LV, left ventricle; PA, pulmonary artery.

gradient to 60 mm Hg with septal thickness >1.8 cm, and no organic MR.[3,17,18] The specific details of the alcohol septal ablation are detailed elsewhere,[6] but the classic hemodynamic abnormalities of the LVOT are abolished when the septum is infarcted, thus failing to contribute to outflow obstruction. Figure 8-20 shows the hemodynamic results of a successful alcohol septal ablation procedure. Note abolition of the LVOT gradient, and spike and dome configuration of the arterial pulse tracing.

Acute procedural success is a reduction of the LVOT gradient ranging from 55% to 75%. Acute procedural success, when defined as a ≥50% reduction in the peak resting or provoked LVOT gradient with a final residual resting gradient of <20 mm Hg, occurs in 80% to 85% of patients. Further reduction in the LVOT gradient over 3 to 6 months after the procedure also occurs due to ventricular remodeling and basal septal thinning. Regression of myocardial mass both at the site of LVOT obstruction and remote from the ventricular septum has been demonstrated using cardiac magnetic resonance imaging.

ATRIAL SEPTAL DEFECTS AND PATENT FORAMEN OVALE CLOSURE

ASDs and patent foramen ovale (PFO) closures are now performed routinely in many labs by experienced operators. The hemodynamics of atrial pressures are not used

as indictors for the procedure but the degree of shunting in some patients makes the case for ASD closure. Because shunt determinations are important as an indication for the procedure, accurate calculations are needed.[19,20] Shunt calculations use oxygen saturation samples obtained during a diagnostic "saturation run," obtaining blood from multiple locations (Table 8-2) in a rapid, organized manner. A standard balloon-tipped Swan-Ganz–type catheter is satisfactory, but a large-bore end-hole or side-hole (multipurpose) catheter performs better rapid sampling. A left-to-right shunt is suggested when oxygen steps up, or increase of oxygen content in a chamber or vessel exceeds that of a proximal compartment. A step-up in oxygen saturation at the PA by more than 7% above the right atrium (RA) saturation is indicative of a left-to-right shunt at the atrial level (Table 8-3). Similarly, the desaturation of arterialized blood samples from the left heart chambers and aorta suggests a right-to-left shunt. In determining the site of the right-to-left shunt, sequential sampling can be made from the pulmonary veins, LA, LV, and aorta.

Mixed venous blood is assumed to be fully mixed PA blood. If there is a left-to-right shunt, mixed venous blood is measured one chamber proximal to the step-up. In the case of an ASD, the mixed venous oxygen content is computed from the weighted average of vena caval blood (i.e., as the sum of three times the superior vena cava plus one inferior vena cava oxygen content and divided by four). When pulmonary venous blood is not collected, Pvo_2

TABLE 8-2 Sample Sites for Oxygen Saturations During Diagnostic Saturation Run

Right side of the heart

  Left PA

  Right PA

  Main PA

  PA_{pv} (above pulmonary valve)

  RV_{pv} (below pulmonary valve)

  RV (mid)

  RV (apex)

  RV_{TV} (tricuspid valve)

  RA_{TV} (tricuspid valve)

  RA (mid)

  SVC (high)

  SVC (low)

  RA (high)

  RA (low)

  IVC (high, just beneath heart, above hepatic vein)

  IVC (low, above renal vein, but below hepatic vein)

Left side of the heart

  Arterial saturation, aortic

  (If possible cross atrial septal defect, pulmonary vein saturation)

  PFO or LA

PA, pulmonary artery; RV, right ventricle; RA, right atrium; SVC, superior vena cava; IVC, inferior vena cava; PFO, patent foramen ovale; LA, left atrium.

(From Kern MJ. Cardiac Catheterization Handbook. 5th ed. Philadelphia: Elsevier; 2010.)

(pulmonary vein) percentage saturation is assumed to be 95%.

SHUNT CALCULATION

The Fick or left-sided indicator dilution methods of CO determination are employed to measure systemic flow. Using the Fick method, the following formulas apply:

Systemic flow,

$$Q_s \ (L/min) = \frac{O_2 \ consumption \ (mL/min)}{(arterial - mixed \ venous) \ O_2 \ content}$$

Pulmonary flow, Q_P (L/min)

$$= \frac{O_2 \ consumption \ (mL/min)}{(pulmonary \ venous - pulmonary \ arterial) \ O_2 \ content}$$

The effective pulmonary blood (EPB) flow

$$Q_{EPB} = \frac{O_2 \ consumption \ (mL/min)}{(pulmonary \ venous - mixed \ venous) \ O_2 \ content}$$

TABLE 8-3 Oxygen Saturation Values for Shunt Detection

Level of Shunt	Significant Step-Up Difference* O_2 % Saturation
Atrial (SVC/IVC to right aorta)	≥7
Ventricular	≥5
Great vessel	≥5

*Difference between distal and proximal chamber. For example, for atrial septal defect: $MVO_2 = (3 \ SVC + 1 \ IVC)/4$ and difference from PA should be ≤7% normally.

SVC, superior vena cava; IVC, inferior vena cava; PA, pulmonary artery pressure.

(From Kern MJ. Cardiac Catheterization Handbook. 5th ed. Philadelphia: Elsevier; 2010.)

Normally the EPB flow is equal to the systemic blood flow. In a left-to-right shunt, the EPB flow is increased (by the amount of the shunt) as follows:

$$Q_{EPB} = systemic \ flow + shunt \ flow \ (left-to-right) \quad (1)$$

In a right-to-left shunt, the EPB flow is decreased (by the amount of the shunt):

$$Q_{EPB} = systemic \ flow - shunt \ flow, \ (right-to-left) \quad (2)$$

The shunt volume is determined by use of Equations (1) and (2).

The ratio of pulmonary to systemic flow (called Q_P/Q_S, where Q is flow, $_P$ is pulmonary, and $_S$ is systemic) for a left-to-right shunt is called the shunt fraction. An ASD with a $Q_P/Q_S > 1.5$ often requires closure.

LEFT AND RIGHT ATRIAL HEMODYNAMICS

The LA pressure is always greater than the right atrial pressure after birth because of the differences in resistances of the two sides of the heart. The RA sees lower resistance of the pulmonary circuit compared to the LA, which fills into a lower compliance systemic circuit. This relationship is evident in a patient with aortic stenosis in whom transseptal LA to RA pressure pullback was recorded showing large LA V waves compared to the lower RA pressure with much reduced A and V waves (Fig. 8-21). However, during various times, and especially during the Valsalva maneuver, the RA pressure can increase above that of the LA pressure and, in the presence of a PFO, produce right-to-left shunting and possible transit of emboli producing clinical sequelae. An example of the pressure changes between the LA and RA can be seen with Valsalva maneuver and is shown on Figure 8-22. It should be recalled that PFO requires no special hemodynamic measurements.

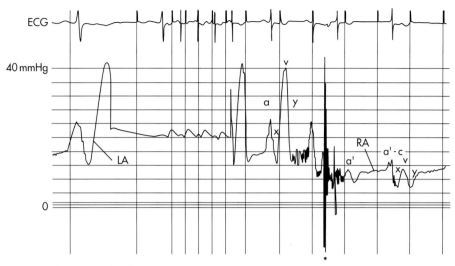

FIGURE 8-21.

Hemodynamic recording of left atrium (*LA*) to right atrium (*RA*) pullback in a patient with aortic stenosis in whom transseptal LA to RA pressure shows large LA V waves compared to the lower RA pressure with much reduced A and V waves. The difference in the pressure waves is a function of different chamber compliance.

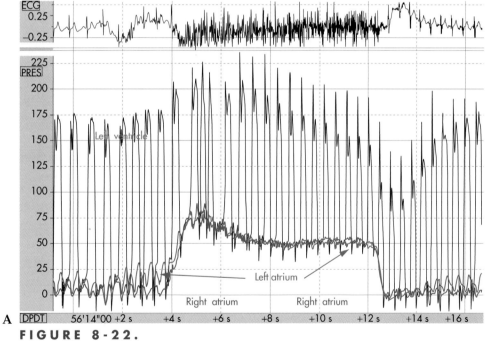

FIGURE 8-22.

A: Hemodynamics of Valsalva maneuver showing elevation of right atrial pressure above left atrial pressure during phase 2 and 3 of the maneuver. Pressure scale 0 to 200 mm Hg. (Courtesy of Dr. Bernard DeBruyne.) *(Continued)*

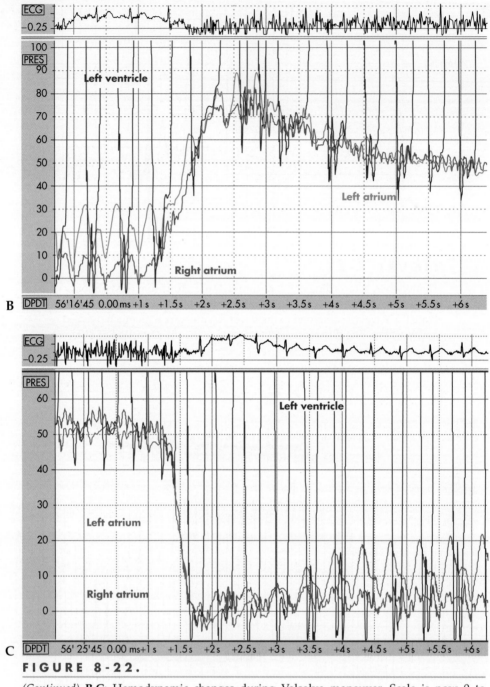

FIGURE 8-22.

(Continued) **B,C:** Hemodynamic changes during Valsalva maneuver. Scale is now 0 to 100 mm Hg. Note increasing right atrial pressure matching and then exceeding left atrial pressure during the beginning of the strain phase at right side of tracing.

CONCLUSION

The hemodynamics associated with SHD for the interventional cardiologist reflect the underlying pathophysiology and its manifestations on the pressure waveforms, cardiac flow, and resolution after mechanical interventions. Careful attention to these changes in pressure wave forms before and after SHD interventions will assist the operators in producing optimal clinical outcomes.

R E F E R E N C E S

1. Kern MJ, Lim MJ, Goldstein J. *Hemodynamic Rounds: Interpretation of Cardiac Pathophysiology from Pressure Waveform Analysis*. 3rd ed. Hoboken, NJ: Wiley-Blackwell; 2009.

2. Kern MJ. *The Cardiac Catheterization Handbook*. 5th ed. Philadelphia: Elsevier; 2010.

3. Kern MJ. *Interventional Cardiac Catheterization Handbook*. 2nd ed. St Louis: Mosby; 2004.

4. Baim DS. *Grossman's Cardiac Catheterization, Angiography, and Intervention*. 7th ed. Philadelphia: Lippincott Williams & Wilkins; 2006.

5. Uretsky BF. *Cardiac Catheterization: Concepts, Techniques and Applications*. Malden, MA: Blackwell Science; 1997.

6. Brogan WC, Lange RA, Hillis LD. Accuracy of various methods of measuring the transvalvular pressure gradient in aortic stenosis. *Am Heart J*. 1992;123: 948–953.

7. Folland ED, Parisi AF, Carbone C. Is peripheral arterial pressure a satisfactory substitute for ascending aortic pressure when measuring aortic valve gradients? *J Am Coll Cardiol*. 1984;4:1207–1212.

8. Carabello BA. Percutaneous therapy for valvular heart disease: A huge advance and a huge challenge to do it right. *Circulation*. 2010;121:1798–1799.

9. Bonow RO, Carabello BA, Chatterjee K, et al. ACC/AHA 2006 guidelines for the management of patients with valvular heart disease: a report of the American College of Cardiology/American Heart Association Task Force on Practice Guidelines (Writing Committee to Develop Guidelines for the Management of Patients With Valvular Heart Disease). *J Am Coll Cardiol*. 2006;48:e1–e148.

10. Hakki AH, Iskandrian AS, Bemis CE, et al. A simplified valve formula for the calculation of stenotic cardiac valve areas. *Circulation*. 1981;63:1050.

11. Grayburn PA. Assessment of low-gradient aortic stenosis with dobutamine. *Circulation*. 2006;113:604–606.

12. Gorlin R, Gorlin SG. Hydraulic formula for calculation of stenotic mitral valve, other cardiac valves, and central circulatory shunts. *Am Heart J*. 1951;41:1–29.

13. Ben-Shachar G, Cohen MH, Sivakoff MC, et al. Development of infundibular obstruction after percutaneous pulmonary balloon valvuloplasty. *J Am Coll Cardiol*. 1985;5:754–756.

14. Lange RA, Moore DM Jr, Cigarroa RG, et al. Use of pulmonary capillary wedge pressure to assess severity of mitral stenosis: Is true left atrial pressure needed in this condition? *J Am Call Cardiol*. 1989;13:825–831.

15. Schoenfeld MH, Palacios IF, Hutter AM Jr, et al. Underestimation of prosthetic mitral valve areas: role of transseptal catheterization in avoiding unnecessary repeat mitral valve surgery. *J Am Coll Cardiol*. 1985;5:1387–1392.

16. Freihage JH, Joyal D, Arab D, et al. Invasive assessment of mitral regurgitation: Comparison of hemodynamic parameters. *Catheter Cardiovasc Interv*. 2007;69:303–312.

17. Sherrid MV, Wever-Pinzon O, Shah A, et al. Reflections of inflections in hypertrophic cardiomyopathy. *J Am Coll Cardiol*. 2009;54:212–219.

18. Geske JB, Sorajja P, Nishimura RA, et al. Evaluation of left ventricular filling pressures by Doppler echocardiography in patients with hypertrophic cardiomyopathy: Correlation with direct left atrial pressure measurement at cardiac catheterization. *Circulation*. 2007;116:2702–2708.

19. Gossel M, Rihal CS. Cardiac shunt calculations made easy: A case-based approach. *Catheter Cardiovasc Interv*. 2010;76:137–142.

20. Kern MJ. Fick Simple-shunt hard: simple shunts commentary. *Catheter Cardiovasc Interv*. 2010;76: 143–144.

CHAPTER 9

The Technique of Transseptal Catheterization

Anita W. Asgar and Raoul Bonan

Transseptal catheterization was pioneered in the 1950s by innovative cardiologists of the day. Initially, this technique was directed toward the diagnosis of valvular and left ventricular pathologies, and it provided invaluable information that furthered our understanding of the hemodynamics of cardiac diseases. As technology and equipment advanced, the role of transseptal catheterization for diagnostic purposes diminished; however, the technique found new purpose in the treatment of mitral stenosis with the advent of mitral valvuloplasty. Although balloon mitral valvuloplasty continues to be performed in many centers in North America, the incidence of rheumatic heart disease has decreased and, with it, the need for transseptal catheterization. Electrophysiologists, however, have embraced the technique and routinely perform transseptal puncture for ablation of left atrial arrhythmias, including atrial fibrillation. Although seemingly forgotten by interventional cardiologists, transseptal catheterization is now making a comeback with the recent explosion in the field of structural heart disease intervention. Modern transcatheter interventions for the left atrial appendage and mitral valve require the ability to safely traverse the interatrial septum and, as such, being able to perform and teach the technique of transseptal catheterization is once again a necessity. As the saying goes, what was old can be new again.

DEVELOPMENT OF THE ATRIAL SEPTUM

The intact atrial septum is formed from fusion of the septum primum and the septum secundum during fetal development. Both septae extend from the roof of the atria toward the endocardial cushions. The septum primum, which is on the left atrial side, develops perforations during development, which become a defect in the septum, the foramen secundum. This defect is eventually covered by the development of the septum secundum, which gradually grows and overlaps part of the foramen secundum, forming an incomplete septal partition as an oval-shaped window. It is this window that becomes the foramen ovale. The septum primum forms a flap-like valve over the foramen ovale, which closes by fusing with the septum secundum after birth and becomes the fossa ovalis.[1]

ANATOMY OF THE ATRIAL SEPTUM

A thorough understanding of the atrial septum anatomy and anatomical relationships is essential to performing a successful and safe transseptal catheterization. The interatrial septum is bordered anteriorly by the aorta, and posteriorly by the posterior wall of the heart (Fig. 9-1). The plane of the septum is oriented obliquely and runs from a right posterior to a left anterior position.

The true interatrial septum occupies only a small part of the atrial walls and can be described more as a septal surface. This surface is a triangular region, which consists of the fossa ovalis and the area of the septum inferior to the fossa near the orifice of the tricuspid valve. Knowledge of the margins of the true septum is important because a puncture directed outside of this area will lead to puncturing outside the heart.

131

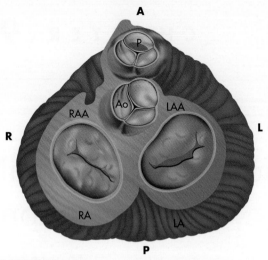

FIGURE 9-1.

Cross-sectional anatomy of the heart depicting the relation of the cardiac structures. The interatrial septum lies between the tricuspid and mitral valves, and is bordered anteriorly by the aorta (*Ao*), and posteriorly by the posterior wall of the heart. **A**, anterior; **L**, left; LA, left atrium; LAA, left atrial appendage; **P**, posterior; P, pulmonary artery; **R**, right; RA, right atrium; RAA, right atrial appendage. (Redrawn from original art by Anita Asgar.)

The septal surface is bordered superiorly by the superior limbus, which is an infolding and fusion of the thicker, more muscular septum secundum and the thinner septum primum. The anterior limbus is the anterior atrial wall that is directly posterior to the ascending aorta, separated only by the transverse sinus of the pericardium. There is frequently a recess in the anterior wall of the right atrium, anterior to the fossa ovalis, that can simulate a position in the fossa. Puncture in this region rather than the fossa can lead to passage into the transverse sinus and then the aorta. The inferior limbus is part of the true septum and extends toward the attachment of the tricuspid valve.[2] When viewed from the right atrial side, the depression of the fossa ovalis surrounded by the muscular ridge of the superior limbus is easily identified as the true septum.

In a normal heart, the atrial septum is located posteriorly at the junction of the mid and lower right atrium running obliquely (Fig. 9-2). In the case of valvular pathology, such as aortic stenosis, dilatation of the aortic root can displace the position of the atrial septum superoposteriorly (Fig. 9-3). In mitral stenosis, with dilatation of the left atrium, the septum is likely to be positioned more inferiorly (Fig. 9-4).

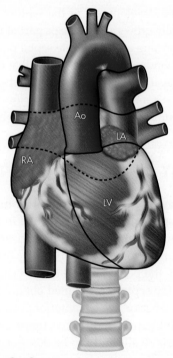

FIGURE 9-2.

Normal relationship of the atrial septum to the other cardiac structures as visualized on anteroposterior radiography. The *dotted line* represents the position of the interatrial septum in a normal heart. Ao, aorta; LA, left atrium; LV, left ventricle; RA, right atrium. (Redrawn from original art by Anita Asgar.)

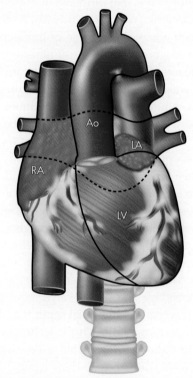

FIGURE 9-3.

Position of the interatrial septum in aortic stenosis: dilatation of the aortic root displaces the septum superoposteriorly. Ao, aorta; LA, left atrium; LV, left ventricle; RA, right atrium. (Redrawn from original art by Anita Asgar.)

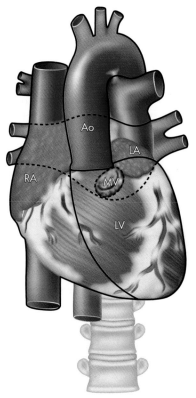

FIGURE 9-4.

Mitral stenosis: dilatation of the interatrial septum displaces the interatrial septum inferiorly with respect to the aorta. Ao, aorta; LA, left atrium; LV, left ventricle; MV, mitral valve; RA, right atrium. (Redrawn from original art by Anita Asgar.)

HISTORY OF TRANSSEPTAL CATHETERIZATION

The initial description of transseptal catheterization was published in 1962 by Brockenbrough, Braunwald, and Ross.[3] Development of the technique in the 1950s was focused on providing a safe, reliable technique to gain access to the left atrium and left ventricle for angiographic and hemodynamic assessment and led to the creation of many of the tools we use today, such as the Brockenbrough needle and transseptal sheath.

In the era of the 1950s and 1960s, the field of cardiac surgery was expanding with the advent of heart and lung machines and valve replacement surgery was becoming a reality. Echocardiography was still in its infancy and transseptal catheterization became an invaluable tool for the evaluation of valvular heart disease. The early research applications of the technique included understanding the pressure volume relationships in heart failure and the phenomenon of obstruction in hypertrophic cardiomyopathy.[4]

The development of the Swan-Ganz catheter and right heart catheterization for wedge pressure measurements and advances in echo led to the decline of the transseptal catheterization as a diagnostic procedure in the 1970s and 1980s. The technique continued to be used, however, for therapeutic procedures such as mitral valvuloplasty. In recent years, the technique has seen resurgence in the field of electrophysiology where transseptal catheterization is routinely performed to gain access to the left atrium for arrhythmia ablation. In addition, the growing field of structural intervention has seen renewed interest in transseptal puncture to perform percutaneous mitral valve and left atrial appendage closure procedures.[5]

The technique of transseptal catheterization has truly had a "50-year odyssey"—one that will continue as the new generation of interventionalists rediscover this skill for the new future of interventional cardiology: structural heart disease intervention.

IMAGING OF THE INTERATRIAL SEPTUM FOR TRANSSEPTAL CATHETERIZATION

As previously described, the true "septum" is a small area of the atria, and a thorough understanding of the anatomy is important to ensure a safe transseptal puncture. The original technique described by Ross and colleagues used only fluoroscopy and anatomic landmarks to localize the region of puncture.[6]

Fluoroscopic-guided transseptal puncture often requires imaging in at least two planes. The anteroposterior (AP) projection is the main working view and a pigtail catheter is placed in the aortic sinuses to provide a landmark for the aortic valve. The transseptal catheter and needle are advanced into the right atrium. The junction of the mid and lower two-thirds of the cardiac silhouette on fluoroscopy is the approximate region of the interatrial septum. In the lateral or right anterior oblique view, the position of the catheter–needle assembly should be posterior to the pigtail, which signifies the aortic valve. In experienced centers, transseptal puncture is routinely performed with fluoroscopy alone.

In the case of difficult transseptal catheterization—such as severe kyphoscoliosis, aortic root dilatation, or therapeutic procedures where puncture in a specific region of the septum is required—or in centers with access to other imaging modalities, transesophageal echocardiography (TEE) or intracardiac echocardiography (ICE) can provide invaluable information on the position of the septum and the transseptal catheter. TEE with multiplanar imaging provides real-time imaging of the atrial septum and transseptal catheter during transseptal catheterization. Tenting of the septum by the transseptal needle can be visualized and the exact position of the septal puncture can be chosen. The availability of three-dimensional (3D) TEE is of additional benefit due to superior resolution and understanding of the 3D anatomy.[7] The only disadvantage to the use of TEE is discomfort to the patient, which usually requires the use of general anesthesia.

An alternative to TEE is ICE. ICE utilizes catheters capable of intracardiac and intravascular ultrasound imaging. These devices provide real-time 360-degree images of the structures surrounding the catheter tip. Because the imaging frequencies are high (10 to 30 MHz in commercially available devices), the spatial resolution is excellent. In addition, imaging with such devices is potentially simpler and less intrusive than either TEE or transthoracic echocardiography because it may be performed by one of the catheterizing team. A feasibility study of this technique using 12.5- and 20-MHz catheters demonstrated that ICE can determine the position of the fossa ovalis in virtually all patients and therefore aid substantially in cases of difficult transseptal puncture.[8]

TRANSSEPTAL CATHETERIZATION TECHNIQUE

The initial description of the technique of transseptal catheterization utilized fluoroscopy and pressure monitoring in a single view with good success.

A thorough understanding of 3D cardiac anatomy and the use of multiple views have enhanced the success of fluoroscopic-guided puncture. Our center uses mainly fluoroscopic guidance in multiple planes for transseptal puncture. In order to perform transseptal catheterization, the material required includes a 5 or 6 French pigtail catheter, a Mullins catheter or other catheter with a 270-degree curve and dilator, a needle (most commonly the Brockenbrough needle), and, finally, a system to monitor intracardiac pressure. The Brockenbrough needle is an 18-gauge hollow tube that tapers distally to 21-gauge. The proximal end of the needle has a flange with an arrow that points to the position of the needle tip (Fig. 9-5).

There are two techniques that can be used to perform transseptal catheterization using fluoroscopy, both of which utilize a pigtail catheter positioned in the aorta. The fossa ovalis is normally located posterior to the aortic valve. The pigtail catheter is advanced via the femoral artery retrograde into the ascending aorta in the noncoronary sinus. This is used to mark the position of the aorta and aortic valve. A Mullins catheter is then advanced over the wire from the right femoral vein into the superior vena cava (SVC), and using the AP projection, the wire is then retracted to advance the Brockenbrough needle. The needle is connected to a pressure transducer and then advanced under pressure flush into the sheath between 5 and 15 mm from the distal end of the sheath with the needle oriented toward the lateral aspect of the SVC (9 o'clock

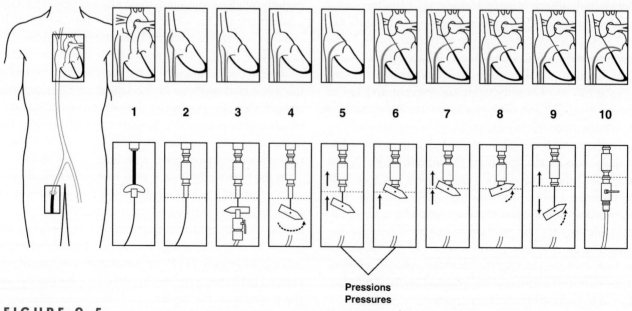

Pressions
Pressures

FIGURE 9-5.

Position of transseptal needle and sheath and orientation of transseptal needle during puncture.

of the needle watch). It is important to ensure that the needle moves freely in the SVC prior to manipulation of the system.

The first technique requires the retraction of the entire system with a posteromedial motion (approximately 45 degrees) to engage the fossa ovalis, see Figures 9-5 and 9-6 (from 9 o'clock to 4 o'clock of the needle watch). This movement is made with the needle on pressure recording the right atrial pressure. Once contact is made with the fossa ovalis, the needle is advanced on pressure monitoring to recognize a change in pressure once the left atrium has been entered. As soon as left atrial pressure is confirmed, the needle is moved to the 3 o'clock position, the entire system is then advanced 10 mm. The dilator and sheath are advanced over the needle into the left atrium and the needle is removed and the system is aspirated. Once needle puncture of the interatrial septum has been achieved, it is important when the left atrium is small to rotate the needle hub about 15 degrees anteriorly (to a position 30 degrees from the horizontal plane) before the needle and catheter are advanced together into the left atrium; this maneuver avoids contact of the posterior wall of the left atrium by the needle.[9] Once in the left atrium, unfractionated heparin is given to reduce the risk of thrombus formation. If difficulties are encountered while engaging the fossa ovalis in the AP projection, the right anterior oblique and lateral can be used to adjust the needle position.

The second technique involves positioning the needle with the flange at 3 o'clock in the SVC. The system is then retracted maintaining a medial-facing needle position. As the needle assembly is retracted, there will be a downward sensation as the system drops into the right atrium. This position is maintained and the system is retracted further until the tip of the dilator catches on the limbus of the foramen ovale. Once contact is made with the foramen ovale, the needle is advanced with pressure monitoring into the left atrium as previously described.

As described by Cheng et al., fluoroscopically guided transseptal puncture is a technique still used by both interventional cardiologists and electrophysiologists alike.[10]

INDICATIONS FOR TRANSSEPTAL CATHETERIZATION

In some centers, transseptal catheterization continues to be performed for diagnostic purposes, such as the evaluation of valvular heart disease. More commonly, however, the technique is used in the setting of interventional procedures.

One of the most frequent uses of transseptal catheterization is in the field of electrophysiology. Diagnostic studies and therapeutic ablations of left atrial pathways or atrial fibrillation require access to the left atrium which can be safely achieved by transseptal puncture. Some of the largest series of transseptal catheterizations have in fact been published by the electrophysiology community using only fluoroscopic guidance.[11]

Following close behind electrophysiology, interventional cardiologists are performing more and more transseptal catheterizations in the context of therapeutic structural heart disease intervention. These interventions include closure of a patent foramen ovale, paravalvular leak closure, left atrial appendage occlusion, and transcatheter mitral valve repair.

COMPLICATIONS OF TRANSSEPTAL CATHETERIZATION

The technique of transseptal catheterization furthered the understanding of the physiology of valvular and myocardial diseases. In the modern era of interventional cardiology, it is now considered an art, as a result of it being practiced at fewer and fewer centers. The major concern of transseptal catheterization remains the risk of complications which can include perforation of surrounding cardiac structures such as the aorta, right or left atrial wall, systemic embolization, and death.

The first published series of transseptal puncture by Ross in 1962 described 156 diagnostic percutaneous transseptal catheterizations in 144 patients. In these, the early days of the experience, there were no fatalities and only three serious complications—inadvertent aortic puncture, one of which required pericardiocentesis. Other complications included transient atrial arrhythmias and unexplained hypotension. Several patients that underwent subsequent surgery were found to have blood-stained pericardial fluid, presumably from unrecognized puncture of the right atrium without significant sequelae.[3]

Thirty-two years later, Roelke et al. published a series of 1,279 patients undergoing transseptal catheterization at Massachusetts General Hospital from 1981 to 1992. The indication for transseptal catheterization was diagnostic purposes in 56.4% of patients, percutaneous mitral valvuloplasty in 39.9%, and anterograde valvuloplasty in 3.6%. A total of 17 major complications

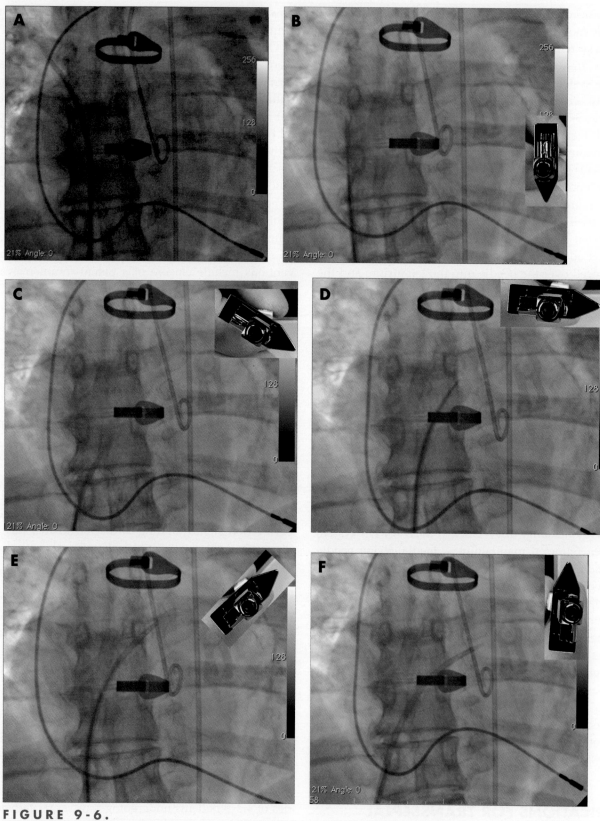

FIGURE 9-6.

Angiographic images of transseptal puncture. **A:** Position of the transseptal sheath in the right atrium. **B:** Transseptal sheath in the right atrium with needle position at 6 o'clock. **C:** Interatrial septum engaged with the needle position at 4 o'clock for puncture. **D:** Needle positioned at 3 o'clock to advance into left atrium. **E:** Transseptal sheath and dilator advanced over needle into left atrium. **F:** Transseptal sheath in place in left atrium.

(1.3%) occurred; one embolic, two aortic, and 13 atrial perforations resulting in cardiac tamponade (1.2%). One death occurred as a result of aortic perforation yielding a mortality of 0.08%.[12] Overall, the rate of complications was low, perhaps explained by the presence of experienced operators in this high-volume center and the use of biplane fluoroscopic guidance.

Although the use of transseptal puncture for diagnostic purposes in most centers has plateaued, there has been an increase particularly among electrophysiologists for the purpose of ablation of left atrial arrhythmias. In fact, in addition to structural interventions, this is likely one of the more common indications for transseptal catheterization. A national survey performed in Italy from 1992 to 2003 among electrophysiologists revealed that over 5,000 transseptal catheterizations were performed for the purpose of electrophysiologic interventions. In 2003 alone, 1,729 procedures were performed with only 14 complications (0.74%). Complications included cardiac perforation with or without tamponade in the majority of cases without any deaths. It is interesting to note that one-third of centers in this survey performed transseptal catheterization without the use of pressure monitoring, ultrasound, or the use of a pigtail in the aorta.[10] These were centers with more experienced operators, and previous work by De Ponti has suggested that a simplified method of transseptal puncture is not associated with increased complications.[13]

Recent studies of left atrial appendage occluders for atrial fibrillation have highlighted the importance of a safe transseptal catheterization. In the PROTECT-AF trial of the Watchman device, serious safety events occurred in 49 patients in the intervention arm. The most common safety event was serious pericardial effusion which occurred in 22 patients (4.8%) and required either pericardiocentesis or surgical intervention.[14] In the absence of obvious perforation of the atrial appendage, it is likely that majority of these complications were related to the transseptal puncture.

For those operators new to the technique of transseptal catheterization, imaging support with TEE or ICE provides valuable information on the location of the fossa ovalis that may help to minimize complications and may be very helpful in the case of distorted anatomy.[15] Despite the prevailing low rates of transseptal complications in the published literature, there has been renewed interest in technology to make this procedure even more user-friendly and safe. A recent review by Babaliaros and colleagues outlined several new technologies to assist transseptal catheterization, including a radio-frequency catheter and laser that may make transseptal catheterization more accessible and safe, particularly in difficult patients.[5]

CONCLUSION

The technique of transseptal catheterization revolutionized hemodynamic assessments in the early days of cardiac catheterization. A thorough understanding of atrial anatomy can ensure that the technique is performed effectively and safely. Fifty years later, this technique is an invaluable skill for the interventional cardiologist in the field of structural heart intervention.

REFERENCES

1. Hara H, Virmani R, Ladich E, et al. Patent foramen ovale: Current pathology, pathophysiology, and clinical status. *J Am Coll Cardiol.* 2005;46(9):1768–1776.
2. Anderson RH, Becker AE. *Cardiac Anatomy: An Integrated Text and Color Atlas.* London: Gower Medical Publishing; 1980.
3. Brockenbrough EC, Braunwald E, Ross J Jr. Transseptal left heart catheterization: A review of 450 studies and description of an improved technic. *Circulation.* 1962;25:15–21.
4. Ross J Jr. Transseptal left heart catheterization: A 50-year odyssey. *J Am Coll Cardiol.* 2008;51(22):2107–2115.
5. Babaliaros VC, Green JT, Lerakis S, et al. Emerging applications for transseptal left heart catheterization: Old techniques for new procedures. *J Am Coll Cardiol.* 2008;51(22):2116–2122.
6. Ross J Jr, Braunwald E, Morrow AG. Left heart catheterization by the transseptal route: A description of the technic and its applications. *Circulation.* 1960;22:927–934.
7. Pushparajah K, Miller OI, Simpson JM. 3D echocardiography of the atrial septum: Anatomical features and landmarks for the echocardiographer. *JACC Cardiovasc Imaging.* 2010;3(9):981–984.
8. Mitchel JF, Gillam LD, Sanzobrino BW, et al. Intracardiac ultrasound imaging during transseptal catheterization. *Chest.* 1995;108(1):104–108.
9. Ross J Jr. Considerations regarding the technique for transseptal left heart catheterization. *Circulation.* 1996;34:391–399.
10. Cheng A, Calkins H. A conservative approach to performing transseptal punctures without the use of intracardiac echocardiography: Stepwise approach with real-time video clips. *J Cardiovasc Electrophysiol.* 2007;18(6):686–689.
11. De Ponti R, Cappato R, Curnis A, et al. Transseptal catheterization in the electrophysiology laboratory

data from a multicenter survey spanning 12 years. *J Am Coll Cardiol.* 2006;47(5):1037–1042.

12. Roelke M, Smith AJ, Palacios IF. The technique and safety of transseptal left heart catheterization: The Massachusetts General Hospital experience with 1,279 procedures. *Catheter Cardiovasc Diagn.* 1994;32: 332–339.

13. De Ponti R, Zardini M, Storti C, et al. Trans-septal catheterization for radiofrequency catheter ablation of cardiac arrhythmias: results and safety of a simplified method. *Eur Heart J.* 1998;19:943–950.

14. Holmes DR Jr, Reddy VY, Turi ZG, et al. Percutaneous closure of the left atrial appendage versus warfarin therapy for prevention of stroke in patients with atrial fi brillation: a randomised non-inferiority trial. *Lancet.* 2009;374:534–542.

15. Cafri C, de La Guardia B, Barasch E, et al. Transseptal puncture guided by intracardiac echocardiography during percutaneous transvenous mitral commissurotomy in patients with distorted anatomy of the fossa ovalis. *Catheter Cardiovasc Interv.* 2000;50: 463–467.

CHAPTER 10

Vascular Access and Closure Issues in Structural Heart Disease Interventions

Ivan P. Casserly

ascular access is necessary for all percutaneous structural heart disease (SHD) procedures. Table 10-1 summarizes the primary vascular access sites used to perform the range of SHD procedures described in this textbook. Clearly, the dominant access sites are the common femoral artery (CFA) and common femoral vein (CFV), with use of upper extremity arterial access and jugular venous access being confined to a small subset of procedures, or in certain unique situations. Successful management of the vascular access is central to the overall success and safety of SHD interventions. This chapter provides a practical overview of vascular access for SHD intervention, focusing on preprocedural planning, execution of the access, and postprocedural management of the access site.

ARTERIAL ACCESS: COMMON FEMORAL ARTERY

Preprocedural Assessment

Clinical assessment of the access site and anatomic assessment of the access site and aortoiliac anatomy using imaging studies are important during the preprocedural assessment for CFA access.

Clinical Assessment

The clinical assessment includes a careful history of symptoms of peripheral artery disease (PAD), prior peripheral artery revascularization procedures (either percutaneous or surgical), and documentation of the femoral and tibial pulses. It is important to understand that calf claudication is the most common symptom of PAD, regardless of the level of disease. However, the presence of buttock or thigh claudication suggests disease at or above the level of the internal iliac and profunda femoral arteries, respectively. Therefore, the presence of claudication in the buttock or thigh suggests disease in an anatomic distribution that is likely to impact either CFA access or the delivery of catheters and interventional devices through the iliac arteries.

Obtaining accurate documentation of prior percutaneous and surgical revascularization procedures is essential, particularly when these involve the aortoiliac and femoral segments. For example, knowing that a patient has had a prior femoral–femoral bypass is insufficient; it is essential to know the direction of flow in this bypass. A left-to-right femoral–femoral bypass will mandate left CFA access, and vice versa. When grafts involve the femoral segment (e.g., aortobifemoral, iliofemoral, femoral-popliteal), it is important to be certain of the touchdown site of the femoral attachment of the graft. In most patients, this will be in the CFA, but in others, the profunda femoral artery may be used. In the case of an aortobifemoral or iliofemoral bypass, the use of the profunda femoral artery as a touchdown site for the graft suggests the presence of significant CFA disease, which will likely preclude CFA access. In terms of prior percutaneous revascularization, it is very rare for CFA access to be compromised by the prior placement of stents. However, placement of stents in the iliac territory is common. The timing of such placement

TABLE 10-1 **Most Commonly Used Access Sites for Structural Heart Disease Interventions**

Structural Heart Intervention	Vascular Access
Aortic valvuloplasty	
Antegrade	Femoral artery
Retrograde	Femoral vein
Aortic valve replacement[a]	Femoral artery
	Subclavian artery[b]
Mitral valve edge-to-edge repair	Femoral vein
Mitral valvuloplasty	Femoral vein
Aortic coarctation	
Device delivery	Femoral artery
Procedure guidance	Brachial/radial artery
Pulmonary valve replacement	Femoral vein
Paravalvular leak repair	Femoral artery
	Femoral vein
Left atrial appendage exclusion	Femoral vein
PFO/ASD closure	Femoral vein
VSD closure	Femoral vein
	Internal jugular vein
	Femoral artery
PDA closure	Femoral vein
	Femoral artery
Alcohol septal ablation	Femoral artery
	Radial artery
	Femoral vein[c]

[a]Retrograde approach.
[b]Via surgical cut down.
[c]Temporary pacemaker insertion.
PFO, patent foramen ovale; ASD, atrial septal defect; VSD, ventricular septal defect; PDA, patent ductus arteriosus.

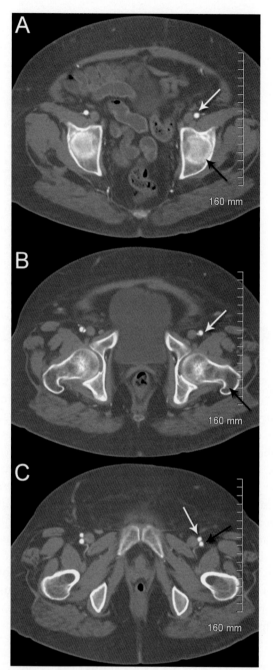

FIGURE 10-1.

Axial computed tomography images demonstrating the precise location of the bifurcation of the common femoral artery (CFA). **A:** Left CFA (*white arrow*) at the level of the top of the femoral head (*black arrow*). **B:** Left CFA (*white arrow*) at level of the bottom of the femoral head (greater trochanter shown by *black arrow*). **C:** Bifurcation of left CFA below the level of the femoral head (*white arrow*, superficial femoral artery; *black arrow*, profunda femoral artery).

should be recorded, as recently implanted stents have a propensity for dislodgement during attempts to delivery large caliber interventional equipment through the iliac arteries. Self-expanding stents are likely to be more prone to this phenomenon compared to balloon-expandable stents.

Femoral pulses should be documented by manual palpation. The absence of a femoral pulse strongly suggests the presence of a proximal occlusion. In markedly obese patients, the accurate documentation of femoral pulses by palpation may be difficult. In this situation, assessment of the popliteal and tibial pulses is helpful, particularly if these pulses are intact.

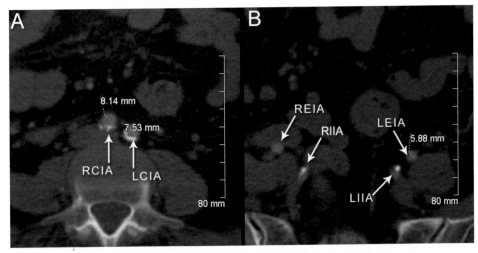

FIGURE 10-2.

Axial computed tomography images showing measurement of iliac artery diameters. **A:** LCIA, left common iliac artery; RCIA, right common iliac artery. **B:** LEIA, left external iliac artery; LIIA, left internal iliac artery; REIA, right external iliac artery; RIIA, right internal iliac artery.

Anatomic Assessment

The gold standard for the anatomic assessment of the CFA access site and aortoiliac anatomy prior to SHD interventions is computed tomographic (CT) angiography (Figs. 10-1 to 10-4). In the case of transcatheter aortic valve implantation (TAVI), this assessment has become mandatory,[1,2] since the dominant contraindication to femoral delivery of the prosthetic aortic valve is related to anatomic issues in the CFA and aortoiliac segment. The chief advantages of CT angiography over magnetic resonance (MR) angiography include improved spatial resolution, speed of image acquisition such that the requirement for patient compliance is minimal, widespread availability, reduced cost, and ability to assess the extent and severity of vessel calcification.[3–6] The major limitation in obtaining CT angiographic data preprocedurally is the need to use iodinated contrast agents in patients with renal insufficiency. In most institutions, 60 to 100 mL of contrast is administered through a peripheral IV during lower extremity CT angiography. Novel strategies have been developed that allow the acquisition of CT data with much smaller volumes of contrast administered through a pigtail catheter in the distal abdominal aorta,[2,7] and should be considered for those patients with significant renal insufficiency.

Most of the information regarding the aortoiliac anatomy is gleaned from the unprocessed axial images. Accurate determination of the diameter of the CFA and the iliac segments is particularly helpful where larger interventional devices need to be delivered

(e.g., aortic valvuloplasty balloon, prosthetic aortic valve) (Fig. 10-2). The location of the CFA bifurcation with respect to the femoral head is easily seen by CT angiography (Fig. 10-1). This has important implications for planning and executing CFA access because a reasonable determination of the appropriate location of the CFA arteriotomy in relation to the fluoroscopic landmark of the femoral head can be made from the CT data. Significant vessel calcification in the CFA influences the ability to successfully deploy suture-mediated closure devices and achieve hemostasis following sheath removal. Severe vessel calcification along the length of the aortoiliac segment predicts a noncompliant vessel that may make device delivery more challenging and increase the risk of iliac injury (Fig. 10-3). The assessment of the degree of tortuosity in the aortoiliac segment can be assessed using the axial images, but three-dimensional (3D) reconstructions and other postprocessing techniques aid in the appreciation of this anatomic issue (Fig. 10-4).

Executing Access

The optimal execution of CFA access achieves a single anterior wall stick in the CFA above the level of the bifurcation of the CFA into superficial and profunda femoral branches and below the level of the inguinal ligament (Figs. 10-5 and 10-6). In most situations, the artery is accessed using the combination of fluoroscopic guidance (i.e., using location of radiopaque hemostat on the skin surface in relation to the head of the femur; Fig. 10-5A) and palpation, with the goal of sticking the

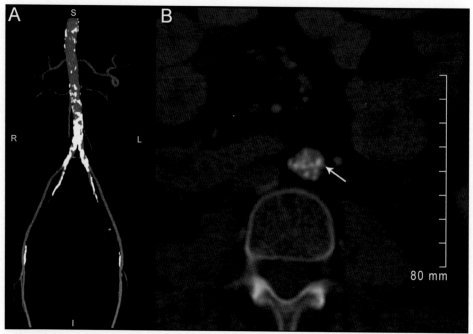

FIGURE 10-3.

Role of computed tomography (CT) imaging in demonstrating aortoiliac vessel calcification. **A:** Three-dimensional volume-rendered CT image showing diffuse severe calcification involving distal abdominal aorta and both common iliac arteries. **B:** Axial CT image from the same patient showing diffuse calcification in the lumen of the distal abdominal aorta (*arrow*).

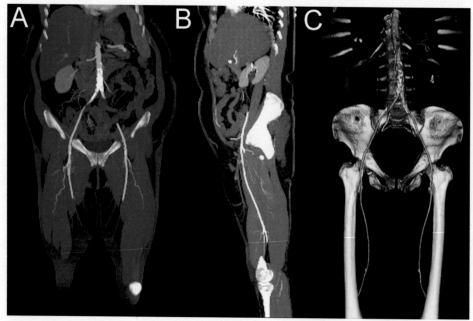

FIGURE 10-4.

Postprocessing display of computed tomography (CT) data to demonstrate anatomy of the aortoiliac and femoral anatomy. **A:** Coronal multiplanar reconstruction (MPR) CT image of the aortoiliac segment. **B:** Sagittal MPR CT image of the femoral segment. **C:** Three-dimensional volume-rendered CT image from this same patient showing straight iliac and femoral vessels without significant tortuosity.

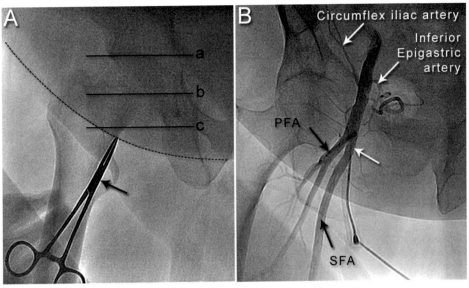

FIGURE 10-5.

Example of low puncture of the common femoral artery in morbidly obese patient. **A:** Fluoroscopic image showing relationship of radiopaque hemostat (*arrow*) to the femoral head: (*a*) proximal margin of femoral head; (*b*) middle of femoral head; and (*c*) inferior margin of the femoral head. The *dashed line* indicates shadow created by pannus from abdominal wall. **B:** Angiogram from the same patient showing arterial anatomy and entry point of the arterial sheath in the proximal segment of the profunda femoral artery (PFA). SFA, superficial femoral artery.

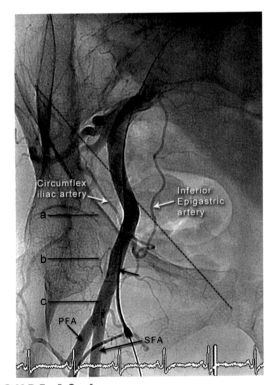

FIGURE 10-6.

Example of correct location of arterial puncture at the level of the middle of the head of the femur (black arrow). Proximal margin of femoral head (*a*). Middle of femoral head (*b*). Inferior margin of the femoral head (*c*). PFA, profunda femoral artery; SFA, superficial femoral artery.

CFA above the level of the middle of the head of the femur. This is based on the fact that the CFA bifurcation is located below this fluoroscopic level in over 96% of individuals.[8–10] The author's practice is to gain CFA access using a 7-cm long, 21-gauge micropuncture needle that allows placement of a 0.018-inch wire in the artery. At this point, repeat fluoroscopy is performed to confirm the appropriate location of the arteriotomy prior to placement of the arterial sheath (Fig. 10-7).

In situations where large caliber sheaths must be placed in the CFA (e.g., aortic valvuloplasty, TAVI), and the use of suture-mediated closure devices is of paramount importance in minimizing hemorrhagic complications, additional strategies may be used to ensure the appropriate location of the CFA arteriotomy. Using information from preprocedural CT angiography or prior invasive angiography, the CFA contralateral to the CFA in which device delivery is planned is accessed. An IM or SOS catheter is then used to engage the opposite common iliac artery (CIA) and a roadmap of the target CFA is performed in the ipsilateral oblique projection (because this view provides optimal visualization of the CFA bifurcation) (Fig. 10-8). The roadmap function is available on all contemporary imaging systems with digital subtraction capabilities, which are standard for performing peripheral angiography.[4,6] During acquisition of a roadmap, the background bony structures are initially

FIGURE 10-7.

Fluoroscopic confirmation of the position of the arteriotomy by inspection of the fluoroscopic level of
the junction of the needle and wire. **A:** Arteriotomy
(*arrow*) located over upper third of the femoral
head. **B:** Arteriotomy (*arrow*) located over middle
of the femoral head.

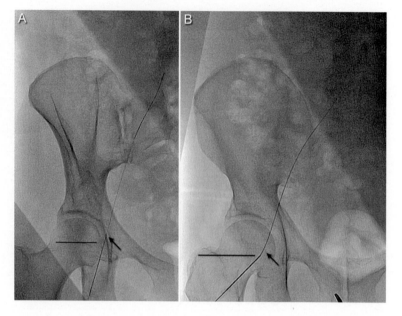

subtracted followed by injection of contrast with continuous image acquisition until the vessel of interest is
completely opacified. The resulting roadmap has a gray
background and a white vessel lumen roadmap that may
now be used to guide subsequent maneuvers in the vessel. Under most circumstances, injection of a total of 5
to 6 mL (3 mL/sec) is sufficient to generate a reasonable
quality roadmap of the CFA with a catheter selectively
engaged at the CIA. In situations where the CFA fills
briskly, a "smartmask" may be generated from a single
image of a routine cine acquisition, and provides similar
functionality to a roadmap. The roadmap or smartmask
is then used to provide direct fluoroscopic guidance of
the CFA puncture (Fig. 10-8B), assuming the patient has
not moved in the interim. In patients with significant calcification of the CFA on routine fluoroscopy that demonstrates the level of the bifurcation, the author will often

puncture the CFA using real-time fluoroscopic guidance,
obviating the need for a roadmap or smartmask.

Ultrasound guidance of the CFA puncture is an alternative method that is used by some operators. A variety of mobile ultrasound systems that provide B-mode
and color Doppler imaging of vascular structures are
available and are suitable for this purpose. In practice,
color Doppler is the primary modality that is used to
visualize the CFA target, and to differentiate it from
the adjacent CFV. The location of the CFA bifurcation is
best examined initially in the longitudinal plane. This
facilitates the acquisition of a cross-sectional image of
the CFA above this level, which is the image that should
guide the arterial puncture. Confirmation of the anticipated level of the arteriotomy site using fluoroscopy is
prudent because the location of the arteriotomy in relation to the level of the femoral head is not provided

FIGURE 10-8.

Roadmap function to guide common femoral arterial
(CFA) access. **A:** Roadmap of right CFA obtained by
injection of contrast through internal mammary
diagnostic catheter introduced through left CFA sheath
and engaged at the origin of the right common iliac artery. **B:** Fluoroscopic image showing guidance of needle
puncture of the right CFA using the road map image.
White arrow indicates the site of the arteriotomy.

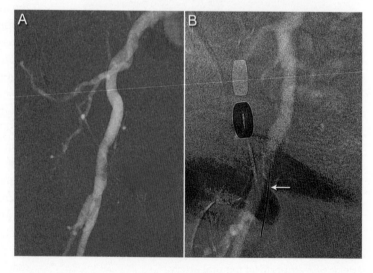

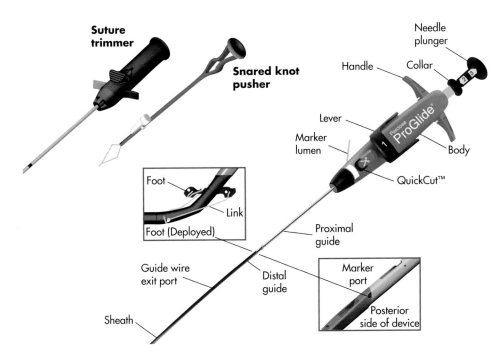

FIGURE 10-9.

Illustration of the Perclose Pro-Glide device (Redrawn from Abbott Vascular, Redwood City, CA).

by ultrasound. One of the frustrations of current ultrasound systems is the difficulty in accurately visualizing the tip of the needle, particularly micropuncture needles. Although there are micropuncture needles that are marketed as having specially adapted echogenic tips,[11,12] the author and others[13] have not found such needles to have significantly improved visibility. Recent software modifications to ultrasound systems purport to provide enhanced needle visualization. The major advantage of ultrasound guidance of the CFA puncture is that no iodinated contrast is required, which makes this strategy attractive in patients with significant renal insufficiency.

Vascular Closure of Arterial Access

The routine use of closure devices to achieve hemostasis at the arteriotomy site in the CFA is controversial. Although a large number of vascular closure devices are commercially available, the Angioseal (St. Jude, St. Paul, MN) and Perclose/ProStar XL (Abbott Vascular, Redwood City, CA) devices that achieve active closure of the arteriotomy are the most commonly used (Figs. 10-9 and 10-10). The former uses a collagen plug deployed in the tract at and above the level of the arteriotomy to achieve hemostasis, whereas the latter uses a suture deployed around the arteriotomy.

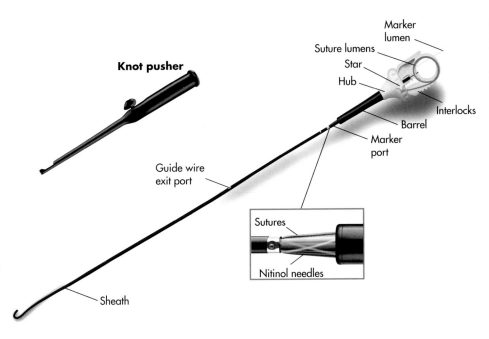

FIGURE 10-10.

Illustration of Prostar XL device (Redrawn from Abbott Vascular, Redwood City, CA).

Almost all of the data regarding the use of vascular closure devices are derived from studies of diagnostic coronary angiography and coronary intervention.[14] Although the anticoagulant and antiplatelet regimens used in SHD intervention are distinct from those used during coronary intervention, there is sufficient overlap such that the findings of coronary intervention studies likely have application in SHD intervention. It should be emphasized that these findings relate to the use of CFA sheath sizes of 6 to 8 French. Overall, the data suggest that, compared to manual pressure, the use of closure devices is associated with a similar rate of vascular complications and a shorter time to ambulation.[15–18]

For the subset of SHD interventions that use large caliber arterial sheaths (i.e., TAVI, aortic valvuloplasty), the use of closure devices is driven by empiric evidence. Given the large caliber of these sheaths, the hemorrhagic risk is significantly increased, such that most operators will elect to use a closure device when technically feasible. In these situations, it is typical to use suture-mediated closure devices exclusively (i.e., Perclose, ProStar XL), and to use a preclose technique, where the sutures are deployed after placement of a 6 to 8 French sheath, prior to placement of the larger sheath (i.e., 12 to 24 French).[19–21] For the largest arterial sheaths, the author typically predeploys two sutures from two separate 6 French Perclose ProGlide devices that are deployed at 180 degrees from one another. One author has reported predeploying three 6 French Perclose ProGlide devices in a modest cohort of patients ($n = 15$) undergoing TAVI. Alternatively, a ProStar XL device may be used that allows simultaneous deployment of two sutures around the arteriotomy. This device requires significant blunt dissection above the level of the arteriotomy to allow delivery of the device, but is probably the most reliable method of achieving closure of the arteriotomy. However, because this device requires retraction of four needles through the wall of the artery (as opposed to two needles for the Perclose ProGlide system), it is more sensitive to failure due to severe vessel calcification. Both devices are limited in morbidly obese patients, and cannot be used where the distance between the arteriotomy and skin surface is greater than the distance between the intra-arterial portion of the marker lumen and the hub of the device.

In the author's experience, achieving hemostasis using predeployed sutures at the completion of SHD interventions is best performed using three operators. One operator secures hemostasis using manual pressure proximal to the level of the arteriotomy. A second operator then removes the arterial sheath over a long (i.e., 160 to 300 cm) wire. When sutures are predeployed using the Perclose ProGlide device, any wire may be used, but the manufacturer recommends the use of a hydrophilic glidewire when sutures are predeployed using the ProStar XL device. The third operator then cinches the suture around the arteriotomy in the usual manner using the knot pusher.

ARTERIAL ACCESS: UPPER EXTREMITY

Preprocedural Assessment

Upper extremity arterial access is rarely used during SHD interventions. Due to the limited diameter of the brachial and radial arteries, it is rare to use these arterial access sites for device delivery. Instead, they tend to be used to provide additional image guidance or aid hemodynamic assessment during procedures such as aortic coarctation stenting. For alcohol septal ablation, radial artery access may be safely used as the primary arterial access.

In terms of the preprocedural assessment for upper extremity access, it is typical to rely on clinical assessment alone, particularly when the plan is to use smaller caliber sheaths and there is no intention for device delivery through these sheaths. Compared to the lower extremity, PAD of the upper extremities is rare.[22] When it occurs, the most common site is the subclavian artery (SCA), with the majority of patients having involvement of the left SCA (~80%).[23] However, even in the presence of a subclavian occlusion, retrograde flow in the ipsilateral vertebral artery into the SCA is usually sufficient to provide adequate arterial flow during upper extremity activity. As a result, the majority of patients with significant SCA disease are entirely asymptomatic.[23] Therefore, although symptoms should be inquired for, the absence of upper extremity claudication does not exclude the presence of proximal disease, and the most accurate method of assessment is documentation of the upper extremity pressures. Significant asymmetry in the pressures (i.e., >20 mm Hg) suggests significant proximal disease.

Palpation of the brachial and radial artery pulses is straightforward, even in obese patients. When radial artery access is planned, documentation of the Allen's test is mandatory. Following compression of the ulnar and radial arteries, the patient is asked to make a fist. On opening the fist, the patient's palm should appear blanched. Release of pressure from the ulnar artery should result in restoration of the color to the palm (i.e., negative Allen's test).[24] Applying a pulse oximeter to the thumb and demonstrating return of a normal waveform following release of pressure from the ulnar artery provides additional reassurance that radial artery occlusion, if it occurs, will be clinically silent.[25]

Anatomic assessment prior to upper extremity access is rarely required. Duplex ultrasound of the radial or brachial arteries is an efficient and accurate method of assessing vessel diameter. CT angiography is the optimal technique for assessing more proximal disease in the SCAs and the anatomy of the aortic arch.

Execution of Access

Brachial Artery

With the refinement in radial artery access techniques over the last decade, brachial artery access should rarely be performed in current practice. In the author's experience, this access site is associated with a significant complication rate. Achieving hemostasis at this site can be difficult and requires meticulous attention with prolonged manual compression (up to 30 minutes). Poor hemostasis technique predisposes to hemorrhage and pseudoaneurysm formation. Severe spasm of the brachial artery is the norm, particularly after the placement of long sheaths. In vulnerable individuals with small caliber vessels, acute ischemia of the limb can occur.

When this access site is used, the author will typically use a 4-cm long, 21-gauge micropuncture needle to achieve a front wall puncture of the brachial artery. Immobilizing the vessel between the index and middle fingers appears to facilitate puncture. For vessels that are not easily palpated, ultrasound guidance is helpful.

The site of vessel puncture should be just proximal to the elbow crease. Puncture more proximal to this location makes subsequent hemostasis more difficult, predisposing to hematoma and pseudoaneurysm formation. Depending of the diameter of the brachial artery, 5 to 7 French sheaths may be placed in the brachial artery. Following sheath insertion, 2 to 3 mg of verapamil and 4,000 to 5,000 units of heparin should be administered. Careful monitoring of the clinical status of the hand (i.e., development of pain, pallor), and the Doppler signals in the radial and ulnar arteries, is required as long as the brachial sheath is in place.

Radial Artery

If upper extremity access is required for SHD interventions, radial artery access is strongly recommended, assuming sheath size is not a limiting factor and a negative Allen's test is documented in the hand. Two basic strategies of radial artery access are employed: a front

wall stick using a 2.5- or 4-cm long, 21-gauge micropuncture needle, and a conventional Seldinger technique using an IV cannula (e.g., SURFLO Teflon IV catheter, Terumo, Somerset, NJ).[10,26] For larger caliber radial arteries that are easily palpable, the front wall stick technique is reasonably successful. However, for more challenging cases, the conventional Seldinger technique is likely associated with a higher success rate. With the latter technique, the typical puncture site is located 1 cm proximal to the level of the head of the styloid process and 1 to 1.5 mL of local anesthetic is administered. The SURFLO catheter is advanced until an arterial flashback is observed in the chamber at the hub of the catheter. At this point, the catheter is advanced forward to puncture the posterior wall of the artery. The needle is removed from the catheter, and the plastic cannula is slowly withdrawn until there is free backflow of blood. A 0.021-inch nitinol wire is then advanced into the radial artery through the cannula. The cannula is removed and a glidesheath is advanced directly over the nitinol wire.

Following sheath insertion, the pharmacologic cocktail used is similar to that following brachial artery access (i.e., 2 to 3 mg of verapamil and 4,000 to 5,000 units of heparin). Hemostasis following radial artery access has been greatly facilitated by the use of dedicated radial artery wrist bands (e.g., TR Band, Terumo, Somerset, NJ) that are applied immediately at the end of the procedure following sheath removal and are left in place for ~3 hours. In contrast to brachial artery access, complications related to radial artery access are very rare.

ARTERIAL ACCESS COMPLICATIONS

The spectrum of arterial access complications that occur during SHD interventions is similar to that observed during coronary artery interventions. These are comprised mainly of hemorrhagic complications (i.e., hematoma, retroperitoneal hemorrhage), and arteriovenous fistula and pseudoaneurysm formation. These specific complications and their management are well described in multiple textbooks on coronary intervention.[10] During SHD interventions involving large caliber delivery catheters (i.e., TAVI, aortic valvuloplasty), a number of serious vascular access complications that are rarely seen during routine coronary intervention can occur. These include perforation of the iliac vessels, flow-limiting dissection of the iliac or femoral arteries, and acute limb ischemia.[20,27–30] The precise incidence of each of these specific complications has varied among series, likely related to variation in patient and anatomic variables, and device-related characteristics.

Perforation

Perforation of the iliac arteries is a potentially life-threatening complication (Fig. 10-11). This is because the iliac vessels communicate with the retroperitoneum, resulting in the loss of large amounts of blood within a short period (seconds to minutes) into the retroperitoneal space if the complication is not recognized promptly. Perforation should be suspected in any patient with unexplained hemodynamic instability, particularly when accompanied by pelvic or lower quadrant discomfort. During TAVI procedures, perforation is typically caused by trauma to the iliac artery by the delivery sheath, and is often seen following removal of the delivery sheath from the femoral artery. For this reason, most operators recommend having contralateral femoral access during all such procedures and performing a completion angiogram of the ipsilateral iliac and femoral arteries using a crossover technique following removal of the delivery sheath and deployment of the closure device(s) in the CFA.

The management of an iliac artery perforation requires prompt recognition, followed by aggressive resuscitation (i.e., reversal of anticoagulation, IV fluids, administration of blood products) and institution of a rapid strategy to seal the perforation. Vascular surgery should be alerted immediately, but, in most circumstances, endovascular techniques are successful in achieving cessation of flow through the perforation and providing definitive treatment.

For perforations of the external iliac artery (EIA), contralateral access that facilitates placement of a crossover sheath in the ipsilateral CIA is optimal. In an ideal situation, a 0.035-inch wire is advanced distal to the perforation, and a peripheral angioplasty balloon

TABLE 10-2 Sample of Standard Angioplasty Balloons and Occlusion Balloons[a]

Standard Balloon	Occlusion Balloons
Agiltrac (Abbott Vascular, Redwood City, CA)	Equalizer (Boston Scientific)
Ultra-thin Diamond (Boston Scientific, Natick, MA)	Coda (Cook Medical, Bloomington, IN)
XXL (Boston Scientific)	Reliant (Medtronic Inc., Minneapolis, MN)
OPTA Pro (Cordis Corporation, Bridgewater, NJ)	
Powerflex (Cordis Corporation)	
Maxi-LD (Cordis Corporation)	
EverCross (ev3, Plymouth, MN)	
Admiral Xtreme (Invatec Inc., Bethlehem, PA)	

[a]*May be used to aid in treatment of aortoiliac and femoral artery perforation.*

(Table 10-2) that is sized to the diameter of the EIA is inflated at 2 to 4 atm across the perforation. Angiography from above through the side arm of the crossover sheath should be performed to confirm occlusion of the vessel and cessation of flow through the perforation. Definitive treatment is typically achieved by deploying a covered stent across the perforation. Currently, there are four covered stent systems available for use in the United States in this clinical situation (Table 10-3). In the author's practice, the iCAST (Atrium Medical, Hudson, NH) and Viabahn (Gore Medical, Flagstaff, AZ) stents have typically been used.

The iCAST stent is a polytetrafluoroethylene (PTFE)-covered stainless steel balloon-expandable stent whose primary advantage is its low profile (i.e., delivered through a 6 to 7 French sheath depending on

FIGURE 10-11.

Iliac artery perforation. **A:** Angiogram of left external iliac artery (EIA) via contralateral access showing large perforation of the EIA with extravasation of contrast into the retroperitoneal space (indicated by *white arrows*). **B:** Angiogram following placement of iCAST (balloon-expandable covered stent; Atrium Medical, Hudson, NH) resulting in effective treatment of the perforation.

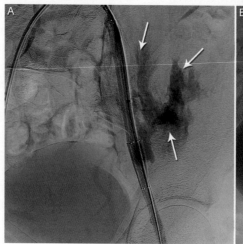
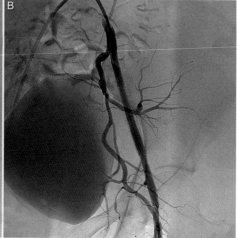

TABLE 10-3 Summary of Covered Stents Available in the United States for Treatment of Aortoiliac Perforation

Stent	iCAST	Viabahn	Flair	aSpire
Company	Atrium Medical, Hudson, NH	Gore Medical, Flagstaff, AZ	Bard, Tempe, AZ	LeMaitre, Burlington, MA
Stent Type	Balloon-expandable	Self-expandable	Self-expandable	Self-expandable
Stent Design	Stainless steel/PTFE	Nitinol/ePTFE	Nitinol/ePTFE	Nitinol/ePTFE
Wire Compatibility (in)	0.035	0.035	0.035	0.018
Stent Diameter (mm)	5–12	5–13	6–9	7
Stent Lengths (mm)	16, 22, 38, 59	25, 50, 100, 150	30, 40, 50	20, 30, 50, 100
Sheath Delivery (French)	6, 7	7–12	9	6–9

ePTFE, expandable polytetrafluoroethylene.

the stent diameter). This stent is extremely stiff, and caution in delivering the stent through a contralateral sheath is warranted. Using a strongly supportive wire (e.g., SupraCore, Abbott Vascular; Amplatzer super stiff, Boston Scientific, Natick, MA) that is placed as far distal as possible (i.e., into the profunda or superficial femoral arteries if possible) will minimize the risk of prolapse of the contralateral sheath into the distal abdominal aorta during attempts to deliver the stent. Because of its stiffness, this stent should be avoided for the treatment of perforations in the distal EIA, because this segment of vessel is subject to significant conformational change. The iCAST stent diameter should approximate the diameter of the vessel in which the perforation occurs.

The Viabahn stent graft is a flexible self-expanding nitinol stent which serves as an exoskeleton for an expanded PTFE (ePTFE) lining (Fig. 10-12). This stent has the advantage of being significantly more flexible than the iCAST stent. Hence, it is more easily delivered from

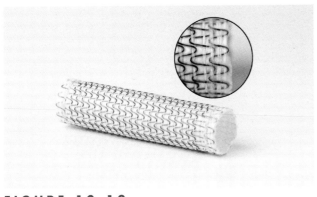

FIGURE 10-12.

Viabahn stent (Gore Medical, Flagstaff, AZ). Inset shows magnified view of the edge of the stent.

the crossover access, through tortuous anatomy, and is suitable for the treatment of perforations in the distal EIA. This stent does have a significantly larger profile compared to the iCAST stent. Sheath sizes of 8 to 11 French are required to deliver stents of 7 to 10 mm in diameter, which reflects the range of typical diameters of most iliac arteries. This needs to be considered when choosing the French size of the crossover sheath. Similar to the iCAST stent, the Viabahn stent should be delivered over strongly supportive 0.035-inch wires. As with all self-expanding stents, it is important to use a stent with a diameter ~1 mm larger than the iliac vessel diameter to ensure appropriate apposition of the stent with the vessel wall.

Perforations of the CIA are most easily approached using a retrograde approach from the ipsilateral CFA. Because this arterial segment is not felt to be subject to significant conformational change, use of either a balloon-expandable or self-expandable covered stent is appropriate. For perforations near the CIA ostium, the balloon-expandable covered stent may be preferred due to the ability to more accurately position these stents. Alternatively, if there is significant size mismatch along a vessel segment, or there is significant vessel tortuosity, a self-expanding covered stent may be preferred.

Perforations of the CFA should ideally be referred for surgical repair, stenting of this vessel that is subject to significant conformational change is generally felt to be contraindicated. Achieving balloon occlusion (as described previously) across the perforation or proximal to the perforation using contralateral access can allow stabilization of the patient prior to surgical repair. In extreme clinical circumstances, a self-expanding covered stent should be used rather than a balloon-expandable stent in this location. It is important to ensure that the stent does not extend to cover the CFA bifurcation.

In situations where it is not feasible to place a balloon across the site of perforation in the iliac or femoral artery, occlusion of flow in the distal abdominal aorta is helpful in achieving hemodyamic stability prior to instituting definitive therapy.[28] Because of the large diameter of the aorta, and the significant inter-individual variation in aortic diameter, a separate class of balloons, referred to as occlusion balloons, are desirable for this indication (Table 10-2). These balloons are highly compliant. As a result, they can accommodate a wide range of vessel diameters and can easily adjust to the anatomy of the vessel in which they are inflated. As these balloons are inflated beyond the diameter of the vessel in which they are inflated, the balloon elongates without applying significant additional radial force on the arterial wall. This shape change in the balloon is used as a marker that occlusion of the artery has been achieved. All of the available occlusion balloons are delivered over 0.035-inch wires, and it is recommended to use very supportive wires for balloon delivery (e.g., Amplatzer super stiff). In addition, the recommended sheath size for delivery and removal of these balloons is large (i.e., 12 to 14 French).

Dissection

Severe flow limiting dissections of the iliac and femoral vessels have been observed in a significant number

TABLE 10-4 **List of Available Noncovered Stents[a]**

Balloon-expandable	Self-expandable
Omnilink (Abbott Vascular, Redwood City, CA)	Absolute (Abbott Vascular)
LifeStent Valeo (Bard, Tempe, AZ)	LifeStent (Bard)
Express LD (Boston Scientific, Natick, MA)	Zilver 518/Zilver 635 (Cook Medical, Bloomington, IN)
Palmaz (Cordis Corporation, Bridgewater, NJ)	SMART (Cordis Corporation)
Visi-Pro (ev3, Plymouth, MN)	Progege (ev3)
	Complete SE (Medtronic Inc.)
Bridge Assurant (Medtronic Inc., Minneapolis, MN)	Supera (IDev Technologies, Webster, TX)

[a]May be used to treat aortoiliac dissection.

of TAVI procedures, but may rarely be observed following other SHD interventions. Dissection of the iliac vessels is most commonly related to trauma from the delivery sheath, whereas dissection of the femoral artery is often related to trauma from the use of closure devices.

Endovascular treatment of iliac artery dissections should be possible in most situations. CIA dissections are best approached using a retrograde ipsilateral CFA approach, whereas EIA dissections are most easily approached using an antegrade approach from

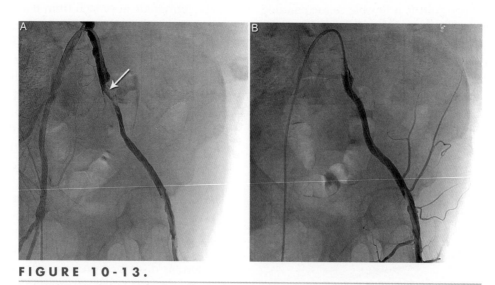

FIGURE 10-13.

Endovascular treatment of flow-limiting dissection of the left external iliac artery (EIA). **A:** Angiography of left iliac artery via contralateral common femoral artery access showing flow-limiting dissection (*arrow*) of the left EIA. **B:** Angiography of left iliac artery following deployment of self-expanding stent (SMART, Cordis Corporation, Bridgewater, NJ) to seal the dissection with restoration of normal antegrade flow.

the contralateral CFA access. The dissection should be crossed with an interventional wire, taking care to confirm the intraluminal position of the wire beyond the dissection. Sealing the dissection with either an uncovered balloon-expandable or self-expandable stent (Table 10-4) will result in restoration of flow (Fig. 10-13).

Flow-limiting dissections of the CFA are more problematic, due to the fact that stents are contraindicated in this location. In the author's experience, most CFA dissections may be treated using endovascular techniques. Prolonged balloon inflation with an angioplasty balloon (Table 10-2) at the site of dissection will often result in restoration of flow. In some cases, removal of the obstructive intimal flap using an atherectomy device (e.g., SilverHawk, ev3, Plymouth, MN) has been performed with success (Fig. 10-14).

Acute Limb Ischemia

Acute limb ischemia (ALI) is the term used to describe an acute loss in perfusion to the limb. The mechanism of ALI following SHD interventions most commonly relates to flow-limiting dissection in the iliac or femoral segments (see previous text), but may also occur as a result of distal thromboembolism from the aortoiliac and femoral segments (Fig. 10-15). The most common site of distal embolism is the popliteal bifurcation. Patients typically complain of a cold limb with associated sensory symptoms. Examination should focus on careful documentation of palpable and Dopplerable pulses to help assess the level of occlusion. If ALI is recognized prior to the patient leaving the catheterization laboratory, angiography using contralateral CFA access is the most expedient method to assess the site and likely etiology of ALI.[31] Treatment of iliac and femoral dissection is as outlined in previous text. Treatment of distal embolization will most commonly require a mechanical approach. Thrombolysis is contraindicated in patients in whom the large bore arterial access sheath has been removed. If the patient has left the catheterization laboratory prior to recognition of ALI, an assessment of the severity of limb ischemia dictates the clinical management. For a viable limb, there is typically time to allow noninvasive techniques (e.g., Duplex ultrasound, CT angiography) to help assess the anatomy of the arterial occlusion and plan an appropriate revascularization strategy. If the limb is threatened (i.e., absent arterial Doppler signals, significant sensory symptoms, any motor symptoms), immediate transfer to the catheterization laboratory for angiography and attempted revascularization is appropriate.

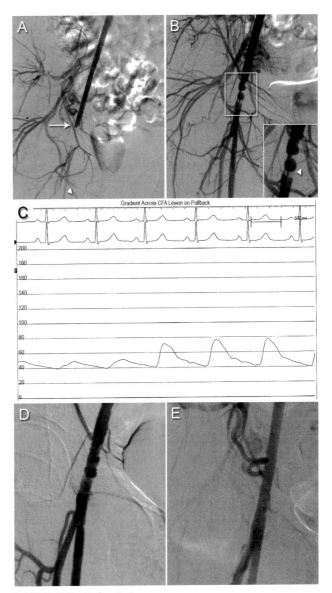

FIGURE 10-14.

Vascular closure device–induced common femoral artery (CFA) dissection. **A:** Angiography of right external iliac artery illustrating complete occlusion of the CFA (*arrow*) with reconstitution of the superficial femoral artery (*arrowhead*) via collaterals. **B,C:** Angiography following angioplasty of occluded CFA demonstrating severe focal stenosis (*arrowhead*) representing a flow-limiting dissection. The stenosis was associated with a significant pressure gradient. **D:** Angiography of CFA following atherectomy. **E:** Repeat angiography 12 hours later. (Reproduced with permission from Klein AJ, Messenger JC, Casserly IP. Contemporary management of acute lower extremity ischemia following percutaneous coronary and cardiac interventional procedures using femoral access—a case series and discussion. *Catheter Cardiovasc Interv.* 2007;70: 129–137.)

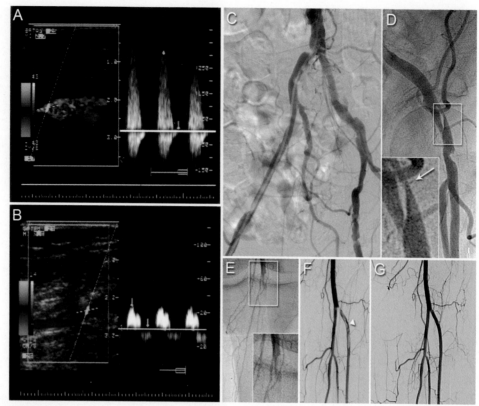

FIGURE 10-15.

Thromboembolic occlusion of popliteal artery from a vascular closure device–induced common femoral artery (CFA) dissection. **A:** Doppler interrogation of the CFA demonstrating high-velocity flow (peak systolic velocity of 298 cm/sec) indicative of a high-grade stenosis with color B-mode indicating turbulent flow. **B:** Doppler interrogation of the popliteal artery demonstrating low-velocity flow indicative of an upstream obstruction. **C:** Pelvic angiography demonstrating a high-grade right common iliac artery stenosis. **D:** Angiogram of left CFA with appearance consistent with dissection (*arrow*). **E:** Left popliteal artery angiogram demonstrating complete thrombotic occlusion. **F:** Left popliteal artery angiogram following rheolytic thrombectomy of the popliteal artery and tibioperoneal trunk. Note persistent thrombus within the anterior tibial artery (*arrowhead*). **G:** Final left popliteal artery angiography following rheolytic thrombectomy of anterior tibial artery.

VENOUS ACCESS

Common Femoral Vein

Preprocedural Planning

When planning CFV access, the clinical history is the most important element of preprocedural planning. A history of iliofemoral deep venous thrombosis should raise the possibility of an occlusion of the femoral vein that would preclude venous access (Fig. 10-16). Prior placement of an inferior vena cava (IVC) filter is important to note because this will warrant special care during delivery of sheaths and/or devices through the IVC (Fig. 10-17). Any prior documentation of anomalous anatomy of the IVC should be confirmed (Figs. 10-18, 10-19, and 10-20). These anomalies are uncommon, but an awareness of the most common types is important.[32] Where an anatomic assessment of the femoral and iliac veins or the IVC is felt to be warranted prior

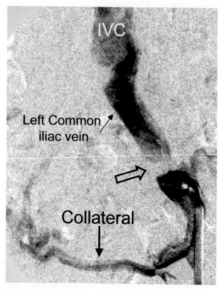

FIGURE 10-16.

Venogram from the left common femoral vein showing occlusion of the left common iliac vein (*hollow arrow*) and prominent collaterals from the left iliac vein to the right iliac vein. IVC, inferior vena cava.

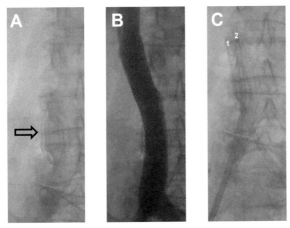

FIGURE 10-17.

Inferior vena cava (IVC) filter placement and venous access. **A:** Fluoroscopic image showing presence of IVC filter (*arrow*). **B:** Venogram performed from common femoral vein access confirming absence of significant thrombus on the IVC filter. **C:** Fluoroscopic image showing two long sheaths (*1, 2*) placed through IVC filter to facilitate patent foramen ovale (PFO) closure procedure (i.e., one sheath to provide access for intracardiac echo catheter and second sheath to allow delivery of the PFO closure device).

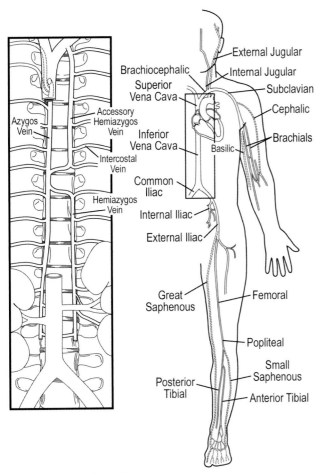

FIGURE 10-18.

Schematic illustration of normal venous anatomy of the body. Inset shows magnified view azygos, hemiazygos, and accessory hemiazygos venous system.

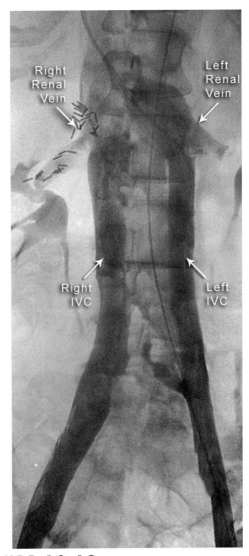

FIGURE 10-19.

Venogram from patient undergoing patent foramen ovale closure showing double inferior vena cava. Schematic illustration of the anomaly is shown in Figure 10-20B. IVC, inferior vena cava.

to an SHD intervention, the study that yields the best data is a magnetic resonance venogram.[33,34]

Execution

Femoral venous access is usually achieved using fluoroscopic guidance and palpation. Using a radiopaque hemostat to assess the skin surface landmark of the femoral head, and palpation to assess the position of the CFA, the femoral vein is typically punctured medial to the femoral artery at the level of the lower third of the femoral head. In situations where the femoral vein is difficult to access using this strategy, color Doppler ultrasound may be used to help identify the location of the CFV and guide its puncture. If a sheath has already been placed in the CFA, this can be used to provide real-time fluoroscopic guidance for CFV access.

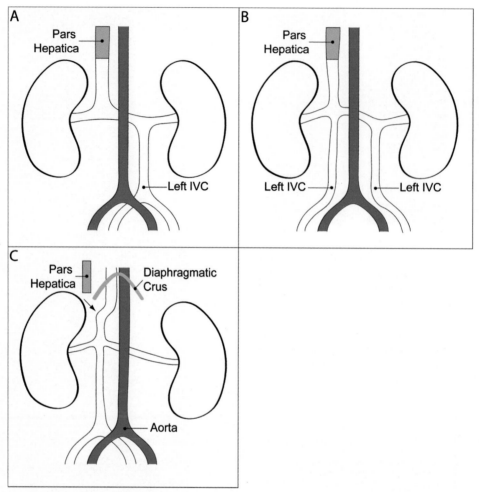

FIGURE 10-20.

Schematic illustration of major anomalies of the inferior vena cava (IVC) that may affect venous access from common femoral vein during structural heart interventions. **A:** Left IVC, where the IVC lies to the left of the aorta and empties into the left renal vein. **B:** Double IVC, where there is an IVC located in the normal position to the right of the aorta and an additional IVC located to the left of the aorta that ends in the left renal vein. **C:** Azygos continuation of the IVC, where the prerenal segment of the IVC (*arrow*) is disconnected from the hepatic segment of the IVC (pars hepatica) and drains into the azygos vein which is enlarged due to the increased venous return.

Closure

Closure of the CFV access site is typically achieved using manual pressure. The only circumstance in which the author's practice varies from this recommendation is when using the MitraClip device (Abbott Laboratories, Abbott Park, IL) to perform percutaneous edge-to-edge mitral valve repair, which currently utilizes a 24 French CFV sheath. In this circumstance, the author and others have predeployed two 6 French Perclose ProGlide devices at 180 degrees prior to placement of the 24 French sheath, which are then used to achieve hemostasis following sheath removal.[35] Because calcification of the CFV does not occur, deployment of the Perclose device is typically straightforward. The

venous pressure is sufficient to generate backflow through the ouflow channel when the device passes beyond the venotomy site. Other authors have described a technique in which a subcutaneous figure-of-eight stitch is used to secure hemostasis following removal of large venous sheaths (Fig. 10-21).[36] The author has used this technique with modest success.

CONCLUSION

Vascular access is an essential component of all SHD interventions. A thorough understanding of appropriate preprocedural evaluation, execution, and

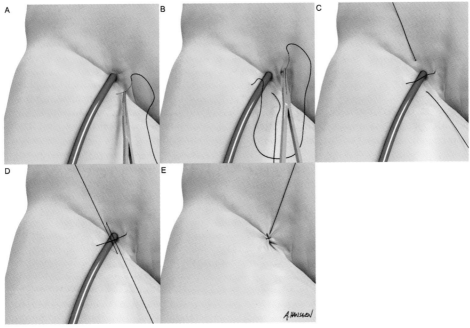

FIGURE 10-21.

Sequential steps to achieve subcutaneous figure-of-eight stitch to achieve hemostasis following removal of large caliber venous sheaths in common femoral vein. **A:** Silk suture is passed under the Mullins sheath and superficial to the vein grabbing a generous amount of subcutaneous tissue. **B:** The suture is then passed through the subcutaneous tissue above the Mullins sheath. **C:** The two ends of the suture are now used to create a figure-of-eight knot, shown in **(D)**. **E:** The knot is tightened as the venous sheath is removed, creating a puckered skin appearance. The suture may be removed approximately 1 to 2 hours later after the effects of anticoagulant have worn off or the day after the procedure.

postprocedural management of arterial and venous access is fundamental to achieving optimal clinical outcomes. Although many considerations for arterial and venous access for SHD interventions overlap those for percutaneous coronary intervention, it is important to be aware of the specific access issues highlighted in this chapter that relate to SHD intervention, which will enhance the overall safety of these procedures.

R E F E R E N C E S

1. Ben-Dor I, Waksman R, Satler LF, et al. Patient selection—risk assessment and anatomical selection criteria for patients undergoing transfemoral aortic valve implantation. *Cardiovasc Revasc Med.* 2010;11:124–136.
2. Leipsic J, Wood D, Manders D, et al. The evolving role of mdct in transcatheter aortic valve replacement: A radiologists' perspective. *AJR Am J Roentgenol.* 2009;193:W214–W219.
3. Fraioli F, Catalano C, Napoli A, et al. Low-dose multidetector-row ct angiography of the infra-renal aorta and lower extremity vessels: Image quality and diagnostic accuracy in comparison with standard dsa. *Eur Radiol.* 2006;16:137–146.
4. Pomposelli F. Arterial imaging in patients with lower-extremity ischemia and diabetes mellitus. *J Am Podiatr Med Assoc.* 2010;100:412–423.
5. Romano M, Mainenti PP, Imbriaco M, et al. Multidetector row ct angiography of the abdominal aorta and lower extremities in patients with peripheral arterial occlusive disease: Diagnostic accuracy and interobserver agreement. *Eur J Radiol.* 2004;50: 303–308.
6. Tang GL, Chin J, Kibbe MR. Advances in diagnostic imaging for peripheral arterial disease. *Expert Rev Cardiovasc Ther.* 2010;8:1447–1455.
7. Joshi SB, Mendoza DD, Steinberg DH, et al. Ultra-low-dose intra-arterial contrast injection for iliofemoral computed tomographic angiography. *JACC Cardiovasc Imaging.* 2009;2:1404–1411.
8. Garrett PD, Eckart RE, Bauch TD, et al. Fluoroscopic localization of the femoral head as a landmark for common femoral artery cannulation. *Catheter Cardiovasc Interv.* 2005;65:205–207.

9. Spector KS, Lawson WE. Optimizing safe femoral access during cardiac catheterization. *Catheter Cardiovasc Interv.* 2001;53:209–212.

10. Turi ZG. Vascular access and closure. In: Mukherjee D, Bates ER, Roffi M, Moliterno DJ, eds. *Cardiovascular catheterization and intervention.* London: Informa Healthcare; 2010: 67–84.

11. Culp WC, McCowan TC, Goertzen TC, et al. Relative ultrasonographic echogenicity of standard, dimpled, and polymeric-coated needles. *J Vasc Interv Radiol.* 2000;11:351–358.

12. Venkatesan K. Echo-enhanced needles for short-axis ultrasound-guided vascular access. *Int J Emerg Med.* 2010;3:205.

13. Phelan MP, Emerman C, Peacock WF, et al. Do echo-enhanced needles improve time to cannulate in a model of short-axis ultrasound-guided vascular access for a group of mostly inexperienced ultrasound users? *Int J Emerg Med.* 2009;2:167–170.

14. Dauerman HL, Applegate RJ, Cohen DJ. Vascular closure devices: The second decade. *J Am Coll Cardiol.* 2007;50:1617–1626.

15. Applegate RJ, Sacrinty MT, Kutcher MA, et al. Propensity score analysis of vascular complications after diagnostic cardiac catheterization and percutaneous coronary intervention 1998–2003. *Catheter Cardiovasc Interv.* 2006;67:556–562.

16. Arora N, Matheny ME, Sepke C, et al. A propensity analysis of the risk of vascular complications after cardiac catheterization procedures with the use of vascular closure devices. *Am Heart J.* 2007;153:606–611.

17. Koreny M, Riedmuller E, Nikfardjam M, et al. Arterial puncture closing devices compared with standard manual compression after cardiac catheterization: Systematic review and meta-analysis. *JAMA.* 2004;291:350–357.

18. Nikolsky E, Mehran R, Halkin A, et al. Vascular complications associated with arteriotomy closure devices in patients undergoing percutaneous coronary procedures: A meta-analysis. *J Am Coll Cardiol.* 2004;44:1200–1209.

19. Kahlert P, Eggebrecht H, Erbel R, et al. A modified "pre-closure" technique after percutaneous aortic valve replacement. *Catheter Cardiovasc Interv.* 2008;72:877–884.

20. Sharp AS, Michev I, Maisano F, et al. A new technique for vascular access management in transcatheter aortic valve implantation. *Catheter Cardiovasc Interv.* 2010;75:784–793.

21. Starnes BW, Andersen CA, Ronsivalle JA, et al. Totally percutaneous aortic aneurysm repair: Experience and prudence. *J Vasc Surg.* 2006;43:270–276.

22. Zimmerman NB. Occlusive vascular disorders of the upper extremity. *Hand Clin.* 1993;9:139–150.

23. Labropoulos N, Nandivada P, Bekelis K. Prevalence and impact of the subclavian steal syndrome. *Ann Surg.* 2010;252:166–170.

24. Peters KR, Chapin JW. Allen's test—positive or negative? *Anesthesiology.* 1980;53:85.

25. Barbeau GR, Arsenault F, Dugas L, et al. Evaluation of the ulnopalmar arterial arches with pulse oximetry and plethysmography: Comparison with the allen's test in 1010 patients. *Am Heart J.* 2004;147: 489–493.

26. Patel T. Puncture technique. In: Patel T, Shah S, Ranjan A, eds. *Patel's atlas of transradial intervention.* 2007: 11–20.

27. Kahlert P, Al-Rashid F, Weber M, et al. Vascular access site complications after percutaneous transfemoral aortic valve implantation. *Herz.* 2009;34: 398–408.

28. Masson JB, Al Bugami S, Webb JG. Endovascular balloon occlusion for catheter-induced large artery perforation in the catheterization laboratory. *Catheter Cardiovasc Interv.* 2009;73:514–518.

29. Tchetche D, Dumonteil N, Sauguet A, et al. Thirty-day outcome and vascular complications after transarterial aortic valve implantation using both edwards sapien and medtronic corevalve bioprostheses in a mixed population. *EuroIntervention.* 2010;5: 659–665.

30. Van Mieghem NM, Nuis RJ, Piazza N, et al. Vascular complications with transcatheter aortic valve implantation using the 18 fr medtronic corevalve system: The rotterdam experience. *EuroIntervention.* 2010;5:673–679.

31. Klein AJ, Messenger JC, Casserly IP. Contemporary management of acute lower extremity ischemia following percutaneous coronary and cardiac interventional procedures using femoral access—a case series and discussion. *Catheter Cardiovasc Interv.* 2007;70:129–137.

32. Bass JE, Redwine MD, Kramer LA, et al. Spectrum of congenital anomalies of the inferior vena cava: Cross-sectional imaging findings. *Radiographics.* 2000;20:639–652.

33. Koizumi J, Horie T, Muro I, et al. Magnetic resonance venography of the lower limb. *Int Angiol.* 2007;26:171–182.

34. Spritzer CE. Progress in mr imaging of the venous system. *Perspect Vasc Surg Endovasc Ther.* 2009;21: 105–116.

35. Mylonas I, Sakata Y, Salinger M, et al. The use of percutaneous suture-mediated closure for the management of 14 french femoral venous access. *J Invasive Cardiol.* 2006;18:299–302.

36. Bagai J, Zhao D. Subcutaneous "figure-of-eight' stitch to achieve hemostasis after removal of large-caliber femoral venous sheaths. *Cardiac Interventions Today.* 2008:22–23.

CLOSURE OF CONGENITAL AND ACQUIRED CARDIAC DEFECTS IN ADULTS

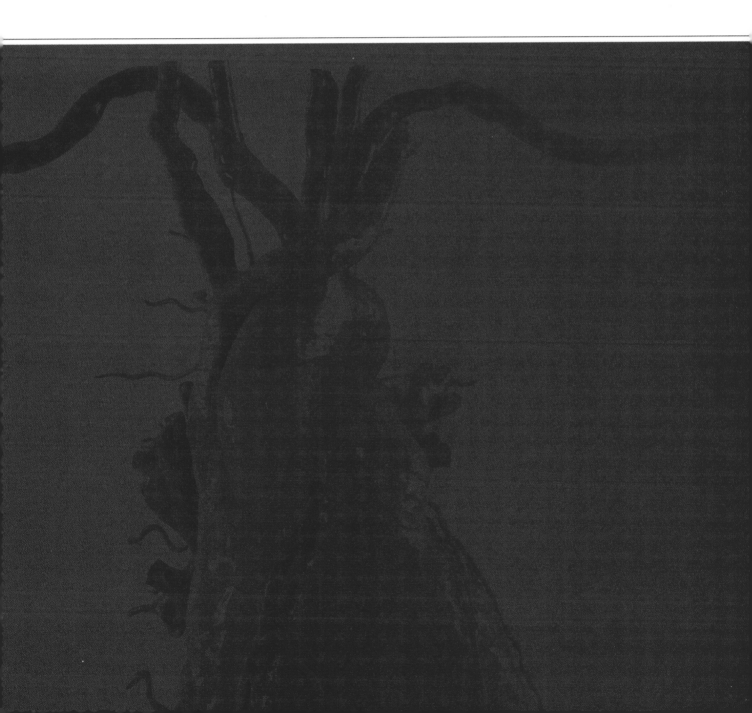

CHAPTER 11

Closure of Patent Foramen Ovale

Paul Poommipanit and Jonathan Tobis

P atent foramen ovale (PFO) has been associated with a variety of clinical disease states, including cryptogenic stroke,[1,2] migraine headaches,[3] platypnea-orthodeoxia,[4] sleep apnea, and decompression illness.[5] In the past, surgical closure was the only means of corrective therapy. More recently, percutaneous septal occluder implantation for PFO closure has been shown to be a safe alternative to surgical closure.[6–10] In the United States, the U.S. Food and Drug Administration (FDA) has not approved the use of any closure device to treat PFO-related conditions because they are waiting for the results of ongoing randomized clinical trials. Despite the lack of FDA approval, the frequency of PFO closure has increased worldwide as implantation techniques have become more refined, making this a safer alternative to surgery. In addition, in the United States, there are devices that are approved for closure of atrial septal defects (ASDs) and these are being used off-label to close PFOs. This chapter reviews the etiology, pathogenesis, and therapies for PFO, with an emphasis on the role of percutaneous PFO closure. The two devices currently available in the United States for closure of ASDs that are being used for off-label PFO closure are the Helex device from Gore Medical (Newark, DE) and the Amplatzer device from AGA Medical (Plymouth, MN). The CardioSEAL device from NMT Medical is currently only approved in the United States for ventricular septal defect (VSD) closure, but is used on an off-label basis for PFO closure. These three devices are discussed, as well as some possible complications.

ETIOLOGY

The foramen ovale is a passageway between the atria formed by the septum secundum superiorly and the septum primum inferiorly. It is present during fetal development and permits the shunting of oxygenated blood from the placenta and the inferior vena cava into the left atrium. This blood effectively bypasses the nonfunctional pulmonary circulation and delivers oxygenated blood directly to the systemic circulation. The oxygen saturation of placental venous blood is only 67%, so if there were no foramen ovale to shunt the blood, it would lose even more oxygen as it traversed the nonaerated lungs and would be insufficient to maintain tissue perfusion. Presumably, this is why the foramen ovale mechanism is preserved in mammalian evolution. After birth, placental circulation ceases and the lungs serve as the means of oxygenating the blood. There is a decrease in the pulmonary vascular resistance and an increase in pulmonary blood flow resulting in decreased pressure in the right atrium compared to the left atrium. This results in functional closure of the foramen ovale and scar tissue formation permanently closes the foramen ovale within the first year of life.[11] In 20% to 25% of the population, the foramen ovale remains patent for reasons that are not known but is genetically determined, in part. The anatomic presence of a PFO was described nearly two millennia ago by the Greek physician Galen, who studied cardiac anatomy in mammals (Fig. 11-1).[12–14]

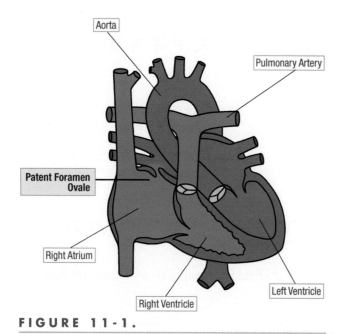

FIGURE 11-1.

Diagram of the heart in cross-section with the presence of a patent foramen ovale. (Courtesy of AGA Medical.)

DIAGNOSIS

The diagnosis of PFO can be made using a number of different imaging modalities. If a rigid and continuously open PFO is present, the blood may flow from the higher pressure left atrium, across the PFO into the right atrium, and then reverse direction with inspiration. This can be visualized by Doppler color flow. When right atrial pressure is abnormally increased, or when the subject strains and transiently increases the right atrial pressure, the blood flow reverses and a puff of blood or contrast agent can be observed to flow from the right atrium, through the PFO, into the left atrium. An intravenous agitated saline injection with transthoracic echocardiography (TTE) has been used to diagnose the presence of a PFO and to quantitate the right-to-left passage of blood. TTE is not as sensitive or specific as transesophageal echocardiography (TEE) for detecting intracardiac shunts.[15] Some patients with a high clinical suspicion of PFO have inconclusive echocardiographic studies, partially from inefficient Valsalva maneuver from sedation and intubation with the TEE probe. In addition, tomographic imaging of the interatrial septum during agitated saline injections may miss small, but clinically significant, right-to-left shunts (RLS). Detection of RLS using transcranial Doppler (TCD) imaging overcomes the limitation of sedation and intubation during TEE while maintaining a high sensitivity rate.[16–18] TCD can identify an RLS, but will not be able to locate the level of the shunt.

Other imaging modalities, such as cardiac computed tomography and magnetic resonance imaging, can detect PFO. These imaging techniques are dependent on imaging plane and timing because PFO flow is transient in nature. This effectively lowers the sensitivity of these tests and decreases their utility in the diagnosis of PFO. Cardiac catheterization can also be used for diagnosis by passing a guidewire across the interatrial septum or by visualizing the shunt with an injection of contrast directed at the atrial septum in the left anterior oblique cranial projection. However, diagnostic catheterization is rarely necessary given the other noninvasive imaging modalities available, but there are cases where the noninvasive imaging studies are inconclusive or incorrect. Our preference for identification of an RLS is to perform a TCD as well as a TEE. This allows for the highest sensitivity of documentation of an RLS, as well as localization of the shunt with the highest specificity.

PATHOGENESIS AND CLINICAL IMPLICATIONS

The amount of blood flow from left to right atrium through the PFO is too small to be hemodynamically significant, unlike an ASD where a large volume of shunted blood may occur. However, a PFO can cause clinical manifestations when RLS occurs. This can happen when the right atrial pressure transiently exceeds left atrial pressure, such as during Valsalva maneuvers or even normal respiratory cycles. The clinical significance of this interatrial opening had long been considered trivial because the degree of hemodynamic shunting is generally minimal. In 1877, however, Julius Cohnheim postulated that the presence of a PFO could result in a paradoxical embolism.[19] A venous thrombosis that appears as an arterial embolus is considered paradoxical because a venous thrombus would not be expected to be able to pass through the pulmonary circulation. By deductive reasoning, it is assumed that the venous embolus could not enter the arterial circulation unless there was an anomalous connection. It is postulated that the passage of thrombus or some other chemicals through a PFO, bypassing the pulmonary "filter," could lead to various clinical manifestations.

PFO has been associated with a number of different clinical manifestations. These include, but are not limited to, cryptogenic stroke,[1,2] migraine headaches,[3] platypnea-orthodeoxia,[4] decompression illness,[5] cerebral fat embolism syndrome after orthopedic surgery,[20] high altitude pulmonary edema,[21] obstructive sleep apnea (OSA) exacerbation,[22] and peripheral emboli including myocardial infarction with normal coronary arteries.[23] The majority of these associations have been made via observational data or case reports.

There has been one published randomized trial assessing medical therapy versus PFO closure for the treatment of migraine headaches. The Migraine Intervention with STARFlex Technology (MIST) trial was a double-blind, sham-controlled trial comparing PFO closure with medical therapy in migraineurs suffering from migraine with aura, five or more headache days per month, and having failed two or more prophylactic medications for migraine headaches. The primary endpoint was migraine headache cessation at 91 to 180 days and the secondary endpoints were change in frequency of headaches, character of headaches, or quality of life. Of the 432 patients with migraine and aura who were screened, 60% had an RLS and 163 patients had a moderate to large RLS; 147 of those patients were randomized. The cessation of migraine headaches was equal in both groups (3/74 implant group, 3/73 sham group). The implant group had a greater reduction in headache days after the exclusion of two outliers.[24] Although the reported success rate for PFO closure was 94%, there is some controversy surrounding this trial.

In the MIST study, the presence of RLS was determined by TTE, which has a lower sensitivity than TEE or TCD. There is also significant controversy concerning the reported success rate of closure. One of the previous coinvestigators, Peter Wilmhurst, has alleged that up to 35% of patients had large residual shunts after the attempted closure procedure. Some of these patients may have had large pulmonary shunts and, in others, the device did not achieve adequate closure. With the intention-to-treat protocol, seven patients were allegedly randomized to the device arm but did not have a PFO at the time of the procedure. With the lack of an independent core lab analyzing the data, these allegations may never be clarified. However, even if one-third of the closure patients had a residual shunt, given what is known from the observational analyses leading to this randomized trial, one would still expect a number of patients to have improvement or resolution of their migraine headaches. Perhaps the patient population analyzed in the MIST trial is fundamentally different from those patients in the observational reports. With these questions surrounding the MIST trial, interested individuals are awaiting the results of the ongoing PREMIUM trial using the Amplatzer PFO occluder by AGA Medical.[25]

With respect to PFO closure for the prevention of recurrent cryptogenic stroke, there are three randomized trials that are in various stages of development. CLOSURE I was a randomized clinical trial assessing medical therapy versus PFO closure using the STARFlex device for the prevention of recurrent strokes or transient ischemic attack (TIA). The preliminary results of this trial indicate that the primary endpoint of the trial, the reduction of stroke and TIA in the device treatment arm compared to medical therapy, was not reached.[26] The preliminary results, reported in 2010 at the American Heart Association Scientific Sessions, demonstrate that an equivalent result of recurrent stroke or TIA occurred in each arm of the study. Concern has been raised about the efficacy of the device, which only had an 86.5% closure rate. It will be important to know whether the 13.5% of patients with large residual shunts were more likely to have recurrent events. In addition, the inclusion of patients with TIA may confuse the issue of stroke because TIA cannot be clinically distinguished from a complex migraine with transient neurologic dysfunction, especially if a headache is not present. Lastly, the risk of atrial fibrillation (AF) after implantation seems to be higher with the STARFlex device than the other available devices. In the CLOSURE I trial, postimplantation AF was found in 5.7% of patients. This is higher than the rate for the Amplatzer device (2.9%) or the Helex device (1.8%) reported in a recent study analyzing the rate of AF following PFO closure. In this study, the incidence of AF for the STARFlex device was 10%, which was significantly higher in comparison to the other two devices. As the rate of AF increases, so does the risk of further neurologic events.[27]

The results of the other two ongoing, randomized trials—the RESPECT trial by AGA Medical and the REDUCE trial by W.L. Gore & Associates—will hopefully clarify the effect of PFO closure for the prevention of cryptogenic stroke. Unfortunately, because many patients can obtain PFO closure off-label outside of the randomized trials, there is concern that the highest risk patients are not being included in these trials. This will diminish the power of the trials and may lead to a type II statistical error.

MEDICAL THERAPY

There are currently no guidelines for medical therapy regarding primary prevention for patients with PFOs. Those patients who have had strokes, peripheral emboli, migraine headaches, or OSA are given medical therapy according to their specific illness. This often includes antiplatelet or anticoagulation therapy for strokes and peripheral emboli, prophylactic or abortive medications for migraine headaches, and positive pressure ventilation for OSA.

INDICATIONS FOR CLOSURE

In the United States, there is no FDA approval for closure of PFO. As discussed previously, there are randomized trials in progress or recently completed to assess the value of percutaneous closure in disease states such as migraine headache (MIST, PREMIUM) and cryptogenic stroke (CLOSURE I, RESPECT, REDUCE). Off-label percutaneous PFO closures have been performed in patients with cryptogenic stroke, migraine headaches, decompression illness, platypnea-orthodeoxia, and myocardial infarction with normal coronary arteries. In Europe, there are multiple devices that have been granted CE mark for PFO closure, and physicians are able to use their judgment as to appropriate criteria for therapy.

PERCUTANEOUS PATENT FORAMEN OVALE CLOSURE

PFO closure is performed in the United States using one of the devices approved by the FDA for ASD or VSD closure. It is important to discuss this with patients before the procedure to ensure that they are fully informed about the procedure, the risks and benefits of PFO closure, as well as acknowledgement of the off-label basis in which these devices are being used. The procedure can usually be done in an outpatient setting with conscious sedation; our preference is to use intravenous midazolam and fentanyl. All patients are premedicated with aspirin 325 mg and clopidogrel 600 mg by mouth.

The closure procedure is usually accomplished with echocardiographic guidance as well as fluoroscopy. In the past, the procedure was performed with TEE but, more recently, studies have described the feasibility of intracardiac echocardiography (ICE). TEE is an uncomfortable procedure for the patient and, in some cases, may require general anesthesia with endotracheal intubation. Some operators prefer to use fluoroscopic guidance exclusively and only perform TEE as part of the preprocedure evaluation.

Hijazi et al. first reported their experience with ICE compared to TEE.[28] The study included patients with either secundum ASDs or PFO. The investigators used the 10 French ACUSON AcuNav ICE catheter

(Siemens Medical Solutions USA Inc., Malvern, PA). For adult patients, the ICE catheter was introduced via a separate 11 French sheath through the same femoral vein as the occluder device. The median diameters of the ASDs by ICE and TEE had a correlation coefficient of 0.97, whereas balloon-stretched diameters had a 0.98 correlation coefficient. The investigators also noted that images of the upper left pulmonary vein and left atrium, which are near field images on TEE due to their proximity to the esophagus, were clearer by ICE. The positions of the wire, catheter, and device in the left atrium were visualized with greater clarity by ICE.

A second study by Koenig et al. reported their experience with ICE-guided transcatheter closure of 111 patients with both secundum ASD ($n = 82$) and PFO ($n = 29$).[29] This study also used the 10 French ACUSON AcuNav catheter. This modality allowed for successful placement of the device in all patients. More recently, an 8 French version of the ICE catheter has become available, which potentially decreases the risk of bleeding. In the United States, the FDA has approved this device to be resterilized up to four times, which significantly reduces the cost of the product.

Although there are variations in the technique for PFO closure, it is usually performed from the right femoral vein. In some instances, fluoroscopic guidance alone can be used; however, it is our practice to perform PFO closure with ICE and fluoroscopic guidance. In rare instances, right femoral vein access is not available. Access via the left femoral vein, the right internal jugular vein, or even the hepatic vein can be used for closure. The transhepatic approach is used in the pediatric cardiac catheterization laboratory[30]; however, it is rarely used in the adult cardiac catheterization laboratory. Access via the right internal jugular vein provides unique challenges given the inferior to superior orientation of the PFO, the difficulty in crossing the PFO with a catheter, and the extra support needed for device delivery. In our experience, an unexposed Brockenbrough needle (Bard, Billerica, MA), a Mullins sheath (Bard), and a Toray stiff guidewire (Toray International America Inc., Houston, TX) have been successful for the deployment of a septal occluder device from the right internal jugular vein (Fig. 11-2).

Our current technique for PFO closure is presented as an example of this procedure, although there is individual operator variation. Two sheaths are placed in the right femoral vein, one of which is for the ICE catheter. Our experience is that an 8 French ACUSON AcuNav ICE catheter provides adequate images through the smallest size sheath. It is preferable to use a longer sheath (30 cm) for the ICE catheter to more easily

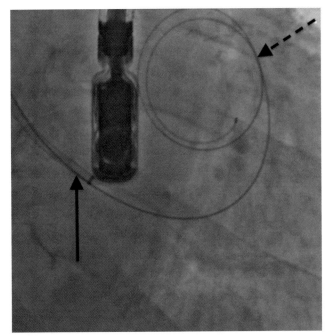

FIGURE 11-2.

Right internal jugular vein access to the left atrium through a patent foramen ovale tunnel with the use of a Mullins sheath (Bard, Billerica, MA), indicated by the *solid arrow*, and a Toray wire (Toray International America Inc., Houston, TX), indicated by the *dashed arrow*. Transseptal atrial or ventricular puncture can also be performed from this position.

negotiate the posterior bends of the iliac vein. The second sheath size varies based on the device that is being used for PFO closure. The three devices currently used in the United States are discussed in the succeeding text.

Helex Device

The Helex septal occluder device by Gore Medical is one of the more complicated devices for an interventional operator to understand mechanistically, yet it is effective and extremely well tolerated by patients. The device is approved by the FDA for closure of ASDs. It is composed of a single nitinol wire covered by expanded polytetrafluoroethylene with a left atrial eyelet, center eyelet, and right atrial eyelet. The locking loop from the left atrial side to the right atrial side holds the device together after deployment (Fig. 11-3). The Helex device comes in various sizes (15, 20, 25, 30, and 35 mm) and comes with a green delivery catheter with the device already extruded from its distal tip. There is a gray catheter attached to the proximal right atrial eyelet, which is used to retract or extrude the device (Fig. 11-4). The mandrel attaches to the left atrial eyelet and contains the locking loop. The mandrel is pulled to release the device and lock it in place (Fig. 11-5).

The sheath size for the delivery catheter varies based on the manufacturer. Most sheath sizes will be 13 French with the use of a guidewire and 10 French without the use of a guidewire. The 11 French Pinnacle sheath (Terumo Medical, Somerset, NJ) is the smallest sheath that will accommodate a 0.035-inch guidewire and the delivery catheter.

Transvenous access is established via the right femoral vein, followed by placement of an 8 and 11 French Pinnacle sheath. Intravenous heparin is given, typically for an activated clotting time between 250 and 350 seconds. A 6 French Multipurpose (MPA) coronary catheter (Cordis Corp, Bridgewater, NJ) is inserted through the 11 French sheath with a 145-cm J-tipped guidewire into the right atrium. The guidewire is removed and the catheter is carefully aspirated and flushed. The 8 French ICE catheter is then carefully inserted into the right atrium. The MPA catheter serves as a guide for the ICE catheter because aggressive advancement can result in venous laceration or puncture. The ICE catheter should not be pushed against resistance for this reason. The use of the 30-cm long sheath eliminates some of this difficulty in advancing the ICE catheter. Bubble studies are performed at rest and with forced expiration into a manometer

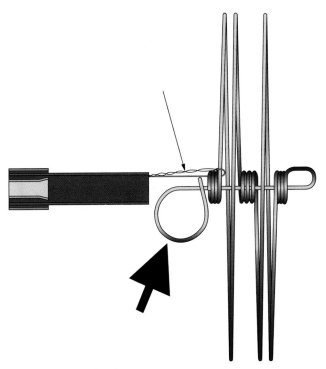

FIGURE 11-3.

Locked Helex nitinol frame prior to final release. The retrieval cord is indicated by the *narrow arrow* and the locking loop is marked by the *wide arrow*. (Courtesy of W.L. Gore & Associates Inc.)

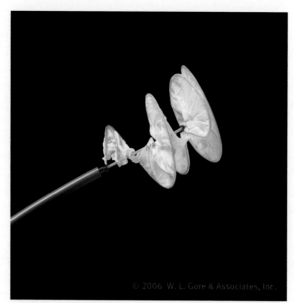

© 2006 W. L. Gore & Associates, Inc.

FIGURE 11-4.

Helex septal occluder device prior to retraction within the delivery sheath. (Courtesy of W.L. Gore & Associates Inc.)

to 40 mm Hg with right atrial pressure measurement through the MPA catheter. If desired, TCD and ICE are utilized to evaluate the grade of RLS. If a Spencer grade 5 TCD shunt is seen at rest, no further bubble studies are necessary.

The short J-tipped guidewire is reinserted and used to cross the PFO, utilizing both fluoroscopic and echocardiographic guidance. The guidewire and catheter

are positioned preferentially into the left superior pulmonary vein. The guidewire is removed and the catheter is aspirated and flushed carefully. Any introduction of air could have adverse consequences. A 0.035-inch J curve 260-cm Amplatzer extra-stiff guidewire is advanced into the left superior pulmonary vein and the MPA catheter is removed (Figs. 11-6 and 11-7). We have switched from using a 260-cm Amplatzer super-stiff guidewire because we had a patient who developed pericardial tamponade from a left atrial puncture with this very stiff guidewire.

The Helex system is prepared in the usual manner recommended by the manufacturer. Both the gray catheter (in line with the green catheter) and the mandrel (at a 60-degree angle to the green catheter) should be locked. The gray catheter can be identified by the red cap holding the white retrieval cord in place. A syringe with heparinized flush is attached to the red cap and the catheter is flushed. After adequate flushing, the gray catheter Luer lock is unscrewed and the device is retracted into the green delivery catheter by pulling back on the gray catheter. Continuous flushing is performed during device retraction. When there is a slight 20- to 30-degree bend at the distal end of the

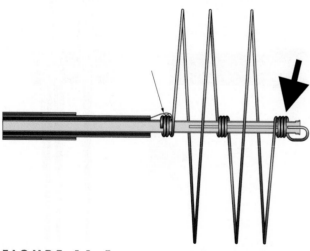

FIGURE 11-5.

Helex nitinol frame with delivery catheter. The right atrium eyelet is identified by the *narrow arrow* and the left atrium eyelet is depicted by the wide *arrow*. (Courtesy of W.L. Gore & Associates Inc.)

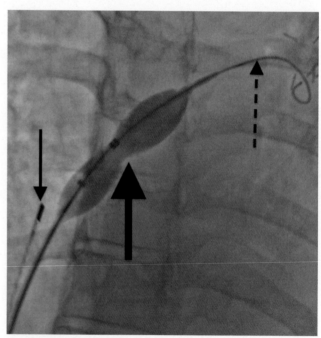

FIGURE 11-6.

Fluoroscopic view of the intracardiac echocardiography catheter (*solid arrow*), Amplatzer extra-stiff guidewire (*dashed arrow*), and a 24-mm Amplatzer sizing balloon (*large arrow*) across a patent foramen ovale (PFO) tunnel. A sizing balloon can be used when there are concerns about the length or width of the PFO tunnel prior to device implantation.

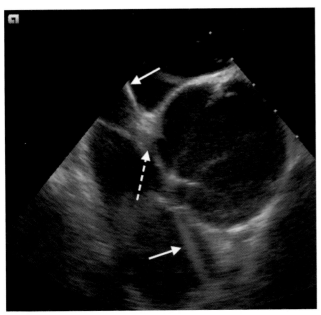

FIGURE 11-7.

Intracardiac echocardiography image of Amplatzer extra-stiff wire (*solid arrows*) across a patent foramen ovale tunnel (*dashed arrow*).

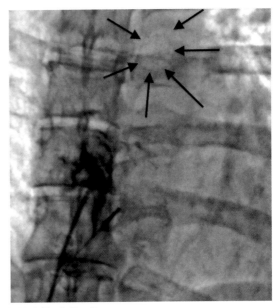

FIGURE 11-9.

Fluoroscopy image of air in the left atrial appendage (*arrows*) introduced through the multipurpose catheter.

device (Fig. 11-8), the mandrel is unscrewed and the device is retracted completely into the green catheter by pulling back on the gray catheter. The Helex device must be withdrawn about 1 cm into the green catheter to allow a guidewire to clear the short monorail at the distal end of the catheter. The catheter is flushed once again to ensure that no air is introduced into the left atrium during placement of the occluder (Fig. 11-9).

The green delivery catheter is placed into the left atrium over the 0.035-inch guidewire. Care is taken not

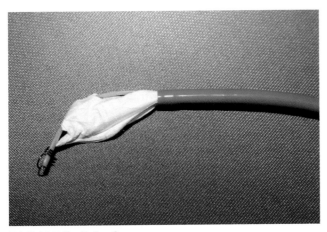

FIGURE 11-8.

Photograph of the appropriate bend on the Helex device prior to loosening of the mandrel and final retraction into the delivery catheter.

to advance the catheter into the left superior pulmonary vein. The guidewire is removed and the left atrial disk is deployed. This is accomplished by the "push-pinch-pull" method. The gray catheter is "pushed" to extrude the device, however, to form the left atrial disk, the gray catheter is "pinched," and the mandrel is "pulled" until its distal end is against the green delivery catheter. This sequence of "push-pinch-pull" is continued until the left atrial disk is formed and flat and the middle eyelet is at the distal tip of the green catheter. Fluoroscopy and ICE ensure that deployment of the device is at the appropriate position within the left atrial chamber. Although the device is the softest of the three devices currently in use in the United States, the Helex delivery system still has the potential to puncture the left atrium with resulting pericardial effusion and tamponade.

Once the left atrial disk is deployed, the gray catheter and mandrel are fixed in relationship to the green delivery catheter and the entire system is pulled back as a unit against the left side of the interatrial septum. Confirmation of this is seen on ICE and fluoroscopy. The gray catheter is held in place to ensure that the left atrial disk remains flush against the interatrial septum, and the green catheter is pulled back until it meets the mandrel. The Helex device is compliant, so any excessive back tension on the gray catheter during this maneuver could result in left atrial disk retraction into the right atrium through the PFO tunnel. The mandrel is locked at this point. The remainder of the device is extruded by pushing the gray catheter into the body while maintaining the placement of the green catheter. The gray catheter Luer lock is then locked to the green catheter.

Confirmation of acceptable placement is done under fluoroscopy and ICE imaging (Fig. 11-10). Fluoroscopy is typically done in a cranial left anterior oblique projection to assess for left and right atrial disk separation across the septum secundum. ICE images confirm right and left atrial disks in the proper location with their superior portions straddling the septum secundum and the interatrial septum visualized between the disks.

When the position of the device is acceptable, the red cap is removed from the gray catheter. The mandrel is loosened and repeat fluoroscopy should demonstrate the eyelets moving closer together. Under fluoroscopic imaging, the mandrel is forcefully and quickly withdrawn from the green catheter. This pulls the distal tip of the mandrel off the left atrial eyelet and deploys the locking loop. Repeat imaging should confirm placement of the locking loop around the right atrial eyelet as well as the eyelets moving closer together. If the device is in proper position, the green

catheter is advanced over the gray catheter up to the device. This acts as a brace for the removal of the gray catheter, which is withdrawn from the green catheter. The white retrieval cord should not be grasped while removing the gray catheter because this could result in withdrawal of the entire device. At any point prior to removal of the gray catheter, the Helex device can be retrieved. Pulling back on the gray catheter while the red cap is attached or while simultaneously holding the white retrieval cord will accomplish device retrieval. The green catheter is removed and final images are obtained (Fig. 11-11).

Our protocol is to administer protamine to partially reverse the anticoagulation and facilitate hemostasis. In over 350 cases with this technique, we have not observed any acute thrombus formation or distal embolization. Both sheaths are removed and a single figure-of-eight stitch is placed in the skin and subcutaneous tissues to obtain hemostasis. The suture is removed 1 to 2 hours later in the recovery area and a frog-leg pressure bandage is applied. The patient is observed for 4 hours, then discharged home with the pressure bandage. This bandage is removed by the patient the following morning.

Amplatzer Devices

The Amplatzer atrial septal occluder (ASO) is a self-expandable, double-disk device with a connecting waist of variable dimensions. The device is made with a nitinol wire mesh (0.004- to 0.0075-inch). Polyester patches are sewn within each disk and serve to occlude blood flow through the device. The occluder is available in multiple sizes (range 4 to 38 mm), which describe the diameter of the waist. This allows the device to self-center within ASDs. The right and left atrial disks are larger than the waist and are of varying sizes depending on the size of the device (the disk diameter is between 8 and 16 mm wider than the waist). The left atrial disk is generally larger than the right atrial disk.

The Amplatzer multifenestrated ASO (cribriform) is a similar self-expanding, double-disk device constructed from nitinol with polyester patches. As opposed to the ASO device, the cribriform device has a thin waist with atrial disks of equal size. It comes in four sizes (18, 25, 30, and 35 mm) and is approved for the closure of multifenestrated secundum ASDs.[31] Both the ASO and the cribriform device have been used on an off-label basis for the closure of PFO. The PREMIUM and RESPECT trials are still ongoing to assess the efficacy of the Amplatzer PFO occluder (Fig. 11-12). The Amplatzer PFO device is not

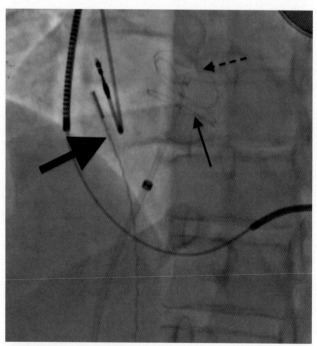

FIGURE 11-10.

Fluoroscopy of Helex device prior to removal of the mandrel. The left atrial disk (*dashed arrow*) and the right atrial disk (*solid arrow*) are seen straddling the septum secundum in the cranial left anterior oblique projection. Pacemaker wires and the intracardiac echocardiography catheter (*large arrow*) are seen to the left of the device.

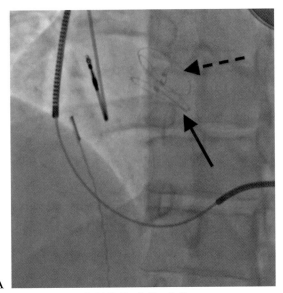
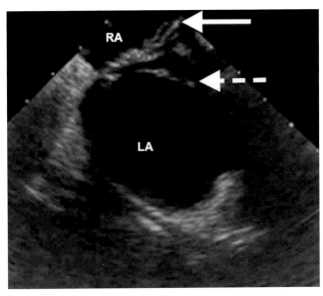

FIGURE 11-11.

A: Fluoroscopy of the Helex device in place across the patent foramen ovale (PFO) tunnel. The left atrial disk (*dashed arrow*) and the right atrial disk (*solid arrow*) are seen straddling the septum secundum in the cranial left anterior oblique projection. **B:** Intracardiac echocardiography image of a typical result from a Helex device implantation for PFO closure. The left atrial disk (*dashed arrow*) and the right atrial disk (*solid arrow*) are seen opposed to the interatrial septum. The left atrium (*LA*) and right atrium (*RA*) are labeled.

approved by the FDA and is only available for patients enrolled in the clinical trials; therefore, it cannot be used off-label in the United States. Device selection is dependent on the length and width of the PFO tunnel.

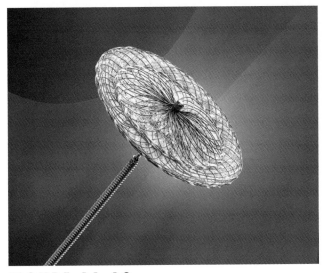

FIGURE 11-12.

Amplatzer patent foramen ovale occluder device. This device is available in Europe. Clinical trials assessing its efficacy are still ongoing. This device has yet to receive FDA approval for use in the United States. (Courtesy of AGA Medical.)

The initial steps for PFO closure using an Amplatzer device are not significantly different than outlined in the previous section. An 8 French sheath is used for ICE and the second sheath is generally 7 or 8 French, depending on the size of implant. The MPA catheter is used to cross the PFO, and a 0.035-inch Amplatzer extra-stiff, J-tipped guidewire is placed in the left superior pulmonary vein. The catheter and sheath are removed.

An appropriate-sized guiding sheath and introducer are prepared by flushing both meticulously. The sheath/introducer unit is then advanced over the guidewire under fluoroscopy into the left atrium. The introducer is parked in the mid left atrium and the sheath is advanced over the introducer into the left atrium. This is done to avoid atrial puncture by the introducer. The introducer and wire are removed and the catheter is aspirated and flushed; the back end is closed with a Luer-lock syringe. This step is important to prevent air from entering the left atrium. The catheter may also be kept below the chest level to make sure that gravity will help drain blood out of the catheter instead of permitting air to enter the catheter while it is in the left atrium. The occluding device is then placed in a water bath and is loaded onto the delivery cable. While the device is still under water, the cable and device are retracted into a 6-inch loading catheter adapted with an O-ring to permit flushing and prevent air from entering into the loading device. Meticulous care is necessary at this point to prevent any air from being introduced into the guiding catheter, which could then embolize if released at the end of the catheter within the left atrium. The device within the loading tube is then attached to the main catheter and advanced within the sheath. The left atrial disk is advanced out of the catheter and expands to its original shape within the left atrium. The catheter and the left atrial disk are retracted as a unit until the left atrial disk abuts against the interatrial septum. This process is visualized both by fluoroscopy as well as ICE guidance. The right atrial disk is then deployed by withdrawing the sheath and simultaneously advancing the cable holding the device. The expanded right atrial disk is readvanced against the septum. It is important to visualize that the pliable interatrial septum is clearly positioned between the right and left atrial disks. Placement of the device is confirmed by fluoroscopy and ICE.

When satisfactory position of the device is confirmed, the device is released from the cable by counterclockwise rotation of the cable. Gentle manual retraction is held on the cable in relationship to the sheath during this release maneuver to prevent the sharp, distal tip of the cable from puncturing other structures. The cable is completely withdrawn after release and final images are obtained (Fig. 11-13). Hemostasis is achieved as previously outlined.

CardioSEAL and STARFlex Devices

The CardioSEAL and STARFlex devices are both self-expanding, double umbrella devices. Each umbrella consists of four arms made out of MP35N, a nickel-cobalt–based alloy covered by Dacron. There are two hinges within each arm to relieve excess stress on the device. Unlike the CardioSEAL device, the STARFlex device has a self-centering mechanism. Both devices come in a range of sizes from 17 to 40 mm in diameter.[32] The CardioSEAL and STARFlex devices are FDA approved for VSD closure and are used on an off-label basis for ASD and PFO closures (Fig. 11-14).

The deployment of these devices proceeds in a manner similar to the Amplatzer device deployment previously described. After the PFO is crossed and the 260 cm Amplatz extra-stiff wire is placed in the left superior pulmonary vein, an 11 French long sheath is placed in the left atrium over a dilator. The sheath is flushed. The appropriate-sized device is loaded into the delivery catheter and advanced through the sheath into the left atrium. Advancing the delivery wire on the delivery sheath exposes the left atrial umbrella. The entire unit is pulled back until the umbrella

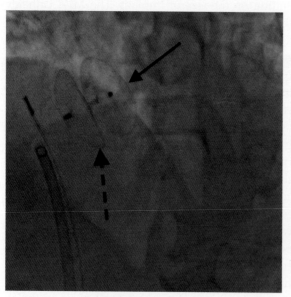
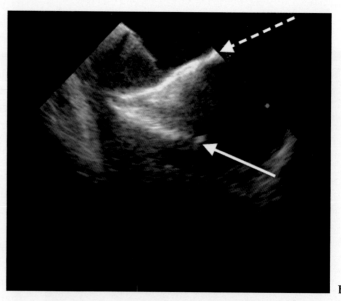

A   B

FIGURE 11-13.

A: Fluoroscopy of an Amplatzer cribriform device through a patent foramen ovale (PFO) tunnel with the left atrial disk (*solid arrow*) and right atrial disk (*dashed arrow*) on either side of the interatrial septum. **B:** Intracardiac echocardiography image of the Amplatzer device through the PFO tunnel with the left atrial disk (*solid arrow*) and the right atrial disk (*dashed arrow*) seen on opposite sides of the interatrial septum.

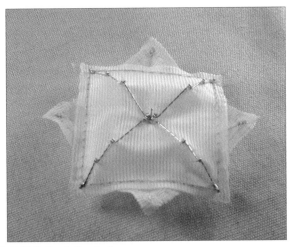

FIGURE 11-14.

CardioSEAL septal repair implant. A double umbrella occlusion device with each umbrella consisting of four arms made out of MP35N, a nickel-cobalt–based alloy covered by Dacron. There are two hinges within each arm to relieve excess stress on the device.

is near the left atrial side of the septum. Unlike the Amplatzer or Helex devices, the umbrella should be near or barely touching the left atrial septum. Further retraction will result in the left atrial arms being pulled through to the right atrial side. When an acceptable position is obtained, the sheath is retracted over the delivery catheter, deploying the right atrial umbrella. The release mechanism is used to separate the delivery catheter and wire from the occluding device. Final confirmation of position is done under fluoroscopy and ICE.[32]

COMPLICATIONS

Percutaneous PFO closure is a relatively safe procedure. There is a small risk of death, hemorrhage requiring blood transfusion, cardiac tamponade, need for surgical intervention, and fatal pulmonary emboli. In a meta-analysis of 1,355 patients treated in the early experience, the combined risk for serious complications was 1.5%. Atrial arrhythmias, heart block, and transient ST elevation are also possible complications during and after device implantation.[33,34] Device embolization is rare for occluders used for PFO closure as compared with ASD occluders because there is more tissue for the device to hold onto. However, embolization has been reported and is device dependent[35,36]; as less bulky devices are developed, the risk of embolization increases.

Each device has a higher propensity for certain complications and will be reviewed in more detail.

The Helex device is the newest of the three devices available in the United States for ASD or off-label PFO closure. It is a well-tolerated device with very few reported complications. Because it is softer than the other devices, it produces less chest discomfort or atrial arrhythmias. The healing process depends on the materials that are used to make the devices. Expanded polytetrafluoroethylene is well tolerated by the body and produces a mild inflammatory response with a thin layer of collagen. Although it may take longer for the Helex device to completely seal a PFO due to the less exuberant expression of fibrous tissue, 90% of PFOs show no residual shunt at 3 months by TCD. The remaining patients have mild, Spencer grade 2 to 3 shunts, and only 2% of patients had shunt grades of 4 or 5 by TCD after 6 months (Gervorgyan and Tobis, unpublished data).

One potential concern with all of the devices is embolization from the atrial septum to the pulmonary circulation, the heart chambers, or the passage through the aortic valve with more remote dislodgement. The Helex device may be more susceptible to embolization because it is softer and more flexible than the other devices. If the right atrial disk is not stable over the limbus of the septum secundum, it may fall into the PFO tunnel and work its way through the PFO into the left atrium. For those operators who are interested in more details, a case of peripheral embolization of a Helex device has been reported and the optimal method of retrieval is described.[37]

The Amplatzer family of septal occluders is also well tolerated. However, the stiffness of the devices makes erosion more of a concern. This was true of the ASD occluders when they were relatively oversized, especially in children. The incidence of erosion with the Amplatzer PFO device is difficult to know, but, as of 2008, the incidence was 0.018%.[38] Current data suggest that there have been six reported cases in about 40,000 devices used. In contrast, there have been no documented cases of erosion with the Helex device. The CardioSEAL family of devices has a low incidence of erosion, which is limited to case reports.[39] The clinical impact of device erosion is dependent on the site of perforation and the communicating structures involved, but typically include hemopericardium, fistula formation, and hemodynamic compromise. Perforation can result in death, which has been reported following the use of the ASD occluder but not with the PFO occluder device.[40]

The efficacy of the CardioSEAL family of devices for PFO closure is a concern to us. If the device is implanted in a foramen ovale that has a relatively long tunnel, the device cannot open completely. The arms can remain at 90 degrees to the septum and actually stent the PFO open so that the shunt is larger than it was before. In addition, as scar tissue forms on this device, if it is not implanted flat and adherent to the septum, we believe that the device may retract with time and increase the shunt. Reisman reported that there was a ≥2-grade increase over time (between month 6 and 12 post-PFO closure) in the mean TCD grade in 6% of patients who received the CardioSEAL device and that 14% of their implants had a grade 4 or 5 shunt at 360 ± 257 days.[41]

The increased incidence of AF with the CardioSEAL family of devices has previously been addressed. Based on published data, the rate of AF with the STARFlex device is reported between 5.7% and 10%.[42] This is much higher than the rate of AF with the Amplatzer device (2.9%) or the Helex device (1.8%).[27] Recurrent stroke or peripheral emboli has been observed as a complication of AF induced by these devices.

The CardioSEAL/STARFlex devices are also relatively more prone to thrombosis. Although complete endothelialization of the implanted devices tends to occur within 3 to 6 months, there are reports of thrombus formation on the device postimplantation. In one study of 593 patients who received one of four devices—Amplatzer PFO Occluder, CardioSEAL, STARFLex, and PFO-Star—the rates of thrombus formation were 0%, 7.1%, 5.7%, and 6.6%, respectively. The difference between the Amplatzer device and the other three was statistically significant. In this study, postprocedural AF and the presence of an atrial septal aneurysm were predictors for thrombus formation.[43] In another single center study of 200 patients, no thrombus formation was seen on an Amplatzer PFO or ASD device. Implantation of the CardioSEAL device was associated with a 23% incidence of thrombus formation on the device documented by TEE at 1 month.[44] The formation of thrombus on the Helex device is limited to rare case reports.[45] We suspect that these observations of thrombus formation on the CardioSEAL devices are clinically important. Reisman reported a late embolic event rate of 3.4%, all of which occurred in the CardioSEAL cases.[41] In contradistinction, there have been no recurrent stroke or peripheral emboli in over 300 of our cryptogenic stroke patients treated with Amplatzer or Helex closure devices.[43]

Antiplatelet therapy may be effective in the prevention of thrombus formation on devices, but there are no randomized trials to prove their necessity or efficacy.[46,47] Our patients are usually maintained on dual antiplatelet therapy for 1 to 3 months and 81 mg aspirin for at least 6 months postimplantation.

The development of infective endocarditis is rare and limited to case reports in the literature. Prophylactic antibiotics are given for any dental work for at least 1 year. Typically, amoxicillin 2 g is given 1 hour prior to dental cleaning or intervention. Other alternatives for penicillin-intolerant patients include clindamycin or azithromycin.

Our patients return for a TEE and TCD at 3 months to evaluate the position of the device and the presence of thrombus. The presence of a significant residual shunt is relatively uncommon in our experience but averages 4% and depends on the device implanted. Initially, we performed a TEE and TCD at 1 month after the procedure, but there was a higher incidence of residual shunts. Most of these shunts closed over the next 3 months, so we currently perform our first follow-up TEE and TCD at 3 months. This allows enough time for the healing process to close the PFO for the current devices. The main risk factors for residual shunts with using the Amplatzer PFO occluder are the presence of an atrial septal aneurysm, redundant atrial septum, or the use of the larger 35-mm device. The incidence of residual shunts with the Amplatzer device is between 6% and 19%[48,49] and is higher with the cribriform device than the PFO or ASD occluder. With the Helex device, it may take longer to completely seal a PFO due to the less exuberant fibrous tissue formation. There is no evidence of significant residual shunt in 90% of PFO at 3 months by TCD. The patients with a residual shunt of grade 3 or more returned for a TCD at 6 months. Only 2% of patients had shunt grades of 4 or 5 by TCD after 6 months (Gevorgyan and Tobis, unpublished data). The STARFlex device appears to have a significantly higher incidence of residual shunts. In the CLOSURE I trial, the incidence of a large residual shunt was 13.5%.[42]

The management of patients with residual shunts usually consists of medical therapy for their underlying disease process. The optimal management of patients with large residual shunts is evaluated on a case-by-case basis. Many of these patients can be safely managed with medical therapy; however, some patients may benefit from implantation of a second closure device. On occasion, it may be necessary to surgically explant a device due to a large residual shunt when placing a second device, but it is not advisable.

Although the risk of explantation is small, it requires open heart surgery, and this should be discussed with the patient when obtaining informed consent. In a multicenter survey, the frequency of surgical explantation of septal occluder devices after closure of PFO was 0.27%. The explantation rate by device is given in Table 11-1. The presence of residual

TABLE 11-1 Type of Device and Number of Implants and Explants Reported [50]

	CardioSEAL	Amplatzer	Helex	Other	Total
Implantations	2,023	9,109	1,201	1,403	13,736
Explantations	16	19	2	1	38
% Explanted	0.79%	0.21%	0.16%	0.07%	0.28%
P value	|----0.00003----| |------ns------|				

shunting or thrombus formation on the device as the reason for explantation was more frequent with the CardioSEAL device than with the other devices. In this survey of close to 14,000 cases, the CardioSEAL device had to be explanted in 1 out of every 126 implants. The Amplatzer device was explanted 1 in 479 times and the Helex was explanted in 1 out of 600 cases.[50]

CONCLUSION

PFO closure, once only amenable to surgical correction, is now routinely performed percutaneously as an outpatient procedure. PFO has been implicated in a number of pathologic states, and there are likely more associations that have yet to be discovered. In addition to the passage of venous blood clots, the RLS of deoxygenated blood or other chemical factors appears to be detrimental. The indications for percutaneous closure are relatively limited at this time and, in the United States, it must be emphasized that there is no FDA approval for PFO closure devices outside of the randomized trials. However, as more information is uncovered, the randomized trials conclude, and newer technologies develop, the field of percutaneous closure has the potential to expand and encompass many more patients who might benefit from PFO closure.

As this chapter was being published, it was announced that NMT Medical, Inc., the company that produced the CardioSEAL and STARFlex, was going out of business. These devices will no longer be available and this will address many of the concerns raised in this chapter.

REFERENCES

1. Lechat P, Mas JL, Lascault G, et al. Prevalence of patent foramen ovale in patients with stroke. *N Engl J Med.* 1988;318:1148–1152.
2. Handke M, Harloff A, Olschewski M, et al. Patent foramen ovale and cryptogenic stroke in older patients. *N Engl J Med.* 2007;357:2262–2268.
3. Azarbal B, Tobis J, Suh W, et al. Association of inter-atrial shunts and migraine headaches: Impact of transcatheter closure. *J Am Coll Cardiol.* 2005;45:489–492.
4. Sorrentino M, Resnekov L. Patent foramen ovale associated with platypnea and orthodeoxia. *Chest.* 1991;100:1157–1158.
5. Moon RE, Camporesi EM, Kisslo JA. Patent foramen ovale and decompression illness in divers. *Lancet.* 1989;1:513–514.
6. Seivert H, Krusdorf U. Transcatheter closure of intracardiac shunts. *Z Kardiol.* 2002;91:77–83.
7. Krumsdorf U, Keppler P, Horvath K, et al. Catheter closure of atrial septal defects and patent foramen ovale in patients with an atrial septal aneurysm using different devices. *J Interv Cardiol.* 2001;14:49–55.
8. Beitze A, Schuchlenz H, Beitze M, et al. Interventional occlusion of foramen ovale and atrial septal defects after paradoxical embolism incidents. *Z Kardiol.* 2002;91:693–700.
9. Post MC, Van Deyk K, Budts W. Percutaneous closure of a patent foramen ovale: single-centre experience using different types of devices and mid-term outcome. *Acta Cardiol.* 2005;60:515–519.
10. Vincent RN, Raviele AA, Diehl HJ. Single-center experience with the HELEX septal occluder for closure of atrial septal defects in children. *J Interv Cardiol.* 2003;16:79–82.
11. Moore KL, Persaud TVN. *The Developing Human, Clinically Oriented Embryology.* 6th ed. Philadelphia: WB Saunders; 1998:394–396.
12. Hagen PT, Scholz DG, Edwards WD. Incidence and size of patent foramen ovale during the first 10 decades of life: an autopsy study of 965 normal hearts. *Mayo Clin Proc.* 1984;59:17–20.
13. Cleveland Clinic. Patent foramen ovale (PFO). Available at: http://my.clevelandclinic.org/disorders/patent_foramen_ovale_pfo/hic_patent_foramen_ovale_pfo.aspx. Accessed May 31, 2011.
14. Galen. De usu partium L. Nicolaus. De usu partium corporis humani, magna cura ad exemplaris Graeci veriritatem [sic] castigatum, universo hominum

geni apprime necessarium. *Parisiis: Ex officina Simonis Colinaei.* 1528; 32:484.

15. Pearson AC, Labovitz AJ, Tatineni S, et al. Superiority of transesophageal echocardiography in detecting cardiac source of embolism in patients with cerebral ischemia of uncertain etiology. *J Am Coll Cardiol.* 1991;17:66–72.

16. Teague SM, Sharma MK. Detection of paradoxical cerebral echo contrast embolization by transcranial Doppler ultrasound. *Stroke.* 1991;22:740–745.

17. Blersch WK, Draganski BM, Holmer SR, et al. Transcranial duplex sonography in the detection of patent foramen ovale. *Radiology.* 2002;225:693–699.

18. Van H, Poommipanit P, Shalaby M, et al. Sensitivity of transcranial Doppler versus intracardiac echocardiography in the detection of right-to-left shunt. *JACC Cardiovasc Imaging.* 2010;3:343–348.

19. Cohnheim J. *Vorlesungen über allgemeine Pathologie: ein Handbuch für Aerzte und Studirende.* Berlin: Hirschwald; 1877.

20. Chen JJS, Ha JC, Mirvis SE. MR imaging of the brain in fat embolism syndrome. *Emerg Radiol.* 2008;15: 187–192.

21. Allemann Y, Hutter D, Lipp E, et al. Patent foramen ovale and high-altitude pulmonary edema. *JAMA.* 2007;296:2954–2958.

22. Shanoudy H, Soliman A, Raggi P, et al. Prevalence of patent foramen ovale and its contribution to hypoxemia in patients with obstructive sleep apnea. *Chest.* 1998;113:91–96.

23. Mehan VK, Wahl A, Walpoth N, et al. Instant percutaneous closure of patent foramen ovale with acute myocardial infarction and normal coronary arteries. *Catheter Cardiovasc Interv.* 2006;67:279–282.

24. Dowson A, Mullen MJ, Peatfield R, et al. Migraine Intervention with STARFlex Technology (MIST) Trial. A prospective, multicenter, double-blind, sham-controlled trial to evaluate the effectiveness of patent foramen ovale closure with STARFlex septal repair implant to resolve refractory migraine headache. *Circulation.* 2008;117:1397–1404.

25. Tobis J. Management of patients with refractory migraine and PFO: Is MIST I relevant? *Catheter Cardiovasc Interv.* 2008;72:60–64.

26. NMT Medical, Inc. NMT Medical announces preliminary results of CLOSURE I PFO/stroke trial. Available at: http://www.snl.com/irweblinkx/file.aspx?IID=4148066&FID=9712903&printable=1. Accessed May 31, 2011.

27. Staubach S, Steinberg DH, Zimmermann W, et al. New onset atrial fibrillation after patent foramen ovale closure. *Catheter Cardiovasc Interv.* 2009;74:889–895.

28. Hijazi Z et al. Transcatheter closure of atrial septal defects and patent foramen ovale under intracardiac echocardiographic guidance: feasibility and comparison with transesophageal echocardiography. *Catheter Cardiovasc Interv.* 2001;52:194–199.

29. Koenig P, Cao QL, Heitschmidt M, et al. Role of intracardiac echocardiographic guidance in transcatheter closure of atrial septal defects and patent foramen ovale using the Amplatzer device. *J Interv Cardiol.* 2003;16:51–62.

30. Ebied MR. Transhepatic vascular access for diagnostic and interventional procedures: techniques, outcome, and complications. *Catheter Cardiovasc Interv.* 2007;69:594–606.

31. AGA Medical Corporation. US instructions for use. Available at: http://www.amplatzer.com/USProducts/USInstructionsforUse/tabid/873/Default.aspx. Accessed May 31, 2011.

32. Pedra C, Piklala J, Lee KJ, et al. Transcatheter closure of atrial septal defects using the Cardio-Seal implant. *Heart.* 2000;84:320–326.

33. Khairy P, O'Donnell CP, Landzberg MJ. Transcatheter closure versus medical therapy of patent foramen ovale and presumed paradoxical thromboemboli: a systematic review. *Ann Intern Med.* 2003;139:753–760.

34. Chessa M, Carminati M, Butera G, et al. Early and late complications associated with transcatheter occlusion of secundum atrial septal defect. *J Am Coll Cardiol.* 2002;39:1061–1065.

35. Braun M, Gliech V, Boscheri A, et al. Transcatheter closure of patent foramen ovale (PFO) in patients with paradoxical embolism. Periprocedural safety and mid-term follow-up results of three different device occluder systems. *Eur Heart J.* 2004;25: 424–430.

36. Braun MU, Fassbender D, Schoen SP, et al. Transcatheter closure of patent foramen ovale in patients with cerebral ischemia. *J Am Coll Cardiol.* 2002;39: 2019–2025.

37. Poommipanit P, Levi D, Shenoda M, et al. Percutaneous retrieval of the locked Helex septal occluder. *Catheter Cardiovasc Interv.* 2010;77:892–900.

38. Amin Z, Hijazi ZM, Bass JL, et al. PFO closure complications from the AGA registry. *Catheter Cardiovasc Interv.* 2008;72:74–79.

39. Motreff P, Dauphin C, Souteyrand G. Cardiac perforation and tamponade 3 months after transcatheter PFO closure by STARFlex device: A case report. *Catheter Cardiovasc Interv.* 2008;71:412–416.

40. Amin Z, Hijazi ZM, Bass JL, et al. Erosion of Amplatzer septal occluder device after closure of secundum atrial septal defects: Review of registry of complications and recommendations to minimize future risk. *Catheter Cardiovasc Interv.* 2004;63:496–502.

41. Harms V, Reisman M, Fuller C, et al. Outcomes after transcatheter closure of patent foramen ovale in patients with paradoxical embolism. *Am J Cardiol.* 2007;99:1312–1315.

42. American Heart Association. CLOSURE I Presentation slides. Available at: http://networking.americanheart.org/files/179. Accessed May 31, 2011.

43. Krumsdorf U, Ostermayer S, Billinger K, et al. Incidence and clinical course of thrombus formation on atrial septal defect and patent foramen ovale closure devices in 1,000 consecutive patients. *J Am Coll Cardiol.* 2004;43:302–309.

44. Slavin L, Tobis JM, Rangarajan K, et al. Five-year experience with percutaneous closure of patent foramen ovale. *Am J Cardiol.* 2007;99:1316–1320.

45. Zaidi AN, Cheatham JP, Galantowicz, et al. Late thrombus formation on the Helex septal occluder

after double-lung transplant. *J Heart Lung Transplant.* 2010;29:814–816.

46. Brandt RR, Neumann T, Neuzner J, et al. Transcatheter closure of atrial septal defect and patent foramen ovale in adult patients using the Amplatzer occlusion device: no evidence for thrombus deposition with antiplatelet agents. *J Am Soc Echocardiogr.* 2002;15:1094–1098.

47. Anzai H, Child J, Natterson B, et al. Incidence of thrombus formation on the CardioSEAL and Amplatzer inter-atrial closure devices. *Am J Cardiol.* 2004; 93:426–431.

48. Zajarias A, Thanigaraj S, Lasala J, et al. Predictors and clinical outcomes of residual shunt in patients undergoing percutaneous transcatheter closure of patent foramen ovale. *J Invasive Cardiol.* 2006;18:533–537.

49. Greutmann M, Greutmann-Yantiri M, Kretschmar O, et al. Percutaneous PFO closure with Amplatzer PFO occluder: predictors of residual shunts at 6 months follow-up. *Congenit Heart Dis.* 2009; 4:252–257.

50. Verma SK and Tobia JM. Explanation of patent foramen ovale devices: a multicenter survey. JACC Cardiovasc Interv. 2011;4:579-585 in press.

CHAPTER 12

Closure of Atrial Septal Defects

Wail Alkashkari, Qi-Ling Cao, and Ziyad M. Hijazi

DEFINITION

An atrial septal defect (ASD) is a miscommunication between the right atrium (RA) and left atrium (LA) due to abnormal septation leading to shunting of oxygenated blood from the LA to RA with potential pathological complications.

EMBRYOLOGY

It is important to know how the atrial septum develops to understand an ASD.[1] During embryological development, the LA and RA are formed with the growth of atrial septum. This dividing wall between the atria originates with the growth of two separate septa: septum primum and septum secundum. The first to be formed is the septum primum, which grows from the superior aspect of the atrial wall inferiorly, toward the endocardial cushion between the atria and ventricles.

In its normal development, the septum primum attaches to the endocardial cushion, with eventually resorption of its superior attachment. Concurrently, a second septum develops slightly to the right of the septum primum, with progressive growth from the superior aspect of the atrium toward the endocardial cushion, but does not reach or attach to this area. Therefore, when developed, the septum primum attaches inferiorly to the floor of atrial cavity and the septum secundum attaches superiorly to the roof of the atria. Together, these two septa overlap to form the basis of

interatrial septum, between which the foramen ovale is formed. The foramen ovale is a flap valve communication between the RA and LA, which in utero allows oxygenated blood from the placenta to preferentially crossover to the left side of the heart and perfuse the upper body. Shortly after birth, the pulmonary vascular resistance drops. Consequently, the left atrial pressure rises above the right atrial pressure, resulting in functional closure of the foramen ovale. In the majority of patients, this leads to fibrosis and scarring with ultimate closure of the flap valve communication.

ANATOMY

There are four types of ASDs:

1. Secundum ASD (75% of cases): It is located at the level of the fossa ovalis. It is caused by a single or multiple defects of the thin flap valve of the fossa ovale. From the RA side, the defect is bordered by the limbus of the fossa ovalis or the C-shaped septum secundum. The limbic septum separates the defect from the atrial walls, orifices of the venae cavae, and atrioventricular (AV) valves. The secundum ASD usually presents as an isolated lesion or can be part of complex congenital heart disease (CHD). The isolated form can be associated with mitral valve prolapse. Valvular pulmonic stenosis is also frequently described in association with ASD.[2,3]
2. Primum ASD (15% to 20%): It is positioned inferiorly near the crux of the heart. Primum ASD is a result

of the deficiency of endocardial cushion tissue. As a form of atrioventricular septal defect (AVSD), the primum ASD is nearly always accompanied by a cleft in the anterior mitral valve leaflet.

3. Sinus venosus ASD (5% to 10%): It is located superiorly near the superior vena caval entry or inferiorly near the inferior vena caval entry. Sinus venosus ASD results from an error in the incorporation of the sinus venosus chamber into the RA. Sinus venosus ASDs are frequently (up to 90%) associated with partial anomalous venous drainage of the right pulmonary veins.

4. Coronary sinus septal defect (less than 1%): The defect is in the wall (roof) separating the coronary sinus from the LA. It causes shunting from the LA to RA through the ostium of the coronary sinus. It may be accompanied by partial or total anomalous pulmonary venous connection and/or a persistent left superior vena cava (SVC) draining to the coronary sinus.

The patent foramen ovale (PFO) is a flap-like communication in which the septum primum covering the fossa ovalis overlaps the superior limbic band of the septum secundum. In some patients, the septum primum or secundum is aneurysmal and may have multiple small fenestrations.

PREVALENCE

ASDs are relatively frequent, accounting for about 10% of all CHDs. Females constitute 65% to 75% of patients with secundum ASDs, but the gender distribution is equal for sinus venosus and ostium primum ASDs.[4]

GENETIC FACTORS

Down syndrome is associated primarily with "AV septal defects or ostium primum defects where AV stands for atrioventricular", but secundum defects also occur with increased frequency. Approximately 40% of subjects with Down syndrome have CHD. Of these, 40% have an AVSD, usually the complete form. Ostium primum ASDs may also be associated with DiGeorge syndrome and Ellis-Van Creveld syndrome. Adults with AVSDs have an approximate 10% risk of recurrence of heart disease in their offspring. ASDs are the most common cardiac manifestation of Holt-Oram syndrome,[4] which has been shown to be caused by mutations of TBX5.3. The familial forms of secundum ASDs have also been associated with GATA4 and NKX2.5 mutations. Conduction abnormalities are very common among them. At present, only the

secundum type is amenable to transcatheter closure and the following discussion focuses on the secundum ASD.

PATHOPHYSIOLOGY

The pathophysiology of an ASD is complex and multifactorial.[4] Flow across the defect occurs in both systole and diastole. In most patients, flow is predominantly left to right, but transient right-to-left shunting is common, particularly with isometric strain. The bulk of the shunt flow occurs during diastole. In this phase, blood in each atrium has two alternative pathways: following the normal route through the AV valve to the ventricle on that side or passing through the ASD to fill the opposite ventricle. The direction of flow across the ASD during diastole is determined by the instantaneous differences in the compliance and the capacity of the two ventricles. Ventricular chamber compliance is determined to a large extent by afterload. (Other factors such as intravascular volume status, myocardial muscle mass, chamber geometry, coronary perfusion, and pericardial and intrathoracic pressures also contribute to the intrinsic distensibility of the chamber.) In an otherwise normal patient, the left ventricle (LV), pumping to the systemic circulation, faces a substantially larger workload than the right ventricle (RV), pumping to the lungs. The LV becomes physiologically hypertrophied, reflecting its level of work, whereas the RV myocardium remains thin. The thick-walled LV will stretch/distend to accept additional volume less readily than the thinner RV. As a result, in the usual ASD patient, the difference in chamber compliance favors a left-to-right shunt because the blood in the LA finds it easier to fill the more compliant RV.

In patients with increased RV afterload resulting from congenital obstructions in the pulmonary arteries or veins, or with high pulmonary vascular resistance resulting from pulmonary parenchymal disease or primary pulmonary hypertension, the RV will be hypertrophied and less compliant. Left-to-right shunting at the ASD may be minimal, reflecting little overall difference between the two ventricles. With more severe RV noncompliance or distensibility, flow across the ASD may be predominantly from right to left. In some patients with reduced RV compliance, the RV may be able to handle a normal cardiac output at rest but will not readily accept additional flow (when cardiac output increases), and a right-to-left shunt may occur only with exertion. Other factors such as a prior RV myocardial infarction, extrinsic compression of the RV, or any associated congenital abnormality that results in

RV or tricuspid valve hypoplasia may reduce the effective RV capacity and impede its filling. When the AV valves are closed, ventricular compliance no longer affects blood flow across the defect at the atrial level.

Several factors determine flow volume and direction in systole. As in diastole, the size of the defect is a critical determinant in the volume but not the direction of flow. The atria may have differential capacities or compliances themselves, which may affect flow direction during systole. In patients with a large left-to-right shunt in diastole, pulmonary venous return will exceed systemic venous return (because $Q_P > Q_S$). Volumes in the two atria tend to equilibrate during systole, resulting in a left to right flow during that phase of the cardiac cycle. AV valve regurgitation may also affect the direction of ASD flow during systole. Significant mitral or tricuspid regurgitation may impede flow across an ASD, increasing or decreasing shunting during systole. Finally, the size of the ASD itself helps to determine the volume of shunting. If the ASD is large, the defect creates little or no resistance to flow. Blood flow across the defect in diastole is determined entirely by the relative properties of the ventricles as previously described. With a smaller, restrictive defect, blood flow is limited by the resistance of the ASD itself, no matter how large the difference in ventricular compliance.

NATURAL HISTORY

In a patient with an ASD, shunt direction and magnitude are variable and age dependent. In fetal life, RV noncompliance, a result of high pulmonary vascular resistance, allows nearly unidirectional right to left flow at the atrial level. Immediately after birth, with RV compliance comparable to that of the LV, there may be little net shunting through an ASD. Over several months, with the physiological fall in pulmonary vascular resistance, the RV thins, compliance falls, and the typical left-to-right shunt develops in children and young adults. As a result of normal physiological changes associated with aging, the LV myocardium tends to become more hypertrophied and less compliant.[5] With similarly sized ASDs, therefore, adults tend to have larger shunts as they age. It is part of the reason why children are rarely symptomatic, but patients in their fourth or fifth decade may begin to develop the symptoms frequently associated with ASD.

Clinical Presentation

In childhood, most children with ASD present with a murmur and are asymptomatic. Occasionally, infants may present with breathlessness, recurrent chest infections, and even heart failure. Failure to thrive is uncommon presentation. In the current era, many children are referred to a pediatric cardiologist for spurious reasons and found to have an ASD on echocardiographic evaluation.

There are four common clinical presentations of ASD in the adult population. Most frequently, adult patients complain of progressive shortness of breath with exertion. Studies have shown a reduction in maximum oxygen consumption in the unrepaired ASD population because of the inherent inefficiency of a continuously preload-reduced LV in combination with a volume overload in the pulmonary circulation. After repair of the ASD, exercise capacity improves within days to weeks.[6,7] Atrial arrhythmias, resulting from stretching of the conduction system, may be the first presenting sign of an ASD. An adult who presents with atrial arrhythmia at a young age should be evaluated for dilatation of the right-side cardiac chambers and evidence of an atrial level shunt. Prevention of long-term atrial fibrillation is one of the reasons for repairing ASD in young asymptomatic patients,[8] although the subsequent development of atrial fibrillation may depend more on the patient's age at intervention and may occur despite surgery in patients older than 25 years of age.[9]

Although both RA and RV volumes are reduced acutely with ASD repair and both chambers return to normal dimensions in children, there appears to be persistent RA enlargement when the ASD is closed in adult patients.[10] This may explain an ongoing, increased risk of atrial fibrillation after adult ASD repairs compared with patients who underwent closure at a younger age.[11] Rarely, a patient with ASD will present with stroke or other systemic ischemic event caused by paradoxical embolization of thrombus through the defect,[12] similar to the PFO. Although most patients have a significant net left-to-right shunt through the defect, virtually all have transient flow reversal with the Valsalva maneuver or other isometric strain. A small number of adult patients may also be identified on echocardiograph when a heart murmur or unrelated cardiac symptoms in the absence of exercise, rhythm, or embolic symptoms bring them to a physician's attention.

Pulmonary hypertension is uncommon with ASD, even in patients with large defects, in part because of the large capacitance of the pulmonary bed. Natural history studies dating to the presurgical and pre-echocardiography eras suggested an incidence of more than 15% in the ASD population.[13] The observations that pulmonary vascular disease may develop in patients with a tiny ASD and that it is absent in the vast majority of patients with large ASDs suggest that the ASD may be an associated marker of pulmonary hypertension but not necessarily causative. More recent reviews suggest a rate of 6% to 9%.[14,15] Once a patient has reached adulthood with normal PA pressures, the natural history is established. They no longer develop significant pulmonary hypertension related to the shunt, but they may have pressure elevation, like any other patient, as a result of the development of pulmonary parenchymal disease, left-sided heart dysfunction, or obstructive sleep apnea. It would be fair to say that the overall risk of and specific risk factors for developing pulmonary vascular disease with an ASD remain unknown.

When severe pulmonary hypertension from any cause results in RV systolic failure, high RV end-systolic volumes impede filling from the RA. With an intact atrial septum, there is systemic venous stasis and symptoms of "classic" right-heart congestive failure (anasarca and low cardiac output) because the LV can pump out only what it receives back from the lungs. In a patient with pulmonary hypertension and an ASD, however, the defect allows decompression of the right heart via a right-to-left shunt. The systemic venous blood does not need to traverse the lungs to reach the LV. It may cross through the ASD, mixing with the pulmonary venous return in the LA, to augment LV preload. These patients are cyanotic from the right-to-left shunt and show minimal response to supplemental oxygen.[16] However, tissue oxygen delivery is often better than in the patient without an ASD because the detrimental reduction in blood oxygen content is far outweighed by the maintenance of a normal or nearly normal cardiac output. For this reason, it is likely that repair of adult patients with ASD and moderate or severe pulmonary hypertension may not improve survival. Similarly, in patients with end-stage primary pulmonary hypertension, the creation of an ASD has been demonstrated to be of benefit in prolonging life and as a bridge to lung transplantation.[17]

Symptoms

Symptoms may include the following:

- Reduced exercise tolerance, tiredness
- Exertional dyspnea
- Palpitations (due to supraventricular arrhythmias, frequent atrial fibrillation/atrial flutter in older age), or syncope for sick sinus syndrome
- Atypical chest pain (right ventricular ischemia)
- Frequent respiratory tract infections
- Signs of right-heart failure

- Paradoxical embolism from peripheral venous or pelvic vein thrombosis, atrial arrhythmias, unfiltered intravenous infusion, or indwelling venous catheters.

Physical Examination

- The patients are usually pink; cyanosis suggests severe pulmonary hypertension with reversed shunting in the presence of a secundum ASD or superior sinus venosus defect; cyanosis can also reflect associated pulmonary stenosis, a coronary sinus defect, or an inferior sinus venosus defect (with a prominent Eustachian valve directing the blood to the LA).
- Right ventricular heave, but the left ventricular impulse is usually normal.
- Wide and fixed split of the second heart sound above the pulmonary artery (PA) (delayed PA valve closure); a loud pulmonary component reflects severe pulmonary hypertension.
- Ejection systolic murmur heard best at the left sternal border (increased blood flow through the PA orifice [relative pulmonary stenosis]); sometimes, a pulmonary ejection click can be heard.
- Diastolic murmur at the lower right sternal border due to increased blood flow through the tricuspid orifice specially if the $Q_P:Q_S$ ratio is more than 2.5:1 (relative tricuspid stenosis).
- Examination should also focus on the status of the left heart pathology; for example, a pansystolic murmur can be heard in the presence of mitral regurgitation on the apex. The clinical findings and auscultation may be completely discrete and unremarkable.

LABORATORY FINDINGS

Chest Radiography

The chest X-ray film is often, but not always, abnormal in patients with significant ASDs.

Cardiomegaly may be present from right heart dilation, and occasionally from left heart dilation if significant mitral regurgitation is present in the patient with an ostium primum ASD. Right heart dilation is better appreciated in lateral films. The central pulmonary arteries are characteristically enlarged, with pulmonary plethora indicating increased pulmonary flow. A small aortic knuckle is characteristic, which reflects a chronically low systemic cardiac output state, because increased pulmonary flow in these patients occurs at the expense of reduced systemic flow.

Electrocardiogram

The electrocardiogram (ECG) may be an important clue to diagnosis. The rhythm may be sinus, atrial fibrillation, or atrial flutter. Inverted P waves in the inferior leads suggest an absent or deficient sinus node, as may be seen in a sinus venosus defect. RA overload is often present. First-degree heart block suggests a primum ASD but may be seen in older patients with a secundum ASD. The QRS axis is typically rightward in secundum ASD, markedly so if pulmonary hypertension is present. The QRS axis is leftward or extremely to the right in ostium primum ASDs. Voltage evidence of RV hypertrophy may be seen in all ASDs, often in the form of "incomplete" right bundle-branch block, with the more extreme forms usually found in patients with pulmonary hypertension. Patients with mitral valve insufficiency may have LV hypertrophy or LA overload.

Crochetage, a notch seen in the QRS in lead II and III, has also been reported in secundum ASD.

Echocardiography

In the adult, transthoracic echocardiography (TTE) may be diagnostic, demonstrating a clearly visible defect in the atrial septum, best seen in the apical four-chamber and subcostal long-axis views. However, it is common to see "echo fallout" in the region of the interatrial septum and this may lead to misdiagnosis of an ASD or incorrectly describing the ASD as echo fallout. Improvements in two-dimensional (2D) echocardiography with harmonic imaging have improved the diagnostic accuracy of echocardiography. It is worth highlighting some key points regarding the use of these imaging modalities:

- Bubble contrast echocardiography with provocation has led to the accurate diagnosis of interatrial communications.
- The stability of the image is checked during provocation maneuvers. These maneuvers are performed to transiently increase RA pressure and to provoke shunting through a potential interatrial communication.
- Typical maneuvers include a sharp nasal sniff, a cough, or the relaxation phase of the Valsalva maneuver.
- A positive test sees the rapid transit of bubbles from the right to the left heart within three to five cardiac cycles.
- The amount or number of bubbles seen is related to the size of the defect. Late transit (>5 cardiac cycles) of bubbles is associated with intrapulmonary shunting.

In addition to demonstrating the defect, TTE can demonstrate the hemodynamic consequences of the left-to-right shunt:

- Dilation of the RA and RV
- Tricuspid valve annular dilation with associated tricuspid incompetence
- Estimation of the peak right ventricular systolic pressure and, in the absence of pulmonary valve stenosis, an estimate of the systolic PA pressure.

Associated lesions of the mitral valve (mitral valve prolapse, mitral stenosis), tricuspid valve (Ebstein anomaly), and anomalous pulmonary venous drainage can also be looked for.

In the current era of percutaneous device closure of interatrial communications, transesophageal echocardiography (TEE) or intracardiac echocardiography (ICE) are mandatory prior to consideration of device closure. Many centers will do this immediately prior to a planned device closure. The key points regarding this include:

- Demonstration of all four pulmonary veins draining to the LA is essential prior to device closure of oval fossa defects.
- Ten percent of secundum ASD have anomalous pulmonary venous drainage, most commonly of the right upper pulmonary vein.
- Exclude a superior sinus venosus defect, in the long axis 90-degree view and at 0 degree.
- Measure the margins of the atrial septum for suitability for device closure.
- A detailed mitral valve assessment is mandatory prior to closure as mitral incompetence is a potential complication of device closure.
- The severity of mitral stenosis and regurgitation are often underestimated in the presence of an ASD.
- Closure of a defect in the context of significant mitral valve disease will likely worsen symptoms rather than improve them.
- Exclude intracardiac thrombus.

The roles of three-dimensional echocardiography and cardiac magnetic resonance imaging (MRI) have yet to be fully evaluated in the assessment of ASDs, although both may have a role in noninvasively defining which patients are suitable for device closure of the defect.

Cardiac Magnetic Resonance Imaging/ Computed Tomography

MRI provides an additional noninvasive imaging modality if findings by echocardiography are uncertain. Direct visualization of the defect and pulmonary veins is possible, RV volume and function can be quantified, and estimates of shunt size can also be obtained

Contrast-enhanced ultrafast cine computed tomography (CT) can also provide diagnostic information, even though the radiation exposure limits its utility in most cases.

Cardiac Catheterization

Diagnostic cardiac catheterization is not required for uncomplicated ASDs in younger patients with adequate noninvasive imaging. It is generally reserved for investigation of coronary artery disease in those patients at risk by virtue of age or family history and for whom surgical intervention is planned, and to assess pulmonary vascular resistance and reactivity in patients with significant pulmonary arterial hypertension (PAH). Catheterization may also be required to evaluate ASD size, pulmonary venous return, and associated valvular disease if noninvasive methods have been unable to provide this information. In most instances, catheterization is now performed in conjunction with device closure of the defect.[18,19]

Exercise Testing

Exercise testing can be useful to document exercise capacity in patients with symptoms that are discrepant with clinical findings or to document changes in oxygen saturation in patients with PAH. However, maximal exercise testing is not recommended in ASD with severe PAH.

MANAGEMENT OF SECUNDUM ATRIAL SEPTAL DEFECT

A hemodynamically significant ASD requiring closure is said to exist if there is right ventricular volume overload. There is no real role for medical management of a hemodynamically significant ASD. In rare circumstances, a diuretic may be used to decrease pulmonary congestion, and afterload-reducing agents have a theoretical role in decreasing systemic relative to pulmonary vascular resistance (thereby decreasing the left-to-right shunt).

INDICATIONS FOR PERCUTANEOUS CLOSURE OF SECUNDUM ATRIAL SEPTAL DEFECT

Large defects with evidence of RV volume overload on echocardiography usually only cause symptoms in the third decade of life or beyond, and closure is usually indicated to prevent long-term complications even if the patient is asymptomatic.

It is of great importance to understand the natural history of unrepaired ASD as mentioned earlier to understand why we are keen to close the hemodynamically significant ASD even in asymptomatic patients. It is mainly to prevent long-term complications,[4] including premature death, atrial arrhythmias, reduced exercise tolerance, hemodynamically significant TR, right-to-left shunting, embolism during pregnancy, overt congestive cardiac failure, or pulmonary vascular disease that may develop in up to 5% to 10% of affected (mainly female) individuals.

The development of symptoms or complications will not preclude the patients with ASD from closure regardless of age. The closure will prevent further deterioration and probably will reverse or normalize some of the complications, especially RV dilatation, RV failure, tricuspid regurgitation, atrial flutter, or atrial fibrillation.[4] Defect closure may be complemented with radio-frequency ablation, ablation of cavotricuspid isthmus, or atrial surgery (Maze procedure). If the patient developed PAH, complete assessment of reversibility of pulmonary vascular disease should be done before closure, and closure may be considered in the presence of net left-to-right shunting, PA pressure less than two-thirds systemic levels, pulmonary valve regurgitation less than two-thirds systemic vascular resistance, or when responsive to either pulmonary vasodilator therapy or test occlusion of the defect. Patients should be treated in conjunction with providers who have expertise in the management of pulmonary hypertensive syndromes.

Closure of an ASD is also reasonable in the presence of paradoxical embolism and documented orthodeoxia-platypnea.[20,21] Closure of an ASD should be considered and discussed with the patients in some cases as prophylaxis, even if the defect is small. Examples being the professional diver and the patient undergoing pacemaker implantation due to their respective risks of decompression illness and paradoxical embolism.[20] Pregnancy and delivery are generally well tolerated, even by patients with an unclosed ASD with a significant left-to-right shunt. However, clinical symptoms may emerge or deteriorate during pregnancy or after childbirth. During pregnancy and delivery, there is an increased risk of paradoxical embolism, regardless of the defect size. It is more appropriate in our opinion to close the defect before planned pregnancy even if it is hemodynamically not significant. Sudden major loss of blood, leading to hypovolemia, systemic vasoconstriction, reduced venous return, increase in the left-to-right shunt, and a decrease in cardiac output, is poorly tolerated. Pregnancy is contraindicated in patients with Eisenmenger syndrome.

CONTRAINDICATIONS FOR PERCUTANEOUS CLOSURE OF SECUNDUM ATRIAL SEPTAL DEFECT

- Small ASDs with a diameter of less than 5 mm and no evidence of RV volume overload do not impact the natural history of the individual and thus may not require closure unless associated with paradoxical embolism.
- An absolute contraindication for percutaneous ASD closure is the development of severe irreversible PAH and no evidence of a left-to-right shunt.

Other contraindications include:

- Poor state of the patient with other serious conditions or comorbidities
- Patients with current systemic or local infection/sepsis within 1 month of device placement
- Patients with bleeding disorder, or with other contraindications to aspirin therapy, unless another antiplatelet drug can be administered for 6 months
- Patients with severe LV dysfunction and elevated left ventricular end-diastolic pressure (>14 mm Hg) is present and the ASD is functioning as a pop-off valve for the systemic ventricle,[4] closure should not be performed unless the LV function is optimized and the hemodynamic data before the ASD closure (balloon test occlusion) prove that the left ventricular end-diastolic pressure will not rise significantly.
- Patients allergic to nickel may suffer an allergic reaction. This is a relative contraindication. Most nickel allergies are contact reactions. It is unclear if intracardiac devices will mount a similar reaction. A consultation with an allergist may be needed.
- Presence of intracardiac thrombus

Surgical closure is indicated in the following conditions:

- Patients with associated cardiac anomalies requiring cardiac surgery
- Patients with other types of ASD (primum ASD, sinus venosus ASD, coronary sinus defect)
- Unsuitable defect anatomy including deficient superior/inferior or posterior rims. Deficient anterior rim is not a contraindication for the use of percutaneous closure devices.

Currently, two devices are approved by the U.S. Food and Drug Administration for the percutaneous closure of secundum ASD: the Amplatzer septal

occluder (AGA Medical, Plymouth, MN) and the Gore Helex septal occluder device (W.L. Gore & Associates, Flagstaff, AZ). Outside the United States, there are multiple other devices that are being used for closure of secundum ASD, including the Amplatzer septal occluder (ASO), the Gore Helex device, the Figulla-Occlutech device, the Cardia Intrasept device, and the Lifetech ASD device. In this chapter, we discuss only the two devices that are approved in the United States.

DEVICE DESCRIPTION

The Amplatzer Septal Occluder

Figure 12-1 demonstrates the two disks and the connecting waist of the ASO.

The ASO is a self-expandable, double-disk device made of nitinol (55% nickel; 45% titanium) wire mesh constructed from a 0.004- to 0.0075-inch nitinol. The ASO is tightly woven into two flat disks. There is a 3 to 4 mm connecting waist between the two disks, corresponding to the thickness of the atrial septum. Nitinol has superelastic properties, with shape memory. This allows the device to be stretched into an almost linear configuration and placed inside a small sheath for delivery and then to return to its original configuration within the heart when not constrained by the sheath. The device size is determined by the diameter of its waist and is constructed in various sizes ranging from 4 to 40 mm (1-mm increments up to 20 mm; 2-mm increments up to the largest device currently available, 40 mm; the 40 mm size is not available in the United

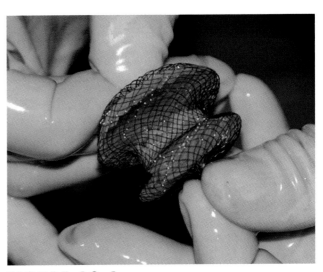

FIGURE 12-1.

The Amplatzer septal occluder device with its two disks and connecting waist.

States). The two flat disks extend radially beyond the central waist to provide secure anchorage.

Patients with secundum ASD usually have left-to-right shunt. Therefore, the LA disk is larger than the RA disk. For devices 4 to 10 mm in size, the LA disk is 12 mm and the RA disk is 8 mm larger than the waist. However, for devices larger than 11 mm and up to 32 mm in size, the LA disk is 14 mm and the RA disk is 10 mm larger than the connecting waist. For devices ≥32 mm, the LA disk is 16 mm larger than the waist and the RA disk is 10 mm larger than the waist. Both disks are angled slightly toward each other to ensure firm contact of the disks to the atrial septum.

A total of three Dacron polyester patches are sewn securely with polyester thread into each disk and the connecting waist to increase the thrombogenicity of the device. A stainless steel sleeve with a female thread is laser-welded to the RA disk. This sleeve is used to screw the delivery cable to the device. For device deployment, we recommend using a 6 French delivery system for devices less than 10 mm in diameter; a 7 French delivery system for devices 10 to 15 mm; an 8 French sheath for devices 16 to 19 mm; a 9 French sheath for devices 20 to 26 mm; a 10 French sheath for devices 28 to 34 mm; a 12 French sheath for the 36 and 38 mm device; and a 14 French sheath for the 40 mm device. Each device, excluding the delivery system, costs $5,000.

Amplatzer Delivery System

The delivery system is supplied sterilized and separate from the device. It contains all the equipment needed to facilitate device deployment. It consists of a delivery sheath of specified French size and length and appropriate dilator; a loading device, used to collapse the device and introduce it into the delivery sheath; a delivery cable (internal diameter [ID], 0.081 inch); a plastic pin vise which facilitates unscrewing of the delivery cable from the device during device deployment; Tuohy-Borst adapter with a side arm for the sheath to act as a one-way stop-bleed valve; and the device is screwed onto its distal end and it allows for loading, placement, and retrieval of the device.

All delivery sheaths have a 45-degree angled tip. The 6 French sheath has a length of 60 cm, the 7 French sheath is available in lengths of 60 and 80 cm, and the 8, 9, 10, and 12 French sheaths are 80 cm long.

The Amplatzer Exchange (Rescue) System

This is made up of the same components as the delivery system with the one exception being that the inner lumen and tip of the dilator can accommodate the delivery cable. It is available in two sizes, 9 French (dilator ID, 0.087 inch) and 12 French (dilator ID, 0.113 inch), with a 45-degree curve and 80 cm length. The distal tip of the delivery cable can screw into the back of another delivery cable. This allows it to become an exchange length cable. The damaged sheath then can be removed and the rescue sheath with its dilator can be inserted over the cable to recapture the device. The exchange system costs $580.

Optional but Recommended Equipment

1. Amplatzer sizing balloon: a double-lumen balloon catheter with a 7 French shaft size. The balloon is made from nylon and is very compliant, making it ideal for sizing secundum ASD by "stop-flow" and without overstretching of the defect. The balloon catheter is angled at 45 degrees and there are radio-opaque markers for calibration at 2, 5, and 10 mm. The balloon catheters are available in three sizes: 18 mm (maximum volume is 20 mL and is used for defects up to 20 mm); 24 mm (maximum volume 30 mL and used to size defects up to 22 mm); and 34 mm (maximum volume 90 mL and used to size defects up to 40 mm).
2. Amplatzer super stiff exchange guidewire 0.035 inch: used to advance the delivery sheath and dilator into the left upper pulmonary vein.

Table 12-1 summarizes all the necessary materials for ASD closure.

Step-by-Step Technique

TRANSCATHETER DEVICE CLOSURE OF SECUNDUM ATRIAL SEPTAL DEFECT MATERIALS AND EQUIPMENT
1. Single or bi-plane cardiac catheterization laboratory
2. TEE or ICE
3. Full range of device sizes, delivery and exchange (rescue) systems
4. Sizing balloon catheters
5. A multipurpose (MP) catheter to engage the defect and the left upper pulmonary vein

TABLE 12-1 Materials/Equipment Required for Transcatheter Procedures

Item	Size	Cost Each ($)
Amplatzer septal occluder	4–40 mm	5,000
Amplatzer delivery system	7–12 French	580
Amplatzer super stiff exchange wire	0.035 inch	45
Multipurpose catheter	6–7 French	10
Amplatzer sizing balloon	18, 24, 34 mm	265
Amplatzer rescue system	9, 12 French	580

6. Super-stiff exchange length wire—we prefer the 0.035-inch Amplatzer super stiff exchange length guidewire with a 1 cm floppy tip, but any extra stiff J-tipped wire may be used.

PERSONNEL

1. Interventional cardiologist appropriately proctored to perform device closure
2. Cardiologist, noninvasive to facilitate TEE or ICE
3. Anesthesiologist, if procedure is performed under TEE guidance
4. Nurse certified to administer medications if procedure is performed under conscious sedation, usually using ICE guidance
5. Catheterization laboratory technologists

Method

PREPROCEDURE

Review all pertinent data relating to the patient and to the defect to be closed and ensure that appropriate devices and delivery systems are available. The procedure and complications should be explained to the patient/family and opportunity given to ask questions. All preprocedure orders should be given to the patient. Aspirin 81 to 325 mg should be started 48 hours prior to the procedure. If allergic to aspirin, clopidogrel 75 mg should be used.

ACCESS

The right femoral vein is accessed using a 7 to 8 French short sheath. An arterial monitoring line can be inserted in the right femoral artery, especially if the patient's condition is marginal or if the procedure is performed under TEE and general endotracheal anesthesia. If the femoral venous route is not available, we advocate the transhepatic approach. If a subclavian or internal jugular venous approach is used, it is very difficult to maneuver the device deployment, especially with large defects.

We administer heparin to achieve an activated clotting time (ACT) of more than 200 seconds at the time of device deployment. Antibiotic coverage for the procedure is recommended. We usually use cefazolin 1 g intravenously—the first dose at the time of procedure and two subsequent doses 6 to 8 hours apart.

Figures 12-2 and 12-3 demonstrate ICE images in a patient during sizing of a large secundum ASD and

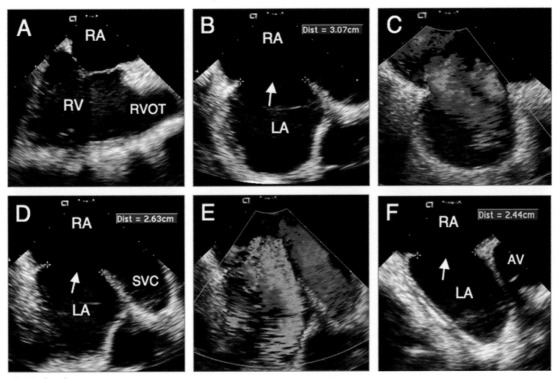

FIGURE 12-2.

Intracardiac echocardiographic images in a patient with a large secundum atrial septal defect (ASD). **A:** Home view demonstrating the right atrium, tricuspid valve, right ventricle, and right ventricle outflow tract. **B:** Septal view, demonstrating the large ASD (*arrow*), the right and left atria, and the superior and inferior rims. **C:** Same view with color Doppler. **D,E:** Caval view with and without color Doppler demonstrating the entire superior rim and the defect (*arrow*). **F:** Short-axis view demonstrating the defect (*arrow*), the aortic root, the deficient anterior rim, acceptable posterior rim, and both atria. AV, aortic valve; LA, left atrium; RA, right atrium; RV, right ventricle; RVOT, right ventricle outflow tract; SVC, superior vena cava.

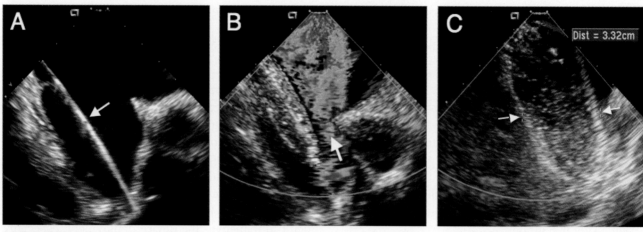

FIGURE 12-3.

Intracardiac echocardiographic images in the patient in Figure 12-2, showing defect sizing. **A:** The exchange wire (*arrow*) across the defect into the left upper pulmonary vein. **B:** Sizing balloon during inflation still showing residual shunt (*arrow*). **C:** Full balloon occlusion occluding the defect. This is the stretched "stop-flow" diameter (*arrows*) of the defect.

the sizing of the defect. Figure 12-4 demonstrates the cineangiographic images appearance in a patient with a secundum ASD.

Routine right-heart catheterization should be performed in all cases to ensure presence of normal pulmonary vascular resistance. The left-to-right shunt can also be calculated.

Echocardiographic assessment of the secundum ASD should be performed simultaneously using either TEE or ICE. A comprehensive study should be performed, looking at all aspects of the ASD anatomy

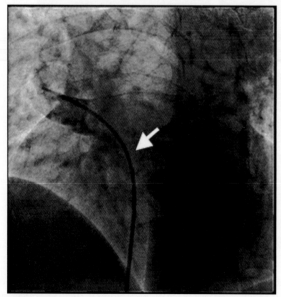

FIGURE 12-4.

An angiogram in the right upper pulmonary vein in the four-chamber view demonstrating left-to-right shunt (*arrow*) via the secundum atrial septal defect.

(location, size, presence of additional defects, and adequacy of the various rims). Figure 12-2 demonstrates the full assessment of the defect by ICE.

RIMS

The important rims to look for are:

- Superior/SVC rim—best achieved using the bicaval view
- Superior posterior/right upper pulmonary vein rim
- Anterior superior/aortic rim—the least important rim; often, patients lack it
- Inferior vena cava (IVC) and coronary sinus rim—an important rim to have
- Posterior rim—seen best in the short-axis view at the aortic valve level.

The rims must not be deficient (<5 mm) except the anterior rim because a deficient anterior rim is not a contraindication to perform the procedure.

HOW TO CROSS THE ATRIAL SEPTAL DEFECT

Use an MP catheter; the MP A2 catheter has the ideal angle. Place the catheter at the junction of the IVC and the RA. The IVC angle should guide the catheter to the ASD. Keep a clockwise torque on the catheter while advancing it toward the septum (posterior). If unsuccessful, place the catheter in the SVC and slowly pull it into the RA; keep a clockwise posterior torque to orient the catheter along the atrial septum until it crosses the defect. TEE/ICE can be very useful to guide the catheter across difficult defects.

Figures 12-4 and 12-5 demonstrate cineangiographic images of the patient in Figure 12-3 during balloon

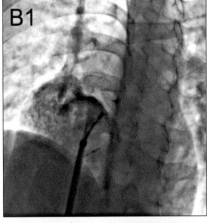

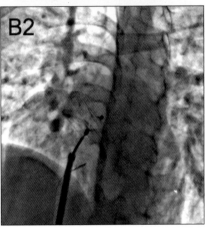

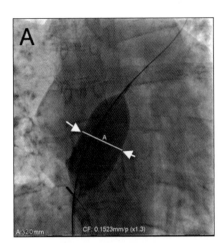

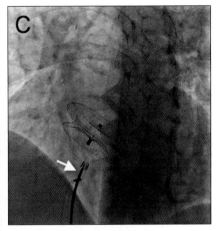

FIGURE 12-5.

A: Cine image during balloon occlusion of the defect (*arrows*). **B1:** Angiogram via the side arm of the delivery sheath demonstrating opacification of the right atrial disk. **B2:** Pulmonary levophase showing only left atrial disk opacifies. **C:** Cine image after the device has been released showing good device position parallel to the atrial septum. Compare profile of the atrial septum in this image with Figure 12-4 profile of the atrial septum.

sizing of the defect, demonstrating the stretched diameter (*arrows*) of the defect.

RIGHT UPPER PULMONARY VEIN ANGIOGRAM

It can be useful to perform an angiogram in the right upper pulmonary vein (Fig. 12-4) in the hepatoclavicular projection (35 degrees, left anterior oblique/35 degrees, cranial). This delineates the anatomy, shape, and length of the septum. This may come in handy when the device is deployed but not released—the operator can position the I/I (tube/flat detector) in the same view of the angiogram and compare the position of the device with that obtained during the deployment.

Figure 12-6 demonstrates ICE images showing device delivery and deployment.

DEFECT SIZING

Position the MP catheter in the left upper pulmonary vein. Prepare the appropriate size balloon according to the manufacturer's guidelines. We prefer to use

the 34-mm balloon since it is longer and during inflation, it sits nicely across the defect. Pass an extra-stiff, floppy/J-tipped 0.035-inch exchange length guidewire (Fig. 12-3A). This gives the best support within the atrium for the balloon, especially in large defects. Remove the MP catheter and the femoral sheath. We advance the sizing balloon catheter directly over the wire without a venous sheath. Most sizing balloons require an 8 or 9 French sheath. The balloon catheter is advanced over the wire and placed across the defect under both fluoroscopic and echocardiographic guidance. The balloon is then inflated with diluted contrast until the left-to-right shunt ceases, as observed by color flow Doppler TEE/ICE (flow occlusion). Once shunt ceases, deflate the balloon slightly until shunt reappears. This is called "stop-flow" technique, and that is what we rely on to select a device size. The best echo view for measurement is to observe the balloon in its long axis (Fig. 12-3B,C). In this view, the indentation

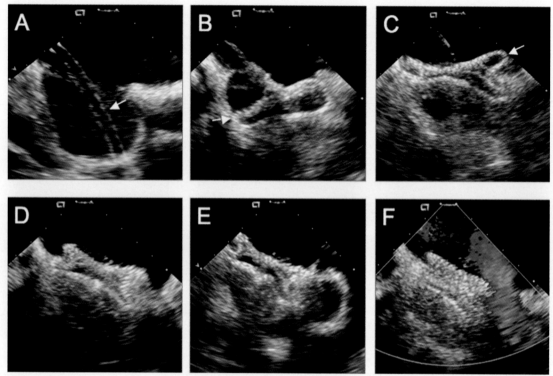

FIGURE 12-6.

Intracardiac echocardiographic images of the patient in Figure 12-2, showing device delivery and deployment. **A:** Delivery sheath (*arrow*) across the defect into the left upper pulmonary vein. **B:** The left atrial disk (*arrow*) deployed in the left atrium. **C:** The right atrial disk (*arrow*) deployed in the right atrium. **D:** The device released, demonstrating good position. Color Doppler **(E)** short-axis view and **(F)** long-axis view, both demonstrating good device position and no residual shunt.

made by the margins of the ASD can be visualized and precise measurement can be made.

FLUOROSCOPIC MEASUREMENT

Angulate the X-ray tube so the beam is perpendicular to the balloon. This can be difficult but the various calibration markers can help. Ensure that the markers are separated and discrete. Measure the balloon diameter at the site of the indentation (or at the middle of the balloon) as per the diagnostic function of the laboratory (Fig. 12-5A). If a discrepancy exists between the echocardiographic and the fluoroscopic measurements, we have found that the echocardiographic measurement is usually more accurate.

Once the size is determined, deflate the balloon and pull it back into the junction of the RA and IVC, leaving the wire in the left upper pulmonary vein.

This is a good time to recheck the ACT and give the first dose of antibiotics.

DEVICE SELECTION

If the defect has adequate rims (>5 mm), select a device 0 to 2 mm larger than the "stop-flow" diameter of

the balloon. However, if the superior/anterior rim is deficient (5 to 7 mm), we tend to select a device 4 mm larger than the balloon "stop-flow" diameter. Note that if the device size chosen is >50% larger than the 2D diameter of the defect, the operator should pause and rethink this size. We have found that oversizing by >50% from the 2D diameter can potentially lead to device erosion.

DEVICE DELIVERY

Once the device size is selected, open the appropriate-sized delivery system. Flush the sheath and dilator. The proper size of delivery sheath is advanced over the guidewire to the left upper pulmonary vein (Fig. 12-6A). Both dilator and wire are removed, keeping the tip of the sheath inside the left upper pulmonary vein. Extreme care must be exercised not to allow passage of air inside the delivery sheath. An alternative technique to minimize air embolism is passage of the sheath with the dilator over the wire until the IVC, at which point the dilator is removed and the sheath is advanced over the wire into the LA while continuously flushing the side arm of the sheath.

The device is then screwed to the tip of the delivery cable, immersed in normal saline, and drawn into the loader underwater seal to expel air bubbles out of the system. A Y connector is applied to the proximal end of the loader to allow flushing with saline. The loader containing the device is attached to the proximal hub of the delivery sheath. The cable with the ASO device is advanced to the distal tip of the sheath, taking care not to rotate the cable while advancing it in the long sheath to prevent premature unscrewing of the device. Both cable and delivery sheath are pulled back as one unit to the middle of the LA. Position of the sheath can be verified using the cine fluoroscopy or TEE/ICE.

DEVICE DEPLOYMENT

The LA disk is deployed first under fluoroscopic and/or echocardiographic guidance (Fig. 12-6B). Caution should be taken not to interfere with the LA appendage. Part of the connecting waist should be deployed in the LA, very close (a few millimeters) to the atrial septum (the mechanism of ASD closure using the ASO is stenting of the defect). While applying constant pulling of the entire assembly and withdrawing the delivery sheath off the cable, the connecting waist and the RA disk are deployed in the ASD itself and in the RA, respectively (Fig. 12-6C).

DEVICE POSITIONING

Proper device position can be verified using different techniques:

1. Fluoroscopy in the same projection as that of the angiogram: Good device position is evident by the presence of two disks that are parallel to each other and separated from each other by the atrial septum. In the same view, the operator can perform the "Minnesota wiggle" (the cable is pushed gently forward and pulled backward). Stable device position manifests by the lack of movement of the device in either direction.
2. TEE/ICE: The echocardiographer should make sure that one disk is in each chamber. The long-axis view should be sufficient to evaluate the superior and inferior part of the septum and the short-axis view for the anterior and posterior part of the disk.
3. Angiography: This is done with the camera in the same projection as for the first angiogram to profile the septum and device using either the side arm of the delivery sheath or a separate angiographic catheter, inserted in the sheath used for ICE or via a separate puncture site. Good device position manifests by opacification of the RA disk alone when the contrast is in the RA and opacification of the LA disk alone on pulmonary levophase (Fig. 12-5B1,B2).

If the position of the device is not certain, or is questionable, after all these maneuvers, the device can be recaptured, entirely or partly, and repositioned following similar steps.

DEVICE RELEASE

Once the device position is verified, the device is released by counterclockwise rotation of the delivery cable using a pin vise. There is often a notable change in the angle of the device as it is released from the slight tension of the delivery cable and it self-centers within the ASD and aligns with the interatrial septum. To assess the result of closure, repeat TEE/ICE (Fig. 12-6D–F), color Doppler, and angiography (optional) in the four-chamber projection in the RA with pulmonary levophase are performed. Patients receive a dose of an appropriate antibiotic (commonly cephazolin 1 g) during the catheterization procedure and two further doses at 8-hour intervals. Patients are also asked to take endocarditis prophylaxis when necessary for 6 months after the procedure, as well as aspirin 81 to 325 mg orally once daily for 6 months. In addition, we have been adding 75 mg clopidogrel for 2 to 3 months. We have observed that the incidence of postclosure headaches is much less in those patients taking the clopidogrel. Full activity, including competitive sports, is usually allowed after 4 weeks of implantation. MRI (if required) can be performed any time after implantation.

POSTPROCEDURE

Once the procedure is complete, recheck the ACT and, if appropriate, remove the sheath and achieve hemostasis. We use a figure-of-eight suture to achieve the hemostasis up to 14 French sheath. If larger sheaths are to be used, we use double per-close technique. Some use protamine sulfate to reverse the effect of heparin if the ACT is above 250 seconds.

PROCEDURE MONITORING

Patients recover overnight in a telemetry ward. Some patients may experience an increase in atrial ectopic beats. Rarely, some patients may have sustained atrial tachycardias. The following day, an ECG, a chest X-ray (posteroanterior and lateral [optional]), and a TTE with color Doppler should be performed to assess the position of the device and the presence of residual shunt.

A repeat chest X-ray 1 week after the procedure to look for device position is recommended but not mandatory.

Recheck ECG, chest X-ray, and TTE/TEE at 6 months postprocedure to assess everything. If device position is good, with no residual shunt, follow-up can be annual for the first 2 years, then every 3 to 5 years. Long-term follow-up of device performance should be assessed and any new information should be communicated to the patient.

The patient is asked not to engage in contact sports for 1 month after the procedure.

PROCEDURE MEDICATION

Aspirin and clopidogrel are given as described previously. Infective endocarditis prophylaxis should be given, when needed, for 6 to 12 months. After 6 to 12 months, if there is no residual shunt, prophylaxis and aspirin can be discontinued.

Troubleshooting

AIR EMBOLISM

Meticulous technique should be used to prevent air entry. The sheath should be positioned at the mouth of the left upper pulmonary vein. Doing so allows free flow of blood into the sheath. Forceful negative pressure should not be applied to aspirate the sheath. If a large amount of air is introduced on the left side, it will usually pool in the right coronary sinus and right coronary artery causing inferior ST segment elevation. This may manifest with bradycardia, asystole, or profound hypotension. If this occurs, immediately place a right coronary catheter in the right coronary sinus and forcefully inject saline or contrast to displace the air and hence reperfuse the right coronary system.

COBRA HEAD FORMATION

This describes the situation when the left disk maintains a high profile when deployed, mimicking a cobra head. This can occur if the left disk is opened in the pulmonary vein or the left atrial appendage, or if the LA is too small to accommodate the device. It can also occur if the device is defective or has been loaded with unusual strain on it. If this occurs, check the site of deployment; if appropriate, recapture the device and remove and inspect it. If the cobra head forms outside the body, use a different device. If the disk forms normally, try deploying the device again. Do not release a device if the left disk has a cobra head appearance.

DEVICE EMBOLIZATION

If a device embolizes, it has to be removed. This can be done surgically or by transcatheter snare and recapture into a long sheath. The transcatheter technique is difficult and should not be performed if the operator is inexperienced in snaring techniques. Furthermore, the catheter laboratory should be equipped with large Mullins-type sheaths (12 to 16 French) and should also have various-sized snares. We use the Amplatzer Goose Neck Snare (ev3, Plymouth, MN) or the Ensnare

(Merit Medical, Salt Lake City, UT). The device should not be pulled across valves because it may damage the chordae and leaflets. Always use a long sheath to pull the device outside the body. To snare a device, we usually use a sheath 2 French sizes larger than the sheath that was used to deliver the device. On rare occasions, if the LA disk cannot be collapsed inside the sheath, another snare is introduced from the right internal jugular vein to snare the stud of the microscrew of the LA disk and stretch it toward the internal jugular vein while the assistant pulls the device with snare toward the femoral vein. This allows the device to collapse further and come out of the sheath in the femoral vein.

PROLAPSE OF THE LEFT DISK ACROSS THE DEFECT DURING DEPLOYMENT[22]

On occasions, especially in patients with large defects with deficient anterior/superior rims, when the left disk is deployed, it opens perpendicular to the plane of the atrial septum and prolapses through the anterior superior part of the defect.

There are several maneuvers that can be done to overcome this problem:

1. Use a device in these cases that is at 4 mm larger than the measured "stop-flow" balloon diameter.
2. If this is not possible, or it does not work, change the angle of the deployment by placing the sheath either in the left or right upper pulmonary vein rather than middle left LA.
   a. For large ASDs with deficient aortic rims, the left upper pulmonary vein technique works well. The delivery sheath is placed into the left upper pulmonary vein; the depth of the sheath should be enough to ensure that the device will temporarily stay in the pulmonary vein when the sheath is withdrawn. The sheath is then withdrawn swiftly all the way into the RA to deploy both disks simultaneously while the delivery cable is kept taut and stable in one location. The left disk springs out of the pulmonary vein and slaps onto the atrial septum. This maneuver keeps the left disk parallel to the atrial septum which prevents the aortic edge of the device from protruding into the RA. If the device does not spring out of the pulmonary vein, a gentle traction on the cable helps in withdrawing the device. Extreme care and caution should be exercised to avoid advancing the device deep into the pulmonary vein because injury to the pulmonary vein can occur.
   b. The LA roof technique works well in patients with deficient posterior rim. In this technique, the delivery sheath is placed near the orifice of

the right upper pulmonary vein. On fluoroscopy (anteroposterior view), the delivery sheath appears parallel to the spine. The device is advanced and the left disk is deployed in the atrial roof while keeping the sheath stable. The deployed left disk is perpendicular to the spine after it is deployed in the atrial roof. The right disk is deployed by withdrawing the sheath. This maneuver keeps the posterior edge of the device inside the LA and away from the posterior rim of the defect while the remainder of the device is deployed. This technique is also applicable in patients who have combined deficiency of aortic and posterior rims.

3. Another potential solution is to use the Hausdorf sheath (Cook Medical, Bloomington, IN), which has two posterior curves at the end. This sine curve can be quite useful in changing the deployment angle.

4. The dilator technique implies the use of a long dilator from the contralateral femoral vein to hold the LA disk in the LA while the assistant/operator deploys the remainder of the device.[23]

5. The balloon-assisted technique is similar to the dilator technique. A guidewire is positioned in the left upper pulmonary vein from the contralateral femoral vein. A balloon is inflated in the RA very close to the septum. The device is deployed in the usual fashion. The presence of the balloon will prevent prolapse of the left disk. Once the device is deployed, the balloon is deflated slowly. After complete deflation, the guidewire is pulled out carefully from the LA.[24]

RECAPTURE OF THE DEVICE

To achieve the smallest sheath size for device delivery, sheath wall thickness should be small, with a resultant decrease in strength. To recapture a device prior to its release, the operator should hold the sheath at the groin with the left hand and with the right hand pull the delivery cable forcefully inside the sheath. In order to achieve the smallest sheath diameter possible for device delivery, sheaths are relatively thin walled and relatively weak. If the sheath is damaged or kinked (accordion effect), use the exchange (rescue) system to change the damaged sheath. First, extend the length of the cable by screwing the tip of the rescue cable to the proximal end of the cable attached to the device. Then remove the sheath or, if the sheath is 9 or 12 French, introduce the dilator of the rescue system over the cable inside the sheath until it reaches a few centimeters from the tip of the sheath. This dilator will significantly strengthen the sheath, allowing the operator to pull back the cable with the dilator as one unit inside it. Then the operator can decide what to do next (change the entire sheath system or the device).

RELEASE OF THE DEVICE WITH A PROMINENT EUSTACHIAN VALVE

To avoid the possibility of cable entrapment during release, advance the sheath to the hub of the right disk. Then release the cable and immediately draw back inside the sheath before the position of the sheath is changed.

CLOSURE OF MULTIPLE SECUNDUM ATRIAL SEPTAL DEFECT[25]

If two defects are present and separated by more than 7 mm from each other, cross each defect separately. Size each one and then leave a delivery system in each defect. Initially deploy the smaller device, then the larger device, and release sequentially, starting with the smaller one.

If there are multiple fenestrations, use the Amplatzer Multi-Fenestrated Septal Occluder–"Cribriform" (these devices are similar in design to the Amplatzer PFO Occluder except that the two disks are equal in size). The device should be deployed in the middle of the septum so that it can cover all fenestrations.

Complications

In the US phase II trial comparing device to open surgical closure, the incidence of complications was 7.2% for device closure, far less than what was encountered when using an open surgical technique (24%). Most complications were related to rhythm disturbance,[26,27] with very few patients requiring long-term medical therapy. These included device embolization (the majority of which were encountered during the early learning curve of the investigators); heart block (rare, and when reported, it is most likely related to the use of an oversized device); atrial arrhythmia (significant increase in atrial arrhythmias following device placement, resolving by 6 months); and headaches occurred in about 5% of patients following device placement, generally resolving within 6 months, and the use of clopidogrel for 2 to 3 months postdevice closure has minimized this complication significantly.

Results

In the US phase II trial, closure rates were similar to those achieved by open surgery results. However, patients who underwent device closure were somewhat older than those who underwent open surgical closure.[26] Furthermore, the cost of device closure was much less than open surgical closure and the length of hospital stay was shorter (1 day) for the device group than the surgical group (3.4 days). In a study by Kim and Hijazi, the mean cost for transcatheter closure was $11,541 and for surgical closure was $21,780.[28]

Helex Septal Occluder Device

The Gore Helex device is a non–self-centering double-disk device of nitinol and expanded polytetrafluoroethylene (ePTFE). The cost of the device is $5,179 and Figure 12-7 demonstrates the device.

The device is designed such that, following introduction across the septum, one disk is constituted on the LA side and the other on the RA side of the septum. The construction of the device consists of a curtain of ePTFE bonded to a single-piece wire frame of 0.012-inch nitinol. The nitinol is prepared in the manner of a helical pattern of opposing rotations which, on full configuration, assumes two parallel disks. The device is delivered through its own composite triaxial 10 French delivery catheter with a workable length of 75 cm. This obviates the need for a long transseptal sheath. For both ASD and PFO, the delivery system can be monorailed through a hole close to its distal end using a wire placed through a diagnostic catheter positioned in one of the left pulmonary veins. The device is available in 15, 20, 25, 30, and 35 mm diameters. The devices are delivered through a short 10 French femoral vein sheath, although if using the monorail technique, a short 11 to 12 French femoral sheath is required.

The Helex device is designed to be flexible and atraumatic, molding itself to the atrial septum and contiguous structures, rendering it particularly appealing for use in a growing heart. Similarly, the proven low thrombogenicity of ePTFE imparts confidence in delivering devices on the systemic side of

the circulation (LA). This is of particular relevance in closure of the PFO where there are implications of thrombotic events to the systemic circulation, producing transient ischemic attacks and strokes. ePTFE has been used in various formats as patches and vascular tubes in the growing heart for almost 30 years now, and thus has proven longevity and biocompatibility with rapid endothelialization characteristics. Studies particular to the Helex device have confirmed this excellent biocompatibility.

Patient Selection

In addition to the recommended indications for percutaneous secundum ASD closure, the Helex occluder is designed to occlude only the central (secundum) type ASDs. The morphology of secundum ASDs is of course variable and multiple fenestrated and aneurysmal defects can be closed using this device. A deficient anterior superior rim, where there is a lack of effacement of the atrial septum at the aorta, can also be accommodated by relative oversizing of the device.

A non–self-centering device up to defect diameter ratio of 1.8:2.0 is recommended for ASDs. With the largest available device being 35 mm, the largest diameter defect closable would be in the region of 18 to 19 mm (balloon size). There is a proviso, however, in that children with large ASDs have a relatively small LAs—experience has shown that the 30 and 35 mm devices do not sit effectively on the LA side of the septum in children weighing less than 25 kg.

For most operators, precardiac catheter closure assessment is usually done using TTE. It is likely, therefore, that defects measuring more than 15 mm on a standard TTE will balloon size to 18 mm or more and will be unsuitable for the Helex device.

Technique of Closure

A fairly standard technique of implantation is employed.

ANESTHESIA

In children, general anesthesia is required usually with endotracheal intubation. In adults, conscious sedation can be used if ICE is used. If TEE is planned, general anesthesia is required.

In our practice, we use ICE exclusively with excellent image quality and avoidance of endotracheal intubation.

ACCESS

Venous access is established through the right femoral vein with a short (15 to 20 cm) 10 to 11 French valved sheath. Another 8 French sheath short or preferably

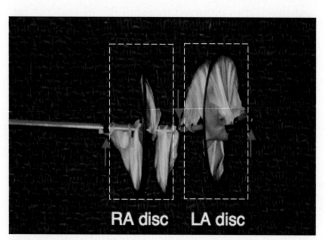

FIGURE 12-7.

The Helex device with its two disks. *Red arrows* indicate the position of the eyelets. RA, right atrium; LA, left atrium.

30-cm long sheath is used for ICE in the same right femoral vein proximal to the first sheath. Invasive arterial pressure monitoring is not required unless general anesthesia is used. Heparin 100 U/kg is administered intravenously. Hemodynamic study will be done to assess the shunt and PA pressure and resistance. Echocardiography is commenced and the morphology of the ASD with respect to size, margins, proximity to the aorta, and AV valves is assessed. At this stage, multiple defects not apparent on TTE may be imaged, as well as fenestrations and aneurysms of the septum.

The same steps performed when using the ASO are used when using the Helex. However, for device size, we use a device size that is 1.8 to 2:1 the size of the balloon diameter.

LOADING THE DEVICE

The Helex device is supplied with its own delivery catheter such that a long Mullins-type sheath is not necessary. The delivery system consists of three distal coaxial components transitioning to a parallel component arrangement at the proximal Y-arm hub: a 10 French green delivery catheter, a gray control catheter, and a tan mandrel (Fig. 12-8). The proximal end of the control catheter exits the Y-arm hub and is terminated by a red retrieval cord cap. The proximal end of the mandrel exits the side port of the Y-arm hub and is terminated by a clear Luer. The control catheter is equipped with a retrieval cord if occluder repositioning or retrieval is deemed necessary. A 0.035-inch guidewire channel is incorporated into the distal end of the delivery catheter.

LOADING THE OCCLUDER INTO THE GREEN DELIVERY CATHETER

Remove the device from the sterile tray. Discard the sterile tray then follow these steps (Fig. 12-8 demonstrates all steps of loading):

1. To reduce the chance of air entrapment in the delivery system, loading the occluder should be conducted with the occluder and catheter tip submerged in a heparinized saline bath.
2. Fill a large volume (20- to 30-mL) syringe with heparinized saline.
3. Attach the syringe to the red retrieval cord cap.
4. Tighten the mandrel Luer.
5. Loosen the control catheter Luer.
6. Flush the control catheter into the bowl or sterile tray.
7. When the initial flushing is completed, draw back on the gray control catheter with the attached syringe until only about 3 cm of the occluder remains outside the delivery catheter and the tan mandrel appears slightly curved.
8. Loosen the mandrel Luer.
9. Complete loading by continuing to draw back on the gray control catheter hub until the entire occluder has been withdrawn into the green delivery catheter.
10. Flush the control catheter into the bowl or sterile tray.

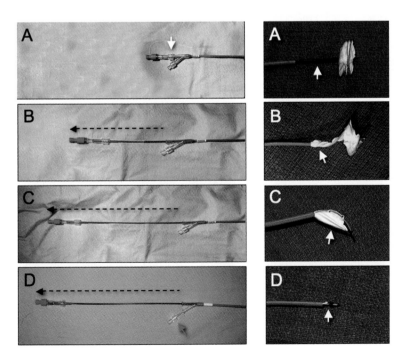

FIGURE 12-8.

Steps of Helex device loading. **A:** The device and delivery catheter once opened from the box showing the device and the gray catheter (*arrow*). **B:** The gray catheter is pulled; this pulls the device inside the green catheter. **C:** Further pulling of the gray catheter until the distal part of the device is "banana shaped" (*arrow*). Then at that time, the Luer of the mandrel is opened, and further pulling of the gray catheter will bring the entire device inside the green catheter (**D**).

11. Keep the flushing syringe attached to the red cap to prevent the entrance of air into the delivery system until the catheter tip is placed inside the introducer sheath.

DEVICE DELIVERY

Load the delivery catheter onto a guidewire through the guidewire port from the luminal surface out and ensure that the occluder is sufficiently withdrawn into the green delivery catheter to avoid interference with the guidewire (monorail system). Load the delivery system into the appropriately sized introducer sheath. At this stage, we remove the flushing syringe. Verify that the red retrieval cord cap affixing the retrieval cord is securely attached to the gray control catheter.

DEPLOYMENT

Figure 12-9 demonstrates an ASD closed under ICE using the Helex device. Figure 12-10 demonstrates the cineangiography images of closure in the same patient as Figure 12-9.

LEFT ATRIAL DISK DEPLOYMENT

1. Under direct fluoroscopic visualization, advance the catheter tip across the ASD until the radio-opaque marker at the tip of the green delivery catheter is positioned within the middle left LA. Verify that the tip of the green delivery catheter is across the defect and away from the left atrial appendage using TEE or ICE.

2. At this stage, the guidewire should be removed before attempting to deploy the occluder.

3. Use the following "push-pinch-pull" method to deploy the LA occluder disk: Push the gray control catheter, moving the occluder into the left atrial chamber off of the septum, but do not push against the atrial wall—or, if the chamber space is adequate, push until the tan mandrel Luer stops against the Y-arm hub (approximately 2 cm). While holding the green delivery catheter to maintain position, pinch the gray control catheter, then pull the tan mandrel back approximately 2 cm or less to form exposed segment of occluder. Repeat the "push-pinch-pull" sequence until the center eyelet exits the green delivery catheter tip demarcated by the radio-opaque marker.

4. Once the LA disk is deployed, hold the entire system as one unit and pull it back until the LA disk is in contact with the atrial septum under echo and fluoroscopy guidance.

FIGURE 12-9.

Atrial septal defect (ASD) closure with Helex guided by intracardiac echocardiography. **A:** Septal view, demonstrating the ASD (*arrow*), the right and left atria, and the superior and inferior rims. **B:** The left atrial disk (*arrow*) deployed in the left atrium. **C:** The right atrial disk (*arrow*) deployed in the right atrium. **D:** The device released, demonstrating good position (*arrow*). RA, right atrium; LA, left atrium.

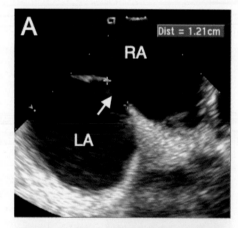
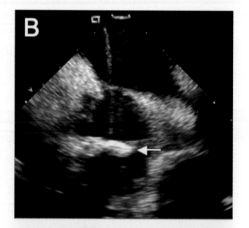
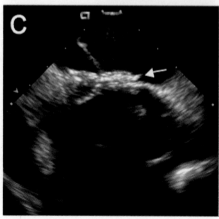
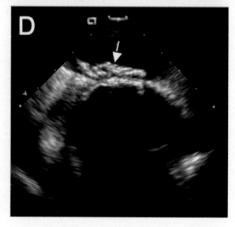

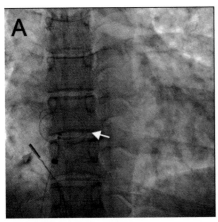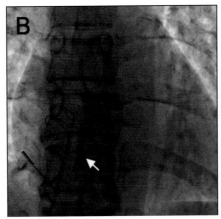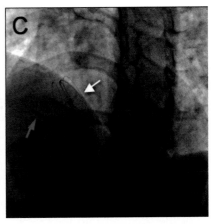

FIGURE 12-10.

Cine angiographic image in the same patient as Figure 12-9 in the straight frontal projection **(A,B)**. **A:** The left atrial disk (*arrow*) deployed in the left atrium, close to the septum. **B:** The right atrial disk (*arrow*) deployed in the right atrium. **C:** Cine image in four-chamber view showing the device (*arrow*) in good position. The *red arrows* indicate the intracardiac echocardiogram catheter (AcuNav, Biosense Webster, Diamond Bar, CA).

RIGHT ATRIAL DISK DEPLOYMENT

1. To prepare for RA disk deployment, hold the gray control catheter in a fixed position and gently expose a portion of the RA side by withdrawing the green delivery catheter until the mandrel Luer stops on the Y-arm hub, then tighten the mandrel Luer.

2. Deploy the RA disk by holding the green delivery catheter in a fixed position with the left hand and pushing the gray control catheter with the right hand until the control catheter Luer contacts the Y-arm hub, then tighten the control catheter Luer.

3. Confirm that both left and right disks appear planar and opposed to the septum with septal tissue trapped between the disks.

4. Confirm proper position using TEE/ICE and at this time, we do angiogram (optional) at left anterior oblique 35 degrees, cranial 35 degrees. If the position is not correct, refer to the repositioning steps later in this chapter.

5. Completely remove the red retrieval cord cap and set it aside.

OCCLUDER LOCK AND RELEASE

1. It is important to note that the occluder can only be repositioned prior to lock release.

2. If position and occlusion are acceptable, loosen the mandrel Luer. Hold the green delivery catheter in a fixed position and release the lock by sharply pulling the tan mandrel at least 2 cm.

3. At the completion of the lock and release step, the occluder is still loosely attached to the gray control catheter by the retrieval cord. If the occluder position is not acceptable, refer to the section "Removing

the Occluder with the Retrieval Cord." Once the delivery system is withdrawn (next step), the occluder cannot be removed using the delivery system.

4. If position is acceptable, remove the entire delivery system as a single unit, making sure the retrieval cord moves smoothly through the control catheter hub.

REPOSITIONING THE OCCLUDER

1. Replace and tighten the red retrieval cord cap and tighten the mandrel Luer.

2. Repeat steps mentioned in the section "Loading the Occluder into the Green Delivery Catheter" in order to bring the occluder back into the catheter.

3. Reposition across the defect.

4. Repeat steps of deployment.

5. During repositioning, if increased force is required to move the catheter components due to abnormal conditions (such as a kinked mandrel, curved mandrel-lock loop, or premature lock release), remove the occluder and delivery system entirely and utilize a new device.

REMOVING THE OCCLUDER WITH THE RETRIEVAL CORD

1. If the lock is released and if the retrieval cord is still attached to the gray control catheter, the occluder can be removed by taking up any slack in the retrieval cord and securely reattaching the red retrieval cord cap.

2. Position the green delivery catheter in the RA. Withdraw the gray control catheter while pulling the occluder into a linear form and drawing the occluder back into the green delivery catheter.

3. Do not use excessive force in an attempt to withdraw all of the occluder into the green delivery catheter. Doing so could cause the retrieval cord to break or result in occluder fracture.

   • Note: Without the mandrel to support the wire frame of the occluder, the operator must ensure that the lock loop and eyelets do not catch on the delivery catheter tip or introducer sheath. If the lock loop or eyelet catch, and the delivery system is forcibly retracted, the retrieval cord or wire frame is at risk of fracture.

4. Normal removal practices withdraw 50% to 100% of the occluder into the green delivery catheter. If a portion of the locked or unlocked occluder remains outside of the delivery catheter, the control catheter and delivery catheter should be withdrawn together. If necessary, remove the introducer sheath and occluder together. If the occluder is removed, it should be disposed of and a new occluder should be used to complete the procedure.

RECAPTURE

1. In the event that the occluder is malpositioned or embolized, it can be recaptured with the aid of a loop snare. A long sheath (10 French or greater) positioned close to the device is recommended for recapture.

2. Place the loop snare around any portion of the occluder frame.

3. Pull the occluder into the sheath using the snare. If a portion of the occluder frame cannot be retracted into the long sheath, it may be necessary to remove the occluder, loop snare, and long sheath as one unit.

4. Bring the recaptured occluder into the sheath to avoid pulling the unlocked device across the valve tissue.

Postprocedure

Same recommendations as mentioned for ASO.

Complications

Serious complications following Helex closure of an ASD are rare. Cardiac perforation and tamponade have not yet been reported. Embolization occurs, but almost always, the device can be retrieved using a snare device and a long 10 French sheath. Wire fractures have been seen in a small percentage of patients (about 5% to 6%) and are usually of no clinical consequence as the wire is held secure by the fabric of the device and its comprehensive endothelialization.

Results

Early experience has demonstrated the ease of use of this device, its complete retrievability, and excellent closure of small to moderate ASDs in children.

Results of the U.S. Multicenter Pivotal Study of the Helex Septal Occluder for Percutaneous Closure of Secundum Atrial Septal Defects[29] showed that closure of ASD with the Helex septal occluder is safe and effective when compared with surgical repair, with reduced anesthesia time and hospital stay. Clinical success was achieved in 91.7% (100 of 109) of device patients and in 83.7% (72 of 86) of surgical control patients. The most common major adverse event for the Helex septal occluder group was device embolization requiring catheter retrieval (1.7%), and in the surgery group, it was postpericardiotomy syndrome (6.3%), including one death due to tamponade.

REFERENCES

1. Lindsey JB, Hillis LD. Clinical update: atrial septal defect in adults. *Lancet.* 2007;369:1244–1246.

2. Rigby M. Atrial septal defect. *Diagnosis and Management of Adult Congenital Heart Disease.* London: Churchill Livingston; 2003.

3. Schreiber TL, Feigenbaum H, Weyman AE. Effect of atrial septal defect repair on left ventricular geometry and degree of mitral valve prolapse. *Circulation.* 1980;61:888–896.

4. Webb G, Gatzoulis M. Atrial septal defects in the adult recent progress and overview. *Circulation.* 2006;114:1645–1653.

5. Booth DC, Wisenbaugh T, Smith M, et al. Left ventricular distensibility and passive elastic stiffness in atrial septal defect. *J Am Coll Cardiol.* 1988;12:1231–1236.

6. Brochu MC, Baril JF, Dore A, et al. Improvement in exercise capacity in asymptomatic and mildly symptomatic adults after atrial septal defect percutaneous closure. *Circulation.* 2002;106: 1821–1826.

7. Giardini A, Donti A, Specchia S, et al. Recovery kinetics of oxygen uptake is prolonged in adults with an atrial septal defect and improves after transcatheter closure. *Am Heart J.* 2004;147:910–914.

8. Silversides CK, Siu SC, McLaughlin PR, et al. Symptomatic atrial arrhythmias and transcatheter closure of atrial septal defects in adult patients. *Heart.* 2004;90:1194–1198.

9. Murphy JG, Gersh BJ, McGoon MD, et al. Long-term outcome after surgical repair of isolated atrial septal defect: follow-up at 27–32 years. *N Engl J Med.* 1990; 323:1645–1650.

10. Kort HW, Balzer DT, Johnson MC. Resolution of right heart enlargement after closure of secundum atrial

septal defect with transcatheter technique. *J Am Coll Cardiol.* 2001;38:1528–1532.

11. Gatzoulis MA, Freeman MA, Siu SC, et al. Atrial arrhythmia after surgical closure of atrial septal defects in adults. *N Engl J Med.* 1999;340:839–846.

12. Berthet K, Lavergne T, Cohen A, et al. Significant association of atrial vulnerability with atrial septal abnormalities in young patients with ischemic stroke of unknown cause. *Stroke.* 2000;31:398–403.

13. Cherian G, Uthaman CB, Durairaj M, et al. Pulmonary hypertension in isolated secundum atrial septal defect: high frequency in young patients. *Am Heart J.* 1983;105:952–957.

14. Vogel M, Berger F, Kramer A, et al. Incidence of secondary pulmonary hypertension in adults with atrial septal or sinus venosus defects. *Heart.* 1999;82:30–33.

15. Steele PM, Fuster V, Cohen M, et al. Isolated atrial septal defect with pulmonary vascular obstructive disease: long-term follow-up and prediction of outcome after surgical correction. *Circulation.* 1987;76: 1037–1042.

16. Frost AE, Quinones MA, Zoghbi WA, et al. Reversal of pulmonary hypertension and subsequent repair of atrial septal defect after treatment with continuous intravenous epoprostenol. *J Heart Lung Transplant.* 2005;24:501–503.

17. Kerstein D, Levy PS, Hsu DT, et al. Blade balloon atrial septostomy in patients with severe primary pulmonary hypertension. *Circulation.* 1995;91:2028–2035.

18. Freed MD, Nadas AS, Norwood WI, et al. Is routine preoperative cardiac catheterization necessary before repair of secundum and sinus venosus atrial septal defects? *J Am Coll Cardiol.* 1984;4:333–336.

19. Shub C, Tajik AJ, Seward JB, et al. Surgical repair of uncomplicated atrial septal defect without "routine" preoperative cardiac catheterization. *J Am Coll Cardiol.* 1985;6:49–54.

20. Bove AA. Risk of decompression sickness with patent foramen ovale. *Undersea Hyperb Med.* 1998;25: 175–178.

21. Cheng TO. Platypnea–orthodeoxia syndrome: etiology, differential diagnosis, and management. *Catheter Cardiovasc Interv.* 1999;47:64–66.

22. Amin Z. Transcatheter closure of secundum atrial septal defects. *Catheter Cardiovasc Interv.* 2006;68: 778–787.

23. Wahab HA, Bairam AR, Cao QL, et al. Novel technique to prevent prolapse of the Amplatzer septal occluder through large atrial septal defect. *Catheter Cardiovasc Interv.* 2003;60:543–545.

24. Dalvi BV, Pinto RJ, Gupta A. New technique for device closure of large atrial septal defects. *Catheter Cardiovasc Interv.* 2005;64:102–107.

25. Cao Q, Radtke W, Berger F. Transcatheter closure of multiple atrial septal defects. Initial results and value of two- and three-dimensional transesophgeal echocardiography. *Eur Heart J.* 2000;21: 941–947.

26. Du ZD, Hijazi ZM, Kleinman CS, et al. Comparison between transcatheter and surgical closure of secundum atrial septal defect in children and adults: results of a multicenter nonrandomized trial. *J Am Coll Cardiol.* 2002;39:1836–1844.

27. Hill SL, Berul CI, Patel HT. Early ECG abnormalities associated with transcatheter closure of atrial septal defects using the Amplatzer Septal Occluder. *J Interv Cardiac Electrophysiol.* 2000;4:469–474.

28. Kim JJ, Hijazi ZM. Clinical outcomes and cost of Amplatzer transcatheter closure as compared with surgical closure of ostium secundum atrial septal defects. *Med Sci Monit.* 2002;8:CR787–CR791.

29. Jones TK. Results of the U.S. multicenter pivotal study of the HELEX septal occluder for percutaneous closure of secundum atrial septal defects. *J Am Coll Cardiol.* 2007;49:2215–2221.

SUGGESTED READINGS

Gore Medical. HELEX Septal Occluder instructions for use. Available at: http://goremedical.com/helex/instructions/. Accessed August 4, 2011

Warnes CA, Williams RG, Bashore TM, et al. ACC/AHA 2008 Guidelines for the Management of Adults with Congenital Heart Disease: a report of the American College of Cardiology/American Heart Association Task Force on Practice Guidelines (writing committee to develop guidelines on the management of adults with congenital heart disease). *Circulation* 2008;118(23):e714–883.

CHAPTER 13

Closure of Ventricular Septal Defects in Adults

Eric M. Horlick, Lee N. Benson, and Mark D. Osten

Ventricular septal defects (VSDs) are among the most common lesions in congenital heart disease. The ease of detection of these lesions in infancy and childhood often leads to definitive care at an early age or a plan of serial follow-up and observation. It is not surprising that percutaneous closure in adults is not a common procedure despite the incidence of these lesions. In the adult catheter lab, we are more frequently called upon to address lesions in modified anatomy. This may consist of leaks around previous surgical patches used for congenital heart disease, after postmyocardial septal rupture repair, or after aortic valve replacement. Acquired VSDs related to unrepaired postmyocardial septal rupture or trauma may also be seen.

This chapter reviews the epidemiology, indications, echocardiographic and angiographic anatomy, and a procedural overview for congenital and acquired VSDs. A separate section within this chapter is dedicated to the treatment of postmyocardial infarction (post-MI) VSDs owing to the unique challenges in their assessment and treatment.

VSD closure is a challenging procedure that consists of more components than most interventions. Operators must be skilled at multimodality imaging for lesion assessment. From a technical point of view, crossing over one or multiple lesions with a catheter and wire from either ventricle and potentially through a transseptal or perventricular approach is critical. The use of snares, work with an arteriovenous loop through the heart, large sheaths, access management, and device deployment and assessment are mandatory components. The potential for harm to the patient both during and following an intervention should not be underestimated and these procedures should be given careful consideration before proceeding.

EPIDEMIOLOGY

Isolated VSD is the most common form of congenital heart disease, accounting for almost 20% of isolated defects.[1] VSD may occur in isolation or in conjunction with other congenital cardiac malformations. In the adult population, a VSD is the second most common congenital heart defect following a bicuspid aortic valve.

The first surgical VSD repair was performed by Lillehei and associates in 1954[1]; surgery has been performed for many years and is considered the gold standard for the treatment of VSD. However, surgery is associated with significant morbidity and mortality, patient discomfort, and permanent scarring.[2] Complications such as redo sternotomy for residual leak and atrioventricular (AV) block have been reported to occur in up to 6% of cases.[2,3] Mortality may occur in 0.5% to 10% of patients. The risk for these events is increased in patients with multiple defects, associated lesions, or when redo surgery is performed in patients with a residual VSD.[4,5] Finally, negative long-term effects on developmental and neurocognitive functions have been reported in children who underwent surgery on cardiopulmonary bypass.[6]

Since the first reported percutaneous VSD closure in 1988 by Lock et al.,[4] various devices and techniques have been used to close isolated muscular, perimembranous, and post-MI VSDs in an attempt to reduce the impact of morbidity, mortality, and psychological stress associated with surgery.

NOMENCLATURE

Before discussing percutaneous solutions to VSD closure, it is important to have an understanding of the anatomic differences between the different types of VSDs (congenital and acquired). VSDs are classified according to their location. The septum is composed of a large muscular portion and a smaller membranous portion and is divided into four components (Figs. 13-1 and 13-2).

The membranous septum is located at the base of the heart between the inlet and outlet components of the muscular septum and below the right and noncoronary cusps of the aortic valve. These defects open into the right ventricle and are related to the aortic root—in the area where the subpulmonary outflow tract turns superiorly above the AV junction. The anatomic hallmark of these defects, as seen from the right side, is fibrous continuity between the leaflets of the aortic and tricuspid valves. Defects of the true membranous

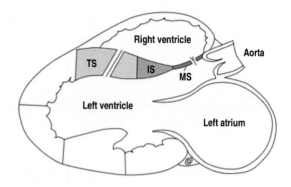

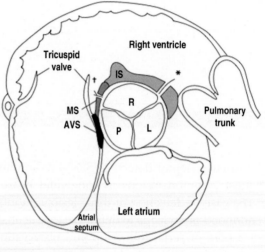

FIGURE 13-2.

Top: Standard parasternal long-axis echocardiographic view showing the membranous septum (*MS*), the infundibular septum (*IS*), and the trabecular muscular septum (*TS*). **Bottom:** Parasternal short-axis view. The *asterisk* indicates supracristal or subarterial ventricular septal defect in the right ventricular outflow tract. In the same basal view, the *dagger* indicates membranous ventricular septal defect in proximity to the tricuspid valve. AVS, atrioventricular septum; L, left; R, right; P, posterior coronary facing sinuses.

septum are surrounded by fibrous tissue without extension into adjacent muscular septum. Defects that extend into the muscular component are called perimembranous VSDs and are the most common type of VSD (80%).

The muscular component of the septum can be divided into the trabecular, inlet, and infundibular. The trabecular septum is the largest part of the interventricular septum. It extends from the membranous septum to the apex and superiorly to the infundibular septum. A defect in the trabecular septum is called muscular when the defect is completely surrounded by a muscular rim (5% to 20% of VSDs).

The infundibular septum separates the right and left ventricular outflow tracts. Infundibular defects,

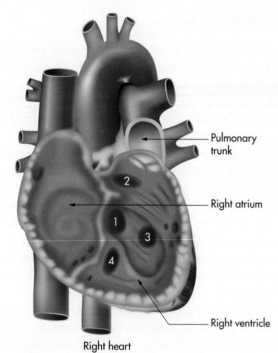

Right heart

FIGURE 13-1.

Positions of different ventricular septal defects seen from the right ventricle. *1*, membranous; *2*, subarterial or supracristal; *3*, muscular or trabecular; *4*, inlet defect.

TABLE 13-1 Echocardiographic Views for VSD Diagnosis

Echo View	Defect Profiled
Parasternal long axis	Anterior defects
Parasternal short axis near mitral tips	Muscular defects: Anterior at 12 to 1 o'clock Mid muscular at 9 to 12 o'clock Inlet at 7 to 9 o'clock
Four-chamber view (at atrioventricular valve level)	Apical, mid muscular, inlet defects
Five-chamber view	Subaortic and mid muscular defects

also called doubly committed defects or subpulmonary defects, occur when part of the border of the defect is formed by fibrous continuity between the two semilunar valves (5% of defects).

The inlet septum is inferoposterior to the membranous septum. It separates the mitral and tricuspid valves formed from the embryonic endocardial cushion. Defects in the inlet septum are called atrioventricular septal defects. The defects are often associated with other abnormalities of the central fibrous body.

Table 13-1 outlines the transthoracic echocardiography (TTE) views best suited to characterize each defect.

PHYSIOLOGIC ASSESSMENT

All VSDs should be assessed for size, location, number of defects, and adjacent cardiac structural abnormalities. For example, the development of aortic insufficiency in the case of infundibular defects as a result of insufficient support apparatus of the aortic valve or, in the case of a perimembranous defect, that can be associated with various degrees of malalignment of the infundibular septum and associated other congenital defects such as tetralogy of Fallot. Although not all perimembranous defects are amenable to percutaneous closure because of associated or adjacent cardiac malformations, congenital muscular defects are usually amenable to closure based on location. The decision to close these defects with transcatheter techniques does not depend on the size and location alone. The primary consideration for closure depends on the hemodynamic consequences of the lesion.

The size of the defect, pressure in the right and left ventricles, and pulmonary vascular resistance (PVR) influence the hemodynamic significance of VSDs. The magnitude of the shunt (in the absence of valvular or

outflow obstruction) is determined primarily by the size of the defect and the PVR.

In patients with pulmonary hypertension, cardiac catheterization is crucial in the decision whether to close the defect. A catheterization to determine candidacy for VSD closure should include a full saturation run on room air, computation of left and right sided flows and $Q_P:Q_S$ by the Fick principle (if oxygen consumption is measured as opposed to estimated, accuracy will be significantly enhanced), measurement of the pulmonary artery pressure and wedge pressure or left atrial pressure, and computation of the PVR and its index. Dynamic studies—where PVR is calculated after challenging the patients with oxygen, 20 to 40 PPM of inhaled nitric oxide, prostaglandins, or other pulmonary vasodilators—may prove to be important in decision making and the opportunity should not be missed for this type of assessment.

For the most part, patients with hemodynamically significant VSD undergo intervention early on in life. However, patients with small-to-moderate-sized VSDs, residual VSD after surgical intervention, and patients who have developed structural complications as a result of the VSD may require intervention.

INDICATIONS

Indications for closure include[5]:

1. The presence of a "significant" VSD (symptomatic; Q_P/Q_S of >2:1; pulmonary artery systolic pressure >50 mm Hg); deteriorating ventricular function due to volume or pressure overload
2. Perimembranous defect with aortic cusp prolapse with at least mild aortic insufficiency*
3. Significant right ventricular outflow tract obstruction (catheter gradient or mean echo gradient >50 mm Hg)*
4. History of recurrent endocarditis may be an indication for closure
5. The requirement for a transvenous pacing system may be an indication for VSD closure

*Denotes surgical closure only.

Pulmonary Hypertension

Closure can be considered for patients with pulmonary hypertension with VSD or after surgical closure with a residual leak if the pulmonary artery pressure is less than two-thirds of systemic pressure; PVR is less than two-thirds of the systematic vascular resistance; and the $Q_P:Q_S$ is >1.5:1. If the PVR is more than two-thirds of systemic pressure and/or the pulmonary artery systolic pressure is more than two-thirds of systematic vascular resistance—and there is a net 1.5:1 shunt or the pulmonary hypertension is reversible by oxygen, vasodilators, or nitrous oxide—then closure may also be considered. Consultation with local experts in pulmonary hypertension is advised in this situation.

CONTRAINDICATIONS TO CLOSURE

Fixed pulmonary vascular obstructive disease resulting in diminution of left-to-right shunting, or even right to left shunting, is an absolute contraindication to VSD closure. In this situation, the VSD acts as a "pop-off valve," allowing right to left flow to bypass the lungs and maintain systemic cardiac output and closure of the defect results in poorer long-term outcome.

Eisenmenger syndrome results from large VSDs with long-term left-to-right shunting. The elevated, irreversible pulmonary artery pressure leads to reversal of the shunt with resultant desaturation, cyanosis, and secondary erythrocytosis and is a contraindication to closure.

ANATOMIC ASSESSMENT

Once the decision has been made to close the VSD based on physiological assessment, the next critical step is to define the anatomy of the VSD to ensure both safe and effective closure. TTE plays an important role in the initial diagnosis and delineation of the location of the VSD. For instance, the left parasternal long-axis view demonstrates perimembranous defects, whereas the short-axis view at the level of the aortic and pulmonary valves is the best view for the exact location of the VSD (Table 13-1, Fig. 13-3). TTE may be limited in the delineation of the size and number of defects in the adult. Transesophageal echocardiography (TEE) and real-time three-dimensional (3D) TEE are useful imaging modalities to assess defect margins, number of defects, and proximity to adjacent cardiac structures. The advent of real-time 3D TEE images obtained before the procedure allow for en face visualization of the defects and measurement of their size, which helps to determine the sizes of the closure devices to be used. Three-dimensional images during the closure procedure allow for visualization of intracardiac catheters and devices throughout their lengths, alignment of the closure devices within the defects, and immediate assessment of procedural results. Increasing availability and expertise in gated multislice computed tomography (CT) and magnetic resonance imaging are also

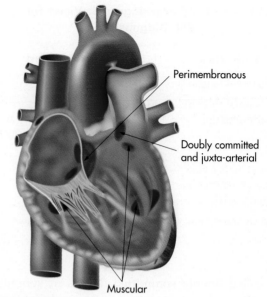

Perimembranous

Doubly committed and juxta-arterial

Muscular

FIGURE 13-3.

The illustration shows the locations of the various phenotypic types of holes permitting shunting between the ventricles as seen from the right ventricle.

useful adjunctive imaging modalities to understand the anatomy and for preprocedure planning of transcatheter closure. During the procedure, angiography provides a crude assessment of the amount of shunting before and after device implantation, but is invaluable in guiding the procedure. We depend on TEE imaging as well as angiography to assess residual shunts post device closure and to verify device stability and alignment.

PERIMEMBRANOUS AND MUSCULAR VENTRICULAR SEPTAL DEFECTS

Transcatheter closure of perimembranous and muscular VSDs has been an alternative to surgery since 1988.[4] The Rashkind and button devices were originally used to close these defects. However, these devices had poor success rates because of complex implantation techniques, the inability to reposition and redeploy the device, and significant residual shunting. After the introduction of the specifically designed Amplatzer muscular and perimembranous VSD occluder devices in 1998 and 2002, respectively, procedures were simplified and repositioning was easily achievable.[7–9] Since then, transcatheter closure has become an acceptable alternative with high closure rates, low mortality, and acceptable complication rates.[7–10]

Perimembranous VSDs are the most common form of VSDs. The Amplatzer membranous VSD occluder

(AGA Medical Inc., Plymouth, MN) is the most commonly used device and has been reported in large series with minimal complications. The most frequent complication associated with the device is complete atrioventricular block (cAVB) (see later text). TEE plays a critical role in patient selection for device closure. The left parasternal long-axis view is used to visualize perimembranous defects. The short-axis parasternal view at the level of the semilunar valves is the best view to delineate the location of the defects. In the short axis, defects seen between 9 and 12 o'clock are membranous defects, whereas defects between 7 and 9 o'clock are termed perimembranous defects. Evidence of associated aortic valve prolapse or a Gerbode defect (left ventricle to right atrial defect) are contraindications to closure.

Muscular VSDs account for 10% to 15% of all VSDs. The most common location of these defects is at the apex of the ventricular septum. There can also be multiple defects, the so-called Swiss cheese septum. Almost all muscular VSDs are congenital. Acquired causes are most often related to post-MI or trauma. From a surgeon's perspective, muscular VSDs are difficult to visualize because of the coarse right ventricular trabeculae, and pose a challenge for the surgical repair. Thus, transcatheter closure has become an acceptable alternative for congenital muscular defects. TEE is the best modality to assess size, number, and location of muscular defects. The parasternal short-axis view is best for delineation of the muscular defects. The four-chamber view will help demonstrate apical and midmuscular defects. In the five-chamber view, anterior muscular defects are well seen. Cardiac CT imaging can also aid in the understanding of the size and location of the defects and to help plan for transcatheter closure.

PROCEDURAL COMPLICATIONS

Procedural complications such as device embolization, air embolization, wire thrombus, and pericardial effusion are rare occurrences and are usually avoidable with meticulous technique, adequate anticoagulation, and experienced TEE imaging at the time of the procedure. Pericardial effusion is usually the result of catheter or guidewire perforation. If device embolization does occur, the device can be snared and retrieved percutaneously, although usually the sheath needs to be upsized to remove the device. A variety of retrieval equipment (snares, bioptomes) and large sheath sizes should be readily available to deal with this complication. AGA devices (AGA Medical Inc.) should be snared by the screw hub for retrieval. Caution should be exercised in extracting embolized devices, especially those with articulations. It is almost certainly better to have a device surgically removed than to damage an AV valve and require valvular replacement as well.

The most common reported complication during perimembranous VSD closure is cAVB. This has been reported to occur up to 5.8% of the time in published series.[11] This complication can happen during device deployment or days after deployment. The exact mechanism is not completely understood, but is thought to be related to myocardial edema. If asymptomatic cAVB occurs, close monitoring and treatment with oral steroids may reverse the block.[12,13] Also, if a permanent pacemaker is not inserted for temporary cAVB, careful monitoring during long-term follow-up is necessary because of the risk of recurrent cAVB.

Other potential rare complications that can occur post device deployment include hemolysis and valvular regurgitation. Tricuspid, aortic, or mitral valve regurgitation can occur due to device impingement on the valvular and subvalvular apparatus. Use of TEE during device placement and deployment can help to avoid this complication.

PROCEDURAL OVERVIEW

Although the vast majority of VSDs are managed with surgical algorithms, several presentations lend themselves to transcatheter device approaches, which include muscular VSDs, so-called postoperative residual defects, perimembranous defects, and post-MI VSDs. The general approach to defect closure is similar between lesions, with minor variations depending on the type of occluder chosen for implantation. Devices available in North America include nitinol wire plugs such as the Amplatzer Muscular VSD occluder or the Amplatzer post-MI muscular VSD occluder (AGA Medical Inc.)[7,14–17] (Fig. 13-3); double-umbrella devices such as the CardioSEAL or STARFlex (NMT Medical Inc., Boston, MA).[18] Nitinol coils that are available outside the United States include the Nit-Occlud VSD (PFM Medical AG, Köln, Germany). Additionally, there is a device designed specifically for perimembranous defects also available only outside of the United States (circa 2011) made by AGA Medical Inc.: the Amplatzer membranous VSD occluder.[19,20] Regardless of the implant used, as noted, the general approach to closure is the same.

Detailed in the following text are the general aspects of closure that can be followed using a muscular VSD closure as a paradigm for the other implants.

THE DEVICES

The Amplatzer Muscular VSD Occluder

This is a self-expanding double-disk design of nitinol wire (Fig. 13-4). There is a 7-mm long tubular connecting waist with symmetrical left and right ventricular disks 8 mm larger than the waist. Dacron polyester patches are sewn into the two disks to enhance thrombosis. The right ventricular disk has a stainless steel screw hub to attach the delivery cable, similar to all Amplatzer line devices. The device sizes correspond to the waist diameter and range from 4 to 18 mm in 2 mm increments. Delivery sheaths ranges from 6 to 9 French, depending on device diameter (Table 13-2).

The Amplatzer postinfarction muscular VSD occluder (AGA Medical Inc.) has a slightly different design with a longer waist (10 mm) and the two disks are each 10 mm larger than the waist. Device sizes range from 16 to 24 mm in 2 mm increments, delivered through 8 to 12 French sheaths.

The CardioSEAL/STARFlex Double Umbrella

This design consists of two opposing, self-expanding umbrellas of Dacron, scaffolded by spring arms. There is an internally suspended nitinol spring wire that

TABLE 13-2 Sheath Size Requirements for AGA Muscular Ventricular Septal Defect Devices

Sheath Size	Device Size
6 French	4, 6 mm
7 French	8–10 mm
8 French	12, 14 mm
9 French	16, 18 mm

contributes to device self-centering within the defect in the STARFlex modification. The CardioSEAL device is available in 23 mm, 28 mm, and 33 mm sizes (diagonal measurement) and an additional 17 mm size for the STARFlex modification. Devices are chosen to be 1.5 to 2 times the estimated diameter of the defect.

The Amplatzer Membranous VSD Occluder

This is a self-expanding, self-centering, retrievable double disk device made of 0.003- to 0.005-inch nitinol wire (Fig. 13-5). The device has a 1.5-mm long waist and a right and left retention disks. The right-sided disk is symmetrical and is 2 mm larger than the diameter of the waist. The left-sided disk is asymmetrical with the aortic end being 0.5 mm larger than the waist and the ventricular end being 5.5 mm larger than the waist. The ventricular end of the left-sided disk has a platinum marker to guide correct device deployment. There is a screw on the right-sided disk with a

FIGURE 13-4.

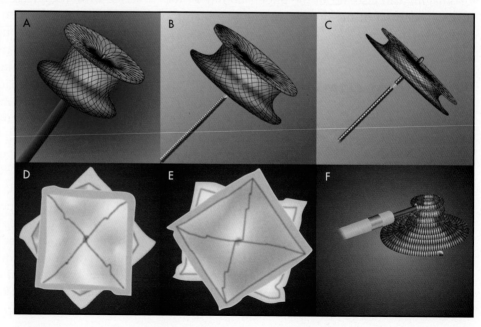

Various ventricular septal defect (VSD) closure devices. **A–C:** The Amplatzer line of implants: postinfarction, muscular, and perimembranous designs (AGA Medical Inc., Plymouth, MN). **D,E:** The STARFlex and CardioSEAL implants from NMT Medical (Boston, MA); note the presence of nitinol wire springs on the STARFlex device used to center the implant within the defect. **F:** The Nit-Occlud coil (PFM Medical AG, Köln, Germany) used for small VSDs.

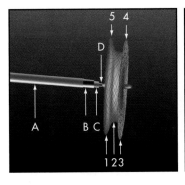
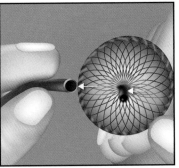

FIGURE 13-5.

The Amplatzer membranous VSD device. *A*, delivery sheath; *B*, pusher cable; *C*, metal capsule of pusher cable; *D*, delivery cable; *1, 5*, right-sided disk; *2*, the waist; *3, 4*, left-sided disk with a platinum marker at *3*.

flat part to help guide the device such that the platinum marker faces toward the ventricular apex when opened. The device is available in sizes ranging from 4 to 18 mm in diameter (diameter of the waist) in 2 mm increments and can be delivered through 6 to 9 French delivery sheaths. The delivery system consists of a delivery cable, sheath and dilator, pusher, loader, and a pin vise. The pusher catheter has a metal capsule at its end and a flat capsule that corresponds to the flat part in the screw of the device. These two flat parts should align with each other. The delivery cable is pushed through the pusher catheter and the device is loaded in the standard fashion. The cable is then pulled back and the flat part of the screw is opposed to the flat part of the capsule. This is an important step to allow the left-sided disk to be delivered in the correct orientation opening toward the ventricular apex. The device and the pusher catheter as a single unit are pulled back into the loader catheter under saline solution.[20]

The PFM VSD Coil (PFM Medical, Köln, Germany)

This device is similar to the PFM PAD coil, the Nit-Occlud (Fig. 13-4). It is made of nitinol coils, shaped in a cone-in-cone pattern, and modified by adding reinforced coil loops on the left and right ventricular sides. Additionally, polyester fibers have been added to the left ventricular cone. Several devices are available in 10 mm by 6 mm diameters up to 18 mm by 8 mm (referring to left ventricular coil/right ventricular diameters).

DEVICE SELECTION

Indications for transcatheter closure vary with lesion location. Generally, the lesions are isolated and amenable to a transcatheter approach, thus avoiding surgical intervention. On the other hand, device implantation may be considered during surgery—so-called hybrid

procedures[20]—when a device is implanted in a defect, which may be difficult to address surgically (e.g., apical muscular defect) during bypass for correction of other defection or perventricular,[21] the device being delivered through the right ventricular wall via a median sternotomy approach on a beating heart (applied primarily in small infants).

For muscular defects, they should be easily demonstrable by echocardiography and the patients symptomatic from the hemodynamic burden. Contraindications include a distance from AV or semilunar valves where the device disks would compromise valve function, pulmonary vascular disease (see previous text), or sepsis.

PLANNING BEFORE THE CATHETERIZATION

Assessment by echocardiography is critical to determine the size, number, and location of the defect(s). Various views are used to demonstrate the location of the lesions (Table 13-1).

PROCEDURAL OVERVIEW (MUSCULAR TYPE)

- General anesthesia preferred with continuous TEE guidance.[22–24]
- Femoral artery and vein access. If the VSD is midmuscular, posterior, or apical the right internal jugular vein can be used for delivery sheath placement. Apical and midmuscular defects can be approached from an atrial transseptal puncture (Figs. 13-6, 13-7, and 13-8).
- Heparinize the patient (activated clotting time >250 seconds), serial monitoring throughout the procedure.
- Standard right and left heart catheterization for shunt calculation and PVR determination.

FIGURE 13-6.

A, top left: A venous end-hole catheter is maneuvered across the atrial septum (natural atrial defect or transseptal puncture) and through the mitral valve into the left ventricle. **A, top right:** Using the end-hole catheter, a wire is passed through the defect into the right ventricle. The wire can be maneuvered in to the pulmonary artery, snared, and exteriorized (as in this illustration) out the jugular vein to direct the device delivery sheath for closure of an apically located defect **(bottom left and right)**. Others have used the femoral vein, particularly in adults (see text). **B:** In this diagram, the defect is crossed from a retrograde arterial approach **(left)**, the end-hole catheter crosses the defect (see text) **(middle)**, and the wire is exteriorized from the internal jugular vein for delivery of the device sheath **(right)**. LV, left ventricle; RA, right atrium; RV, right ventricle.

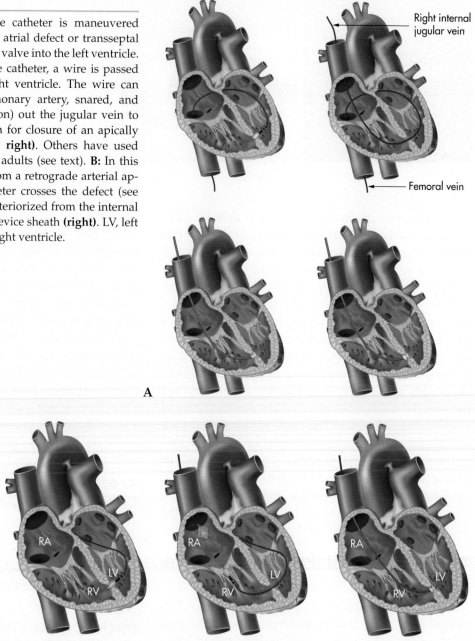

- Left ventriculography in the hepatoclavicular (left anterior oblique, 35 degrees/cranial, 35 degrees) or long-axis oblique (left anterior oblique, 60 degrees/cranial, 20 degrees) projections to define the location and number of defects. The projection will vary according to VSD position in the septum; the hepatoclavicular view is useful for midmuscular, apical, or posterior defects, and long-axis oblique projection is useful for anterior and perimembranous defects (Fig. 13-7).
- The device (in this case, an Amplatzer muscular VSD device) is chosen to be 1 to 2 mm greater than the defect diameter as measured by angiography or echocardiography at end diastole.

- A variety of catheters may be used to cross the defect from the left ventricular side using an end-hole Judkins, Cobra, or Amplatzer curve. The defect is crossed from the left ventricular side assisted with a 0.035-inch guidewire (a Terumo glidewire is most effective; Terumo Medical Corporation, Somerset, NJ). Once the defect is crossed, the wire is maneuvered into a branch pulmonary artery (the left pulmonary artery is most often entered) and, using a snare technique, the wire is exteriorized (see later text). For apical defects, a catheter course from the superior vena cava allows a gentle curve for the delivery sheath (most often applied in children) but

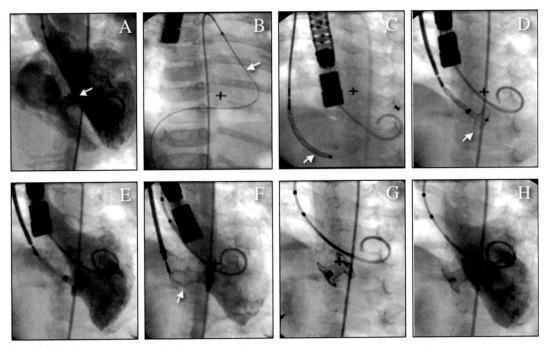

FIGURE 13-7.

Fluoroscopic and angiographic steps in the closure of a muscular ventricular septal defect (VSD). **A:** Left ventricle angiogram demonstrates the presence of a single midmuscular VSD. **B:** The wire is across the VSD from the left ventricle. **C:** The delivery sheath is in the left ventricle from the right internal jugular vein and the device is being advanced. **D:** The left-sided disk is advanced into the left ventricle. **E:** Left ventricle angiogram performed to confirm the position of the left ventricular disk. **F:** The right disk is deployed in the right ventricle. **G:** The device is released from the delivery cable. **H:** Left ventricle angiogram shows complete closure of the muscular VSD. The *arrow* in **A** indicates the muscular vsd on angiography. The *arrow* in **B** indicates a catheter in the left ventricle with a wire being passed from it through the defect. The *arrow* in **C** shows advancement of the VSD device in the sheath. The *arrow* in **D** shows the device's left sided disk deployed and being pulled into position. The *arrow* in **F** indicates deployment of the right ventricular disk. (From Hijazi ZM, Sandhu SK. Ventricular septal defect closure: state of the art. Available at: http://www.fac.org.ar/ccvc/llave/c007/hijazi.php. Accessed June 1, 2011, with permission.)

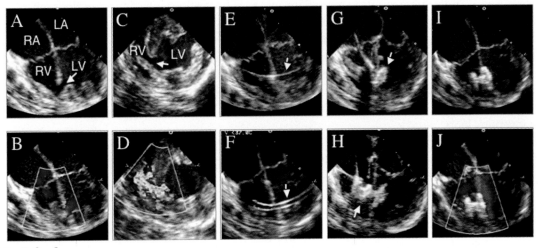

FIGURE 13-8.

Transesophageal echocardiography images of muscular ventricular septal defect (VSD) closure with an Amplatzer muscular VSD device. **A:** Apical four-chamber view of a muscular VSD. **B:** Color Doppler flow across the VSD. **C:** The muscular VSD in the short-axis view. **D:** Color Doppler flow across the muscular VSD in the short-axis view. **E:** Wire across the VSD. **F:** Sheath across the VSD. **G:** The left ventricular disk is deployed in the left ventricle. **H:** The right ventricular disk is deployed in the right ventricle. **I:** The device is released from the delivery cable. **J:** There is no residual shunt across the VSD by color Doppler. LA, left atrium; LV, left ventricle; RA, right atrium; RV, right ventricle. (From Hijazi ZM, Sandhu SK. Ventricular septal defect closure: state of the art. Available at: http://www.fac.org.ar/ccvc/llave/c007/hijazi.php. Accessed June 1, 2011, with permission.)

may not be necessary in the adult especially with the advent of braided kink-resistant sheaths (Fig. 13-6). The cut tip of a Judkins left coronary artery curve may help in crossing anterior defects. Rarely, the defect cannot be crossed with a Judkins-shaped catheter and an end-hole balloon-tipped wedge catheter may be tried for curving the catheter in the left ventricle and inflating the balloon. Crossing the defect from the right ventricular side may be difficult due to the presence of right ventricular trabeculations which complicate the maneuver and can result in the catheter being caught in the trabeculations.

- When positioning the snare to retrieve the wire, it is important to place the snare guide catheter in the pulmonary artery over a guidewire positioned through an end-hole balloon catheter. This avoids inadvertently entrapping a tricuspid valve cord which would entangle the device delivery sheath upon entry to the right ventricle.

- Once the wire traverses the defect, the left ventricular guide catheter can be advanced into the right ventricle to assist placement of the wire into the pulmonary artery. Once the wire is in the pulmonary artery, the retrograde catheter is advanced over it to the pulmonary artery. At that juncture, an extra long exchange wire is placed through the catheter into the pulmonary artery (extra long exchange or Amplatzer "noodle wire"; AGA Medical Inc.).

- The pulmonary artery wire can then be snared and exteriorized with any variety of snare devices; the most often used is a 3D snare (Entrio snare, Bard, Murray Hill, NJ), or Amplatzer Goose Neck Snare (AGA Medical Inc.). When exteriorizing the wire, the left ventricle to right ventricle to pulmonary artery catheter should be brought across the tricuspid valve into the inferior vena cava. This avoids trauma to the heart as the wire is pulled out to form the arteriovenous loop.

- Over the exteriorized wire, an appropriate-sized delivery sheath–dilator complex is then advanced from the femoral vein to the tip of the catheter in the vena cava. With the tips together, the device delivery catheter is maneuvered through the right ventricle across the defect and into the left ventricle. Some operators place the delivery sheath into the aorta. The dilator and wire are removed carefully, flushing to avoid air entering the system. Occasionally, the delivery sheath may kink when the dilator is removed and compromise passage of the device during placement. To overcome this problem, a 0.018-inch glidewire (Terumo) can be placed in the sheath and in the left ventricle or outside the arterial

side, thereby creating an arteriovenous loop. This may allow the sheath to straighten when the device passes and allow easier crossing of the defect should the delivery sheath and device pull through the defect. Once the device is in place and stable, the "safety wire" can be removed.

- The device is loaded on the delivery cabled and de-aired in the standard fashion. Under fluoroscopic guidance, the device is advanced to the sheath tip.

- Some operators deploy the left ventricular disk in the aorta before the sheath is pulled into the left ventricle (primarily for anterior defects to avoid the sheath from pulling back into the right ventricle). For those where the sheath is in the left ventricle, the left ventricular disk is extruded in the middle of the cavity while monitored by echocardiography and fluoroscopy. Imaging of the mitral valve apparatus to ensure that this is not entrapped by the device and, if so, it must be recaptured and redeployed.

- The full assembly is withdrawn to the left ventricular side of the septum and, with retraction of the sheath, the core of the device opened in the defect.

- Once positioning is confirmed by echocardiography, the right ventricular disk can be deployed. Some operators perform a left ventricular angiogram to confirm positioning before exposing the right ventricular disk.

- Once appropriate positioning is confirmed, the device is released with counterclockwise rotation of the cable.

- Echocardiography and angiography can be repeated to confirm positioning once the device is released, function of the AV valve, the characteristics of any residual shunting, and any additional lesions can be reexamined. If there are further defects, the procedure can be repeated.

POSTMYOCARDIAL INFARCTION VENTRICULAR SEPTAL DEFECT

Post-MI ventricular septal rupture (VSR) is among the most feared complications of acute MI. Prior to the era of reperfusion therapy with thrombolytics, VSR complicated 1% to 3% of infarcts. The Gusto-I trial demonstrated that, with reperfusion, the rate of VSR could be reduced to 0.2%.[21] The predictors of VSR were advanced age, female sex, anterior localization, left anterior descending artery territory, and nonsmoking status. The patients in Gusto-I had poor outcomes with an overall 30-day mortality of 74%—of those who had surgery, mortality was 47%, whereas those who were treated medically had a 94% 30-day mortality. Fifty-five of 939 patients in the shock trial had VSR and these patients had an 87% mortality overall.[22] The patients who had surgery had an 81% mortality and those treated medically had a 96% mortality. Both of the studies noted a survival advantage with surgery; however, it is important to note that not all patients had surgery. All surgical series and their results are subject to a selection bias where those patients offered surgery have better outcomes than those treated medically.

Patients with VSR are a heterogeneous group. Cummings compared patients with MI with and without VSR and found that those patients with VSR with either anterior or inferior MI had greater degrees of right ventricular involvement.[23] About 50% of patients with VSR have simple through-and-through defects, whereas 50% have serpiginous tears of great complexity.

Patients with VSR are best managed in the coronary intensive care unit environment. Patients may present similarly to acute free wall rupture with hypotension and often with some worsening chest discomfort. A pansystolic murmur is present often with a thrill. About 15% of these patients have coexistent severe mitral insufficiency. Echocardiography provides the most rapid access to diagnosis. In the past, a 10% step-up in oxygen samples from superior vena cava to pulmonary artery using a pulmonary artery catheter was diagnostic. Care should be taken to sample the pulmonary artery proximally to avoid contamination from severe mitral insufficiency which may confound the diagnosis. V waves may be noted in the wedge tracing—these are typically later than the V waves that occur with severe mitral insufficiency. The V waves reflect the heightened venous return to the left ventricle in the presence of a closed mitral valve.

There is a long standing dogma that the $Q_P:Q_S$ must be optimized to improve outcome. In fact, it is the absolute Q_S alone that helps to perfuse the organs and improves outcome. Reducing $Q_P:Q_S$ does not always translate into improved Q_S, and increasing $Q_P:Q_S$ may result in improved absolute Q_S.

Methods to optimize systemic flow include afterload reduction with a highly titratable agent such as nitroprusside. Fifty to 70% of this population have multivessel disease and caution should be exercised to avoid hypotension and diminished coronary perfusion. An intra-aortic balloon pump is an effective therapy to both decrease afterload and improve coronary filling. Small experiences exist using the Impella device (left ventricular assist device; ABIOMED, Danvers, MA), as well as the TandemHeart device (Cardiac Assist Inc.,

Pittsburgh, PA) as a bridge to definitive therapy or transplant.[24,25]

The American College of Cardiology/American Heart Association and European Society of Cardiology guidelines both recommend urgent or emergent surgery for VSR.[26] The operation of choice is usually the infarct exclusion technique whereby a patch (usually bovine pericardium) is sewn from viable muscle to viable muscle, excluding the VSD to the right ventricular side of the heart. This operation has been associated with survival of 79% at 30 days and actuarial survivals of 59% at 8 years.[27] Unfortunately, these results are exceptional and not the rule. In reality, many patients are found not to be candidates for surgical repair because of age, comorbidity, or end-organ dysfunction.

The role of percutaneous intervention in patients with post-MI VSR is yet to be clarified. Applying what we know about congenital VSD closure is misleading. Clearly, from a technical standpoint, a device can be placed in the lesion. The presence of a jagged, non–geometric-shaped lesion that is usually large often leads to incomplete closure. Worse, because these defects are irregular, a device may place undue tension on the septum and encourage further tearing and defect expansion postprocedure.

Treatment of the acute patient (within days of presentation) without prior surgery has a poor outcome in a population of patients who have been evaluated for and turned down for surgery. This is the same population in whom 30-day survival is measured in single digits. Should the treatable population be expanded to all comers in geographies where it has been decided that surgery too has a poor outcome, it is possible to find additional patients who are not physiologically compromised with smaller defects that might benefit from primary device therapy. There are a handful of patients in the literature who have survived acute post-MI VSD intervention.

The situation becomes quite different if we examine two other populations of patients: (1) those treated medically after VSR who have survived 6 weeks; and (2) those who have had surgery and have developed residual VSR. This second group of patients has a much more favorable response to therapy and it is quite possible to achieve excellent outcomes. Once the defect has had a chance to organize and healing has occurred, the risk of expansion of the defect during or after therapy is substantially reduced. Certainly, patients who have survived their infarcts without intervention with a VSR represent a small percentage of all those presenting with VSR; however, they do have an improved overall survival. Patients who have had surgical patch repair who have residual defects may also be addressed readily in the catheter lab. Although those patients with multiple leaks may be difficult to address, closing the largest of multiple defects often has very therapeutic effect with a reduction in symptoms. The treatment of residual leaks may serve as destination therapy or as a bridge to further recovery and surgical revision.

Timing of intervention is always challenging. As far as primary surgical repair is concerned, there seems little impetus to defer urgent operation, unless the perceived morbidity and mortality is such that surgery will only be undertaken if the patient survives the acute period. The decision to intervene early is to prevent the inevitable multisystem organ dysfunction which often ensues. A 12- to 24-hour period of stabilization with afterload reduction and balloon counterpulsation is often warranted but further delay is often of little point.

If device therapy is anticipated, it may be prudent to obtain additional imaging to define the anatomy clearly to help define whether device therapy is applicable. We and others have used gated CT scanning to define margins, complexity, and size in different imaging planes. We find this to be complimentary to the echo assessment which is often obtained bedside in the intensive care unit. The preoperative or preprocedure echocardiogram should provide in-depth analysis of the size and morphology of the defect, the type (through and through or complex), proximity to the AV valves, the presence of a pericardial effusion or contained rupture, and the state of the mitral valve in addition to the usual information obtained.

Procedural Notes

The procedural technique for post-MI VSR is similar to that for congenital VSD with a few notable modifications. We prefer that all of these patients be under a general anesthetic—this facilitates the use of TEE for procedural monitoring. The use of TEE not only reduces the amount of contrast required but may be helpful in identifying reversible complications during the procedure. TEE generally offers a reasonable assessment of device placement and stability as well as residual leaks; however, angiography should not be discounted for its value in this regard.

Although, for the most part, crossing the defect from the left ventricular side is favored because of its ease and familiarity, the presence of an acquired lesion such as aortic stenosis may mandate transseptal access to the left ventricle. If a patent foramen ovale is present, this technique is greatly facilitated. Great care should

be taken in establishing the arteriovenous loop. It must not put any traction on the VSD, especially with a wire and even when the wire is covered by a catheter. Uncovered wires should never be left passing through the heart in this situation because the fragile infarcted myocardium may easily be cut during manipulation of catheters.

Although many have commented on their preference for the internal jugular vein access for apical VSR, we use the femoral access for all defects. With the use of braided kink-resistant sheaths, an atrial loop from the femoral approach mimics the internal jugular approach closely and avoids the less familiar and inconvenient neck approach.

The CardioSEAL/STARFlex device, as well as the AGA post-MI VSD device, has been used for this application predominantly. The CardioSEAL/STARFlex and AGA platforms are previously discussed. The STARFlex device has the notable addition of nitinol self-centering springs. As these devices are not readily retrievable in case of maldeployment despite their low profile design and ability to self-center without causing undo septal tension, they are favored by few as primary therapy. We have found the use of other devices (PDA, ASD, etc.) less well suited to this application.

A major consideration in these procedures is device size selection. We avoid using a sizing balloon for fear of further damage to the septum. In the acute unoperated population that we traditionally have dealt with, the patients have been turned down for surgery and have large defects causing them to be hemodynamically unwell. Because of the complexity of these defects, multiple exit points are the rule as opposed to the exception, and we usually regret selecting a device smaller than the largest available. Gated CT scanning before these procedures has improved our understanding of these defects and will often be of use in deciding whether a procedure is to be successful. Clearly, in a patient who has survived 6 weeks postinfarct in a compensated hemodynamic state, there is much more flexibility in choosing a smaller device or balloon sizing. Both echocardiography and angiography can be helpful in device selection in the subacute phase of the illness. The same can be said of those treated 6 weeks postsurgery.

As alluded to previously, we routinely leave either a coronary wire or other 0.018-inch wire alongside the device in the sheath traversing the defect as we are preparing to deploy. If the device is pulled through the defect during positioning, it can be recaptured and the sheath maneuvered gently through the defect so that reforming the arteriovenous loop is not required. A minimal amount of stability testing should be performed once the device is in place to avoid disrupting the septum—a gentle push and tug is advised to ensure stability. At this point during the procedure, we interrogate the septum carefully with TEE and angiography. It is rare to have a minimal shunt in the acute setting both because of anatomy and because of the anticoagulation to support the procedure. If the perception is that the device is stable, and a significant part of the shunt has been occluded, it is reasonable to release the device—if not, a further attempt at repositioning can be made or the defect can be recrossed. If a device cannot be positioned appropriately, it should be removed as opposed to "hoping for the best." The safety wire is removed before the device is released.

CONCLUSION

This chapter reviews the epidemiology, indications, essential imaging before and during percutaneous VSD closure, as well as a procedural overview and a special section on post-MI VSD closure. It is difficult to believe that one would be able to complete these procedures without mentoring and training. Although the urgency of a post-MI VSR may make it seem like even the uninitiated should try to be a part of the solution, that is most certainly ill advised. VSD closure in the catheter laboratory is highly technical and this chapter provides a starting point or a refresher for those interested in the technique.

REFERENCES

1. Lillehei CW, Cohen M, Warden HE, et al. The results of direct vision closure of ventricular septal defects in eight patients by means of controlled cross circulation. *Surg Gynecol Obstet.* 1955;101(4):446–466.
2. Roos-Hesselink JW, Meijboom FJ, Spitaels SE, et al. Outcome of patients after surgical closure of ventricular septal defect at young age: longitudinal follow-up of 22–34 years. *Eur Heart J.* 2004;25(12):1057–1062.
3. Nygren A, Sunnegardh J, Berggren H. Preoperative evaluation and surgery in isolated ventricular septal defects: a 21 year perspective. *Heart.* 2000;83(2):198–204.
4. Lock JE, Block PC, McKay RG, et al. Transcatheter closure of ventricular septal defects. *Circulation.* 1988;78(2):361–368.
5. Silversides CK, Dore A, Poirier N, et al. Canadian Cardiovascular Society 2009 Consensus Conference on the management of adults with congenital heart disease: shunt lesions. *Can J Cardiol.* 2010;26(3):e70–e79.
6. Visconti KJ, Bichell DP, Jonas RA, et al. Developmental outcome after surgical versus interventional closure of secundum atrial septal defect in children. *Circulation.* 1999;100(suppl 19):II145–II150.
7. Thanopoulos BD, Tsaousis GS, Konstadopoulou GN, et al. Transcatheter closure of muscular ventricular septal defects with the amplatzer ventricular septal defect occluder: initial clinical applications in children. *J Am Coll Cardiol.* 1999;33(5):1395–1399.
8. Hijazi ZM, Hakim F, Al-Fadley F, et al. Transcatheter closure of single muscular ventricular septal defects using the amplatzer muscular VSD occluder: initial results and technical considerations. *Catheter Cardiovasc Interv.* 2000;49(2):167–172.
9. Hijazi ZM, Hakim F, Haweleh AA, et al. Catheter closure of perimembranous ventricular septal defects using the new Amplatzer membranous VSD occluder: initial clinical experience. *Catheter Cardiovasc Interv.* 2002;56(4):508–515.
10. Fu YC, Bass J, Amin Z, et al. Transcatheter closure of perimembranous ventricular septal defects using the new Amplatzer membranous VSD occluder: results

of the U.S. phase I trial. *J Am Coll Cardiol.* 2006;47(2):319–325.
11. Zuo J, Xie J, Yi W, et al. Results of transcatheter closure of perimembranous ventricular septal defect. *Am J Cardiol.* 2010;106(7):1034–1037.
12. Walsh MA, Bialkowski J, Szkutnik M, et al. Atrioventricular block after transcatheter closure of perimembranous ventricular septal defects. *Heart.* 2006;92(9):1295–1297.
13. Butera G, Gaio G, Carminati M. Is steroid therapy enough to reverse complete atrioventricular block after percutaneous perimembranous ventricular septal defect closure? *J Cardiovasc Med (Hagerstown).* 2009;10(5):412–414.
14. Al-Kashkari W, Balan P, Kavinsky CJ, et al. Percutaneous device closure of congenital and iatrogenic ventricular septal defects in adult patients. *Catheter Cardiovasc Interv.* 2011;77:260–267.
15. Holzer R, Balzer D, Cao QL, et al. Device closure of muscular ventricular septal defects using the Amplatzer muscular ventricular septal defect occluder: immediate and mid-term results of a U.S. registry. *J Am Coll Cardiol.* 2004;43(7):1257–1263.
16. Chessa M, Carminati M, Cao QL, et al. Transcatheter closure of congenital and acquired muscular ventricular septal defects using the Amplatzer device. *J Invasive Cardiol.* 2002;14(6):322–327.
17. Martinez MW, Mookadam F, Sun Y, et al. Transcatheter closure of ischemic and post-traumatic ventricular septal ruptures. *Catheter Cardiovasc Interv.* 2007;69(3):403–407.
18. Knauth AL, Lock JE, Perry SB, et al. Transcatheter device closure of congenital and postoperative residual ventricular septal defects. *Circulation.* 2004;110(5):501–507.
19. Pedra CA, Pedra SR, Esteves CA, et al. Percutaneous closure of perimembranous ventricular septal defects with the Amplatzer device: technical and morphological considerations. *Catheter Cardiovasc Interv.* 2004;61(3):403–410.

20. Thanopoulos BV, Rigby ML, Karansios E, et al. Transcatheter closure of perimembranous ventricular septal defects in infants and children using the Amplatzer perimembranous ventricular septal defect occluder. *Am J Cardiol.* 2007;99(7):984–989.

21. Crenshaw BS, Granger CB, Birnbaum Y, et al. Risk factors, angiographic patterns, and outcomes in patients with ventricular septal defect complicating acute myocardial infarction. GUSTO-I (Global Utilization of Streptokinase and TPA for Occluded Coronary Arteries) Trial Investigators. *Circulation.* 2000;101(1):27–32.

22. Menon V, Webb JG, Hillis LD, et al. Outcome and profile of ventricular septal rupture with cardiogenic shock after myocardial infarction: a report from the SHOCK Trial Registry. Should we emergently revascularize Occluded Coronaries in cardiogenic shocK? *J Am Coll Cardiol.* 2000;36(suppl 3A):1110–1116.

23. Cummings RG, Reimer KA, Califf R, et al. Quantitative analysis of right and left ventricular infarction in the presence of postinfarction ventricular septal defect. *Circulation.* 1988;77(1):33–42.

24. Patane F, Grassi R, Zucchetti MC, et al. The use of Impella Recover in the treatment of post-infarction ventricular septal defect: a new case report. *Int J Cardiol.* 2010;144(2):313–315.

25. Gregoric ID, Bieniarz MC, Aora H, et al. Percutaneous ventricular assist device support in a patient with a postinfarction ventricular septal defect. *Tex Heart Inst J.* 2008;35(1):46–49.

26. Antman EM, Hand M, Armstrong PW, et al. 2007 Focused Update of the ACC/AHA 2004 Guidelines for the Management of Patients With ST-Elevation Myocardial Infarction: a report of the American College of Cardiology/American Heart Association Task Force on Practice Guidelines: developed in collaboration With the Canadian Cardiovascular Society endorsed by the American Academy of Family Physicians: 2007 Writing Group to Review New Evidence and Update the ACC/AHA 2004 Guidelines for the Management of Patients With ST-Elevation Myocardial Infarction, Writing on Behalf of the 2004 Writing Committee. *Circulation.* 2008;117(2):296–329.

27. David TE, Armstrong S. Surgical repair of postinfarction ventricular septal defect by infarct exclusion. *Semin Thorac Cardiovasc Surg.* 1998;10(2):105–110.

CHAPTER 14

Closure of Coronary Artery Fistula, Pulmonary Arteriovenous Malformation, and Patent Ductus Arteriosus

Thomas K. Jones

TRANSCATHETER CLOSURE OF CORONARY ARTERY FISTULA

Incidence and Clinical Impact

Coronary artery fistula (CAF) is a rare congenital vascular malformation of the coronary artery tree that creates a direct vascular connection to a cardiac chamber, the great cardiac vein, or pulmonary artery. CAF is the most common congenital coronary artery anomaly incidentally identified in approximately one in 500 adult coronary angiograms. Over one-half of all CAF originate from the right coronary artery and 92% drain into the right side of the heart.[1] The size of the CAF determines its clinical impact. Small, hemodynamically insignificant CAF do not require treatment.[2] Once diagnosed, especially in a young patient, small CAF should be monitored long term as some may enlarge and become clinically important over time.[3]

Large CAF produce an important left-to-right shunt and cause a steal phenomenon that allows blood flow to bypass the distal myocardium. In children, CAF commonly present as a continuous heart murmur with cardiac enlargement and, occasionally, congestive heart failure. Large CAF in adult patients may present with exertional angina, thrombosis, endocarditis, myocardial infarction, heart failure, or even coronary aneurysm rupture with hemopericardium.

Occasionally, CAF can be acquired as a result of repeated myocardial biopsy, coronary artery bypass grafting, or cardiac surgery. The same indications for intervention apply as they do for patients with congenital CAF: Small CAF can be followed conservatively, whereas large CAF should be considered for treatment.

Indications for Closure and Guideline Recommendations

Transcatheter or surgical closure of CAF should be considered in all patients with large CAF regardless of symptoms (class I, level of evidence C).[4] Transcatheter embolization of CAF is by far the most widely practiced approach to this condition. In addition to being much less invasive than surgical ligation, transcatheter embolization offers superior imaging of the structure of the CAF including the exact site of drainage and the size and source of the feeding arterial vessels.

Preprocedure Evaluation and Imaging

Patients with larger CAF typically exhibit a continuous murmur similar to patent ductus arteriosus. Echocardiography demonstrates dilated and occasionally tortuous proximal coronary arteries. Often, the drainage site into a cardiac chamber, the coronary sinus, or a pulmonary artery can be demonstrated with color Doppler flow mapping (Fig. 14-1). Typically, echocardiographic

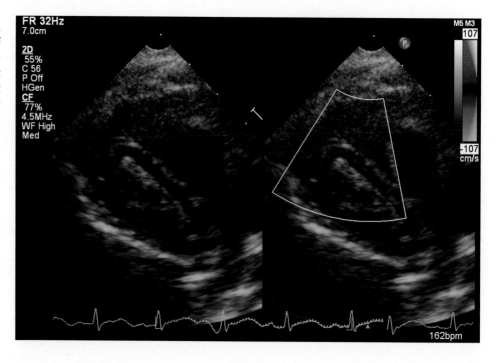

images are of adequate diagnostic quality to render a working diagnosis sufficient to warrant cardiac catheterization and angiographic assessment. For those patients who are incidentally discovered to have a small CAF without proximal coronary artery dilation or symptoms, the echocardiogram study alone is usually sufficient to guide conservative treatment and long-term follow-up. For those patients with large fistulae for whom transcatheter closure is being considered, computed tomography (CT) or magnetic resonance (MR) angiography can be useful in procedural planning. The location of the drainage site or sites, the size and course of the feeding arteries, and the presence of severely aneurysmal vessels can all be determined in advance. Otherwise, aortic root and selective coronary arteriography remains the definitive imaging modality to both diagnose and assess the results of transcatheter intervention.

Angiographic assessment of CAF must include a careful assessment of the entire coronary artery tree. Occasionally, CAF may be associated with ipsilateral or contralateral stenoses or atresias of the proximal coronary artery (Fig. 14-2).

Closure Techniques

Once initial angiographic assessment is complete, the operator is then able to determine the most suitable approach to close the fistula. The choices include cannulation of the arterial feeding vessel to deposit embolization coils or vascular plug, or retrograde access from the venous side of the circulation to occlude the exit site of the fistula at its drainage site typically into the right atrium or right ventricle. There are several important advantages to this latter approach. By closing the defect at its most distal single drainage point, the risk of occluding normal upstream myocardial perfusing branches is minimized. Additionally, prolonged cannulation of the distal coronary arteries with the attendant risk of thrombosis or vascular injury is avoided. Other times, direct retrograde cannulation of the feeding coronary vessels using micro coils delivered through a dedicated delivery catheter and supported coaxially through a coronary guide catheter will yield a very satisfactory result. Regardless of which approach is used, repeat selective coronary angiograms performed during the embolization procedure will inform the operator as to the completeness of the embolization procedure. Patience may be required during this process as cessation of flow may take some time, especially with larger CAF. The goal of complete occlusion may require the placement of several micro coils packed tightly together. Vascular plugs, if properly sized, will typically lead to complete closure with time even when the immediate postdeployment angiogram suggests residual shunt flow through the device.

In the adult patient, the procedure can normally be performed with conscious sedation. Once femoral venous and arterial access is obtained, systemic anticoagulation (heparin 100 U/kg) is provided and the activated clotting time is maintained within the therapeutic range. Aortic root angiography or selective

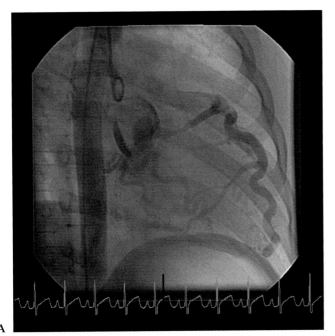
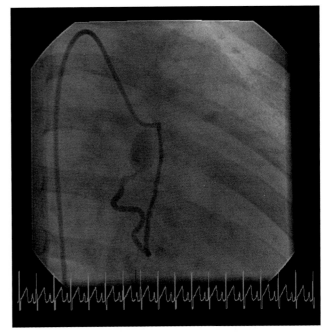

A   B

FIGURE 14-2.

Aortic root angiogram **(A)** demonstrates dilated proximal left coronary arteries with multiple feeding vessels entering a saccular entrance into the anterior right ventricular outflow tract. A selective right coronary artery angiogram **(B)** reveals a hypoplastic proximal vessel with distal total occlusion beyond the single feeding vessel entering the dilated distal portion of the fistula.

coronary arteriography using appropriate angulated views to define the entire coronary circulation is essential. Anatomic details of the location, size, and shape of the drainage site are important, especially if retrograde venous access and closure of the drainage site is being considered. Closure of the drainage site of a CAF from the venous approach can occasionally be accomplished by direct catheter manipulation into the drainage site. Other times, an arteriovenous guidewire loop is required. After retrograde arterial catheter placement is performed, a soft-tipped flexible guidewire can be advanced through the fistula, snared, and exteriorized through the venous sheath. Care must be taken when advancing and maintaining the guidewire through the proximal coronary vessels to avoid injury. This guidewire can then be used to advance a coil delivery catheter or a delivery sheath for a vascular plug from the venous side a short distance beyond the drainage site and into the fistula. Typically, the drainage site is a single narrowed mouth with proximal dilated segment that is ideal for embolization with coils or a vascular plug (Fig. 14-3).

In those instances where the arterial approach is used, the use of a supporting coronary guide catheter is essential and provides the necessary support to safely enter the distal feeding coronary arteries in a coaxial fashion with the coil delivery catheter. The choice of coil delivery catheter and therefore the coronary guide catheter is dependent on the operator's choice of embolization coil; 0.035-inch coils such as the Gianturco or Tornado coils (Cook Inc., Bloomington, IN) (Fig. 14-4) require a 4 or 5 French delivery catheter and a 7 or 8 French guiding catheter. If 0.018-inch micro coils such as the VortX-18 coils (Boston Scientific Corp, Natick, MA) are used, a smaller 6 French guide catheter can be selected. Alternatively, a triaxial delivery system using an 8 French guide, 5 French end-hole catheter, with a 3 French micro coil delivery catheter is very effective and provides extra support to minimize dislodgement of the coil delivery catheter as the coils are pushed forward and out of the distal end of the catheter. A particularly useful micro coil delivery catheter is the Progreat catheter (Terumo Medical Corp, Somerset, NJ) that includes a preloaded integral hydrophilic guidewire that extends beyond the tip of the delivery catheter (Fig. 14-5). This system allows the 3 French coil delivery catheter to be advanced forward into the distal coronary vessels along with the guidewire, eliminating the additional step of having to thread and advance the delivery catheter over a previously placed floppy coronary guidewire all the way from the hub of the guide catheter to the distal coronary artery bed. The coil diameter selected should be approximately 20% larger than the vessel diameter

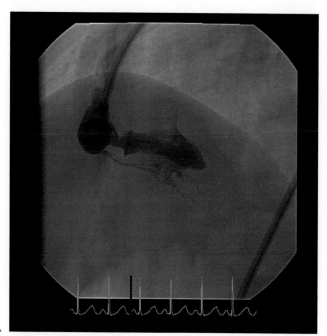
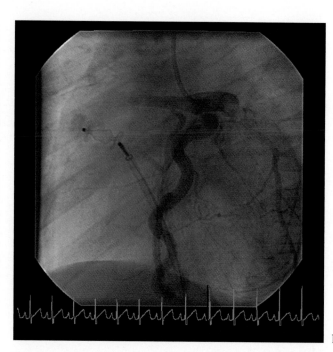

A   B

FIGURE 14-3.

Examples of occluder devices deployed within the distal drainage site of coronary artery fistula. **A:** Prograde delivery of an Amplatzer muscular ventricular septal defect occluder (AGA Medical Inc., Plymouth, MN) into a fistula arising from the proximal right coronary artery and entering the right atrium. Contrast injected through the delivery sheath demonstrates the occluder in appropriate position with contrast passing through the device shortly after deployment. **B:** Retrograde delivery of an Amplatzer vascular plug II (AGA Medical Inc.) into a fistula draining into the right ventricle. After snaring and exteriorizing a guidewire in the right ventricle introduced through the fistula from the left coronary artery, a 4 French delivery sheath is introduced from the femoral vein and into the distal saccular portion of the fistula shown in Figure 14-2. A selective left coronary artery angiogram demonstrates closure of the fistula even before device release.

targeted for embolization. Once an initial coil is placed as a scaffold, smaller diameter coils can be delivered into the original coil in an attempt to interlock the coil mass in place.

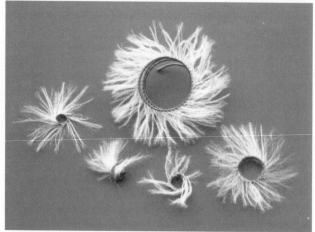

FIGURE 14-4.

Examples of Gianturco embolization coils (Cook Inc., Bloomington, IN). The coils have polyester fibers embedded in the spring coil wire that promotes thrombosis and eventual fibrosis of the vessel lumen.

Occasionally, the length of a CAF can be very short between the arterial entrance and the venous drainage site. This is especially true with fistulae between the circumflex coronary artery and coronary sinus. In such cases, covered coronary artery graft stents to seal the arterial feeding vessel have been successful.[5]

Complications of Transcatheter Treatment

Complications of CAF embolization can be severe, including coil migration into the venous circulation or coil misplacement or dislodgement resulting in occlusion of normal vascular supply to the myocardium. In such cases, transient ST-T wave changes may be observed or, if the obstruction involves a larger portion of myocardium, myocardial infarction can occur. Coronary artery spasm, thrombosis, air embolization, dissection, rupture, and hemopericardium have all been reported. Care with guidewire and catheter manipulations, knowledge and experience with arteriovenous guidewire loops and snare catheters, adequate anticoagulation, and patience are required to optimize patient outcomes.

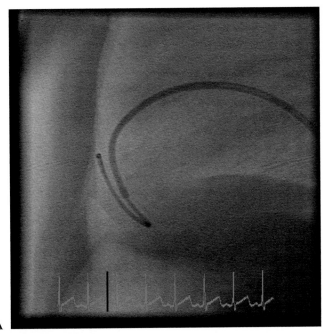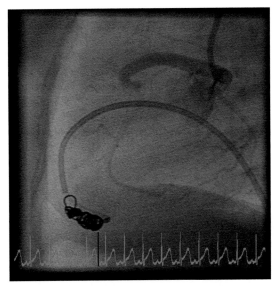

FIGURE 14-5.

A: Retrograde placement of a Progreat catheter (Terumo Medical Corporation, Somerset, NJ) introduced coaxially through a 4 French guiding catheter into the distal feeding vessel arising from the left anterior descending coronary artery and entering the right ventricular apex. **B:** Following embolization of vessel with multiple 0.018 micro coils, no flow through the fistula is noted on selective left coronary artery angiography.

Alternative Therapy

Occasionally, CAF are detected in the setting of other congenital or acquired cardiac disease that requires surgical repair. In such cases, surgical repair of the fistula can be performed in the same setting.[6] When long-standing CAF are discovered in adults, especially in instances where the feeding vessel arises from the distal circumflex coronary artery, there may be a spectacular degree of proximal coronary artery dilation. Such gross enlargement of the coronary vessels may predispose the patient to thrombosis of the entire proximal dilated coronary artery after closure of the distal fistula with resultant myocardial infarction. In such instances, closure must be carefully considered and, if undertaken, aggressive anticoagulation beginning immediately after the procedure should be considered.[7]

Postprocedural Care and Follow-up

Patients should be admitted for observation in a unit capable of continuous electrocardiographic monitoring. Anticoagulation with an antiplatelet agent should be started shortly before the procedure and continued indefinitely following embolization as long as persistent coronary artery dilation is present. In most adult patients, the proximal coronary arteries remain dilated, although some remodeling can occur over time. In cases of grossly dilated proximal coronary arteries, more aggressive anticoagulation with warfarin is preferable. Because there is limited data available on the long-term outlook for adult patients following CAF embolization, continued regular follow-up with assessment of myocardial reserve seems prudent. Stress echocardiography or other forms of myocardial perfusion imaging should be considered at baseline before embolization and periodically during long-term follow-up to assess for any late changes associated with this therapy.

TRANSCATHETER CLOSURE OF PULMONARY ARTERIOVENOUS MALFORMATION

Incidence and Clinical Impact

Pulmonary arteriovenous malformation (PAVM) is a rare congenital vascular malformation occurring within the lung circulation. Although PAVM can exist as an isolated condition, it is commonly associated with a hereditary condition known as hereditary hemorrhagic telangiectasia (HHT). This autosomal dominant disorder, referred to in the past as Rendu-Osler-Weber syndrome, can include clinically important vascular malformations in other organs including the brain, kidney, and nasal mucosa and skin. Affected individuals and their first-degree relatives should be screened for both the presence of PAVM and, especially, cerebral AVM that may be clinically silent until presenting with cerebral hemorrhage.[8]

PAVMs produce an intrapulmonary right-to-left shunt. PAVMs tend to progress over time resulting in important clinical sequelae associated with right-to-left shunting including hypoxemia with dyspnea and exercise intolerance, paradoxical embolization with stroke or transient ischemic attack, and pulmonary hemorrhage with massive hemoptysis or hemothorax.[9]

Indications for Closure and Guideline Recommendations

Transcatheter embolization of PAVM is indicated for relief of symptoms associated with the effects of a large right-to-left shunt including hypoxemia and dyspnea. Treatment is also indicated for prevention of pulmonary hemorrhage and paradoxical embolic events including stroke, transient ischemic attack, or myocardial infarction.

Preprocedure Evaluation and Imaging

Patients commonly present with cyanosis and polycythemia in early adulthood due to large and long-standing intrapulmonary right-to-left shunting. Often, there is a history of exertional dyspnea dating back to childhood. Occasionally, the presenting symptoms are related to paradoxical embolization with stroke or systemic embolic events. Plain chest radiographs may suggest the presence of PAVM, but CT or MR angiography provide important details to inform subsequent catheter-based treatment including the location, number and size of the arterial feeding vessels, and the presence of multiple, smaller malformations.

Contrast echocardiography along with pulse oximetry or arterial blood gas monitoring during 100% oxygen challenge can serve as a useful screening technique for all patients presenting with resting cyanosis.[10] Patients with a fixed intrapulmonary right-to-left shunt will exhibit only a small increase in saturation or Pao_2, whereas patients with pulmonary disease will demonstrate a significant rise with oxygen administration. Saline contrast echocardiography is also a helpful screening technique that can identify the source of right-to-left shunt as intrapulmonary when there is a delay of at least three to five heart beats between

the appearance of saline contrast "bubbles" in the left atrium after a systemic venous injection.[11]

Closure Techniques

Selective pulmonary angiography will define the location, size, and number of arterial feeder vessels; the size and shape of the aneurysmal sac; and the number and location of the draining veins. The most common form of PAVM, the simple type, occurs in 80% of patients.[12] The simple type has a single arterial feeding vessel and draining vein. The aneurysmal sac is nonseptated. The less common complex form has multiple feeding vessels, septated aneurysmal sacs, and may have more than one draining vein (Fig. 14-6). The aneurysmal sac of PAVMs are very thin and prone to rupture and bleeding. Therefore, the goal of closure is to occlude the arterial feeding vessel or vessels as close to the sac as possible while minimizing catheter or guidewire manipulations within the sac. Care should be taken to also avoid embolizing the feeding vessel at a more proximal location that could occlude the blood supply to normal lung. This is especially true when multiple PAVMs are present and multiple indiscriminate proximal occlusions could result in a significant reduction in pulmonary vascular bed.

By far the most common approach to closing PAVM is with pushable fibered embolization coils delivered through coaxial catheters (Fig. 14-7). The use of coaxial or triaxial catheters allows for precise coil delivery and reduces the risk of proximal coil malposition. The use of a guiding catheter to support the delivery catheter also allows smaller coils to be positioned within a

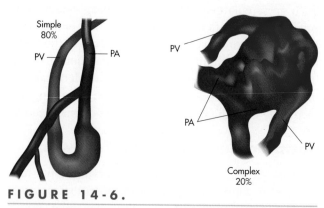

FIGURE 14-6.

Angiographic classification of pulmonary arteriovenous malformations. PA, pulmonary artery; PV, pulmonary vein. (Adapted from Sievert H, Qureshi S, Wilson N. *Percutaneous Interventions for Congenital Heart Disease.* London: Informa Healthcare; 2007. p. 419.)

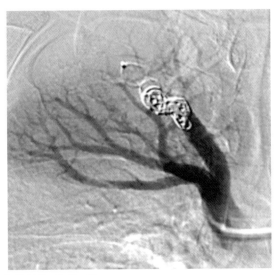

FIGURE 14-7.

Nest of fibered embolization coils densely packed within the arterial feeding vessel of a large right upper lobe pulmonary arteriovenous malformation. Note no residual flow through the embolized vessel and preserved blood flow to unaffected adjacent arterial segments.

larger anchor or scaffold coil. It is important to achieve complete cross-sectional closure at the time of the procedure as delayed closure using embolization coils is uncommon because of the brisk blood flow through larger PAVMs. Care should also be exercised to avoid air or thrombus embolization during catheter and guidewire manipulations along with periprocedural systemic heparinization.

Following pulmonary artery pressure recording and angiography, an 80-cm 7 French guiding catheter is positioned close to the arterial feeding vessel. A 100-cm 5 French end-hole coil delivery catheter can then be advanced beyond the guide catheter to the site of coil placement. The added support provided by the guiding catheter prevents the coil delivery catheter from backing out of the target area during embolization, thereby allowing the coils to be delivered more precisely and in a tighter mass. The initial coil can be delivered initially into a small side branch with the remainder of the coil positioned in the larger feeding artery. This so-called anchor technique provides a stable scaffold for additional coils to be deposited within the original coil.[13]

Alternatively, the Amplatzer family of vascular plugs (AGA Medical Inc., Plymouth, MN) can be used to occlude the feeder vessel and is especially useful for larger or short length arterial feeders. The original Amplatzer vascular plug I (AVP I) is available in diameters up to 16 mm. The newer generation Amplatzer vascular plug II (AVP II) is available in sizes up to 22 mm. The second-generation device has a finer and denser nitinol wire frame along with a multisegmented design that produces rapid and complete closure even in very large PAVMs (Fig. 14-8). The smaller plugs can be delivered through a 5 French sheath, whereas a 7 or 8 French sheath is required for the larger devices. Another advantage of the AVPs is the ability to reposition or retrieve the device prior to unscrewing it from the flexible delivery cable. In a recent large series, 75% of all PAVMs were successfully treated with AVP alone, whereas the balance of smaller or more tortuous feeding vessels were occluded with coils.[14]

Complications of Transcatheter Treatment

Complications reported after transcatheter intervention include pleuritic chest pain, bleeding, infection, pulmonary infarction, pleural effusion, and paradoxical embolization of occluder devices or thrombus resulting in stroke.[15] Following PAVM embolization, low-dose aspirin has been suggested for short-term prevention of stroke.[16]

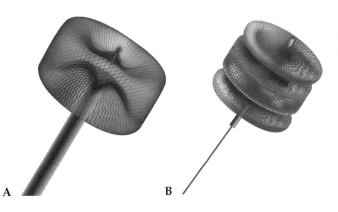

FIGURE 14-8.

A: Amplatzer vascular plug I (AGA Medical Inc., Plymouth, MN). **B:** Amplatzer vascular plug II (AGA Medical Inc.).

Alternative Therapy

Surgical resection of affected lung segments was the standard of care before the early 1980s, but is rarely performed today. On occasion, complex or diffuse PAVM cannot be safely or completely occluded. In such instances, a reduction in the volume of right-to-left shunting by partial or staged transcatheter closure may help reduce cyanosis and alleviate symptoms. Stroke reduction risk may be positively affected, although not eliminated. Such patients may benefit from long-term anticoagulation.

Postprocedural Care and Follow-up

Most patients can be discharged following outpatient treatment on low-dose aspirin therapy. Routine long-term follow-up with annual pulse oximetry, contrast echocardiography, and chest radiography is recommended for the early detection of PAVMs due to enlarging untreated lesions or recanalization of those previously treated. For those patients found to have HHT on preprocedural screening, lifelong follow-up for other long-term manifestations of HHT is important.[17]

TRANSCATHETER CLOSURE OF PATENT DUCTUS ARTERIOSUS

Incidence and Clinical Impact

The ductus arteriosus is a vital structure during fetal life, allowing blood to bypass the lung circulation through a tubular communication between the main pulmonary artery and the proximal descending aorta. Normally, the ductus arteriosus constricts in response to rising arterial oxygen saturations following delivery and closes completely within 24 to 48 hours of life. When the ductus arteriosus fails to close completely, it is termed a patent ductus arteriosus (PDA) and allows a continuous left-to-right shunt from the high resistance systemic circulation into the low resistance pulmonary circulation. The caliber of the PDA is the primary determinant of the volume of blood flowing through this communication.

Persistence of the arterial duct beyond infancy is not uncommon and accounts for approximately 10% of all congenital heart disease. Most adolescent and adult patients are outwardly asymptomatic with smaller diameter PDA (<3.5 to 4.0 mm). The diagnosis in these patients is typically made with the discovery of a continuous murmur. Patients with larger diameter PDA can present with congestive heart failure, recurrent pulmonary infections, or pulmonary hypertension.

Indications for Closure and Guideline Recommendations

Closure of hemodynamically significant PDA is indicated in adult patients to eliminate the considerable long-term risk of bacterial endarteritis and to relieve chronic pulmonary overcirculation and left ventricular volume overload (class I, level of evidence C). Patients with pulmonary arterial hypertension, but with an overall left-to-right shunt, should also be considered for transcatheter closure in the setting of ongoing medical management of their pulmonary hypertension (class IIa, level of evidence C). Patients with severe pulmonary hypertension and pure right-to-left shunt (Eisenmenger syndrome) cannot safely undergo PDA closure (class III, level of evidence C).[4]

Preprocedure Evaluation and Imaging

Complete echocardiographic assessment is often all that is required to guide a recommendation for cardiac catheterization evaluation and transcatheter closure. The PDA size and shape, the volume and direction of shunt, and the effects on chamber volume can all be assessed. Echocardiographic images in some adult patient may fail to adequately define the relevant ductal, aortic arch, and pulmonary artery anatomy. In those instances, CT or MR angiography can be very helpful in guiding the planned intervention. With age, the PDA may undergo aneurysmal enlargement or become calcified. Also, the location of the PDA can change with age as the aortic arch "rolls" forward into the more kyphotic elderly chest shape. The aortic orifice of the PDA will migrate forward arising from the inferior aspect of the transverse aortic arch (Fig. 14-9).

Aortic angiography at the time of transcatheter closure provides anatomic detail needed to determine the most appropriate closure device. In addition to the minimal diameter of the PDA, the length and shape of the PDA are also measured. An angiographic classification system developed in 1989 is still widely used to describe the shape of the PDA.[18] Over 75% of PDA are the familiar conical-shaped type A PDA (Fig. 14-10).

Closure Techniques

The goal of transcatheter closure is to achieve complete closure at the time of the procedure. Embolization coils have been used in an off-label fashion for this purpose since 1992 and are useful for smaller PDA (less than 2.5 to 3.0 mm).[19] Gianturco coils or the detachable Flipper coils (Cook Inc.) are most commonly used and can be delivered either from a pulmonary artery or, more

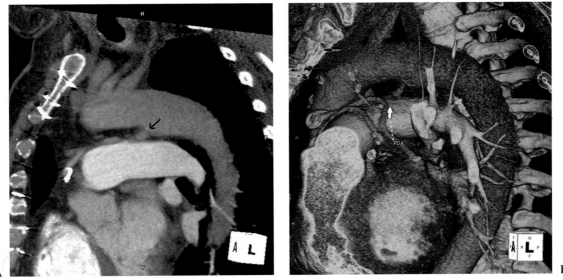

FIGURE 14-9.

Computed tomography (CT) angiogram of persistent patent ductus arteriosus (PDA) in an elderly patient. Kyphotic change in shape of chest and aortic arch leads to migration of the PDA into a more transverse arch location. **A:** CT tomogram, *arrow* indicates PDA. **B:** Three-dimensional CT rendering of aortic arch in the same patient.

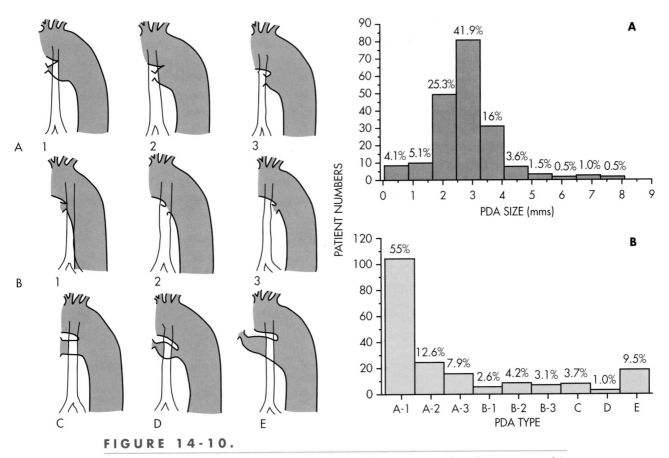

FIGURE 14-10.

A: Krichenko patent ductus arteriosus (PDA) classification system based on angiographic appearance from a lateral view descending aortogram. **B:** Distribution of PDA types. The type A conical form is most common.

commonly, a retrograde aortic approach (Fig. 14-11). A purpose-built nitinol coil for PDA closure, the pfm Nit-Occlud PDA occlusion system (PFM Medical AG, Köln, Germany), makes it possible to close most PDA less than 3.5 mm in diameter using a small and flexible delivery catheter of 4 or 5 French diameter (Fig. 14-12). This useful design is currently not approved in the United States.

Clinically significant PDA in the adult is typically larger than 3.5 to 4.0 mm in diameter. These larger defects are most safely and practically closed using the Amplatzer Duct Occluder (AGA Medical Inc.). The Amplatzer Duct Occluder was first successfully used in 1998. The device consists of a nitinol wire frame with polyester fabric sewn within the interior of the wire frame. The tapered shape of the occluder is designed to conform to the common conical-shaped form of the PDA (Fig. 14-13). The device should be approximately 2 to 3 mm larger than the narrowest portion of the PDA. The occluder is threaded on a flexible delivery cable and advanced through a delivery catheter previously positioned in the descending aorta and across the PDA from the pulmonary artery side. The cable is advanced, allowing the aortic retention skirt to open up in the descending aorta. The entire delivery system is brought back to snug the occluder into the PDA. At this point, the delivery sheath is gently brought back, deploying the remainder of the device across the narrowest portion of the PDA as it enters the main pulmonary artery. The occluder can be recaptured and repositioned at any point prior to device release. After appropriate device position is confirmed by aortography, the device is released by unscrewing the delivery cable (Fig. 14-14).

Occasionally, it is necessary to advance a guidewire across the PDA from the aortic side and snare this wire

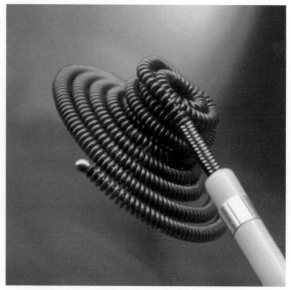

FIGURE 14-12.

Nit-Occlud patent ductus arteriosus (PDA) occlusion system (PFM Medical AG, Köln, Germany). The conical-shaped nitinol coil is designed to conform to the typical shape of small-moderate PDA. The delivery system allows precise coil positioning before release.

in the main pulmonary artery. This guidewire can then be exteriorized from the femoral vein. The resulting arteriovenous guidewire loop provides excellent support to advance the delivery sheath through the right heart and main pulmonary artery, across the PDA, and into the descending aorta.

Very large PDA with pulmonary hypertension creates a special challenge because device dislodgement and embolization is more likely when pulmonary artery pressures are elevated. The Amplatzer Muscular Ventricular Septal Defect Occluder (AGA Medical

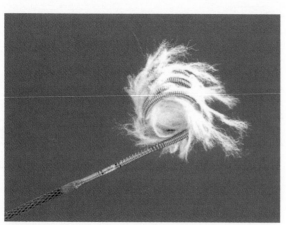

FIGURE 14-11.

Flipper detachable embolization coil (Cook Inc., Bloomington, IN). Coil is retrievable and repositionable.

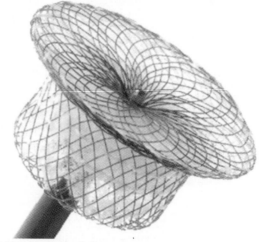

FIGURE 14-13.

Amplatzer Duct Occluder (AGA Medical Inc.).

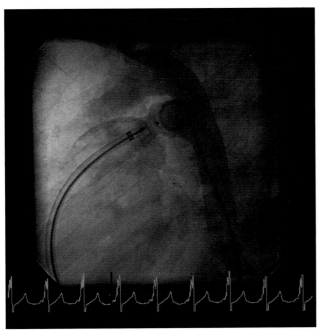
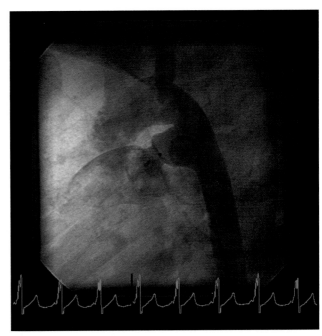

A   B

FIGURE 14-14.

A: 12/10 Amplatzer duct occluder (AGA Medical Inc., Plymouth, MN) appropriately deployed across a large patent ductus arteriosus (PDA). Device is still attached to the delivery cable. **B:** Following device release, the occluder remains well-positioned within the PDA. Note some residual shunt flow through the fabric of the occluder shortly after release. Shunt flow was confirmed to resolve on follow-up color Doppler echocardiogram.

Inc.), a device approved for transcatheter closure of congenital defects in the muscular portion of the interventricular septum, can be used to successfully close these hypertensive PDA. This occluder has the advantage of having two retention skirts, one on either side of a central waist. Once deployed across the PDA, the proximal retention skirt in the main pulmonary artery provides a counterforce to the retention skirt deployed on the aortic side of the PDA and keeps the occluder secure within the PDA, even when the pulmonary artery pressure is significantly elevated.

Complications of Transcatheter Treatment

Complications of transcatheter closure of PDA occur largely at the time of the procedure or in the early time following closure. Embolization of the occluder device can occur due to improper device sizing or maldeployment. With patience, most embolized PDA occluders can be safely removed percutaneously. Skill with snare techniques and a suitable inventory of retrieval equipment is required to safely manage this complication. Residual shunts are uncommon with the occluder devices compared to embolization coils. Residual shunts following device closure

of PDA have been associated with hemolysis and endocarditis.[19]

Alternative Therapy

Very small PDA discovered incidentally that are not associated with a cardiac murmur or chamber enlargement do not need to be closed. Surgical treatment is not commonly performed in the modern era unless there are complications such as a large ductal aneurysm. In such cases, cardiopulmonary bypass is typically required.

Postprocedural Care and Follow-up

Most patients can be discharged following outpatient treatment. A predischarge imaging study (chest radiographic, limited echocardiogram) will confirm that the implanted device position is stable and appropriate. For routine cases, low-dose aspirin therapy following closure is not needed. Endocarditis prophylaxis is advised for the first 6 months after closure until complete endothelial healing has occurred. Occasional follow-up visits, especially in the first year following device closure, are recommended, although the long-term results of catheter closure of PDA are reassuring with extremely low rate of late complications.[20,21]

REFERENCES

1. McNamara JJ, Gross RE. Congenital coronary artery fistula. *Surgery.* 1969;65(1):59–69.

2. Sherwood MC, Rockenbacher S, Colan SD, et al. Prognostic significance of clinically silent coronary artery fistulas. *Am J Cardiol.* 1999;83(3):407–411.

3. Takahashi M, Lurie PR. Abnormalities and diseases of the coronary arteries. In: Adams FH, Emmanouilides GC, Riemenschneider TA, eds. Heart Disease in Infants, Children and Adolescents. 4th ed. Baltimore: Williams & Wilkins; 1989:627–647.

4. Warnes CA, Williams RG, Bashore TM, et al. ACC/AHA 2008 Guidelines for the management of adults with congenital heart disease: executive summary: a report of the American College of Cardiology/American Heart Association Task Force on Practice Guidelines (Writing Committee to Develop Guidelines for the Management of Adults With Congenital Heart Disease). *J Am Coll Cardiol.* 2008;52(23):1890–1947.

5. Kilic H, Akdemir R, Bicer A, et al. Transcatheter closure of congenital coronary arterial fistulas in adults. *Coron Artery Dis.* 2008;19(1):43–45.

6. Cebi N, Shulze-Waltrup N, Frömke J, et al. Congenital coronary artery fistulas in adults: concomitant pathologies and treatment. *Int J Cardiovasc Imaging.* 2008;24(4):349–355.

7. Gowda ST, Latson LA, Kutty S, et al. Intermediate to long-term outcome following congenital coronary artery fistulae closure with focus on thrombus formation. *Am J Cardiol.* 2011;107(2):302–308.

8. Bayrak-Toydemir R, Mao R, Lewin S, et al. Hereditary hemorrhagic telangiectasia: an overview of diagnosis and management in the molecular era for clinicians. *Genet Med.* 2004;6(4):175–191.

9. Khurshid I, Downie GH. Pulmonary arteriovenous malformation. *Postgrad Med J.* 2002;78(918):191–197.

10. Kjeldsen AD, Oxhøj A, Andersen PE, et al. Pulmonary arteriovenous malformations: screening procedures and pulmonary angiography in patients with hereditary hemorrhagic telangiectasia. *Chest.* 1999;116(2):432–439.

11. Parra JA, Bueno J, Zarauza J, et al. Graded contrast echocardiography in pulmonary arteriovenous malformations. *Eur Respir J.* 2010;35(6):1279–1285.

12. White RI Jr, Mitchell SE, Barth KH, et al. Angioarchitecture of pulmonary arteriovenous malformations: an important consideration before embolotherapy. *AJR Am J Roentgenol.* 1983;140(4):681–686.

13. White RI Jr. Pulmonary arteriovenous malformations: how do I embolize? *Tech Vasc Interv Radiol.* 2007;10(4):283–290.

14. Hart JL, Aldin Z, Braude P, et al. Embolization of pulmonary arteriovenous malformations using the Amplatzer vascular plug: successful treatment of 69 consecutive patients. *Eur Radiol.* 2010;20(11):2663–2670.

15. Gupta P, Mordin C, Curtis J, et al. Pulmonary arteriovenous malformation: effect of embolization of right-to-left shunt, hypoxemia, and exercise tolerance in 66 patients. *AJR Am J Roentgenol.* 2002;179(2):347–355.

16. Felix S, Jeannin S, Goizet C, et al. Stroke following pulmonary arteriovenous fistula embolization in a patient with HHT. *Neurology.* 2008;71(24):2012–2014.

17. Faughnan ME, Palda VA, Garcia-Tsao G, et al. International guidelines for the diagnosis and management of hereditary hemorrhagic telangiectasia. *J Med Genet.* 2011;48:73–87.

18. Krichenko A, Benson LN, Burrows P, et al. Angiographic classification of the isolated, persistently patent ductus arteriosus and implications for percutaneous catheter occlusion. *Am J Cardiol.* 1989;63(12):877–880.

19. Cambier PA, Kirby WC, Wortham DC, et al. Percutaneous closure of the small (less than 2.5 mm) patent ductus arteriosus using coil embolization. *Am J Cardiol.* 1992;69(8):815–816.

20. Choi DY, Kim NY, Jung MJ, et al. The results of transcatheter occlusion of patent ductus arteriosus: success rate and complications over 12 years in a single center. *Korean Circ J.* 2010;40(5):230–234.

21. Lee CH, Leung YL, Chow WH. Transcatheter closure of the patent ductus arteriosus using an Amplatzer duct occluder in adults. *Jpn Heart J.* 2001;42(4):533–537.

CHAPTER 15

Closure of Paravalvular Leaks

Yuriy Dudiy, Vladimir Jelnin, and Carlos E. Ruiz

A paravalvular leak (PVL) may occur due to a dehiscence of native tissue around the implanted valve's sewing ring which results in paravalvular regurgitation. It is a well-known complication after surgical valve replacement. Abnormal pressure forces or tractions after the surgery, particularly in the setting of endocarditis or heavy calcification of the annulus, may result in the generation of PVLs.[1] The reported incidence of PVLs is 2% to 10% for prosthetic valves in the aortic position[2,3] and 7% to 17% for prosthetic valves in the mitral position.[2–4] The incidence of PVLs is higher with mechanical prostheses compared to biologic prostheses.[2] Although most PVLs are diagnosed within the first year after the surgery, some may emerge more than 20 years after the valve replacement.[2,5] PVL may be single or multiple and localized anywhere around the sewing ring of the prosthesis.

CLINICAL MANIFESTATION

The majority of patients with PVLs are asymptomatic; however, 1% to 5% of patients[6] may present with symptoms of congestive heart failure and/or hemolysis. Congestive heart failure results from volume overload caused by the regurgitation through the PVL, and it is proportional to the size of the defect. On the other hand, hemolysis, which is caused by sheer stress on red blood cells when passing through the defect, may be significant even with small leaks, especially, if multiple leaks are present.

PHYSICAL EXAMINATION

Physical examination of a patient with aortic PVL may reveal the presence of an early diastolic, decrescendo murmur that can be heard at the second to third intercostal spaces and all accompanying signs of congestive heart failure seen in patients with aortic insufficiency.

Patients with a mitral PVL may also present with classical findings of congestive heart failure and the presence of a mitral regurgitation murmur that is high pitched, pansystolic, and best heard at the cardiac apex with radiation to the axilla. An S3 gallop can be present if a patient develops left ventricle (LV) dysfunction. If there is increased stroke volume of the LV due to volume overload, an ejection systolic flow murmur may also be present when auscultating the aortic area.

LABORATORY STUDIES

All patients with clinically symptomatic PVLs should have blood tests to determine the degree of hemolysis. Serial complete blood count, haptoglobin, lactate dehydrogenase, and free hemoglobin levels should be obtained. Less frequently, thrombocytopenia can be observed. In addition, the trending of NT-pro BNP (N-terminal of the brain natriuretic peptide) may be helpful to assess changes in congestive heart failure.

IMAGING

Echocardiography

Echocardiography is the gold standard procedure for diagnosis of the PVL.[7,8] The severity of the leak can be defined by the same criteria that are used to define the severity of valvular regurgitation by the American Society of Echocardiography.[9] These include the area of the color Doppler regurgitant jet in the proximal chamber (e.g., the mitral regurgitant jet in the left atrium), the narrowest diameter of the leak jet (vena contracta), the magnitude of the proximal isovelocity surface area, and the regurgitant volume and fraction obtained by spectral Doppler volumetric methods. Two-dimensional (2D) transesophageal echocardiography (TEE) is sensitive in accurately identifying the presence of a PVL (sensitivity approaches 88%)[10]; however, pinpointing the exact location using 2D imaging modalities can be difficult.

Currently available three-dimensional (3D) real-time echocardiography addresses the shortcomings of 2D echocardiography and facilitates demonstration of anatomical location, number, size, and shape (round, linear, crescent, irregular) of the PVLs.[11] With the use of the 3D zoom modality, the entire mitral prosthesis can be seen en face and the paravalvular orifices identified and analyzed (Fig. 15-1C).

The full volume modality (which is not real-time acquisition) allows the demonstration of Doppler color flow through the leak site, as well as normal and abnormal flow patterns through the valve (Fig. 15-1D). Because of the aortic valve plane, 3D real-time TEE images of aortic valve prosthesis may not be as effective in characterizing the leaks, but it can still provide valuable information when compared with 2D images.

Computed Tomographic Angiography

Electrocardiography-gated computed tomographic angiography (CTA) prior to the intervention can be a great additional imaging tool to improve accuracy of the description of these defects. Helical acquisition

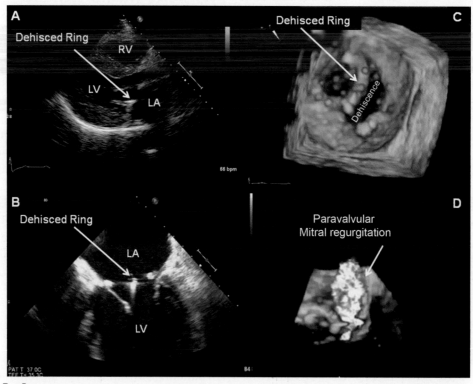

FIGURE 15-1.

Echocardiographic evaluation of mitral ring dehiscence. **A:** Parasternal long-axis view from a transthoracic echocardiogram (TTE) demonstrating mitral annuloplasty ring dehiscence. The posterior aspect of the ring is seen and appears to be possibly separated from the elevated native mitral annulus. **B:** Two-dimensional transesophageal echocardiographic image, obtained at 0 degree. The ring is clearly dehisced, appearing in the middle of the mitral annulus. **C:** Real-time three-dimensional (3D) image obtained using the 3D zoom mode. The mitral ring is viewed en face from the left atrial perspective. The dehisced segment is clearly seen and its shape, size, and location are easily defined. **D:** Image obtained using full-volume, color Doppler acquisition. Significant mitral regurgitation is seen originating from around the ring through the dehisced segment. LA, left atrium; LV, left ventricle; RV, right ventricle.

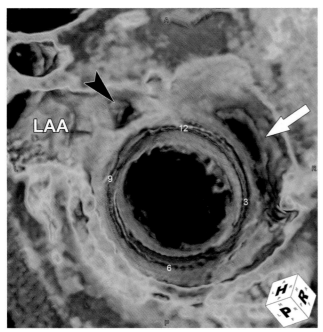

FIGURE 15-2.

Three-dimensional volume-rendered computed tomographic angiography reconstruction. Large, crescent-shape mitral paravalvular leak located between 1 and 3 o'clock (*white arrow*); small, round shape leak at 11 o'clock (*black arrowhead*). LAA, left atrial appendage.

with retrospective electrocardiography-gated reconstruction of multiple phases in 6.25% to 5.0% RR-interval increments allows four-dimensional (4D) reconstruction (time factor), which helps to simulate actual heart movements. Dynamic anatomic interrelations, which are critical in the evaluation process of percutaneous interventions, can therefore be evaluated.

CTA with 3D/4D volume rendering is also helpful in procedural planning of the percutaneous intervention. Based on the information obtained from the CTA (Fig. 15-2), the size of the closing device, approach, and best fluoroscopy view planned are determined by the operator before the procedure.

DIFFERENTIAL DIAGNOSES

PVLs should be differentiated from intravalvular leaks, which can be caused by prosthesis malfunction mechanically (pannus formation, thrombus, etc.) and biologically, especially when there is dehiscence of the leaflet sutures at the level of the posts. Although valvular regurgitation is easy to recognize, dehiscence at the post creates a jet that may be falsely interpreted as a PVL (Fig. 15-3). Therefore, examination of the PVL by an experienced cardiologist-echocardiographer is essential prior to the procedure.

NOMENCLATURE OF ANATOMICAL LOCATION OF PARAVALVULAR LEAKS

We use our own adaptation of the accepted surgical nomenclature[1,12] using the clock-face reference to describe the anatomic location of the leaks. We compare each valve to a clock so there are two clocks; one is in aortic valve position and the second is in mitral valve position as seen from a cephalad position. The 12 o'clock in both clocks corresponds to the mitral-aortic fibrous continuity, and from there, we name each location in a clockwise fashion (Fig. 15-4).

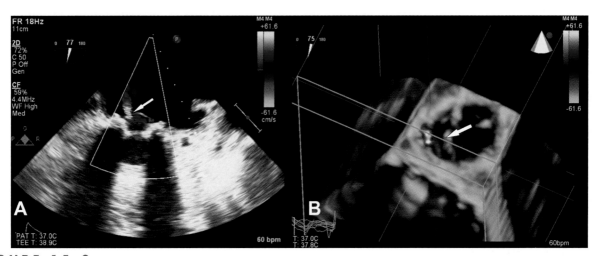

FIGURE 15-3.

Mild mitral intravalvular regurgitation. Two-dimensional transesophageal echocardiographic image, obtained at 0 degrees (**A**). Full-volume, color Doppler acquisition (**B**), obtained at 75 degrees. Defect at the level of posts (*white arrow*).

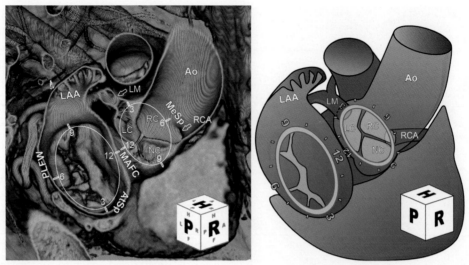

FIGURE 15-4.

Surgical view (computed tomography angiography). Three-dimensional volume–rendered reconstruction of the heart showing the mitral and aortic complexes from a posterior view. Mitral valve: The mitral-aortic fibrous continuity (*MAFC*) is 12 o'clock in both clocks; atrial septum (*AtSp*) is 3 o'clock; posterolateral free wall (*PLFW*) is 6 o'clock; and left atrial appendage (*LAA*) is 9 o'clock. Aortic valve: Left coronary sinus (*LC*) is between 11 and 3 o'clock; right coronary sinus (*RC*) is between 3 and 7 o'clock; and noncoronary sinus (*NC*) is between 7 and 11 o'clock. Ao, aorta; LA, left atrium; LCA, left coronary artery; MeSp, membranous septum; MuSp, muscular septum; RCA, right coronary artery.

For the aortic valve, the left coronary cusp is located between 11 and 3 o'clock, the right coronary cusp between 3 and 7 o'clock, and the noncoronary cusp between 7 and 11 o'clock. The highest rate of PVLs, in our experience, are found at the right coronary cusp (between 7 and 11 o'clock), which corresponds to the membranous septum and the right trigone.[5]

For the mitral valve, the 3 o'clock corresponds to the area of the atrial septum, the 6 o'clock corresponds to the posterolateral free wall, and the 9 o'clock corresponds to the region of the left atrial appendage (LAA). In our series, mitral PVLs were most frequently located between 10 and 2 o'clock, which corresponds to the mitral-aortic fibrous continuity, and between 6 and 10 o'clock, which corresponds to posterior wall.[5]

MANAGEMENT

The management of a patient with a PVL includes the routine medical management of treating congestive heart failure and correction of the anemia in addition to the closure of the defect. Defect closure has been shown to improve quality of life and decrease long-term mortality.[4]

Surgical Treatment

Surgical treatment, still considered the gold standard, and may include a redo valve replacement or patching

the defect. These procedures are associated with higher risk of recurrence of the PVLs (20% after first reoperation and 42.1% after second reoperation)[13] and carry higher mortality rate compared to the initial surgery (7.3% first reoperation, 17.3% second reoperation, 40% third reoperation).[13–15]

Percutaneous Closure

Since the first attempted percutaneous closure of PVL by Hourihan et al. in 1992,[16] it has become an attractive alternative, especially for the patients who are at high surgical risk or are not suitable for open heart surgery. Percutaneous PVL closure is a technically demanding procedure and may require long radiation exposures (the average fluoroscopy time reported for "large series" is between 31 and 62 minutes[6,17,18]). The procedures are commonly performed under general anesthesia and require an experienced operative team of echocardiographer, anesthesiologist, structural interventional cardiologist, and nurses.

The success of percutaneous closures depends on the anatomy of the defect, planning of the procedure, and the devices available.

Guiding the Intervention

1. *Echocardiography*: TEE and intracardiac echocardiography (ICE) have both been used to guide the procedure. ICE is better tolerated by the patient

but requires frequent repositioning and only offers one single plane. On the other hand, multiplanar 2D TEE provides high-resolution images with relatively high frame rate. However, since catheters move in three planes, the entire length and extent of the catheters, especially their tips, often cannot be accurately tracked. Although 3D imaging has a lower frame rate, the entire intracardiac portion of all the catheters can be visualized. The relation between the tip of the wire, the surrounding structures, and the PVL can be better evaluated; furthermore, the direction of the wire can be modified according to this information throughout the procedure, therefore providing a better imaging feedback for faster procedural times and better results (Fig. 15-5). Ultimately, whether the wire crosses through the valve or through the leak can be confirmed. In fact, since 3D TEE became commercially available, it has become our default option to confirm wire passage through the defect, evaluate interference with the prosthesis, look for residual leak, and rule out complications.

2. *CTA:* 4D volume rendered images of the CTA can be used to facilitate the crossing of the defect with hydrophilic wires. In our catheterization laboratory, 4D images are displayed on a separate screen, side-by-side, concurrent with live fluoroscopy. The CTA images are rotated and angulated according to the movement of the fluoroscopy image intensifier, allowing the CTA and the fluoroscopy images to be congruent throughout the procedure. Once the defect is located on the CTA image, a landmark is established that can be extrapolated and tracked by the operator on the fluoroscopy image. This method expedites localization of the leak on fluoroscopic image and adds some additional comfort to the operator (Fig. 15-6).

Interventional Techniques

Prophylactic antibiotics should be given to every patient prior to the procedure. Anticoagulation throughout the procedure should be done in a routine manner maintaining the activated clotting time above 150 seconds.

Retrograde Approach

Using arterial access and different coronary catheters, an angled or straight hydrophilic guidewire is directed through the aorta toward the defect. Once the defect is crossed, the guidewire is exchanged for an extra support wire (Lunderquist extra stiff wire, Cook Medical Inc., Bloomington, IN) and a hydrophilic delivery sheath (Shuttle SL 90 cm, Cook Medical Inc.) is inserted over the wire. Using Amplatzer-type devices, the distal disk of the device is expanded and the device is then deployed within the defect. Special attention must be paid to the function of the prosthetic valve prior to release of the device to ensure that the device does not interfere with valve function, especially with those devices that have double disks.

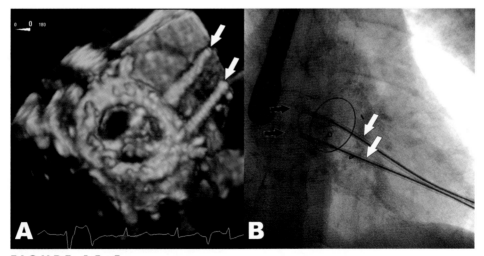

FIGURE 15-5.

Simultaneous deployment of two closure devices using double direct left ventricle (transapical) access. **A:** Three-dimensional transesophageal echocardiogram. Two delivery sheaths (*white arrows*) advanced through the leak at 1 to 3 o'clock. **B:** Fluoroscopy. Two delivery sheaths (*white arrows*) advanced through the paravalvular leak, two 10/8 Amplatzer duct occluder (AGA Medical Inc., Plymouth, MN) devices (*black arrows*) are deployed.

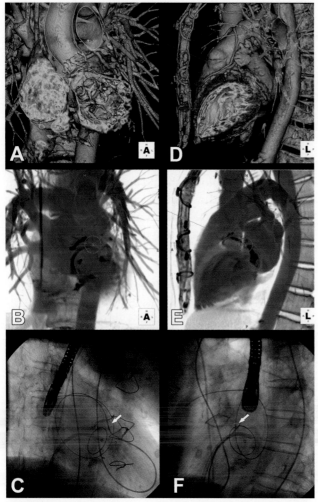

FIGURE 15-6.

Straight anteroposterior view demonstrates a landmark placement at the location of mitral paravalvular leak (*red bull's-eye* and *white arrow*) on a volume-rendered three-dimensional image with contrast subtraction **(A)**, location of the same "mark" on the fluoro-like view **(B)**, and fluoroscopy with catheter advance through the paravalvular leak **(C)**. **D–F:** Three-dimensional volume rendering, fluoro-like view, and fluoroscopy in left anterior oblique view, respectively.

Transseptal Approach

The transseptal approach is accomplished by "standard" transseptal puncture with a Brockenbrough needle and a Mullins sheath, as previously described.[19] After access to the left atrium is established, the leaks can be crossed using multiple preshaped catheters including movable tip catheters in combination with glidewire. After the defect is crossed, the catheter is advanced over the wire into the LV and the wire is exchanged for an extra support wire such as the Amplatzer super stiff (AGA Medical Inc., Plymouth, MN) or Lunderquist extra stiff wire (Cook Medical Inc.). However, if this does not provide the required support to advance the delivery system through, an arteriovenous rail can be established, thereby snaring the wire from the arterial side (Fig. 15-7).

Transapical Approach

Transapical puncture is carefully planned prior to the procedure with 4D CTA reconstruction and is monitored by 3D real-time TEE. A precise point of access on the chest wall toward the most perpendicular plane of the prosthetic valve is chosen and in the prevailing number of cases is within the anterior wall of the LV between the two papillary muscles and away from any major epicardial vessels. A 21-gauge needle and 0.018-inch guidewire are used to enter the LV and a 5 French sheath is advanced. The PVL can then be crossed with a hydrophilic glidewire through a short Berenstein catheter. Then the wire is exchanged for an extra support wire such as the Inoue wire (Toray International America Inc., Houston, TX). The appropriate delivery sheath is advanced over the wire across the defect and an Amplatzer-type occlusive device is placed in similar fashion as previously described across the defect. If the delivery system is 6 French or larger, the transapical access site of the LV is also closed with a 6 to 4 mm Amplatzer-type duct occluder device. In our own

FIGURE 15-7.

Diagram showing the formation of the arteriovenous rail **(A)**, venous-ventricular rail **(B)**, and atrioventricular rail **(C)**. PVL, paravalvular leak; TS, transseptal.

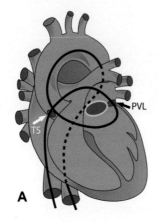

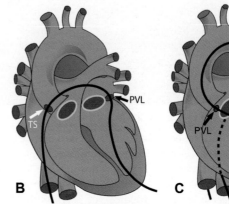

experience of over 30 transapical cases using delivery systems of up to 12 French for closure of mitral PVL, this approach has resulted in significant decrease in procedural time and lower fluoroscopy dose by more than 35% with no major complications.[20]

AVAILABLE DEVICES

There is no device approved by the U.S. Food and Drug Administration for PVL closure; as a result, all devices currently employed in the United States are being utilized "off-label." The Rashkind double umbrella device (USCI Angiographics, CR Bard, Billerica, MA) was used for the first cases of percutaneous closure of the PVL by Hourihan et al.[16] Since then, there have been reported use of CardioSEAL clamshell device (Nitinol Medical Technologies, Boston, MA), Amplatzer family (Amplatzer septal occluder [ASO], Amplatzer duct occluder [ADO], Amplatzer muscular ventricular septal defect occluder [MVSD], vascular plug III [outside of the United States], AGA Medical Inc.), and vascular occlusion devices and coils (Gianturco, Cook Medical).[5,21–25]

The ADO and the MVSD are the preferred devices for leak closure in our laboratory in the absence of the Amplatzer vascular plug III (not available in the United States) because the waist of the ASO (3 to 4 mm) is shorter than the waist of the MVSD occluder (7 mm) and of the ADO occluder (5 to 8 mm), and the length of the disk(s) perimeter to the perimeter of the waist (5 to 8 mm for the ADO and MVSD) is smaller than for the ASO (up to 12 to 14 mm).[9] Coils are useful for smaller leaks or for repeated interventions (residual leaks). The Amplatzer vascular plug III, available outside of the United States, is the device that, perhaps, will adapt best to a larger type of defects.

PLANNING OF THE PROCEDURE

The procedure must be carefully planned beforehand, using information obtained from echocardiography and CTA.

Aortic Paravalvular Leaks

Most aortic PVLs can be easily crossed with the wire using the retrograde approach; however, if unable to advance the delivery sheath through the defect because of tortuosity, calcification, and so forth, a transapical approach can be used to create an atrioventricular rail, followed by retrograde or antegrade-transapical delivery of the closure device. A transseptal arteriovenous rail can also be used with special attention paid to avoid mitral valve damage. Use of devices without proximal anchor disk such as ADO is preferred as this may decrease the risk of interference with aortic valve function when deployed retrogradely.

Mitral Paravalvular Leaks

For mitral PVLs located between 6 and 9 o'clock, the antegrade transseptal approach is very efficient. However, when leaks are located between 1 and 4 o'clock, the transseptal approach may be more cumbersome, given the angulations that the delivery systems must take, and the transapical approach is a preferred route. Leaks located between 10 and 1 o'clock corresponding to mitral-aortic fibrous continuity can also be crossed transapically or retrogradely. When a large crescent-shape leak is present, it is preferable to use two simultaneously deployed smaller devices in order to cover most of the defect rather than use a single larger device (Figs. 15-5 and 15-8).

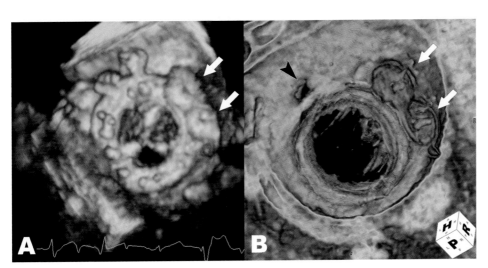

FIGURE 15-8.

Percutaneous closure of crescent-shape leak. Three-dimensional transesophageal echocardiogram **(A)** and volume rendered computed tomographic angiography **(B)**. Two closure devices at the paravalvular leak at 1 to 3 o'clock (*white arrows*); small unclosed paravalvular leak at 11 o'clock (*black arrowhead*).

COMPLICATIONS

Most complications are common to other percutaneous procedures and related to the manipulation of many different catheters, wires, and devices. They include, but are not limited to:

- *Access site related complication:* Vascular complications such as bleeding, thromboembolism, vessel dissection or rupture and rarely pseudoaneurysm, arteriovenous fistula, and infection. Complications for the transseptal approach include cardiac perforation and tamponade, hemothorax, tear of the interatrial septum, conduction abnormalities, and arrhythmias. Transapical complications include tamponade, hemothorax, coronary arterial damage, and myocardial infarction.
- *Device related complications:* Acute or subacute embolization of the occlusive devices after the deployment, device interference with the prosthetic valve, air embolization, and device erosion.
- *Other:* Cerebrovascular complications, including transient ischemic attack and stroke due to thromboembolism/air-embolism, calcium detachment and embolization, and hemorrhage as a consequence of procedural heparinization. Endocarditis is rare but potentially lethal and therefore prophylactic antibiotic is recommended. Persistence or development of the new hemolysis caused by residual leaks around the closure device or shunt through the device itself may persist for several months, until complete endothelialization occurs.

FOLLOW-UP

All patients undergoing percutaneous closure of the PVL require careful long-term follow up by the cardiologist. In most cases, symptoms of congestive heart failure improve within the first month. Hemolysis, on the other hand, may persist or even worsen after closure; therefore, close monitoring of hemoglobin and lactate dehydrogenase levels is warranted. We recommend at least 6 months before any further procedures, surgical or interventional, are contemplated and consider minimizing blood transfusions using erythropoietin injections as needed. A follow-up echocardiogram should be repeated every 6 to 12 months to exclude the developing of new PVLs or embolization of closure device, as has been reported.[26]

CLINICAL RESULTS

Experience with transcatheter PVL closure is still limited, published series are scarce and short, and therefore overall results of these interventions are yet not well defined. Currently available results of short series are presented in Table 15-1.

We recently reported our experience on 57 closure attempts of 47 defects (38 mitral and 11 aortic leaks) in 42 patients.[5] This is the largest presented series to date. Overall procedural success was 86% and clinical success among patients with successful deployed device was 89%. Most procedural failures were due to inability to cross the defect with guidewire, followed by device interference with valve function. There was one procedure-related death (2.3%). Freedom from cardiac-related death after 18 months was 91.9%.

Cortés et al.[27] presented a series where they analyzed the probability of success in relation to the location of the leak and found that crossing the leak was unsuccessful in two of the three patients with PVL in the lateral internal region of the ring and in three of six patients with anterior or lateral external leaks. In contrast, 83% of the leaks in the posterior ring could be successfully closed. Clinical status improved in 59% of the patients with a successful implanted device. Adverse events were also carefully reported in this series and are presented in Table 15-1. At 1 month postprocedure, regurgitation grade had improved in 8 of 17 successfully treated patients.

In the series by Pate et al.,[6] complete closure of the PVL was finally achieved in 5 of 10 patients—four patients had required two procedures. Furthermore, despite successful device deployment in 2 additional patients, residual leak persisted. Similarly, in spite of a success rate of 95% reported in the series by Hein et al.[17] (Table 15-1), three patients required a second procedure because of residual leak with hemolysis, and significant shunt was reported in 45% of the patients at the end of the observation period (14 ± 12 months). In this same study, during the initial procedure, the closure device had to be replaced for a smaller one in five patients due to interference with the valve or device instability.

Sorajja et al.[18] have achieved 81% success rate in 21 separate attempts to close 19 leaks in 16 patients, but significant regurgitation persisted in four patients—in two through additional leaks, in one patient adjacent to the implanted device, and in one additional patient because only an undersized device could be deployed. This group reported four deaths in a follow-up of 3.1 ± 2.6 months: two due to progressive heart failure, one due to pneumonia, and a sudden death 4 weeks after the procedure.

TABLE 15-1 Published Series on Transcatheter Paravalvular Leak Closure

Author	Patients	Mitral	Aortic	Devices	Failure	Success	Complications
Hourihan (1992)[16]	4	0	4	Rashkind	1 not attempted	2	1 hemolysis + migration
Pate (2006)[6]	10	9	1	ASO, ADO, coils	2 failures to cross guidewire; 1 device interference	7	1 device dislodgement + surgery; 2 persistent hemolysis; 1 retroperitoneal bleeding
Hein (2006)[17]	21	13	8	ASO, ADO, VSD	1 failure to cross guidewire	20	1 endocarditis; 1 surgery due to interference and 2 due to hemolysis
Sorajja (2007)[18]	16	14	2	ASO, ADO	1 failure to cross guidewire		1 hemothorax
Cortes (2008)[27]	27	27	0	ADO	10 failure to cross		1 ventricular arrhythmia + electric shock; 1 transient asystole; 5 bleeding events; 2 cerebrovascular events; 1 pericardial effusion
Alonso-Briales (2009)[28]	8	4	4	ADO	1 failure to cross delivery system	7	3 residual shunts; 1 surgery due to shunt
García-Borbolla (2009)[29]	8	8	0	ADO	1 failure to cross guidewire; 2 device interference	5	1 massive stroke + death
Nietlispach (2010)[25]	5	4	1	AVP-III	None	5	2 pericardial bleeding
Ruiz (2010)[5]	43	33	10	ADO ASD VSD AVP-II	4 failure to cross with guidewire; 1 device interference; 1 wire entrapment	37	2 acute embolization; 2 cardiac perforations; 1 iliac dissection; 1 procedure-related death

ASO, Amplatzer septal occluder; ADO, Amplatzer duct occluder; VSD, Amplatzer ventricular septal defect occluder; AVP, Amplatzer vascular plug (AGA Medical Inc, Plymouth, MN).

REFERENCES

1. De Cicco G, Russo C, Moreo A, et al. Mitral valve periprosthetic leakage: Anatomical observations in 135 patients from a multicentre study. *Eur J Cardiothorac Surg.* 2006;30:887–891.
2. Hammermeister K, Sethi GK, Henderson WG, et al. Outcomes 15 years after valve replacement with a mechanical versus a bioprosthetic valve: Final report of the veterans affairs randomized trial. *J Am Coll Cardiol.* 2000;36:1152–1158.
3. Ionescu A, Fraser AG, Butchart EG. Prevalence and clinical significance of incidental paraprosthetic valvar regurgitation: A prospective study using transesophageal echocardiography. *Heart.* 2003;89:1316–1321.
4. Genoni M, Franzen D, Vogt P, et al. Paravalvular leakage after mitral valve replacement: Improved long-term survival with aggressive surgery? *Eur J Cardiothorac Surg.* 2000;17:14–19.
5. Ruiz CE, Kronzon I, Dudiy Y, et al. Percutaneous closure of paravalvular leaks–techniques and clinical outcomes. In press. *J Am Coll Cardiol.* 2011.
6. Pate GE, Al Zubaidi A, Chandavimol M, et al. Percutaneous closure of prosthetic paravalvular leaks: Case series and review. *Catheter Cardiovasc Interv.* 2006;68:528–533.
7. Meloni L, Aru GM, Abbruzzese PA, et al. Localization of mitral periprosthetic leaks by transesophageal echocardiography. *Am J Cardiol.* 1992;69:276–279.
8. Movsowitz HD, Shah SI, Ioli A, et al. Long-term follow-up of mitral paraprosthetic regurgitation by transesophageal echocardiography. *J Am Soc Echocardiogr.* 1994;7:488–492.
9. Zoghbi WA, Chambers JB, Dumesnil JG, et al. Recommendations for evaluation of prosthetic valves with echocardiography and doppler ultrasound: A report

from the American Society of Echocardiography's guidelines and standards committee and the task force on prosthetic valves, developed in conjunction with the American College of Cardiology cardiovascular imaging committee, cardiac imaging committee of the American Heart Association, the European Association of Echocardiography, a registered branch of the European Society of Cardiology, the Japanese Society of Echocardiography and the Canadian Society of Echocardiography, endorsed by the American College of Cardiology Foundation, American Heart Association, European Association of Echocardiography, a registered branch of the European Society of Cardiology, the Japanese Society of Echocardiography, and Canadian Society of Echocardiography. *J Am Soc Echocardiogr.* 2009;22:975–1014; quiz 1082–1014.

10. Matsumoto M, Inoue M, Tamura S, et al. Three-dimensional echocardiography for spatial visualization and volume calculation of cardiac structures. *J Clin Ultrasound.* 1981;9:157–165.

11. Kronzon I, Sugeng L, Perk G, et al. Real-time 3-dimensional transesophageal echocardiography in the evaluation of post-operative mitral annuloplasty ring and prosthetic valve dehiscence. *J Am Coll Cardiol.* 2009;53:1543–1547.

12. De Cicco G, Lorusso R, Colli A, et al. Aortic valve periprosthetic leakage: Anatomic observations and surgical results. *Ann Thorac Surg.* 2005;79:1480–1485.

13. Exposito V, Garcia-Camarero T, Bernal JM, et al. Repeat mitral valve replacement: 30-years' experience. *Rev Esp Cardiol.* 2009;62:929–932.

14. de Almeida Brandao CM, Pomerantzeff PM, Souza LR, et al. Multivariate analysis of risk factors for hospital mortality in valvular reoperations for prosthetic valve dysfunction. *Eur J Cardiothorac Surg.* 2002;22:922–926.

15. Echevarria JR, Bernal JM, Rabasa JM, et al. Reoperation for bioprosthetic valve dysfunction. A decade of clinical experience. *Eur J Cardiothorac Surg.* 1991;5:523–526; discussion 527.

16. Hourihan M, Perry SB, Mandell VS, et al. Transcatheter umbrella closure of valvular and paravalvular leaks. *J Am Coll Cardiol.* 1992;20:1371–1377.

17. Hein R, Wunderlich N, Robertson G, et al. Catheter closure of paravalvular leak. *EuroIntervention.* 2006;2: 318–325.

18. Sorajja P, Cabalka AK, Hagler DJ, et al. Successful percutaneous repair of perivalvular prosthetic

regurgitation. *Catheter Cardiovasc Interv.* 2007;70: 815–823.

19. Roelke M, Smith AJ, Palacios IF. The technique and safety of transseptal left heart catheterization: The massachusetts general hospital experience with 1,279 procedures. *Cathet Cardiovasc Diagn.* 1994;32: 332–339.

20. Jelnin V, Einhorn BN, Dudiy Y, et al. Clinical experience with percutaneous left ventricular transapical access for interventions in structural heart defects: A safe access and secure exit. In press. *JACC Cardiovasc Interv.* 2011.

21. Eisenhauer AC, Piemonte TC, Watson PS. Closure of prosthetic paravalvular mitral regurgitation with the gianturco-grifka vascular occlusion device. *Catheter Cardiovasc Interv.* 2001;54:234–238.

22. Martinez CA, Rosen R, Cohen H, et al. A novel method for closing the percutaneous transapical access tract using coils and gelatin matrix. *J Invasive Cardiol.* 2010;22:E107–E109.

23. Pate G, Webb J, Thompson C, et al. Percutaneous closure of a complex prosthetic mitral paravalvular leak using transesophageal echocardiographic guidance. *Can J Cardiol.* 2004;20:452–455.

24. Piechaud JF. Percutaneous closure of mitral paravalvular leak. *J Interv Cardiol.* 2003;16:153–155.

25. Nietlispach F, Johnson M, Moss RR, et al. Transcatheter closure of paravalvular defects using a purpose-specific occluder. *JACC Cardiovasc Interv.* 2010;3:759–765.

26. Ussia GP, Scandura S, Calafiore AM, et al. Images in cardiovascular medicine. Late device dislodgement after percutaneous closure of mitral prosthesis paravalvular leak with amplatzer muscular ventricular septal defect occluder. *Circulation.* 2007;115: e208–e210.

27. Cortes M, Garcia E, Garcia-Fernandez MA, et al. Usefulness of transesophageal echocardiography in percutaneous transcatheter repairs of paravalvular mitral regurgitation. *Am J Cardiol.* 2008;101:382–386.

28. Alonso-Briales JH, Munoz-Garcia AJ, Jimenez-Navarro MF, et al. Closure of perivalvular leaks using an amplatzer occluder. *Rev Esp Cardiol.* 2009;62: 442–446.

29. Garcia-Borbolla Fernandez R, Sancho Jaldon M, Calle Perez G, et al. Percutaneous treatment of mitral valve periprosthetic leakage. An alternative to high-risk surgery? *Rev Esp Cardiol.* 2009;62:438–441.

CHAPTER 16

Left Atrial Appendage Occlusion

Daniel H. Steinberg, Stefan Bertog, Jennifer Franke, Jens Wiebe,
Nina Wunderlich, and Horst Sievert

A trial fibrillation affects more than 3 million patients in Europe alone. The overall prevalence of atrial fibrillation is approximately 0.4% with a strong association with age and male sex. The age-adjusted incidence approaches 5% per year in patients older than 80 years of age, and prevalence in this population is approximately 9%. The lifetime risk of developing atrial fibrillation is approximately one in four.[1]

Mechanistically, atrial fibrillation is characterized by uncoordinated and uncontrolled activation of atrial tissue. Although numerous classification schemes exist, for the sake of simplicity and consistency, the currently employed classification system centers on the timing and duration of the arrhythmia (Fig. 16-1). Once first detected, if atrial fibrillation occurs again, it is classified as recurrent. If it self-terminates within 7 days, it is considered paroxysmal; however, if it continues beyond 7 days, it is considered persistent. If refractory to cardioversion (or if cardioversion is not attempted), the atrial fibrillation is classified as permanent.[1]

TREATMENT AND PREVENTION

Medical Therapies

Treatment strategies for atrial fibrillation center around two concepts: symptomatic management and prevention of complications. Regarding symptomatic management, treatment can either aim to control heart rate or the rhythm itself. Rate control medications include beta-blockers, calcium channel blockers, digoxin, and, in refractory cases, atrioventricular node ablation with pacemaker implantation. Rhythm control strategies include medical therapies such as sotalol, dofetilide, amiodarone, dronedarone, electrical cardioversion, or catheter ablation.

Regardless of the treatment strategy for rate or rhythm control, treatment efforts must also focus on prevention of thromboembolic events. Atrial fibrillation increases the risk of cerebral ischemic events fivefold across the entire spectrum of age, and it accounts for approximately 1.5% of events in patients under age 50 to more than 20% of events in patients older than age 80.[2] Regardless of whether it is paroxysmal or permanent, the annual rate of cerebral ischemic events in patients with atrial fibrillation approaches 4.5% per year.[3]

Although the overall risk of cerebral ischemic events in patients with atrial fibrillation is understood on the population level, it is both practical and important to make attempts at individualizing the risk for a particular patient. A number of risk models have been proposed. The most commonly used is the $CHADS_2$ score.[4] In this model, a patient is assessed according to five established risk factors (Table 16-1) including age older than 75, history of hypertension, history of congestive heart failure, diabetes, and prior embolic event. Each risk factor is worth one point with the exception of a prior embolic event, which is worth two points. The

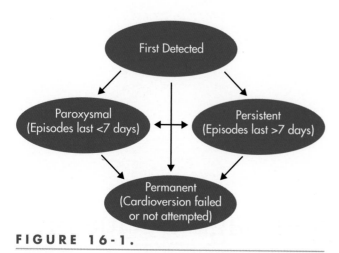

FIGURE 16-1.

Classification of atrial fibrillation

resultant score ranges from 0 to 6 and corresponds to a significant increase in risk for each incremental score. The absolute risk varies by series. In one study of 1,733 patients with atrial fibrillation not on warfarin, the annualized risk of cerebral ischemic events ranged from 1.9% for a CHADS$_2$ score of 0 to 18.2% for a CHADS$_2$ score of 6.[4] In another, larger series of 11,526 patients with atrial fibrillation not on warfarin, the annualized risk of events ranged from 0.49% for a CHADS$_2$ score of 0 to 6.9% for a CHADS$_2$ score of 6.[5] Although these

two studies highlight variability in cerebral ischemic event risk across different populations, the unifying concept that higher CHADS$_2$ scores portend higher event risk remains true.

Although the CHADS$_2$ score is the most commonly applied scoring system by current standards, there exists some controversy as to whether low-risk patients are adequately stratified by this score. This point is highlighted by the fact that even low-risk patients (those with CHADS$_2$ scores of 1) can benefit from oral anticoagulation with warfarin or even the novel agent dabigatran (discussed later).[6] Furthermore, greater emphasis on certain risk factors and the addition of other known risk factors for cerebral ischemic events may further refine risk stratification. The CHA$_2$DS$_2$VASc score (Table 16-2) is a 9-point scale incorporating the factors in the CHADS$_2$ system (congestive heart failure, hypertension, age >75, diabetes, and prior stroke) placing increased emphasis on age (65 to 74 merits 1 point whereas age >75 merits 2 points). Additionally, it adds vascular disease and female gender as risk factors. Based on an analysis of 1,084 patients, Lip et al. validated this risk model and demonstrated incremental risk of embolic events with a rising score (Table 16-2).[7] This score has been further validated in a trial of over 7,000 patients.[6]

TABLE 16-1 CHADS$_2$ Score and Associated Cerebral Event Risk

CHADS$_2$ Score	Annual Risk of Cerebral Events (695% CI)	Treatment Recommendation
0	0.49% (0.30–0.78)[5] 1.9% (1.2–3.0)[4]	Aspirin 325 mg daily
1	1.52% (1.19–1.94)[5] 2.8% (2.0–3.8)[4]	Aspirin 325 mg daily
2	2.50% (1.98–3.15)[5] 4.0% (3.1–5.1)[4]	Warfarin – target INR 2–3
3	5.27% (4.15–6.70)[5] 5.9% (4.6–7.3)[4]	Warfarin – target INR 2–3
4	6.02% (3.90–9.29)[5] 8.5% (6.3–11.1)[4]	Warfarin – target INR 2–3
5	6.88% (3.42–13.84)[5a] 12.5% (8.2–17.5)[4]	Warfarin – target INR 2–3
6	6.88% (3.42–13.84)[5a] 18.2% (10.0–27.4)[4]	Warfarin – target INR 2–3

Risk factors include: Age >75 years old, diabetes, hypertension, and congestive heart failure (1 point each) and prior thromboembolic event (2 points) for a total score of 0 to 6.

[a]In this study, patients with CHADS$_2$ scores of 5 and 6 were grouped together.[5]

TABLE 16-2 CHA$_2$DS$_2$VASc Score and Associated Cerebral Event Risk (n = 1,084)[7]

CHA$_2$DS$_2$VASc Score	Annual Risk of Cerebral Event (695% CI)	Treatment Recommendation
0	0% (0–0)	Aspirin alone or nothing
1	0.6% (0–3.4)	Aspirin or oral anticoagulation
2	1.6% (0.3–4.7)	Oral anticoagulation
3	3.9% (1.7–7.6)	Oral anticoagulation
4	1.9% (0.5–4.9)	Oral anticoagulation
5	3.2% (0.7–9.0)	Oral anticoagulation
6	3.6% (0.4–12.3)	Oral anticoagulation
7	8.0% (1.0–26.0)	Oral anticoagulation
8	11.3% (0.3–48.3)	Oral anticoagulation
9	100% (2.5–100)	Oral anticoagulation

Risk factors include: Prior embolic event (2 points), age >75 (2 points), age 65 to 74 (1 point), congestive heart failure (1 point), hypertension (1 point), diabetes (1 point), vascular disease (1 point), female gender (1 point); P = .003 for trend.

TABLE 16-3 Anticoagulation Options for Patients with Atrial Fibrillation[8-10,16]

Anticoagulation Strategy	Comparison Group	Cerebral Events Risk	Comments
Aspirin	Placebo	Relative risk reduction 22% (CI 2–38)	Superiority of aspirin over placebo
Warfarin	Placebo	Relative risk reduction 62% (CI 48–72)	Superiority of warfarin over placebo
	Aspirin	Relative risk reduction 36% (CI 14–52)	Superiority of warfarin over aspirin
Dual antiplatelet (aspirin and clopidogrel)	Warfarin	Relative risk 1.44 (95% CI 1.18–1.76)	Trial stopped early due to benefit with warfarin
	Aspirin	Relative risk 0.72 (95% CI 0.62–0.83)	Bleeding risk 1.57 (95% CI 1.29–1.92)
Dabigatran 110 mg twice daily	Warfarin	Relative risk 0.91 (95% CI 0.74–1.11)	Bleeding risk lower with dabigatran
Dabigatran 150 mg twice daily	Warfarin	Relative risk 0.66 (95% CI 0.53–0.82)	Bleeding risk similar between groups

Although the CHA$_2$DS$_2$VASc score may represent a more comprehensive system, it should be noted that small numbers at either end of the risk spectrum may underestimate or overestimate absolute risk.

In terms of anticoagulation strategies to prevent cerebral ischemic events, multiple agents have been studied (Table 16-3), including aspirin, clopidogrel, warfarin, and a novel factor Xa inhibitor, dabigatran. Both aspirin and warfarin have been compared to placebo. In 1999, Hart et al. published a meta-analysis of studies comparing aspirin to placebo, warfarin to placebo, and aspirin to warfarin in patients with atrial fibrillation.[8] Across all studies comparing aspirin to placebo with the primary end point of cerebrovascular accident, therapy with aspirin resulted in a relative risk reduction of 22% and an absolute risk reduction of 1.5% per year, respectively, for primary prevention and 2.5% per year for secondary prevention. In the studies comparing warfarin to placebo, warfarin resulted in a relative risk reduction of 62% with absolute reductions of 2.7% per year for primary prevention and 8.4% per year for secondary prevention. In five studies comparing aspirin to warfarin, warfarin resulted in a 34% relative risk reduction, proving superior to aspirin in the reduction of cerebral events; however, it should be noted that the risk of both intracranial and extracranial hemorrhage was higher with warfarin compared to aspirin.[8]

Clopidogrel has also been studied in patients with atrial fibrillation. The Atrial Fibrillation Clopidogrel Trial with Irbesartan for Prevention of Vascular Events (ACTIVE) trials evaluated the efficacy and safety of dual antiplatelet therapy in patients with atrial fibrillation. The ACTIVE W trial evaluated dual antiplatelet therapy versus warfarin in 6,726 patients with atrial

fibrillation and at least one other risk factor for thromboembolic events with a primary end point of cerebral events, noncerebral embolic events, myocardial infarction, or vascular death.[9] This study was stopped early, as therapy with dual antiplatelet therapy was associated with a significantly higher event rate (relative risk 1.44, 95% CI 1.18–1.76, $P = .003$) compared to warfarin alone.[9]

In the ACTIVE A trial, 7,554 patients with atrial fibrillation at increased risk of stroke deemed unsuitable candidates for warfarin therapy were randomized to aspirin plus clopidogrel versus aspirin alone. Over a mean of 3.6 years of follow-up, patients treated with dual antiplatelet therapy had a significantly lower risk of the composite primary end point consisting of cerebral event, noncerebral embolic event, myocardial infarction, or vascular death (relative risk 0.89, 95% CI 0.81–0.98, $P = .01$) at the cost of an increased risk of bleeding (relative risk 1.57, 95% CI 1.29–1.92, $P < .01$).[10] As a result of these and other studies, dual antiplatelet therapy has not gained widespread acceptance for thromboembolic prevention in patients with atrial fibrillation except for patients in whom warfarin is contraindicated.

Although long-term anticoagulation with warfarin is efficacious, there exist numerous drawbacks to such therapy. The narrow therapeutic window of warfarin forces a delicate balance between lack of efficacy and a significantly elevated risk of bleeding, therefore requiring frequent blood tests. Additionally, numerous food and drug interactions exist, thus making chronic management of multisystem disease difficult. Finally, in patients at risk for falling, anticoagulation itself may incur more risk than the thromboembolic event it is prescribed to prevent.

To highlight these issues, warfarin therapy has been associated with bleeding rates upward of 10% per year, leading to a regulatory "black box warning."[11] Additionally, up to 40% of patients with atrial fibrillation have contraindications to anticoagulation therapy.[12] Furthermore, warfarin is often underutilized or associated with difficulties finding appropriate dosage. Among patients who are at moderate or high risk for ischemic stroke and considered good candidates for warfarin therapy, it is prescribed in only 40% of patients,[13] and even in the controlled Stroke Prevention Using and Oral Thrombin Inhibitor in Atrial Fibrillation (SPORTIF III and V) trial settings, up to 30% of patients where subtherapeutic and 15% supratherapeutic on warfarin.[14]

Despite this information, warfarin continues to be the mainstay of medical thromboembolic prevention in atrial fibrillation, particularly in patients at elevated risk of thromboembolism. Balancing the individualized risk of cerebral events in patients with atrial fibrillation and the risks of chronic therapy with warfarin, patients at low risk for cerebral events ($CHADS_2$ score of 0 to 1 or a CHA_2DS_2VASc score of 0) can be treated with full dose aspirin alone whereas those at higher risk should be treated with oral anticoagulation unless otherwise contraindicated due to excessive bleeding risk.[15]

Of particular interest is an emerging alternative in the form of the oral direct thrombin inhibitor, dabigatran. The Randomized Evaluation of Long-term Anticoagulation Therapy (RE-LY) trial evaluated 18,113 patients with atrial fibrillation and an increased risk of stroke (mean $CHADS_2$ score of 2) to therapy with warfarin or dabigatran (110 or 150 mg twice daily) with a primary end point of cerebral events or embolic event in a noninferiority design.[16] Both doses of dabigatran proved noninferior to warfarin; however, dabigatran at 150 mg twice daily proved superior to warfarin with regard to both the primary end point (relative risk 0.66, 95% CI 0.53–0.82, $P < .001$) as well net clinical benefit, including the primary end point, bleeding, and death (relative risk 0.91, 95% CI 0.82–1.00, $P = .04$).[16] This benefit appears to be even greater in patients with poor anticoagulation control with warfarin, but it should be noted that medication discontinuation rates were significantly higher with either dose of dabigatran than with warfarin at both 1 year (14.5% dabigatran 110 mg; 15.5% dabigatran 150 mg; 10.2% warfarin, $P < .01$) and 2 years (20.7% dabigatran 110 mg; 21.2%, dabigatran 150 mg; 16.6% warfarin, $P < .01$).[17]

Mechanical Therapies

When thromboembolic events occur in patients with atrial fibrillation, the majority of thrombi originate in the left atrial appendage (LAA). More than 90% of all thrombi in patients with nonrheumatic atrial fibrillation originate in the LAA.[18] In view of the numerous issues with anticoagulation therapy and the relative simplicity of this anatomical target, exclusion of the LAA, either by surgical or percutaneous means, has garnered interest in recent years.

Anatomic Considerations

The LAA is an embryonic remnant of the left atrium. This often multilobed structure is located anterolaterally in the atrioventricular groove and is lined with trabeculated pectinate muscles. There are wide variations in its shape, number of lobes, length, volume, and orifice diameter.[19] Veinot et al. reported in an autopsy study of 500 normal hearts that the LAA was commonly bent or spiral in shape, and 54% of LAA had two lobes, whereas 23% had three lobes and another 20% had only one lobe.[20] Volumes ranged from 0.7 to 19.2 mL, length ranged from 16 to 51 mm, and orifice diameter ranged from 10 to 40 mm.[20]

Given the wide variation in LAA anatomy, it stands to reason that imaging techniques must adequately visualize the LAA in order to successfully occlude it. Direct surgical visualization is certainly possible, as is noninvasive visualization with transesophageal or intracardiac echocardiography, computed tomography, and magnetic resonance imaging. With regard to procedural guidance, transesophageal echocardiography (TEE) remains the primary modality for assessment of anatomic variation, device positioning, assessment of successful deployment, and monitoring of complications.

Surgical Left Atrial Appendage Exclusion

As an operative procedure, surgical exclusion of the LAA dates back to the 1940s. However, in recent years, the procedure has become increasingly common when patients with atrial fibrillation undergo otherwise indicated cardiac surgery. Interestingly, there exist little published data to support this practice. The only randomized trial to date is the Left Atrial Appendage Occlusion Study (LAAOS) published in 2005.[21] In this trial, 77 patients with atrial fibrillation and risk factors for cerebral events undergoing coronary artery bypass surgery were randomized 2:1 to LAA exclusion or no treatment. Of the 52 patients randomized to exclusion, 44 underwent repeat TEE. Only 5/11 (45%) of patients who had the LAA closed with sutures had successful closure on follow-up TEE, whereas 24/33 (72%) of patients who underwent combined suture and staple closure had complete closure.[21] The study was not powered to assess events, but the results suggest a significant learning curve and suboptimal closure rates despite the employment of multiple techniques.

A more recently published meta-analysis evaluated the conglomerate literature on surgical LAA closure.[22] Specifically examining five clinical trials, including the previously referenced LAAOS trial, the authors concluded that there currently is insufficient evidence to support routine closure of the LAA. In fact, of these five trials, only one showed benefit, while there were neutral and one showed harm. The authors suggest that incomplete closure (average 55% to 65%) may account for the discouraging results.[22] This point is especially relevant as surgical LAA occlusion renders the patient at risk due to increased procedural time and incomplete closure still renders the LAA a potential origin for thromboembolic events.

Percutaneous Left Atrial Appendage Occlusion

The principle downside to surgical LAA occlusion is that it holds little attraction as a stand-alone procedure. Indeed, the trials investigating its utility included only patients undergoing cardiac surgery for another indication. Percutaneous means to occlude the LAA are intuitively attractive as they may potentially be equally (or more) effective with substantially less physiologic insult to the patient and an overall improved safety profile compared to surgical closure or, for that matter, medical therapy. Two devices have thus far been developed specifically for occlusion of the LAA: the percutaneous left atrial appendage occluder (PLAATO; ev3, Inc., Plymouth, MA) and the Watchman LAA system (Atritech, Inc., Minneapolis, MN). Additionally, Amplatzer atrial septal defect and ventricular septal defect devices (AGA Medical Corporation, Plymouth, MN), originally not intended to occlude the LAA, have been utilized to occlude the LAA. The Amplatzer cardiac plug, specifically developed for atrial appendage occlusion, has recently become available in a number of countries. Finally, the transcatheter patch (Custom Medical Devices, Athens, Greece) and has a CE mark, although it has yet to be studied in a formal trial.

Technical Aspects

Regardless of the particular device deployed, procedural aspects related to percutaneous LAA occlusion are similar. First, the LAA should be evaluated by TEE for existing thrombus (Fig. 16-2). If thrombus does exist, the procedure should be postponed. Once the appendage is "cleared," standard transseptal puncture techniques are used to gain access to the left atrium. At this point, a sheath is placed across the septum and a pigtail catheter is inserted in the LAA where multiple fluoroscopic and echocardiographic measurements are made to accurately define the diameter, angle, and

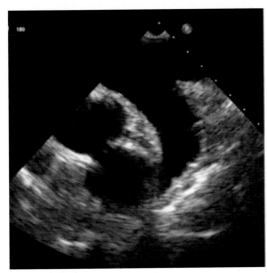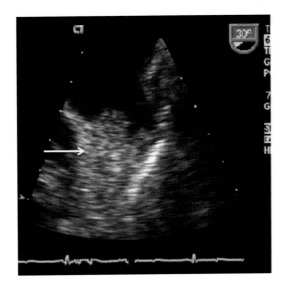

FIGURE 16-2.

Left atrial appendage. **Left:** Transesophageal echocardiographic image of a normal left atrial appendage. **Right:** Left atrial appendage with significant thrombus (*arrow*).

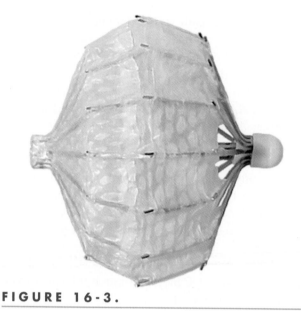

FIGURE 16-3.

PLAATO device (ev3, Plymouth, MA).

depth of the atrial appendage. Once the appropriate size is determined, the device is positioned in the LAA, and the delivery sheath is retracted, thus deploying the device. Upon determination of successful deployment, the delivery sheath is detached from the device. At this point, the sheath is withdrawn into the right atrium. Details pertaining to each individual device are discussed in the following text.

PLAATO

The PLAATO (Fig. 16-3) device, although no longer in production, was the first successfully implanted LAA occlusion device in humans.[23] The device consisted of a self-expandable nitinol cage 18- to 32-mm in diameter and was coated with expanded polytetrafluoroethylene. In 2005, Ostermayer et al. presented the results of a nonrandomized multicenter trial in 111 patients with nonrheumatic atrial fibrillation of at least 3 months duration who had contraindications to therapy with warfarin.[24] The PLAATO system was successfully implanted in 97.3% of patients (108/111). Four patients experienced pericardial effusions or cardiac tamponade and, in three of these patients, pericardiocentesis was necessary. One patient experienced a hemothorax and another a pleural effusion. At 6 months follow-up, successful LAA occlusion was demonstrated in 98% of the patients with a TEE. One patient developed a laminar thrombus on the device, and this was detected routinely 6-month follow-up. During a follow-up period of 91 patient-years, two patients had a stroke, leading to an annual stroke rate of 2.2% after successful LAA occlusion. This was a 65% relative risk reduction

compared to a CHADS$_2$ score predicted stroke rate of 6.3% in this patient cohort.[24] Extending results out to 5 years, Block et al. reported on 64 patients entered into the North American cohort of this study.[25] Over 239 patient years of follow-up, the annualized cerebral events rate in this population (mean CHADS$_2$ score of 2.6) was 3.8% compared to an expected rate of 6.6%.[25]

Watchman

The Watchman (Fig. 16-4) implant consists of a self-expanding nitinol frame covered by a 160-mcm polyester membrane on its left atrial side. Fixation barbs around the mid-perimeter secure the occluder to the wall of the LAA. The device is available in diameters from 21 to 33 mm. Sick et al. reported the initial experience with the Watchman device in 2007.[26] It was successfully implanted in 66/75 patients (88%) with 93% complete sealing of the LAA at 45 days. Device embolization occurred in two of the initial patients, leading to redesign of the fixation barbs with no further instances of embolization. Additional adverse events included cardiac tamponade in two patients, air embolism in one patient, and delivery wire fracture requiring surgery in one patient. Four patients developed a flat layer of thrombus on the device at 6 months, and both resolved with additional anticoagulation. Two patients experienced a transient ischemic attack and there were no cerebral events during follow-up.[26]

In the PROTECT AF trial, 707 patients with atrial fibrillation and a CHADS$_2$ score of ≥1 were randomized 2:1 to LAA occlusion with the Watchman device and planned discontinuation of warfarin after 45 days versus continued therapy with warfarin.[27] The study had a noninferiority design with a composite primary efficacy end point of cerebral events, cardiovascular death, and embolic event. The primary safety end point was

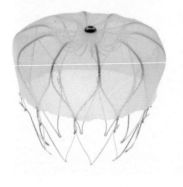
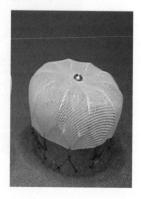

FIGURE 16-4.

Watchman device (Atritech, Minneapolis, MN).

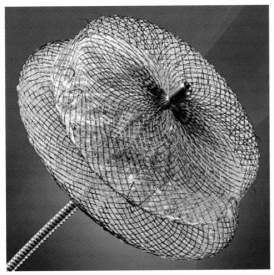

FIGURE 16-5.

Amplatzer cardiac plug (AGA Medical, Plymouth, MN).

a composite of hemorrhagic, pericardial effusion, and device embolization. The device was successfully implanted in 88% (408/463) of intended patients, and at 45 days, 86% of these patients were able to discontinue warfarin. At 1,065 patient-years of follow-up (mean follow-up 18 ± 10 months), the primary efficacy event rate was 3.0/100 patient years in the Watchman group versus 4.9/100 patient years in the warfarin group, with a probability of noninferiority >99%. Safety events were more common in the Watchman group (RR 1.69, 95% CI 1.01–3.19), with a 4.8% occurrence of pericardial effusions requiring drainage. Interestingly, the rate of optimally controlled warfarin therapy (target INR 2.0–3.0) was only 66%.[27] The overall results suggest that LAA occlusion with the Watchman device

may be a reasonable alternative to warfarin therapy in patients with atrial fibrillation and elevated risk of cerebral events.

Amplatzer Devices

LAA occlusion has also been performed using the Amplatzer septal occluder. Meier at al. reported on 16 patients who underwent LAA occlusion with this device.[28] The procedure was successful in 15 patients, with one patient experiencing device embolization. During follow-up, complete occlusion was noted in all 15 patients with no further complicating events.[28]

The Amplatzer cardiac plug (ACP; Fig. 16-5), was developed specifically for atrial appendage occlusion. It consists of a distal lobe with a proximal disk connected by a flexible central waist. The distal lobe is positioned within the LAA, and the proximal disc can be angled to fully cover the orifice of the LAA. Six pairs of hooks are attached to the distal body to engage the occluder to the wall of the LAA. The device is fully repositionable and recapturable. Device sizing refers to the distal lobe and ranges from 16 to 30 mm in 2-mm increments. The proximal disks are 4 mm larger for lobe sizes 16 to 22 mm and 6 mm larger for lobe sizes 24 to 30 mm. Appropriate sizing is 10% to 20% larger than the minimum appendage orifice measurement by TEE (Table 16-4).

The ACP was recently evaluated in 143 European patients with atrial fibrillation.[29] Device implantation was successful in 132/137 (96%) attempted implants. Serious adverse events within 24 hours occurred in 10 (7%) of patients. These events included three cerebral events, two device embolizations, and five pericardial effusions requiring drainage.[29] Longer term data regarding efficacy and safety are anticipated.

TABLE 16-4 Technical Aspects of Watchman and ACP

	Watchman	**ACP**
Device Design	Self-expanding nitinol frame with polyester membrane on left atrial side	Self-expanding nitinol with distal lobe and proximal disc connected by flexible waist
Device Size	21–33 mm	16–30 mm
Delivery Sheath	12 French inner diameter, 14 French outer diameter	9–13 French (depending on size)
Anatomic Inclusion	LAA depth ≥19 mm	LAA depth ≥10 mm
	LAA width 17–31 mm	LAA width ≤28 mm
Sizing	Based on achieving 8%–20% compression device	10%–20% larger than minimum LAA diameter
Positioning	Fluoroscopic and TEE	Fluoroscopic and TEE
Repositionable	Yes (prior to release)	Yes (prior to release)

LAA, left atrial appendage; TEE, transesophageal echocardiography.

FUTURE DIRECTIONS

From both a surgical and percutaneous perspective, a number of device reiterations and new technologies for LAA exclusion are at various stages of investigation. Regarding surgical techniques, there are two separate phase 2 studies sponsored by AtriCure (Westchester, OH) in its ongoing evaluation of the recently U.S. Food and Drug Administration–approved AtriClip device. The LAAOS II trial will be a randomized trial evaluating surgical LAA exclusion and aspirin versus warfarin with embolic events and bleeding as end points. The Evaluation of the Cardioblate Closure Device in Facilitating Occlusion of the Left Atrial Appendage is a phase 2 trial evaluating an occlusion band in patients undergoing cardiac surgery for indications other than atrial fibrillation.

From a percutaneous standpoint, a number of device reiterations as well as novel platforms are in varying stages of development or clinical investigation. Although approved in Europe, the Watchman device has not yet gained approval in the United States, and its design continues to evolve. Additionally, two percutaneously implanted epicardial devices are under early investigation.

CONCLUSION

As the most common cardiac rhythm disorder, atrial fibrillation affects millions of patients worldwide. Thromboembolic cerebral events are the most significant complication of atrial fibrillation, and the LAA is the most common site of thrombus origination. Depending on the risk of thromboembolic cerebral events in a particular patient, anticoagulation therapy with either aspirin or warfarin effectively prevents cerebral events in many patients; however, anticoagulation therapy has important limitations. Even as novel anticoagulation strategies are forthcoming, mechanical occlusion or exclusion of the LAA has potential advantages over anticoagulation therapy. To this end, a number of surgical and percutaneous techniques to accomplish LAA occlusion or exclusion are evolving. Many questions regarding optimal selection of patients, techniques, or devices, maximal safety and long-term efficacy remain unanswered. With further study, the ultimate role of chronic anticoagulation, percutaneous LAA occlusion, and surgical LAA exclusion in patients with atrial fibrillation will be further defined.

REFERENCES

1. Estes NA 3rd, Halperin JL, Calkins H, et al. ACC/AHA/Physician Consortium 2008 Clinical Performance Measures for Adults with Nonvalvular Atrial Fibrillation or Atrial Flutter: a report of the American College of Cardiology/American Heart Association Task Force on Performance Measures and the Physician Consortium for Performance Improvement (Writing Committee to Develop Clinical Performance Measures for Atrial Fibrillation) Developed in Collaboration with the Heart Rhythm Society. *J Am Coll Cardiol.* 2008;51:865–884.
2. Lloyd-Jones D, Adams RJ, Brown TM, et al. Heart disease and stroke statistics—2010 update: a report from the American Heart Association. *Circulation.* 2010;121:e46–e215.
3. Hart RG, Pearce LA, Rothbart RM, et al. Stroke with intermittent atrial fibrillation: incidence and predictors during aspirin therapy. Stroke Prevention in Atrial Fibrillation Investigators. *J Am Coll Cardiol.* 2000;35:183–187.
4. Gage BF, Waterman AD, Shannon W, et al. Validation of clinical classification schemes for predicting stroke: results from the National Registry of Atrial Fibrillation. *JAMA.* 2001;285:2864–2870.
5. Go AS, Hylek EM, Chang Y, et al. Anticoagulation therapy for stroke prevention in atrial fibrillation: how well do randomized trials translate into clinical practice? *JAMA.* 2003;290:2685–2692.
6. Camm AJ, Kirchhof P, Lip GY, et al. Guidelines for the management of atrial fibrillation: The Task Force for the Management of Atrial Fibrillation of the European Society of Cardiology (ESC). *Eur Heart J.* 2010;31:2369–2429.
7. Lip GY, Nieuwlaat R, Pisters R, et al. Refining clinical risk stratification for predicting stroke and thromboembolism in atrial fibrillation using a novel risk factor-based approach: the euro heart survey on atrial fibrillation. *Chest.* 2010;137:263–272.
8. Hart RG, Benavente O, McBride R, et al. Antithrombotic therapy to prevent stroke in patients with atrial fibrillation: a meta-analysis. *Ann Intern Med.* 1999;131:492–501.
9. Connolly S, Pogue J, Hart R, et al. Clopidogrel plus aspirin versus oral anticoagulation for atrial fibrillation in the Atrial fibrillation Clopidogrel Trial with Irbesartan for prevention of Vascular Events (ACTIVE W): a randomised controlled trial. *Lancet.* 2006;367:1903–1912.
10. Connolly SJ, Pogue J, Hart RG, et al. Effect of clopidogrel added to aspirin in patients with atrial fibrillation. *N Engl J Med.* 2009;360:2066–2078.
11. Wysowski DK, Nourjah P, Swartz L. Bleeding complications with warfarin use: a prevalent adverse effect resulting in regulatory action. *Arch Intern Med.* 2007;167:1414–1419.

12. Bungard TJ, Ghali WA, Teo KK, et al. Why do patients with atrial fibrillation not receive warfarin? *Arch Intern Med.* 2000;160:41–46.

13. Brass LM, Krumholz HM, Scinto JM, et al. Warfarin use among patients with atrial fibrillation. *Stroke.* 1997;28:2382–2389.

14. White HD, Gruber M, Feyzi J, et al. Comparison of outcomes among patients randomized to warfarin therapy according to anticoagulant control: results from SPORTIF III and V. *Arch Intern Med.* 2007;167:239–245.

15. Gage BF, van Walraven C, Pearce L, et al. Selecting patients with atrial fibrillation for anticoagulation: stroke risk stratification in patients taking aspirin. *Circulation.* 2004;110:2287–2292.

16. Connolly SJ, Ezekowitz MD, Yusuf S, et al. Dabigatran versus warfarin in patients with atrial fibrillation. *N Engl J Med.* 2009;361:1139–1151.

17. Wallentin L, Yusuf S, Ezekowitz MD, et al. Efficacy and safety of dabigatran compared with warfarin at different levels of international normalised ratio control for stroke prevention in atrial fibrillation: an analysis of the RE-LY trial. *Lancet.* 2010;376:975–983.

18. Blackshear JL, Odell JA. Appendage obliteration to reduce stroke in cardiac surgical patients with atrial fibrillation. *Ann Thorac Surg.* 1996;61:755–759.

19. Hara H, Virmani R, Holmes DR Jr, et al. Is the left atrial appendage more than a simple appendage? *Catheter Cardiovasc Interv.* 2009;74:234–242.

20. Veinot JP, Harrity PJ, Gentile F, et al. Anatomy of the normal left atrial appendage: a quantitative study of age-related changes in 500 autopsy hearts: implications for echocardiographic examination. *Circulation.* 1997;96:3112–3115.

21. Healey JS, Crystal E, Lamy A, et al. Left Atrial Appendage Occlusion Study (LAAOS): results of a randomized controlled pilot study of left atrial appendage occlusion during coronary bypass surgery in patients at risk for stroke. *Am Heart J.* 2005;150:288–293.

22. Dawson AG, Asopa S, Dunning J. Should patients undergoing cardiac surgery with atrial fibrillation have left atrial appendage exclusion? *Interact Cardiovasc Thorac Surg.* 2010;10:306–311.

23. Sievert H, Lesh MD, Trepels T, et al. Percutaneous left atrial appendage transcatheter occlusion to prevent stroke in high-risk patients with atrial fibrillation: early clinical experience. *Circulation.* 2002;105:1887–1889.

24. Ostermayer SH, Reisman M, Kramer PH, et al. Percutaneous left atrial appendage transcatheter occlusion (PLAATO system) to prevent stroke in high-risk patients with non-rheumatic atrial fibrillation: results from the international multi-center feasibility trials. *J Am Coll Cardiol.* 2005;46:9–14.

25. Block PC, Burstein S, Casale PN, et al. Percutaneous left atrial appendage occlusion for patients in atrial fibrillation suboptimal for warfarin therapy: 5-year results of the PLAATO (Percutaneous Left Atrial Appendage Transcatheter Occlusion) Study. *JACC Cardiovasc Interv.* 2009;2:594–600.

26. Sick PB, Schuler G, Hauptmann KE, et al. Initial worldwide experience with the WATCHMAN left atrial appendage system for stroke prevention in atrial fibrillation. *J Am Coll Cardiol.* 2007;49:1490–1495.

27. Holmes DR, Reddy VY, Turi ZG, et al. Percutaneous closure of the left atrial appendage versus warfarin therapy for prevention of stroke in patients with atrial fibrillation: a randomised non-inferiority trial. *Lancet.* 2009;374:534–542.

28. Meier B, Palacios I, Windecker S, et al. Transcatheter left atrial appendage occlusion with Amplatzer devices to obviate anticoagulation in patients with atrial fibrillation. *Catheter Cardiovasc Interv.* 2003;60:417–422.

29. Park JW, Bethencourt A, Sievert H, et al. Left atrial appendage closure with amplatzer cardiac plug in atrial fibrillation—Initial European experience. *Catheter Cardiovasc Interv.* 2010;77:700–706.

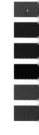

TRANSCATHETER THERAPY FOR VALVULAR DISEASE

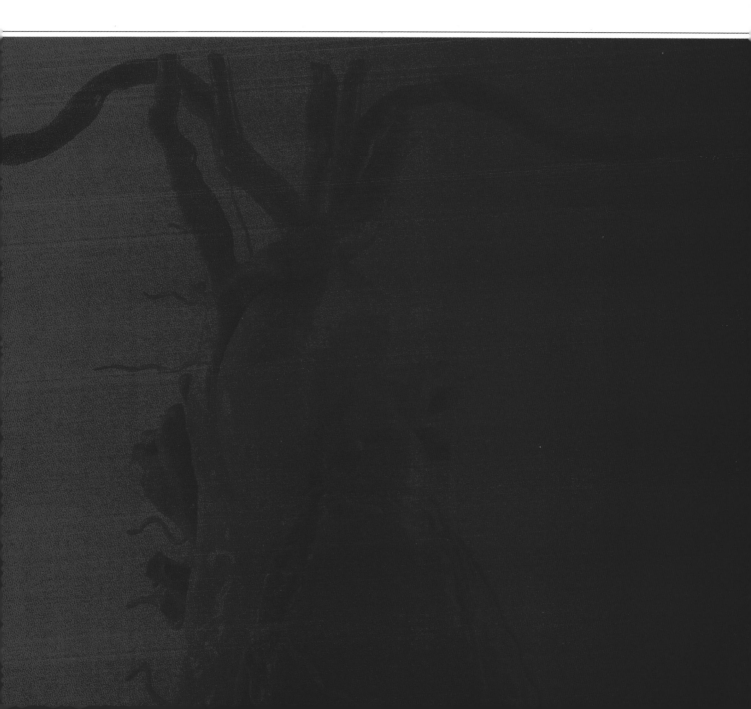

CHAPTER 17

Balloon Aortic Valvuloplasty: Technical Aspects and Clinical Role

Alain Cribier, Christophe Tron, and Helene Eltchaninoff

Aortic stenosis (AS) is the most common form of adult-acquired valvular heart disease in developed countries and its prevalence increases with age. Consequently, the number of AS patients is predicted to double within 15 years. Moderate to severe AS is observed in 4.6% of patients older than 75 years of age.[1] For symptomatic AS patients, aortic valve replacement (AVR) has been the standard of care for decades, associated with a mortality rate of 3% to 4% as reported by the 1998–2005 Society of Thoracic Surgeons database[2] in the ideal candidate, with a return of lifespan to that of general population. However, the operative mortality and morbidity increase with age, combined bypass surgery, depressed ejection fraction, renal failure, diabetes, and comorbidity.[3] These factors are considered one of the main reasons for which one-third of patients with symptomatic AS are not referred for surgery.[4]

For this subset of patients whose prognosis is dreadful without intervention with an average survival of 2 to 3 years,[5] interventional cardiology techniques have been developed. Percutaneous aortic valve intervention has entered an exciting phase since 2002[6] with the onset of transcatheter aortic valve implantation (TAVI), which is considered one of the most important developments in cardiology since angioplasty and which is on the way to become widely applicable. Prior to TAVI, balloon aortic valvuloplasty (BAV) had emerged in the 1990s[7] as a less invasive method to palliate the symptoms in a population of patients considered at that time too old or too sick for undergoing AVR. After having generated an enthusiastic response, there was a gradual loss of interest over the subsequent 15 years due to the temporary benefit in symptoms and the lack of survival benefit.[8] However, to date, this technique is clearly reemerging.

In 2010, BAV remains a viable alternative for the management of selected elderly patients for whom AVR or TAVI are not considered appropriate, providing symptomatic relief and improving the comfort of life. In the field of TAVI, it plays also a crucial role for patient selection and valve implantation.

This chapter describes the current technique of BAV, highlighting the modifications in the technique and materials, reviews the current BAV results, and discusses its important role in the era of TAVI.

INSIGHTS IN THE MECHANISM OF BALLOON AORTIC VALVULOPLASTY

The goal of the procedure is to achieve a nearly 100% increase in aortic valve area, which is a determinant of prognosis.[9] The predominant role of balloon inflation is to fracture the calcium deposits (Fig. 17-1), thereby improving leaflet mobility that allows increased blood flow during left ventricular (LV) contraction.[10] This requires attention to obtaining the maximum pressure exerted on the valve leaflets during balloon inflation, proper balloon sizing, and optimal contact with the valve structures. Improper techniques may explain the disparity of the results in the literature. Late restenosis, within several months, mainly results from a healing process with fibrosis and ossification.[11] Early restenosis,

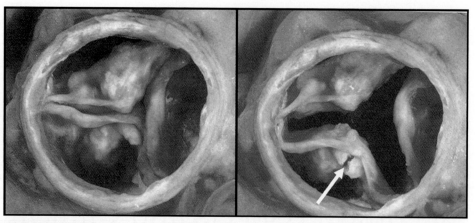

FIGURE 17-1.

Effect of a 23-mm balloon inflation on the native calcific aortic valve. After balloon inflation, the aortic orifice was slightly enlarged and a calcific nodule (*arrow*) appeared fractured.

after hours or days, can be the result of an early recoil following stretching of the elastic components of the valve structures and annulus, or of an inappropriate balloon diameter (due to size or insufficient inflation). Overstretching can result in tearing or rupture of the leaflets, annulus, or adjacent myocardium,[12] leading to aortic insufficiency.

When patients develop recurrent symptoms, BAV can be repeated, usually after an interval of 12 to 24 months, and the dilations can be done serially[13] even though the degree and duration of beneficial effect are less. In some cases, the patient may be "bridged" to AVR or TAVI.[14]

TECHNIQUES OF BALLOON AORTIC VALVULOPLASTY

BAV is regularly performed using the retrograde approach first described by our group in adults in 1986.[7] In rare cases, the antegrade transeptal approach, as initially reported by Block,[15] can be used in case of deficient arterial access due to peripheral vascular disease.[16] For both approaches, we typically perform the baseline hemodynamic study to confirm the presence of severe AS at the same setting as the planned BAV intervention.

The Retrograde Approach

Using our current technique for the retrograde approach, the procedure can be safely performed in less than 1 hour. Understanding and applying the technical "tips and tricks" that we have learned is helpful to make the procedure fast and safer in these critically ill, fragile, elderly patients.

Patient Preparation

The procedure is performed under conscious sedation, using intravenous (IV) midazolam, and local anesthesia. Unfractionated heparin is given IV (3,000 to 5,000 IU) at the start of the procedure.

Femoral arterial and venous access are obtained with a 6 French and 8 French sheath, respectively. Coronary angiography is obtained and, if indicated, coronary intervention performed in the same session, usually after BAV. Right heart catheterization is performed using a Swan-Ganz thermodilution catheter. If the patient is being considered for TAVI, a supra-aortic angiogram is obtained in shallow left anterior oblique projection, followed by abdominal aortic and pelvic vessel angiography.

Retrograde Crossing of the Native Aortic Valve

We use a standard Amplatz left 2 catheter (AGA Medical Inc., Plymouth, MN) in the majority of cases. An Amplatz left 1 catheter may be preferred in case of a nondilated vertical root (Fig. 17-2). A straight tip 0.035-inch guidewire is positioned at the tip of the catheter. In the 40-degree left anterior oblique projection, the catheter tip is positioned at the upper rim of the valve. The catheter is slowly pulled back while maintaining firm clockwise rotation to direct the catheter tip toward the center of the valve plane. The guidewire is carefully moved in and out of the catheter tip, sequentially mapping the valve surface and exploring for the valve orifice. Once the wire crosses the valve, the catheter is advanced over the wire in the right anterior oblique projection and positioned in the middle of the LV (Fig. 17-3). The transvalvular gradient is obtained

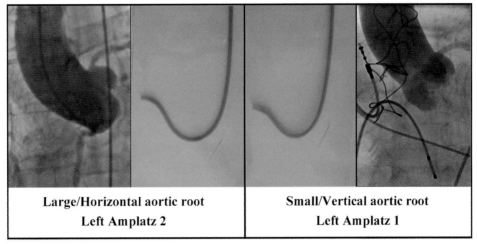

Large/Horizontal aortic root	Small/Vertical aortic root
Large/Horizontal aortic root **Left Amplatz 2**	**Small/Vertical aortic root** **Left Amplatz 1**

FIGURE 17-2.

An Amplatz 1 or 2 left coronary catheter (AGA Medical, Plymouth, MN) is generally selected for crossing the aortic valve, depending on the angulation of the aortic root.

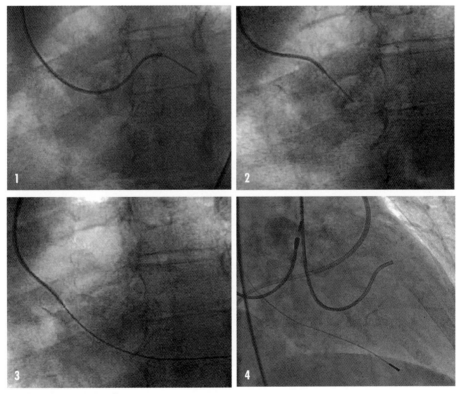

FIGURE 17-3.

Aortic valve crossing with the Amplatz catheter (AGA Medical, Plymouth, MN) and a
0.035-inch straight guidewire. From the upper rim of the valve **(1)**, the catheter is slowly
pulled back **(2)** while maintaining a firm clockwise rotation and the valve is mapped
with the wire (left anterior oblique 40-degree view). After crossing **(3)**, the Amplatz catheter is carefully pushed to the mid left ventricle in the right anterior oblique view **(4)**.

using the sidearm of the femoral sheath to record aortic pressure. Ice cold saline is used to obtain thermodilution cardiac output using a Swan-Ganz catheter positioned in the pulmonary artery. The aortic valve area is calculated using the Gorlin formula.[17]

Exchange of Guidewire and Arterial Sheath

An extra stiff Amplatz 0.035-inch, 270-cm length guidewire (Cook, Bjaeverskov, Denmark) is used to perform all catheter exchanges, and to assist in stabilizing the valvuloplasty balloon during inflation, deflation, and withdrawal. Prior to inserting the wire into the LV, a large pigtail-shaped curve is formed at its distal flexible end using a dull instrument to prevent ventricular perforation and decrease ectopy (Fig. 17-4).

The 6 French arterial sheath is replaced over the extra stiff wire with a 10 French, 12 French, or 14 French sheath, depending on the balloon catheter required. Reduction in sheath profile has considerably reduced local complications at the femoral artery puncture site, which was previously the most common adverse effect reported.[18] Until recently, we used 12 to 14 French sheaths, facilitating hemostasis by preclosing with a 10 French Prostar device (Abbott Vascular, Redwood City, CA). Currently, because a 10 French sheath is generally required, we are able to close the arteriotomy site using an 8 French Angioseal device (St. Jude Medical, Belgium) at the end of the procedure.

BALLOON CATHETERS

The majority of our experience was obtained with specifically designed balloon catheters for BAV: the double-sized Cribier-Letac catheters.[19] When the production of those catheters was discontinued, we used the Z-Med II balloon catheter (NuMED Inc., Hopkinton, NY), compatible with a 12 French or 14 French sheath. Currently, we use the lower profile Cristal balloons (Balt Extrusion, Montmorency, France), which are compatible with a 10 French sheath. The 20-mm and 23-mm diameter balloons are 45 mm in length, and the 25-mm diameter balloon is 50 mm in length. In general, we start with a 23-mm balloon. A 20-mm balloon is preferred if the valve is densely calcified or the aortic annulus is small (<19 mm by echo). In up to 25% of the cases, the 25-mm diameter balloon size can be required to achieve better results if the aortic annulus diameter is larger than 24 mm. For Edwards SAPIEN prosthetic heart valve implantation, the native valve is predilated with the RetroFlex balloon provided by the company (Edwards LifeSciences, Irvine, CA), and a 30-mm long balloon with an external diameter of 20 or 23 mm is used, according to the size of the prosthesis (23 or 25 mm) (Fig. 17-5).

A short extension tubing with a three-way stopcock attached is connected to a handheld 30-mL luer-lock syringe filled with 15%:85% contrast/saline solution to reduce viscosity in order to facilitate the inflation/deflation cycles.

RAPID VENTRICULAR PACING

Stabilizing the balloon across the aortic valve during inflation has been an issue for a long time. In 2000, we developed rapid ventricular burst pacing (RVP) to solve the problem, after having unsuccessfully tested in animals other ways to reduce the blood flow (balloon occlusion of the femoral vein,

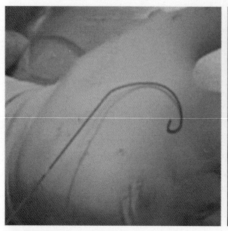 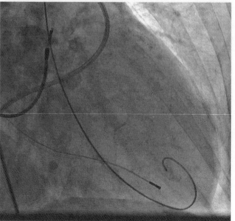

FIGURE 17-4.

The flexible distal segment of the extra stiff Amplatz 0.035-inch, 270-cm length guidewire (Cook, Bjaeverskov, Denmark) is preshaped before use **(left)**. Optimal position of the wire within the left ventricle **(right)**.

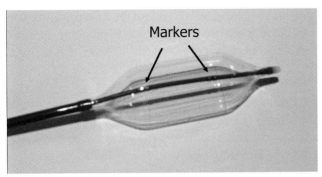

FIGURE 17-5.

The 30-mm long, 23-mm in diameter RetroFlex balloon dilatation catheter (Edwards LifeSciences, Irvine, CA) used for aortic valve predilatation before transcatheter aortic valve implantation.

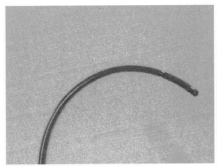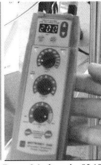

Pacer Medtronic 5348

FIGURE 17-6.

Left: The Medtronic 6 French soloist bipolar pacing lead (Medtronic, Minneapolis, MN) preferentially used for rapid ventricular burst pacing (RVP) in our institution. **Right:** The Medtronic pacer 5348 provides instantaneous RVP at a rate of 220 beats per minute.

atropine, or fast acting beta-blockers). This technique has been shown to provide an excellent and controlled decrease in blood pressure, reduction in transvalvular blood flow, and cardiac motion during balloon inflation. It is regularly used to date during BAV and TAVI.

Through the 8 French venous line, a 6 French temporary bipolar pacing lead is positioned in the right ventricular posterior wall and connected to a pulse generator capable of pacing at up to 220 beats per

minute (bpm) (Fig. 17-6). Pacing threshold is determined. The blood pressure response to pacing at 200 bpm is then evaluated. RVP must cause a precipitous fall of blood pressure to at least 40 to 50 mm Hg to be effective. If this is not achieved at a rate of 200 bpm, then the response is checked again at 220 bpm. If 2:1 conduction block is seen, or in case of loss of ventricular capture (Fig. 17-7), then RVP can be reduced to 180 bpm, or the lead position modified. The pacer is set on

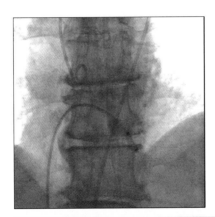

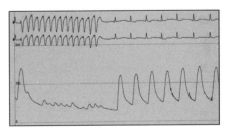

RVP: 180 to 220 bpm
150 bpm in case of severe LV depression

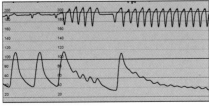

Loss of capture

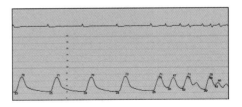

2:1 capture

FIGURE 17-7.

Optimal position of the pacing lead at mid part of the right ventricle's posterior wall **(upper left)**. Immediate drop in blood pressure must be obtained during rapid ventricular burst pacing with 1:1 capture **(upper right)**. Loss of capture and 2:1 capture must be avoided **(lower left and right)**. LV, left ventricle; RVP, rapid ventricular burst pacing.

demand mode at 80 bpm, serving as a backup in the event that a vagal episode or interruption of atrioventricular conduction occurs resulting in bradycardia or asystole in response to balloon inflations.

Balloon Positioning and Balloon Inflations

The diagnostic catheter is removed from the LV over the extra stiff wire and the 8 French sheath is replaced by the 10 French sheath.

While applying negative pressure on the balloon port, the balloon catheter is advanced into the aorta, letting it rest above the aortic valve. The balloon is then inflated and deflated one or more times to completely de-air it. De-airing the balloon in the ascending aorta has the advantage of maintaining the lowest balloon profile while crossing the aortic arch, thus decreasing the risk of atheromatous plaque dislodgement and embolization. The balloon catheter is advanced across the aortic valve, centering the valve between the two markers (Fig. 17-8). Before using RVP, the inflated balloon had a trend to "pop" into the LV, striking the apex with a risk of ventricular perforation, or to be ejected into the aorta with the possibility of disrupting atheromatous plaque that could embolize.

A clear communication between the operators manipulating the balloon catheter and the pacing device is essential. RVP is turned on and maximal balloon inflation is quickly obtained (Fig. 17-8). After 2 to 3 seconds of inflation, the balloon is rapidly deflated and retrieved into the aorta and the pacer turned off. Restoration of antegrade flow is rapidly observed. Rapid balloon deflation and restoration of blood flow is important to minimize the time of hypotension and hypoperfusion in these hemodynamically compromised patients. It is important to allow time for the heart rate and blood pressure to return to preinflation parameters before deciding to inflate the balloon again.

Assessment of the Results

If the balloon does not appear to be fully expanded, or there is no hemodynamic improvement, then repeat inflations are usually carried out before remeasuring the transaortic gradient. The simple observation of the aortic pressure curve allows a first evaluation of the result. An increase in systolic pressure and an improvement in the pressure slope are suggestive of a successful procedure. The lack of pressure recovery, a sudden change in wave form with loss of the dicrotic notch, or falling diastolic blood pressure can indicate the presence of severe aortic regurgitation.

After careful removal of the deflated balloon catheter from the sheath, the transvalvular pressure gradient can be measured after placement of a pigtail catheter into the LV. If there is a significant gradient, the next larger size balloon may be chosen, and the sequence is repeated. A pullback gradient is also obtained after the final balloon inflation. The residual gradient is then obtained by simultaneous measurement of the pressure in the LV and aorta (Fig. 17-4). For assessing the aortic valve area, the pacing lead is removed and replaced with the thermodilution Swan-Ganz for cardiac output measurement. An optimal result is considered to be doubling of the valve area or decreasing the gradient by at least 50% compared to the baseline value.

Supra-aortic angiography to determine the presence and or severity of aortic regurgitation may be performed. If contrast cannot be used, assessment of the presence of aortic regurgitation and its severity may be obtained by transthoracic echocardiography.

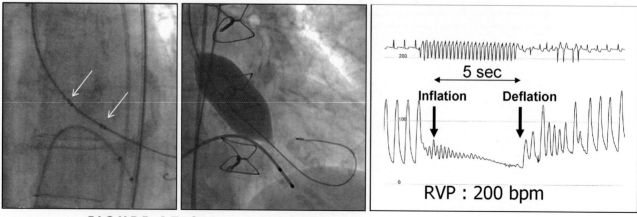

FIGURE 17-8.

Position of the balloon before inflation. **Left:** The valve is centered between the two markers (*arrows*). The balloon is then fully inflated under rapid ventricular burst pacing (RVP) **(middle and right)**.

Immediate Post–Balloon Aortic Valvuloplasty Management

Arterial hemostasis is achieved with the closure device. In case of technical failure, a pneumatic pressure device is used (FemoStop II Plus, Radi Medical Systems AB, Uppsala, Sweden). In absence of complication, the patient is usually discharged within 2 days. However, when BAV is performed in patients with severely impaired LV function or cardiogenic shock, hemodynamic monitoring with inotropic support is usually required in the intensive care unit.

The Antegrade Transseptal Approach

In our center, this approach is used when there is no satisfactory arterial access. Other investigators used it preferentially in the majority of cases on the basis of large sheath access and ease to cross the aortic valve and promote the use of an Inoue balloon for dilating the valve.[16]

Patient Preparation and First Steps of the Procedure

The patient is given mild IV sedation and local anesthesia at the access sites. Femoral venous access is obtained bilaterally, with an 8 French sheath in the right femoral vein, and a 6 French sheath in the left femoral vein. Through a 6 French sheath in the femoral artery if possible or in the brachial (or radial) artery, coronary angiography is performed when indicated, and a pigtail catheter is placed above the aortic valve for monitoring blood pressure and as a reference marker for the transseptal puncture. Using the left femoral vein access, a pacing catheter is positioned in

the right ventricle and RVP is assessed as described previously.

Transseptal Catheterization and Crossing the Aortic Valve

Transseptal catheterization is performed from the right femoral vein, using an 8 French Mullins sheath and Brockenbrough needle to cross the septum in the left lateral view (Fig. 17-9). When entry into the left atrium is confirmed, heparin 5,000 IU is administered intravenously. A 7 French Swan-Ganz catheter with an inner lumen compatible with a 0.035-inch guidewire (Edwards LifeSciences) is advanced through the Mullins sheath across the mitral valve into the LV. The transaortic gradient is determined with the Swan-Ganz catheter and the pigtail catheter in the aorta and the aortic valve area calculated using the Gorlin formula. The balloon catheter is then directed to the aortic valve under fluoroscopic guidance. Incomplete balloon inflation of the Swan-Ganz catheter and the use of a straight hydrophilic 0.035-inch guidewire can facilitate crossing the valve. With its balloon inflated, the catheter is advanced into the descending aorta and an Amplatz 0.035-inch, 360-cm long extra stiff guidewire (Cook) is advanced through the catheter lumen to the iliac bifurcation. The Swan-Ganz catheter is then removed.

Keeping a large loop of the guide wire within the LV is important at each step of the procedure. Straightening of the guidewire between the mitral valve and the aortic valve can open the mitral valve, creating severe mitral regurgitation with hemodynamic deterioration. The 8 French venous sheath is replaced with a 10 French sheath for the

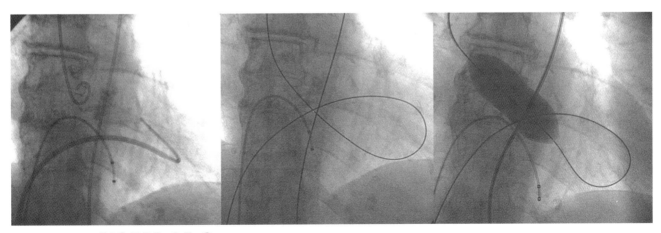

FIGURE 17-9.

Three phases of BAV using the antegrade approach. **Left:** Crossing the valve with the Swan-Ganz catheter after transseptal catheterization. **Middle:** Passage of the extra stiff guidewire from the femoral vein to the lower abdominal aorta. **Right:** Balloon inflation.

subsequent balloon dilations using the Cristal balloon catheter (12 French or 14 French if NuMED balloons are used).

Atrial Septostomy

The atrial septum is dilated with an 8-mm diameter balloon catheter through the 10 French sheath in the right femoral vein. Diluted solution of contrast media/saline (15:85) is used with a 10-mL syringe for at least two balloon inflations of 30 seconds each.

Antegrade Balloon Aortic Valvuloplasty

The same balloon catheters as for the retrograde approach are advanced through the 10 French sheath and positioned across the aortic valve while the loop in the LV is maintained carefully. The balloon has been purged of air prior to use. BAV is then performed as described previously using RVP for stabilization during balloon inflations.

It is not feasible to measure the gradient after inflations of each diameter of balloon with this technique and the results are assessed on the aortic pressure waveform. When the inflations using the largest selected balloon size are completed, usually after two inflations, the balloon catheter is removed. A 6 French pigtail catheter is advanced over the extra stiff wire and positioned over the arch so that the wire can be removed shielded by the catheter, avoiding injury to the aorta or mitral valve. The final gradient is obtained with the pigtail catheter in the LV, and another catheter in the aorta. Supra-aortic angiograms may be obtained. Hemostasis is obtained with manual compression of the femoral artery and vein after sheath removal. Post-BAV management is similar to that described previously.

RESULTS USING CONTEMPORARY BALLOON AORTIC VALVULOPLASTY TECHNIQUES

The recent results obtained in our center in a series of 141 consecutive patients with severe AS who underwent BAV (with the exception of patients undergoing percutaneous heart valve implantation) between January 2002 and April 2005[20] using the updated techniques can be compared with the large Mansfield[18] and NHLBI multicenter registry[21] from the late 1980s. Technical and procedural improvements have resulted in better hemodynamic results and decrease in complications despite an increasingly aged and sicker population of patients.

In our series, the frequency of clinically apparent stroke was less than 2%. This compares favorably with the incidence of cerebrovascular events in a series of retrograde catheterizations of the aortic valve without intervention.[22] We give heparin prior to crossing, and then use a technique that minimizes trauma to the aortic valve structure during attempted crossing. Since many of these patients have concomitant cerebrovascular disease, hypotension and hypoperfusion during balloon inflation can also result in a neurologic event. Minimizing the duration of RVP and balloon inflation are important technical issues, and maintaining optimal heart rate and blood pressure during the procedure are crucial. Preventing, recognizing, and treating vagal reactions expeditiously is also important to avoid the possible neurologic consequences of hypotension.

Valvular restenosis remains constant and is one of the main limitations of BAV and is regularly reported to be in the range of 80% at 1 year.[23] Repeat BAV is less efficient in terms of results and symptomatic improvement with subsequent procedures. The effect of external beam radiation has been shown to decrease the restenosis rate to 30% at 1 year in the RADAR study,[24] but these results should be confirmed on larger series.

If the beneficial effect of BAV on symptomatic improvement is regularly reported, its role in improving the survival has not been demonstrated and it does not alter the natural history of AS. One- and 2-year survival averaged 65% and 35%, respectively.

CURRENT PERSPECTIVES OF BALLOON AORTIC VALVULOPLASTY

BAV has no class I or class IIa recommendation in the recently updated American College of Cardiology/American Heart Association guidelines for the management of patients with valvular heart disease.[24] The class IIb recommendation applies to patients at high risk for AVR because of hemodynamic instability, those who are candidates for "a bridge to surgery," and those for whom BAV is indicated as a palliative procedure because of severe comorbid condition that preclude AVR. All elderly patients who are suitable candidates should have surgical AVR. However, in the elderly frail patient with comorbidities, the perioperative complication risk, the individual patient preferences, ethical, and economic factors should be taken into consideration when considering AVR or a less invasive option. Another potential indication for BAV is for the management of patients with critical symptomatic AS and

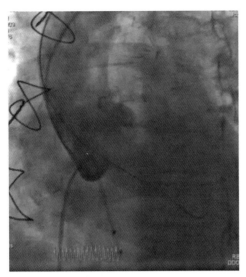

FIGURE 17-10.

In transcatheter aortic valve implantation, aortography during valve predilatation is used for final prosthetic valve sizing and assessment of the risk of left main occlusion and paravalvular leak (none of these risks occurred in this example).

needing urgent noncardiac surgery with the goal of decreasing the risk of general anesthesia. BAV can be used to determine the contributing role of AS to dyspnea in patients with concomitant severe lung disease in order to gauge the potential improvement and risks to undergo AVR or TAVI. Finally, AVR can be considered the most appropriate way to assess the myocardial contractility reserve in patients with low gradient/low ejection fraction in whom associated cardiomyopathy

is questionable. Patients with no demonstrated contractile reserve can have a perioperative mortality as high as 62%.[25] The indication of AVR or TAVI in those patients can be clarified 2 to 3 weeks after BAV if marked improvement of the LV ejection occurs.

Finally, BAV is the first step of any TAVI procedure and this largely explains the current return of interest in this procedure. Aortic valve predilatation must be obtained before placement of the heart valve prosthesis. The balloon sizes used are generally smaller by 2 mm than the annulus size. It is possible to correlate the diameter of the inflated balloon with the aortic annulus size, and thus use BAV as a final way of sizing the prosthesis. Simultaneous aortography at maximal balloon inflation can also usefully assess the risk of paravalvular leak and coronary occlusion at the time of TAVI (Fig. 17-10).

CONCLUSION

In 2010, BAV has become a simpler and safer procedure. However, in spite of several technologic improvements, its benefit remains modest and transient. BAV remains a viable palliative modality in a population of elderly patients with severe comorbidity for whom AVR or TAVI are not considered appropriate and can be used in the management of selected patients as a bridge to TAVI, AVR, or urgent noncardiac surgery. Interventional cardiologists and surgeons should become familiar with this technique that plays an important role as part of TAVI.

REFERENCES

1. Nkomo VT, Gardin JM, Skelton TN, et al. Burden of valvular heart diseases: a population-based study. *Lancet.* 2006;368(9540):1005–1011.
2. Brad CA, Ronald GK, Brockton H, et al. Mortality after aortic valve replacement: results from a nationally representative database. *Ann Thorac Surg* 2000;70:1939-1945.
3. Langanay T, De Latour B, Ligier K, et al. Surgery for aortic stenosis in octogenarians: influence of coronary disease and other comorbidities on hospital mortality. *J Heart Valve Dis.* 2004;4:545–552.
4. Iung B, Baron G, Butchart EG, et al. A prospective survey of patients with valvular heart disease in Europe: the Euro Heart Survey on Valvular Heart Disease. *Eur Heart J.* 2003;24:1231–1243.
5. Turina J, Hess O, Sepulcri F, et al. Spontaneous course of aortic valve disease. *Eur Heart J.* 1987;5:471–483.
6. Cribier A, Eltchaninoff H, Bash A, et al. Percutaneous transcatheter implantation of an aortic valve prosthesis for calcific aortic stenosis: first human case description. *Circulation.* 2002;106:3006–3008.
7. Cribier A, Savin T, Saoudi N, et al. Percutaneous transluminal valvuloplasty in acquired aortic stenosis in elderly patients: an alternative to valve replacement? *Lancet.* 1986;1:63–67.
8. NHLBI Balloon Valvuloplasty Registry. Percutaneous balloon aortic valvuloplasty: acute and 30-day follow-up results in 674 patients from the NHLBI Balloon Valvuloplasty Registry. *Circulation.* 1991;84:2383–2397.
9. O'Neill WW. Predictors of long term survival after percutaneous aortic valvuloplasty: report of the Mansfield scientific balloon aortic valvuloplasty registry. *J Am Coll Cardiol.* 1991;17:193–198.
10. Letac B, Gerber L, Koning R. Insight in the mechanism of balloon aortic valvuloplasty of aortic stenosis. *Am J Cardiol.* 1988;62:1241–1247.
11. Feldman T, Glagov S, Carroll J. Restenosis following successful balloon valvuloplasty: bone formation in aortic valve leaflets. *Catheter Cardiovasc Interv.* 1993;29:1–7.

12. Lembo NJ, King SB, Roubin GS. Fatal aortic rupture during percutaneous balloon valvuloplasty for valvular aortic stenosis. *Am J Cardiol.* 1987;60:733–737.

13. Agarwal A, Kini AS, Attani S, et al. Results of repeat balloon valvuloplasty for treatment of aortic stenosis in patients aged 59 to 104 years. *Am J Cardiol.* 2005;95:43–47.

14. Bonow RO, Carabello BA, Chatterjee K, et al. ACC/AHA 2006 guidelines for the management of patients with valvular heart disease: a report of the American College of Cardiology/American Heart Association Task Force on Practice Guidelines (Writing Committee to Develop Guidelines for the Management of Patients with Valvular Heart Disease). *J Am Coll Cardiol.* 2006;48:e1–e148.

15. Block PC, Palacios IF. Comparison of hemodynamic results of antegrade versus retrograde percutaneous balloon aortic valvuloplasty. *Am J Cardiol.* 1987;60:659–662.

16. Sakata Y, Syed Z, Salinger MH, et al. Percutaneous balloon aortic valvuloplasty: antegrade transseptal vs. conventional retrograde transarterial approach. *Catheter Cardiovasc Interv.* 2005;64(3):314–321.

17. Gorlin R, Gorlin SG. Hydraulic formula for calculations of the area of the stenotic mitral valve, other cardiac valves, and central circulatory shunts. *Am Heart J.* 1951;41:1–29.

18. McKay RG. The Mansfield Scientific Aortic Valvuloplasty Registry: overview of acute hemodynamic results and procedural complications. *J Am Coll Cardiol.* 1991;17:485–491.

19. Letac B, Cribier A, Koning R, et al. Results of percutaneous transluminal valvuloplasty in 218 patients with valvular aortic stenosis. *Am J Cardiol.* 1988;62:1241–1247.

20. Agatiello C, Eltchaninoff H, Tron C, et al. Balloon aortic valvuloplasty in the adult. Immediate results and in-hospital complications in the latest series of 141 consecutive patients at the University Hospital of Rouen (2002–2005). *Arch Mal Coeur.* 2006;99:195–200.

21. [No authors] Percutaneous balloon aortic valvuloplasty. Acute and 30-day follow-up results in 674 patients from the NHLBI Balloon Valvuloplasty Registry. *Circulation.* 1991;84(6):2383–2397.

22. Omram H, Schmidt H, Hackenbroch M, et al. Silent and apparent cerebral embolism after retrograde catheterization of the aortic valve in valvular stenosis: a prospective, randomized study. *Lancet.* 2003;361:1241–1244.

23. Letac B, Cribier A, Eltchaninoff H, et al. Evaluation of restenosis after balloon dilatation in adult aortic stenosis by repeat catheterization. *Am Heart J.* 1991;122:55–60.

24. Pedersen WR, Van Tassel RA, Pierce TA, et al. Radiation following percutaneous balloon aortic valvuloplasty to prevent restenosis (RADAR pilot trial). *Cathet Cardiovasc Interv.* 2006;68(2):183–192.

25. Roques F, Nashef SA, Michel P, et al. Risk factors and outcome in European cardiac surgery: analysis of the EuroSCORE multinational database of 19030 patients. *Eur J Cardiothorac Surg.* 1999;15:816–822.

CHAPTER 18

Implantation of the SAPIEN Aortic Valve: Technical Aspects

Stefan Toggweiler and John G. Webb

Percutaneous transcatheter aortic valve implantation (TAVI) was first accomplished in man by Cribier in Rouen in 2002. The transvenous technique required transseptal access to the left heart and antegrade passage through the mitral and then aortic valve.[1] The more reproducible transarterial retrograde procedure as widely used today was subsequently developed in Vancouver in 2005.[2] Subsequently, other approaches including transapical, iliac, axillary, and direct aortic have been described.

THE VALVE

The first-generation Cribier-Edwards valve (Edwards Lifesciences Inc., Irvine, CA) consisted of a stainless steel balloon-expandable stent frame to which was sewn equine pericardial leaflets. An external seal was provided by a synthetic fabric cuff attached to the ventricular end of the stent.[1-3] Subsequently, the Edwards SAPIEN valve featured more durable bovine pericardial leaflets and a larger sealing cuff.[4] The most recent iteration, the SAPIEN XT transcatheter heart valve (THV), incorporates a redesigned cobalt chromium, tubular, slotted frame that allows the struts to be thinner without loss of radial strength and despite a lower crimped profile (Fig. 18-1). The bovine pericardial leaflets, redesigned with a geometry that is similar to surgical heart valves with reduced leaflet stress, improved coaptation of a partially open valve design. The pericardium is processed with the same

anticalcification treatment utilized in surgical valves. The bottom two-thirds of the frame is covered with a fabric designed to seal against the aortic annulus and minimize paravalvular leakage. Currently, the valve is available in 20-, 23-, 26- and 29-mm diameters. Respective heights are 14, 17, and 19.5 mm when expanded. The valve shortens a few millimeters once expanded with final heights ranging from approximately 14 to 18 mm. In vitro accelerated wear testing demonstrates durability out beyond 10 years, comparable to surgical valves.

The hemodynamic performance of the SAPIEN family of valves is comparable or better than that of most surgical heart valves. Mean systolic gradients are uniformly less than 10 to 15 mm Hg. Effective orifice area is generally between 1.2 and 1.8 cm^2, depending on prosthesis size. The hemodynamic benefits of TAVI are reflected by early and sustained favorable affects on left ventricular function, hypertrophy, and brain natriuretic peptide. With small numbers of patients now beyond 5 years, late structural valve failure has yet to be reported.

All biological valves can be expected to deteriorate with time. Limited experience with THV implantation within degenerated surgical valves demonstrates the feasibility and potential of a valve-in-valve approach to bioprosthetic failure. Early experience with damaged or incorrectly positioned THVs, confirms that a second transcatheter valve can be implanted within the first with a good functional result. To some degree

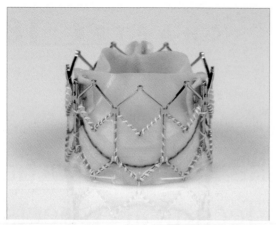

FIGURE 18-1.

The SAPIEN XT (Edwards Lifesciences Inc., Irvine, CA) is a balloon-expandable transcatheter heart valve that incorporates bovine pericardial leaflets and a fabric sealing cuff sewn to a cobalt chromium tubular frame.

TAVI, like percutaneous coronary intervention, may be a repeatable therapeutic strategy.

DELIVERY SYSTEM

Each size of valve is supplied with a matched delivery system, which incorporates a 30-mm long appropriately sized noncompliant high-pressure balloon. The valve is tightly crimped onto the balloon shaft utilizing a specialized manual crimping tool. The original RetroFlex transarterial delivery systems (generations 1, 2, and 3; Edwards Lifesciences Inc.) incorporated a stiff deflectable catheter that covered the deployment balloon shaft and facilitated steering the balloon-mounted valve around the aortic arch and through the stenotic aortic valve.[5] The widely utilized RetroFlex 3 system requires a 22 French sheath for the 23-mm valve and a 24 French sheath for the 26-mm SAPIEN valve.

The current generation NovaFlex catheter (Edwards Lifesciences Inc.) is utilized with the newer SAPIEN XT valve (Fig. 18-2). The low-profile valve is crimped onto the balloon catheter shaft. Only after introduction through the arterial sheath is the valve moved onto, and aligned with, the deployment balloon.[6] The NovaFlex system requires an 18 French sheath for the 20- and 23-mm valve and a 19 French sheath for the 26-mm SAPIEN XT valve.

PATIENT EVALUATION

Patient Selection

From a technical standpoint, almost all patients with severe aortic stenosis are at least potential candidates for TAVI. TAVI is relatively newer than open surgical valve replacement, and there is less information as to clinical outcomes and durability. Consequently, it has been mainly utilized in patients who are considered to be poorly suited to surgery. The Society of Thoracic Surgeons' estimated 30-day mortality risk of >10% or a logistic EuroSCORE of >20% are often utilized to define "high risk." Online risk calculators are readily available. Although useful in a general way, these risk calculators are limited in that they do not account for many surgical risk factors such as porcelain aorta, the need for multivalve surgery, liver disease, frailty, malnutrition, or immobility. In general, a surgical consensus incorporating the "look test" is often the best way to define a high surgical risk patient. Randomized data strongly support TAVI in patients who declined surgery. Registry data suggest favorable outcomes in high-risk surgical candidates. A potential role for TAVI in lower risk surgical candidates has not been evaluated.

Basic evaluation of a potential TAVI candidate consists of a careful history, a clinical examination, a transthoracic echocardiogram, cardiac catheterization,

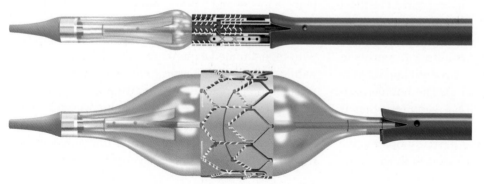

FIGURE 18-2.

The NovaFlex catheter (Edwards Lifesciences Inc., Irvine, CA) used for transarterial implantation of the SAPIEN XT transcatheter heart valve.

aortic angiography, and/or computed tomographic (CT) angiography.

Echocardiography

Transthoracic echocardiography is utilized to assess aortic valve, morphology, vegetations, calcification, restriction, transaortic gradient, regurgitation, and orifice area. Hypertrophy, subaortic obstruction, left ventricular volume and function, and the presence of other cardiac lesions should be evaluated. The presence of multivalvular disease needs to be assessed. Bulky aortic valve leaflets in close proximity to the coronary ostia may require evaluation for potential of coronary obstruction.

Unlike surgery, where the aortic annulus can be physically measured, the interventionalist is dependent on less direct means. The aortic annulus diameter is, by convention, measured at the point of leaflet insertion in the parasternal long-axis view (Fig. 18-3). Importantly, this measurement is not equivalent to the more commonly reported left ventricular outflow tract measurement. Although transthoracic echocardiography is useful for screening, most groups ultimately depend on transesophageal echocardiographic (TEE) measurements. These vary but are, on average, 1 to 2 mm larger.[7] It is the current practice to routinely oversize the prosthesis by 10% to 20% above the annulus diameter as measured by TEE to facilitate secure fixation and paravalvular sealing. Generally, an annulus as measured by TEE at 17 to 20 mm, 18 to 22 mm, 22 to 25 mm, or 25 to 28 mm would be considered

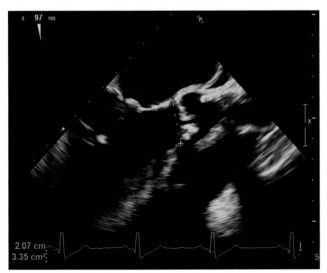

FIGURE 18-3.

The diameter of the annulus is measured at the point of leaflet attachment. On average, transesophageal echocardiography estimates exceed transthoracic estimates by 1 to 2 mm.

appropriate for a 20-, 23-, 26-, or 29-mm diameter prosthesis, respectively.

Cardiac Catheterization

Coronary anatomy needs to be defined to determine the potential for ischemia and possible need for revascularization. In many cases, two or three views of the left and one or two of the right coronary may be adequate for procedural planning and minimize contrast exposure. Right heart catheterization may be helpful to assess for the presence of clinically important pulmonary hypertension or measure cardiac output if invasive assessment of the aortic valve area is required. Ventricular angiography is rarely of value.

Aortic Root Angiography

With the SAPIEN valves, the goal is primarily to assess the aortic valve and root, rather than the ascending aorta or arch. Consequently, high magnification is generally used and a pigtail is placed directly on the noncoronary cusp of the aortic valve with a contrast injection of 20 mL over 1 second. Ideally, the aortogram is done in a projection perpendicular to the plane of the aortic valve. In most patients, the plane of the aortic valve is tilted down anteriorly and to the right. This means that, on average, the plane is around 10 degrees caudal in the anterior projection and 10 degrees cranial as the image detector moves to 20 degrees lateral. Of course, this is highly variable, but we find an anteroposterior caudal angulation is a reasonable initial angulation for aortography.

Ideally, the aortogram will show all three cusps in a single plane. If not, then repeating the aortogram in a slightly different projection may be considered in preparation for later valve implantation. Alternatively, preprocedural CT angiography or intraprocedural three-dimensional (3D) reconstruction (e.g., DynaCT, Siemens Inc., Munich, Germany) can be used to determine optimal projections (Fig. 18-4). The aortic valve is examined for calcification, which might be useful as a landmark at the time of stent positioning. Confirmation that the leaflets are calcified and their motion is restricted can be helpful to confirm the severity of aortic stenosis in low-gradient patients. Bulky calcified leaflets, shallow sinuses, and a low origin of the left coronary ostium (<13 mm from leaflet insertion to left main ostia) may raise concerns about a risk of coronary obstruction. An extremely unfolded or horizontal aorta may increase the difficulty of navigating the stenotic native valve and positioning the prosthesis.

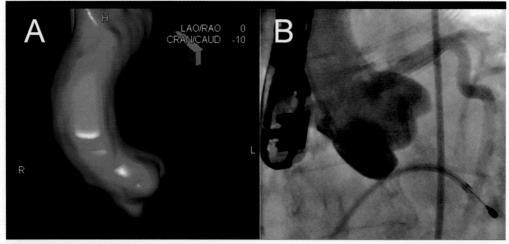

FIGURE 18-4.

A: In-lab three-dimensional reconstruction (DynaCT, Siemens, Munich, Germany) can be used to determine the optimal angle for implantation. In this example, an implantation angle of posteroanterior 0 degrees caudal 10 degrees was chosen. **B:** The corresponding root injection shows all three cusps lined up.

Descending Aortography

We place a calibrated pigtail (Beacon Tip Royal Flush Plus High-Flow Catheter, Cook Inc., Bloomington, IN) in the abdominal aorta just above the bifurcation. With an injection of 30 to 40 mL over 2 seconds and brisk panning of the table, both the iliac and femoral arteries can be imaged (Fig. 18-5). It is important to assess the

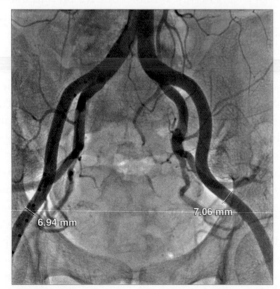

FIGURE 18-5.

Femoral angiography to visualize both iliac and femoral arteries. The minimal diameter is measured on both sides. In cases like this, where there is no circumferential calcification, we consider a minimal diameter of 6.0 and 6.5 mm to be adequate for the 23- and 26-mm valves, respectively.

common femoral artery at the site of intended puncture. Localized femoral disease, calcification of a high femoral bifurcation, may influence the site of puncture and reliability of closure.

The minimal diameter of both iliac and femoral arteries should be determined. The outer diameter of an 18 French sheath is just over 7 mm. Ideally, the entire length of the artery that must be traversed is larger than the sheath that must pass through it. However, in the absence of calcification, particularly circumferential calcification, short segments of artery are relatively compliant. A typical cutoff is an arterial diameter of >6 mm for an 18 French sheath or >6.5 mm for a 19 French sheath, so long as the stenotic segment is not long, calcified, or tortuous (Table 18-1).

Computed Tomographic Angiography

CT is helpful to visualize the aortic valve and the aortic root.[8,9] The aortic annulus is typically oval and both a long and short axis can be measured. Both are typically larger than the reported annulus diameter as determined in echocardiographic long-axis views. The reliability of these measurements for selecting the optimal size of SAPIEN implant has yet to be determined. The risk of left coronary obstruction by a displaced native leaflet may be dependent on the distance between the left coronary ostium and the annulus, the length of the leaflets, and the distribution and bulkiness of calcium (Fig. 18-6).[10] It has been suggested that an annulus to left main distance of ≤12 mm may be a risk factor for coronary obstruction.

TABLE 18-1 Arterial Access[a]

Annulus Diameter	Valve	Delivery System	Sheath Size	Sheath External Diameter (mm)	Minimal Artery Diameter (mm)
18–22 mm	23 mm SAPIEN	RetroFlex 3	22 French	8	7
22–25 mm	26 mm SAPIEN	RetroFlex 3	24 French	9	8
17–20 mm	20 mm SAPIEN XT	NovaFlex	18 French	7	6
18–22 mm	23 mm SAPIEN XT	NovaFlex	18 French	7	6
22–25 mm	26 mm SAPIEN XT	NovaFlex	19 French	7.5	6.5

[a]*The recommended minimal femoral artery diameter varies according to the annular size and valve required, delivery system utilized, and the presence of arterial tortuosity and calcification.*

CT 3D reconstructions may be very helpful in identifying the plane of the native valve and allowing prediction of optimal fluoroscopic angulation for subsequent aortic root injections and actual valve implantation (Fig. 18-7). This may be of particular help when the aorta is tortuous and the orientation of the valve is unusual.

Extensive calcification of the ascending aorta may be a relative contraindication to conventional surgery. Extremely severe aortic tortuosity of the aorta itself may predict technical difficulties with transaortic access. Aortic aneurysms are not necessarily a contraindication to careful transaortic access.

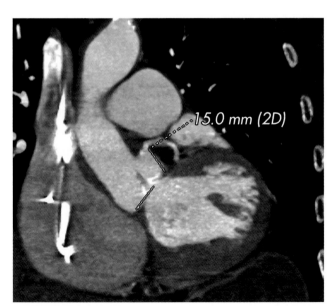

FIGURE 18-6.

Computed tomography is most accurate in measuring the distance between the coronary ostia and the annulus, the length of the leaflets, and the distribution and bulkiness of calcium. A distance of ≤12 mm from leaflet insertion to the left coronary ostium is often considered to be a marker of increased risk of coronary obstruction.

The most important role of CT is in the assessment of vascular access. The minimal diameter of the iliofemoral system from the femoral puncture site to the aorta should be determined from contrast-enhanced axial images which allow accurate assessment of luminal diameter. The degree of tortuosity and calcification needs to be considered in addition to artery diameter. Calcification reduces the ability to dilate a small or stenotic artery, particularly if calcification is circumferential (best evaluated on noncontrast images). Similarly, a tortuous artery will usually straighten with stiff wires and sheaths, unless combined with severe calcification.

THE PROCEDURE

Setup and Equipment

Procedures can be performed in a cardiac catheterization laboratory or hybrid operating room with high-quality imaging. Valve implantation and the potential need for arterial repair warrant a high level of sterility. An interdisciplinary team including interventional cardiologist, cardiac surgeon, vascular surgeon, cardiac anesthesia, perfusionists, and skilled nursing are necessary for a successful transcatheter program.[11] Bailout material for pericardiocentesis, and for coronary and peripheral interventions including occlusion balloons and vascular stents, should be readily available. Rarely, ischemic left ventricular dysfunction may require peripheral cardiopulmonary support.

Patients are generally premedicated with aspirin, clopidogrel, and prophylactic antibiotics. A general anesthetic and endotracheal intubation are generally used to increase patient safety and comfort and to facilitate TEE. However, some groups favor conscious sedation for stable transarterial procedures. Heparin is administered during the procedure and generally not reversed. Central venous access from the neck and a radial

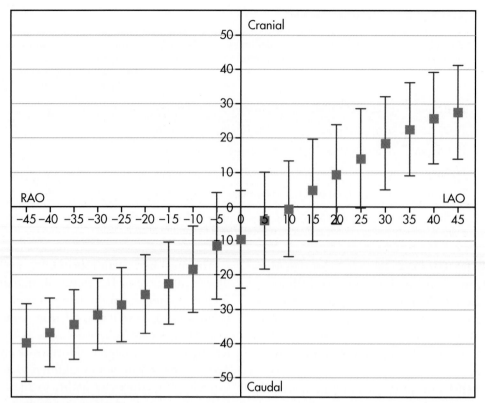

FIGURE 18-7.

The "line of perpendicularity." The graph represents the mean caudal or cranial angulation needed at the spectrum of right anterior oblique (RAO) to left anterior oblique (LAO) projections to achieve valve perpendicularity to the X-ray beam for a large cohort of patients. Individual patients will vary.

arterial line are generally advisable. Radiolucent defibrillation pads are placed on the chest. After the procedure, patients should be extubated rapidly, typically on the table after a transarterial procedure and in the postoperative care unit after transapical access. Intensive care unit observation is common for a day, followed by early mobilization and telemetry for 2 to 3 days.[10]

Vascular Access

The common femoral artery is punctured over the femoral head where it is compressible and above the bifurcation into the deep and superficial femoral arteries (Fig. 18-8). Because this bifurcation typically is below the middle of the femoral head fluoroscopic, confirmation prior to arterial puncture should be routine. When there are concerns related to a high femoral bifurcation, obesity, atheroma, or calcification, angiography utilizing a catheter placed from the contralateral femoral artery or use of a micropuncture system can be very helpful. Typically, "preclosure" is performed using either the 10 French Prostar or two 6 French ProGlide percutaneous sutures (Abbott Vascular Inc., Redwood City, CA).

A specially designed hydrophilic 35-cm long arterial access sheath is carefully advanced under fluoroscopic guidance to the thoracic aorta over a stiff wire. Large dilators supplied with the sheath can be utilized if there is resistance. The NovaFlex system currently requires an 18 French or 19 French internal diameter sheath. However, expandable 16 French and 18 French sheaths are becoming available, which offer the advantage of a low insertion profile with the ability to expand as needed to facilitate valve insertion.

The sheath is removed shortly after successful valve implantation. Rarely, a ruptured artery may only become apparent at the time of removal of the occlusive sheath as a sudden drop in blood pressure. If perforation is suspected, contrast injection through the sheath or through a contralaterally placed catheter may be diagnostic. We routinely leave a wire over which the sheath, dilator, or an occlusion balloon can be quickly placed to tamponade any bleeding. If necessary, an occlusion balloon can also be advanced to, or above, the bleeding site from the contralateral femoral artery. Fortunately, with newer, smaller delivery systems, such concerns are increasingly rare. As the sheath is

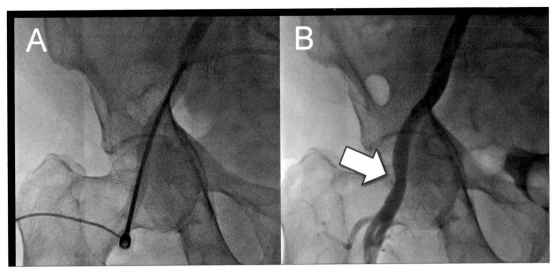

FIGURE 18-8.

A: The common femoral artery puncture is ideally below the peritoneal inferior epigastic artery and over the femoral head (where it is compressible), above the bifurcation into the deep and superficial femoral arteries (to reduce the chance of arterial injury), and on the side with the least calcification and atheroma. **B:** A contralateral injection is carried out after closure with two ProGlide sutures (Abbott Vascular Inc., Redwood City, CA) documents patency of the artery and the absence of a leak. Note the minor residual stenosis of the artery (*arrow*).

removed, the artery is manually compressed and the previously placed suture knots are advanced to the arterial puncture site to achieve hemostasis.

Pacing

A temporary transvenous pacemaker is placed in the right ventricle. Burst pacing at a rate of 180 to 200 per minute at a high-energy output is used to reduce cardiac output, transvalvular flow, and cardiac motion during balloon valvuloplasty and valve expansion.[12] If reliable 1:1 capture cannot be accomplished, burst pacing is reattempted with the rate reduced incrementally by 20 per minute. It is important to minimize the ischemic stress of burst pacing. Ideally, pacing should only be initiated when the blood pressure is optimized with a systolic above 100 mm Hg and limited to episodes of <20 seconds. Time for hemodynamic recovery should be allowed between episodes. In the absence of new atrioventricular block, it is generally safe to remove the transvenous pacemaker shortly after valve implantation.

Wire Placement

The valve is crossed with a straight 0.035-inch soft tip or hydrophilic guidewire using an appropriately angled catheter, such as an Amplatzer left 1 (or Amplatzer left 2 for a horizontal aorta; AGA Medical Inc., Plymouth, MN). However, Judkins right,

multipurpose, or pigtail catheters can be used. The tip of the straight wire should be carefully aimed at the apex of the fluoroscopically visible calcified valve. The wire is gently advanced. If the wire is deflected down the surface of a valve leaflet, it is withdrawn and the catheter is slightly repositioned. Forceful probing does not contribute to crossing and may risk atheroembolization. Once the valve is crossed, the straight wire is exchanged through the diagnostic catheter for an Amplatzer extra stiff or super stiff 0.035-inch guidewire with a manually formed exaggerated J curve on the distal end. The wire is advanced as far as possible into the ventricle, thereby forming a gentle curve without entrapment in the mitral valve apparatus or resulting in excessive ectopy. The right anterior oblique view can be helpful to avoid the foreshortening of the ventricular cavity (which is typically worst in the left anterior oblique view). Great care must be exercised to ensure the wire is not withdrawn until after the valve prosthesis is implanted.

Valvuloplasty

Predilation is desirable to facilitate crossing and positioning of the prosthesis. A balloon slightly smaller in diameter than the aortic annulus is selected to reduce the risk of leaflet dehiscence. We typically use a 4-cm long, 20- to 22-mm diameter balloon that matches the size of the annulus. Use of longer balloons or dumbbell-shaped balloons may be useful to increase stability during expansion. Dilute contrast (10% to 20%) reduces viscosity and inflation–deflation time. The balloon is advanced across the valve, burst pacing is initiated, and when 1:1 capture is confirmed (with a fall in systolic pressure below 60 mm Hg and a reduction in pulse pressure), the balloon is rapidly inflated, deflated, pacing terminated, and the balloon withdrawn from the valve to allow hemodynamic recovery.

Careful observation of the balloon during expansion is important. In the presence of septal hypertrophy, constriction at the level of the sinotubular junction, or a mitral prosthesis extending into the left ventricular outflow tract, the balloon may be displaced during inflation. This should raise concerns about possible interference with balloon expansion during valve deployment resulting in malposition of the prosthesis. Aortic angiography during valvuloplasty is useful to assess the risk of left main obstruction or to assist in annular sizing and prosthesis selection (Fig. 18-9).

Implantation of the Valve

The prosthesis is typically prepared and mounted on the delivery system by a technician or assistant. Before the delivery system is introduced into the sheath, it is important to check that the valve is mounted correctly on the catheter. The prosthesis should be mounted so that the sealing cuff will be implanted in the ventricle and the open cells in the aorta. The orientation of the

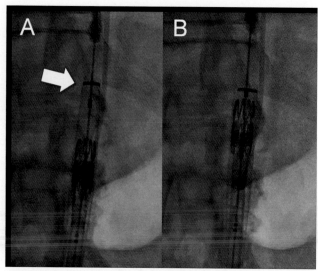

FIGURE 18-10.

A: The SAPIEN XT valve (Edwards Lifesciences Inc., Irvine, CA) is mounted onto the shaft of the balloon catheter. Once this is passed through the sheath and into the aorta, the valve can be advanced onto the bulkier balloon. The *arrow* points at the radiopaque end of the sheath. **B:** In this case, alignment of the valve between the two radiopaque balloon markers has been accomplished prior to exiting the expandable sheath.

prosthesis on the balloon catheter is opposite for the retrograde transarterial and antegrade transapical procedures.

The delivery system is introduced into the sheath and passed into the thoracic aorta. The deployment balloon is then pulled into the prosthesis. Subsequent rotation of an alignment wheel on the handle of the device allows fine adjustment until the valve lies between the two radiopaque balloon markers. This procedure can be performed inside the sheath if an expandable sheath is used (Fig. 18-10). As the valve travels around the aortic arch, rotation of a deflection wheel on the handle bends the distal portion of the delivery catheter to improve tracking. A left anterior oblique view provides the best view during passage around the aortic arch. However, the previously determined view perpendicular to the native valve provides the best view for implantation.

The prosthesis is then placed in the left ventricle and the outer portion of the NovaFlex pusher/deflector catheter is withdrawn from the balloon and prosthesis. The valve is positioned using fluoroscopy, aortography with a pigtail catheter placed on the native noncoronary leaflet, and TEE. Ideally, the prosthesis should extend to the tips of the calcified native valve with over 50% extending into the left ventricle below the angiographic basal hinge point of the native valve.

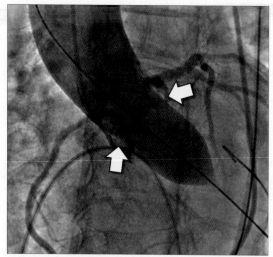

FIGURE 18-9.

This contrast injection at the time of balloon valvuloplasty visualizes the cusps (*arrows*) and shows that the left main artery is unlikely to be obstructed by the native leaflets when they are displaced by the prosthetic valve.

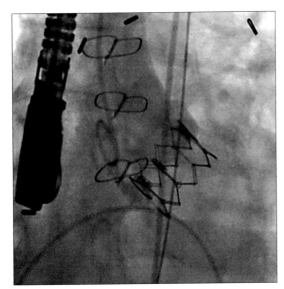

F I G U R E   1 8 - 1 1 .

Aortic root angiography after implantation of the SAPIEN valve (Edwards Lifesciences Inc., Irvine, CA). Approximately one-half to one-third of the valve should be below the most basal leaflet attachment to accommodate effective sealing.

Once the valve is ideally positioned, the balloon is expanded during rapid pacing as with the earlier balloon valvuloplasty. Positioning and the presence and degree of paravalvular leak are assessed with TEE and aortic root injection (Figs. 18-11 and 18-12).[13]

Transapical Access

This technique has become a routine procedure in recent years. The left ventricular apex is readily accessible through a small anterolateral intercostal thoracotomy.[14–16] Pledgeted sutures are placed in a nonfatty portion of the apical left ventricle (typically not in the true apex, which is often fatty and thin). Following left ventricular puncture with an arterial needle, a standard arterial sheath is advanced over a wire into the ventricular cavity. Fluoroscopy is used to advance an extra support wire through the stenotic aortic valve distally into the descending aorta. Balloon valvuloplasty with burst pacing is usually performed. The small diameter sheath is exchanged for a larger 24 to 26 French sheath. The prosthesis is crimped onto an Ascendra delivery catheter (Edwards Lifesciences), which is positioned under fluoroscopic and echocardiographic guidance and deployed during rapid ventricular pacing. The apex and thoracotomy are surgically closed and a chest tube is placed.

The apical approach, in comparison with a transarterial approach, may offer a reduced risk of iliofemoral injury, arch atheroembolism, difficulty crossing the stenotic native valve, noncoaxial positioning, and movement during deployment. Disadvantages include a thoracotomy and chest tube, greater risk of ventricular or chordal injury, bleeding, general anesthesia, postprocedural chest discomfort, respiratory compromise, and late apical pseudoaneurysms. Patient selection requires balancing these advantages and disadvantages. Most groups default to a transarterial approach in the absence of severe iliofemoral disease because outcomes have generally been more favorable.[17]

Valve-in-Valve Implants

Early reported experience with valve-in-valve implantation in aortic, mitral, pulmonary, and tricuspid degenerated surgical bioprostheses has been favorable.[18] The surgical valve facilitates positioning and paravalvular sealing and may shield the atrioventricular conduction system. However, many surgical valves may be too small for a valve-in-valve implant. The most widely used 21-mm surgical tissue aortic valve has an internal diameter of 17 mm, which means that a SAPIEN valve will be underexpanded, thereby resulting in moderate stenosis and reduced durability. Early experience with damaged, incorrectly positioned, or undersized SAPIEN valves confirms that a second valve can be implanted within the first with a good functional result.

Postprocedural Management

Femoral sheaths and the temporary pacemaker are removed on completion of the procedure. If there is new

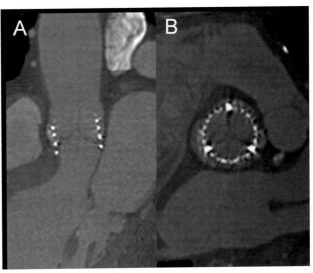

F I G U R E   1 8 - 1 2 .

Multislice computed tomography of an implanted SAPIEN valve (Edwards Lifesciences Inc., Irvine, CA). **A:** Three-chamber view. **B:** Axial view of the valve.

atrioventricular conduction block, the pacemaker is left in place until this is resolved or a permanent pacemaker implanted. Intubated patients are ideally extubated immediately following the procedure. A radial arterial line and internal jugular line are typically left in place until the following morning. In the absence of data, the standard approach to preventing late valve thromboembolism has been long-term aspirin use and 1 to 3 months of clopidogrel. However, in the presence of additional risk factors such as atrial fibrillation, warfarin may be indicated. Antibiotic prophylaxis is recommended for procedures that might be associated with bacteremia for a period of 6 months.

AVOIDANCE AND MANAGEMENT OF COMPLICATIONS

Management of Hypotension during the Procedure

Frequently, patients develop a progressive fall in arterial pressure during percutaneous valve implantation.[19] Rapid pacing, ventricular ectopy, radiographic contrast, balloon valvuloplasty, preexisting left ventricular dysfunction, coronary artery disease, and general anesthesia predispose to myocardial ischemia and reduced contractility. Untreated hypotension can rapidly deteriorate into hemodynamic collapse in patients with severe aortic stenosis. Hypotension should be managed aggressively to avoid a downward spiral of myocardial ischemia, left ventricular depression, and worsening hypotension. Maintaining a systolic blood pressure of above 100 mm Hg often requires low-dose inotropic and vasoconstrictor support (e.g., norepinephrine and phenylephrine). Chronotropic drugs may exacerbate ischemia in the presence of aortic stenosis. Unexpected hypotension should prompt consideration of arterial perforation, catheter-related right or left heart perforation, coronary obstruction, vagal stimulation, iatrogenic mitral regurgitation, severe aortic regurgitation, or generalized myocardial ischemia.[19,20]

Vascular Injury

Although sheath size has now decreased from 24 to 18 French outside of the United States, vascular complications such as perforation, dissection, or thrombosis are still a concern. These complications can be minimized with proper patient selection, precise vascular access, and careful use of closure devices. Nevertheless, it is important to have ready access to equipment suitable for the management of large vessel dissection

or perforation. Dissection or vessel occlusion can usually be managed percutaneously. However, perforation is of greater immediate concern. Unexplained hypotension after sheath placement or shortly following sheath removal may be the initial clue to vascular perforation. Aortic or iliac angiography with a pigtail inserted through the large sheath or through a contralateral sheath should be considered. Contralateral arterial access should be maintained until satisfactory hemostasis following large sheath removal is assured. If arterial perforation is suspected, hemostasis can usually be temporarily accomplished by reinsertion of the sheath or placement of a compliant occlusion balloon upstream to the suspected bleeding site. Once stabilized, the bleeding site can then be controlled with implantation of a covered stent or surgical repair.[19]

Paravalvular Regurgitation

Mild-to-moderate paravalvular regurgitation is common after TAVI, but generally well tolerated. Undersizing, incomplete expansion, or implantation either too high or low within the annulus are the major contributors to leaks.[19] In case of a more severe paravalvular leak, balloon inflation can be repeated to ensure full expansion of the prosthesis. The rare case of severe paravalvular regurgitation due to implantation of a prosthesis too aortic or too ventricular may require implantation of a second overlapping valve so as to extend the paravalvular seal further. However, aortic regurgitation, valvular and paravalvular combined, is generally not increased and is often reduced after TAVI.[21]

Atrioventricular Block

Compression of the atrioventricular conduction system as it travels through the interventricular septum adjacent to the aortic valve may be associated with new atrioventricular block.[22] The rate of new pacemaker insertion associated with the SAPIEN valve ranges from 3% to 12%, depending on local practice. Risk factors for new heart block may include advanced age, preexisting right bundle branch block or atrioventricular delay, low implantation, and prosthesis oversizing.[23-25] Because the onset of complete heart block may be delayed, we recommend telemetric monitoring for at least 48 hours following TAVI.

Stroke

Reported rates of stroke with percutaneous aortic valve replacement vary from 0% to 9% in the high-risk elderly patients undergoing this procedure.[2,4,26,27] However, it appears that stroke rates are falling with improved equipment and expertise. To put this in perspective, the recent large postmarketing SOURCE registry reported a stroke rate of 2.4%, whereas the monitored PARTNER B trial found a major stroke (permanent disability) rate of 5.0% (both with an early generation large profile delivery system). Intraprocedural stroke most often occurs because of embolization of friable calcific debris from the native aortic valve leaflets or atheroma from the ascending aorta. Investigational devices designed to reduce cerebral embolization include membranes placed over the roof of the aortic arch to deflect emboli peripherally as well as carotid filters designed to capture emboli. Screening for, and exclusion of, patients with bulky aortic arch atheroma may be reasonable. However, it appears that the most marked reductions in stroke rate may come from meticulous technique, minimal manipulation within the proximal aorta, the development of less traumatic delivery catheters, and appropriate anticoagulation.

CONCLUSION

Percutaneous aortic valve implantation has evolved into a reproducible procedure with outcomes that compare favorably with conventional surgery in high-risk patients and are demonstrably superior to medical therapy in nonsurgical patients. Hopefully, outcomes will continue to improve, allowing application in a wider spectrum of patients.

REFERENCES

1. Cribier A, Eltchaninoff H, Bash A, et al. Percutaneous transcatheter implantation of an aortic valve prosthesis for calcific aortic stenosis: first human case description. *Circulation.* 2002;106:3006–3008.

2. Webb JG, Chandavimol M, Thompson CR, et al. Percutaneous aortic valve implantation retrograde from the femoral artery. *Circulation.* 2006;113:842–850.

3. Cribier A, Eltchaninoff H, Tron C, et al. Early experience with percutaneous transcatheter implantation of heart valve prosthesis for the treatment of end-stage inoperable patients with calcific aortic stenosis. *J Am Coll Cardiol.* 2004;43:698–703.

4. Webb JG, Pasupati S, Humphries K, et al. Percutaneous transarterial aortic valve replacement in selected high-risk patients with aortic stenosis. *Circulation.* 2007;116:755–763.

5. Webb JG, Chandavimol M, Thompson C, et al. Percutaneous aortic valve implantation retrograde from the femoral artery. *Circulation.* 2006;113:842–850.

6. Webb JG, Altwegg L, Masson JB, et al. A new transcatheter aortic valve and percutaneous valve delivery system. *J Am Coll Cardiol.* 2009;53:1855–1858.

7. Moss RR, Ivens E, Pasupati S, et al. Role of echocardiography in percutaneous aortic valve implantation. *JACC Cardiovasc Imaging.* 2008;1:15–24.

8. Wood DA, Tops LF, Mayo JR, et al. Role of multislice computed tomography in transcatheter aortic valve replacement. *Am J Cardiol.* 2009;103:1295–1301.

9. Leipsic J, Wood D, Manders D, et al. The evolving role of mdct in transcatheter aortic valve replacement: a radiologists' perspective. *AJR Am J Roentgenol.* 2009;193:W214–W219.

10. Tops LF, Wood DA, Delgado V, et al. Noninvasive evaluation of the aortic root with multislice computed tomography implications for transcatheter aortic valve replacement. *JACC Cardiovasc Imaging.* 2008;1:321–330.

11. Lauck S, Mackay M, Galte C, et al. A new option for the treatment of aortic stenosis: percutaneous aortic valve replacement. *Crit Care Nurse.* 2008;28:40–51.

12. Webb JG, Pasupati S, Achtem L, et al. Rapid pacing to facilitate transcatheter prosthetic heart valve implantation. *Catheter Cardiovasc Interv.* 2006;68:199–204.

13. Webb JG, Pasupati SJ, Humphries K, et al. Percutaneous transarterial aortic valve replacement in selected high risk patients with aortic stenosis. *Circulation.* 2007;116:755–763.

14. Ye J, Cheung A, Lichtenstein SV, et al. Transapical transcatheter aortic valve implantation: follow-up to 3 years. *J Thorac Cardiovasc Surg.* 2010;139:1107–1113.

15. Ye J, Cheung A, Lichtenstein SV, et al. Six-month outcome of transapical transcatheter aortic valve implantation in the initial seven patients. *Eur J Cardiothorac Surg.* 2007;31:16–21.

16. Lichtenstein SV, Cheung A, Ye J, et al. Transapical transcatheter aortic valve implantation in humans: initial clinical experience. *Circulation.* 2006;114:591–596.

17. Webb JG, Altwegg L, Boone RH, et al. Transcatheter aortic valve implantation: impact on clinical and valve-related outcomes. *Circulation.* 2009;119:3009–3016.

18. Webb JG, Wood DA, Ye J, et al. Transcatheter valve-in-valve implantation for failed bioprosthetic heart valves. *Circulation.* 2010;121:1848–1857.

19. Masson JB, Kovac J, Schuler G, et al. Transcatheter aortic valve implantation: review of the nature, management and avoidance of procedural complications. *JACC Cardiovasc Intervent.* 2009;2:811–820.

20. Kapadia SR, Svensson L, Tuzcu EM. Successful percutaneous management of left main trunk occlusion during percutaneous aortic valve replacement. *Catheter Cardiovasc Interv.* 2009;73:966–972.

21. Leon MB, Smith CR, Mack M, et al. Transcatheter aortic-valve implantation for aortic stenosis in patients who cannot undergo surgery. *N Engl J Med.* 2010;363;1597–1607.

22. Sinhal A, Altwegg L, Pasupati S, et al. Atrioventricular block after transcatheter balloon expandable aortic valve implantation. *JACC Cardiovasc Interv.* 2008;1:305–309.

23. Baan J Jr, Yong ZY, Koch KT, et al. Factors associated with cardiac conduction disorders and permanent pacemaker implantation after percutaneous aortic valve implantation with the corevalve prosthesis. *Am Heart J.* 2010;159:497–503.

24. Avanzas P, Munoz-Garcia AJ, Segura J, et al. Percutaneous implantation of the corevalve self-expanding aortic valve prosthesis in patients with severe aortic stenosis: early experience in Spain. *Rev Esp Cardiol.* 2010;63:141–148.

25. Godin M, Eltchaninoff H, Furuta A, et al. Frequency of conduction disturbances after transcatheter implantation of an Edwards Sapien aortic valve prosthesis. *Am J Cardiol.* 2010;106:707–712.

26. Grube E, Buellesfeld L, Mueller R, et al. Progress and current status of percutaneous aortic valve replacement: results of three device generations of the corevalve revalving system. *Circ Cardiovasc Interv.* 2008;1:167–175.

27. Grube E, Schuler G, Buellesfeld L, et al. Percutaneous aortic valve replacement for severe aortic stenosis in high-risk patients using the second- and current third-generation self-expanding corevalve prosthesis: Device success and 30-day clinical outcome. *J Am Coll Cardiol.* 2007;50:69–76.

CHAPTER 19

Implantation of the CoreValve Aortic Valve

Jean-Claude Laborde and Stephen J.D. Brecker

Some background of the design concept, functioning, and characteristics of the Medtronic CoreValve ReValving system (Medtronic, Minneapolis, MN) device is required to fully appreciate the technical aspects of CoreValve implantation. Design conception and iterative prototyping of the CoreValve ReValving system took place during 1997 to 2002 with technical preclinical, animal, and cadaver work completed by early 2004. A first-in-human clinical feasibility study was conducted during 2004. Since this first device, the concept of a long, self-expanding, multilevel, nitinol frame with three different levels of potential anchoring on the patient anatomy—outflow tract, valve leaflets, and ascending aorta—proved sound. Despite unexpectedly low implantation of the valve in the left ventricular outflow tract (LVOT), early in the learning curve, valve migration into the left ventricle (LV) cavity never occurred, severe paravalvular leaks have been rare, and emergent conversion to surgery has now all but disappeared.

The first 25 French device, incorporating a trileaflet bovine pericardial tissue valve, was implanted in 14 patients, demonstrating robust valve durability with the longest follow-up being 5.5 years. The prosthesis rapidly evolved with safety and efficacy studies conducted during 2005 and 2006 with two subsequent device generations (Fig. 19-1). The delivery catheter was downsized from 25 French with the first generation to 21 French with the second generation (2005), and 18 French with the third-generation (2006) prosthesis, which is currently used. This major improvement resulted mainly from extension of the valve leaflets' attachment higher on the nitinol prosthesis structure. A significant reduction of the stress on the leaflets during valve functioning resulted, demonstrated nicely by the "suspended bridge" concept (Fig. 19-2), which is important in enhancing valve durability (Fig. 19-3).

Mechanical factors and stress could be the major causes of surgical aortic valve degeneration and explain the propensity of certain sites of the valve to calcify.[1] By reducing the stress on the valve leaflets, thinner biological material can be used without jeopardizing long-term durability. Bovine pericardium, used in the first-generation device, was replaced by porcine pericardium. The thinner porcine pericardium with higher points of attachment on the frame allowed a reduction of the delivery catheter diameter down to 18 French with the third-generation device, enabling a truly percutaneous femoral approach for valve delivery in November 2006. This approach has been used in more than 90% of the 20,000 patients treated with Medtronic CoreValve prosthesis to date. A 16 French next-generation device is under development. In order to appreciate the technical aspects of valve implantation, it is necessary to better understand this 18 French prosthesis.[2,3]

PROSTHESIS CONSIDERATIONS

Support Frame and Bioprosthesis

At the center of the system is a multilevel self-expanding and fully radiopaque nitinol frame with a diamond

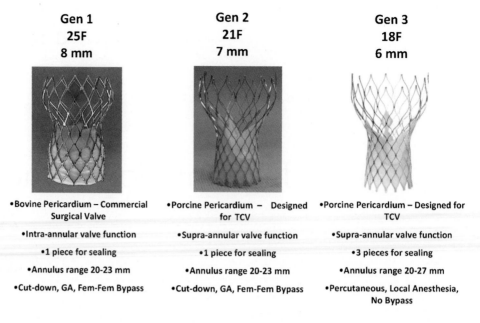

Gen 1
25F
8 mm

Gen 2
21F
7 mm

Gen 3
18F
6 mm

• Bovine Pericardium – Commercial Surgical Valve

• Intra-annular valve function

• 1 piece for sealing

• Annulus range 20-23 mm

• Cut-down, GA, Fem-Fem Bypass

• Porcine Pericardium – Designed for TCV

• Supra-annular valve function

• 1 piece for sealing

• Annulus range 20-23 mm

• Cut-down, GA, Fem-Fem Bypass

• Porcine Pericardium – Designed for TCV

• Supra-annular valve function

• 3 pieces for sealing

• Annulus range 20-27 mm

• Percutaneous, Local Anesthesia, No Bypass

cell configuration that holds the tissue leaflets and anchors the device. This noncylindrical frame incorporates three different levels into a single construct with varying diameter, degrees of radial, and hoop strength and function (Figs. 19-4 to 19-6).

The (lower) inflow level exerts high radial force and functions solely for anchoring on the annulus and native valve leaflets. Constant outward force reduces recoil and allows the frame to adjust to the native annulus size and shape within its size design limitations. This level is 12 mm high and is covered with a skirt composed of a single layer of porcine pericardium that creates a seal in order to prevent paravalvular aortic

regurgitation. At the lowest part, the outer diameter of the frame is 26 mm for the small valve and 29 mm for the large valve.

The center portion of the frame is constrained to resist size and shape deformation (features high hoop strength) and contains the valve leaflets. Its concave apposition to the sinus avoids the coronaries and allows both unimpeded coronary blood flow and coronary catheter access postimplant. The hourglass frame design avoids the need for rotational positioning because the upstroke of the valve commissures always remain away from the coronaries. At the nadir of the valve, the outer frame diameter is 23 mm for the small

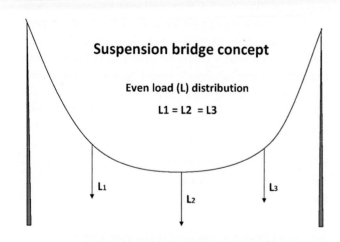

Suspension bridge concept

Even load (L) distribution

L1 = L2 = L3

L₁

L₂

L₃

• **Load absorbed equally by each point on leaflet commissures**
• **NO frame flexing under load: static frame**

FIGURE 19-2.

CoreValve (Medtronic, Minneapolis, MN) design element 1.

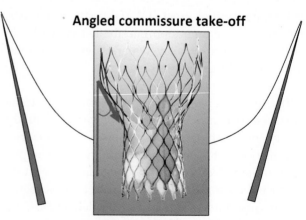

Angled commissure take-off

Angled take-off reduces stress and optimizes leaflet motion

FIGURE 19-3.

CoreValve (Medtronic, Minneapolis, MN) design element 2.

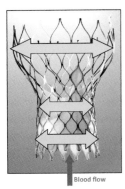

Differing circumferential dimensions:

- Largest dimension for ascending aorta contact

- Smallest dimension to preserve coronary blood flow and avoid coronary jailing

- Flared intra-annular dimension adapting to a range of annulus sizes

FIGURE 19-4.

Self-expanding multilevel frame; diameter varies.

Different radial forces & hoop strengths:

- Orients the valve to blood flow regardless of angle of delivery
- Optimal valve geometry and valve function regardless of annular anatomy
- Intra-annular and native valve anchoring and adaptation to different annulus sizes and shapes

FIGURE 19-5.

Self-expanding multilevel frame; radial forces vary.

valve and 25 mm for the large valve. If properly positioned, this portion of the implanted valve faces the mid-level of the coronary sinuses (Fig. 19-7) allowing the valve to function supra-annularly.

The (upper) outflow level features the largest frame diameter to accommodate the ascending aorta and exerts only low radial force. Its primary function is to assure optimal alignment of the prosthesis to blood flow. The superior rim features two loops that serve to load the valve into the delivery catheter. The outer diameter is 40 mm for the small 26-mm valve and 43 mm for the large 29-mm valve. Uncoupling the anchoring (skirt area) and functional (leaflets) elements of the valve that has lower the valve profile resulted in a bioprosthesis that is *implanted intra-annularly* but that *functions supra-annularly.* The supra-annular function is also an important contributor to superior hemodynamic function of the valve.

The CoreValve bioprosthesis is currently available in two sizes. The 26-mm inflow model is intended for a patient annulus between 20 and 23 mm and the 29-mm inflow model is intended for a patient annulus between 23 and 27 mm. In the near future (estimated 2011), a 23-mm inflow model (16 French delivery catheter) will be added for patient annulus between 18 and 20 mm and a 31-mm inflow model (18 French) will be added for annulus sizes between 27 and 29 mm.

18 French Delivery Catheter System

The CoreValve delivery system (Fig. 19-8) is an over-the-wire catheter and accommodates a 0.035-inch wire. The distal part of the catheter features an 18 French housing capsule that accommodates the bioprosthesis. The proximal part of the catheter shaft steps down to 12 French immediately behind the valve

Radial Force (R): Physical property that has the ability to bring about change in shape/diameter of structure

R > H

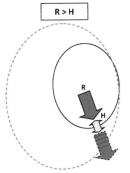

Radial Force (R) overcomes hoop strength resulting in changed structure

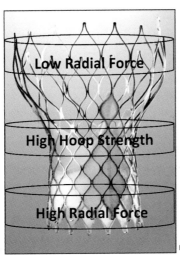

Hoop Strength (H): Physical property that has the ability to resist change in shape/diameter of structure

R < H

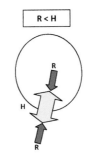

Hoop Strength (H) overcomes radial force resulting in no change to structure

FIGURE 19-6.

Radial force and hoop strength.

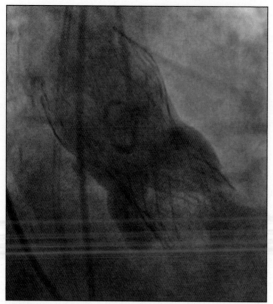

FIGURE 19-7.

CoreValve (Medtronic, Minneapolis, MN) proper position.

during the valve delivery procedure (both inside and outside the catheter).

Catheter Loading System

CoreValve's third-generation loading system is fully disposable (Fig. 19-10). It serves to load the bioprosthesis *into* the catheter housing cone in a consistent and nontraumatic manner. It comprises five individual elements (inflow cone, inflow tube, outflow cone, outflow cap, and outflow tube) that are applied in sequence by a single loader operator. During the loading procedure, the bioprosthesis must be precompressed. The compression procedure is performed during submersion of the loading system, delivery catheter tip, and bioprosthesis in cold saline (approximately 0°–8° C) and must be performed under strict sterile conditions.

Anatomical Considerations

Prosthesis dimensions along with anatomical features and measurements are key considerations in selecting the valve size and optimal positioning.[4] The most important relationship is between the lower portion (skirt) of the prosthesis and base of the aortic root (LVOT, annulus, valve leaflets). The prosthesis skirt is 12 mm in length irrespective of the valve size. This portion of the prosthesis plays a major role in valve anchoring and sealing. In calcific aortic valve disease, anchoring of the implanted valve is ensured by the native valve leaflets, which compress the frame at the lower part of the coronary sinus. Anchoring is also obtained at the subannular level (maximum with severe LV hypertrophy and a small outflow tract, none with a dilated LV cavity with a large outflow tract) and the ascending aorta (upper level of the frame). This is significant with

housing capsule and assures easy navigation through the vasculature and access into the native aortic valve without the need for steerability or flexion elements. The proximal catheter handle features two control elements (Fig. 19-9): a rotating knob (microknob) for slow progressive sheath movement and a slide knob (macroslide) for rapid sheath movement. Both controls are able to make the sheath move backward or forward and are used interchangeably during valve loading and valve delivery; however, the macroslide is not used during valve delivery. The catheter tip is radiopaque and the distal part of the housing capsule features an additional positioning marker. The bioprosthesis frame is at all times fluoroscopically visible

FIGURE 19-8.

Delivery catheter.

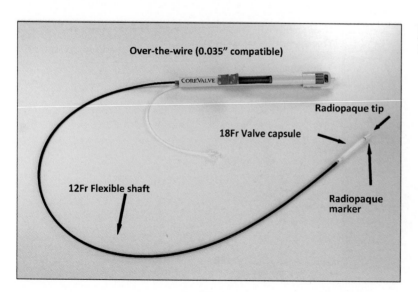

Over-the-wire (0.035" compatible)

COREVALVE

Radiopaque tip

18Fr Valve capsule

12Fr Flexible shaft

Radiopaque marker

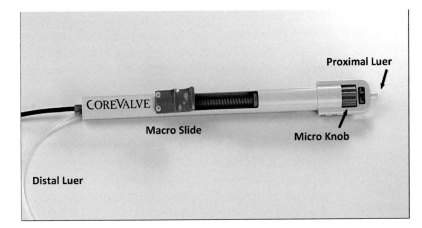

FIGURE 19-9.

Delivery catheter handle.

a small diameter ascending aorta, reduced with a larger diameter and none with an aorta with a diameter larger than the frame (above 40 and 43 mm for the 26-mm and 29-mm devices, respectively). The sealing effect follows the same general rules in regard to the anatomy of the patient involving the LVOT, annulus, and valve leaflets.

The annulus diameter is paramount and the accuracy of this measurement is crucial. The respective role of transthoracic echocardiography (TTE), transesophageal echocardiography (TEE), and multislice computed tomography (CT) is still subject of debate. As the annulus is oval rather than circular,[2-4] three-dimensional (3D) imaging such as multislice CT may give more accurate measurements.[5] Correct prosthesis–patient match is imperative to avoid valve embolization or paravalvar regurgitation due to undersizing. The CoreValve device is purposely oversized to create enough radial force to anchor within the aortic root. A 26-mm valve is intended for a patient annulus of 20 to 23 mm and a 29-mm valve for an annulus of 23 to 27 mm.

The second important relationship is between the center portion (valve leaflets) of the prosthesis and the coronary sinuses to evaluate the potential risk of compromising the coronary artery ostia. Risk assessment is based on: (a) diameter of the sinus of Valsalva, (b) height of the coronary artery orifice from the base of the native aortic leaflet, and (c) degree of aortic valve calcification and thickness. A narrow sinus of Valsalva, low-lying coronary arteries, large aortic valve leaflet, and/or severe leaflet calcifications can act in concert to increase the risk of coronary obstruction. An empty space of 2 mm surrounding the central waist of the valve is recommended (minimum sinus of Valsava diameter 27 mm and 29 mm for the 26-mm and 29-mm valves, respectively.) In addition, a 15-mm coronary sinus height is required to guard against coronary obstruction if the 12-mm skirt is implanted too high. Despite these recommendations, it remains difficult to completely rule out the risk of coronary obstruction.

The final relationship between the prosthesis and patient anatomy is to analyze the upper portion of the prosthesis and the ascending aorta above the sinotubular junction. The potential risk of compromising a coronary bypass graft ostium should take into consideration the height of the prosthesis (~50 mm), although this complication has not been reported. More important is the potential risk of valve embolization if the anatomy is too large (e.g., large ascending aorta, large aortic root, and native valve leaflets with little calcification). The minimum diameter of the ascending aorta has been defined at 40 and 43 mm for implantation of the 26- and 29-mm devices, respectively.

Model - CLS-3000-18Fr

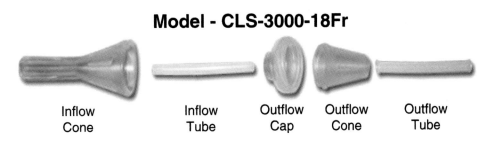

FIGURE 19-10.

Disposable loading system.

Inflow Cone   Inflow Tube   Outflow Cap   Outflow Cone   Outflow Tube

In the ideal position, the ventricular end of the implanted valve is 4 mm (1/2 diamond) below the base of the aortic root with the nadir of the valve 8 mm (1 diamond) above the base of the aortic root allowing a supra-annular functioning of the valve. In the case of a small aortic root with small coronary sinuses, the valve should be implanted slightly lower inside the LVOT to decrease the potential risk of coronary obstruction, irrespective of the increased risk of conduction disorders. In the case of a very large aortic root, the valve will be voluntarily implanted slightly higher. Deep implantation is a key factor increasing the risk of conduction disturbances. The His bundle and left bundle branch emerge superficially around 6 mm below the noncoronary sinus just below the membranous septum.[6]

MATERIAL CONSIDERATIONS

Guidewires

Guidewire choice and handling should not be under estimated, as it can mean the difference between a safely performed successful procedure without complication and death of the patient due to ventricular perforation. Most guidewires are constructed with an inner core and an outer layer in the form of a coil. The stiff inner core tapers distally and ends before the tip of the guidewire, allowing for a flexible and atraumatic distal coil tip. It is important that all but the distal portion of the wire be stiffer than a typical guidewire so as to facilitate easy delivery of the delivery system through tortuous peripheral vessels. The distal tip, however, should be floppy to allow preshaping so that the distal portion of the wire lies coiled within the ventricle in an atraumatic manner.

The most common wire used has been the Amplatz Super Stiff guidewire (Boston Scientific Inc., Natick, MA). This 0.035-inch, 260-cm long wire has a stainless steel core and polytetrafluoroethylene coating and a 1-, 3-, or 6-cm floppy straight or J tip. The floppy tip of the guidewire should be preshaped into a pigtail type configuration. Other guidewires which have been used include the Amplatz Extra Stiff (Cook Medical Inc., Bloomington, IN), Lunderquist Extra Stiff (Cook Medical Inc.), and the Amplatz Ultra Stiff (Cook Medical Inc.) guidewires. These wires have a stiffer mandrel (core) while maintaining tip flexibility.

As important as the choice of guidewire is the appreciation of how important it is to control the guidewire at all times. This depends critically on the interaction between the first and second operators. This may often involve a second operator who may not be as familiar with guidewire handling techniques. By maintaining tip stability and having a preshaped curve on the wire, the risk of ventricular perforation, pericardial effusion, and tamponade can be minimized but not eliminated.

Introducers

The distal nose cone of the CoreValve delivery system requires an 18 French sheath for delivery of which there are two in common clinical use. These are the St. Jude Medical Ultimum EV Hemostatic Introducer 30-cm length sheath (St. Jude Medical Inc., St. Paul, MN) or the Cook sheath (Cook Medical Inc.). Both sheaths can be used from either the femoral or subclavian approach although small differences may be used to advantage in particular clinical situations. The St. Jude sheath has a very slightly lower profile and may be advantageous in vessels of borderline diameter (e.g., 6 mm). The more kink resistant Cook sheath may be better in more tortuous anatomy, particularly from the subclavian approach. Valve retrieval into the St. Jude sheath may be more difficult, requiring that the valve be withdrawn into the common iliac or subclavian artery where the patient's own anatomy can be used to compress the valve prior to retrieval into the sheath. Severely calcified arteries may compromise this maneuver and dictate implantation of the valve in the abdominal aorta in case of femoral access or the ascending aorta in the case of axillary access.

In order to insert the sheath, it is necessary to have a stiff wire to straighten any tortuous anatomy. A particular tip is to place a curve on the distal third of the sheath. By rotational movement of the sheath, with gentle forward pressure, the preshaped sheath can usually be easily advanced, even through tortuous anatomy, along a stiff wire.

Valvuloplasty Balloons

The choice of balloon with which to perform the preimplantation balloon valvuloplasty has been the subject of some debate. All that is required is that an adequate orifice is produced safely to allow full deployment of the transcatheter aortic valve. It is not necessary to obtain a perfect hemodynamic result. Valvuloplasty may not be necessary if performed in the previous 3 months, if a valve is placed within a degenerative xenograft, or in cases of pure aortic regurgitation. It has been common to use valvuloplasty balloons such as the TyShack (NuMED Inc., Hopkinton, NY), the Z-MED (NuMED Inc.), and the Cristal (BALT, Montmorency, France) balloons. These balloons share the characteristic of straight sides and tend to be ejected during inflation from the aortic valve into the aorta unless cardiac output is significantly reduced by rapid ventricular pacing before the advent of transcatheter aortic valve implantation (TAVI), valvuloplasty operators like these balloons because of their ability to achieve full dilatation of the valve.

The Nucleus balloon (NuMED Inc.) is frequently used and engineered for maximal steering and tracking. The coaxial shaft design provides enhanced column strength and pushability combined with a flexible distal tip. This balloon inflates in a dog bone configuration and will center itself on the aortic annulus during inflation. It is still necessary to perform inflation during rapid ventricular pacing although the rate of pacing need not be as high. Balloon inflation without rapid ventricular pacing is recommended only in special circumstances. The balloon material is thin and has a lower deflated profile; however, a low-rated burst pressure can be exceeded. There are reported cases of fragments of the balloon dehiscing from the shaft following balloon rupture. The rated burst pressure for the 22- and 25-mm balloons is 4 atmospheres and for the 28-mm balloon, it is 2 atmospheres. The volume of contrast placed within the balloon should not exceed that in the instruction guide or else the risk of balloon rupture is significant.

The choice of balloon size will depend on which type of balloon is being used. If a straight sided balloon is being used, then it is advised that the size be slightly less than the annulus dimension as measured by TEE. A 22-mm Nucleus balloon should be used with a small-sized CoreValve (26-mm inflow) and a 25-mm Nucleus balloon with a large-sized CoreValve (29-mm inflow). It should be noted that the Nucleus balloon will achieve a waist diameter less than reported size at nominal volume. It is necessary only to inflate the balloon to nominal volume.

Access Strategy

Since 2006, percutaneous femoral arterial access has been established as the access of choice for the Core-Valve prosthesis. However, the device is still relatively bulky and this, coupled with the high incidence of peripheral vascular disease in elderly patients, has driven the search for alternative routes of delivery to treat a wider range of patients. Currently, access options for CoreValve implantation include the common femoral arteries, axillary/subclavian arteries, and transaortic arteries. Transapical access and the carotid approach have been too limited with CoreValve to draw conclusions about their potential.

Femoral Access

Assessing the feasibility and safety of the femoral route is the first consideration when considering a patient for TAVI.[7] Complex femoral anatomy requires a highly individualized, thoughtful approach. No simple algorithm exists, and skill levels in managing peripheral vascular disease vary. Assessing the feasibility and safety of the femoral route requires a complete analysis of all the steps of a procedure and their potential complications:

- Peripheral arterial disease below the common femoral artery to assess for risk of distal ischemia, as in patient with previous occlusion of the superficial femoral artery.
- Femoral puncture site for the risk of occlusion or prolonged bleeding in a calcified or small artery.
- Iliac arteries for the risk of arterial rupture in very calcified vessel.
- Thoracic and abdominal aorta for the risk of distal emboli in case of valve retrieval for misplacement at the time of implantation.
- Angulation and calcification of the aortic arch and native valve for the risk of valve misplacement, stroke, aortic dissection, and cardiac tamponade.

For femoral puncture, the common femoral artery should be ≥6.0 mm in diameter with ≥15 mm length between the superficial epigastric artery and the femoral bifurcation and avoidance of severe calcification. Compliance with this minimum requirement makes for a safe puncture and a high success rate with the use of the 10 French ProStar (Abbott Vascular Inc., Redwood City, CA) for vessel closure. Accurate assessment of those criteria is equally provided by either an angiogram with the use of a graduated pigtail, CT, or magnetic resonance imaging (MRI).

The second step is to assess the feasibility and safety of advancing the 18 French introducer through the iliac arteries.[7] The risk of arterial rupture is directly related to three major features: small arterial diameter, severe tortuosity, and heavy calcification. Thus, if the iliac arterial diameter is <6.0 mm with external iliac artery tortuosity and circumferential arterial calcification, then the femoral approach should be avoided. The third step is to assess the feasibility and safety to advance the 18 French CoreValve catheter through the descending aorta, ascending aorta, crossing of the native valve leaflets in order to ensure safe and accurate implantation of the valve, and, if needed, a safe retrieval of the partially expanded valve. Advancement of the 18 French CoreValve catheter through the 18 French introducer up to the native aortic valve is almost always successful. Rarely, severe angulation and calcification of the horizontal aorta associated with a severe angulation of the aortic root can compromise the progression of the 18 French catheter. This difficulty can be overcome with the use of a "goose-neck" snare catheter to deflect the tip of the delivery system, but the resulting tension on the catheter can potentially compromise the smooth release of the valve.

Axillary/Subclavian Access

The axillary artery, often free of atheroma, is usually large enough to accommodate the 18 French introducer and CoreValve delivery system and therefore offers an alternative route of access for patients with significant peripheral vascular disease. Vessel criteria that exclude the axillary approach due to the potential risk of subclavian dissection, perforation, or vessel rupture include artery diameter <6 mm, severe tortuosity, and severe or circumferential calcification.

Neither the presence of a pacemaker nor a patent left interior mammary artery (LIMA) graft are absolute contraindications to a subclavian approach, but additional expertise is required. In case of patent internal mammary artery graft, the criteria for assessing the safety of the axillary approach are the following:

- Diameter artery of more than 6.5 mm from origin of subclavian artery to the ostia of graft (LIMA or right interior mammary artery [RIMA]).
- Lack of severe tortuosity.
- No circumferential calcification or atherosclerotic disease of the subclavian artery proximal to the graft (risk of dissection).
- No atherosclerotic subclavian artery lesions that might require balloon angioplasty.

When right axillary access is considered, the route of the innominate artery should be assessed using similar criteria as for the left axillary access. From the right axillary approach, because the 18 French sheath and delivery catheter are stiff, the catheter will tend to align vertically and this may lead to difficulty in deploying the valve, particularly if the aorta lies horizontally. As a rule, angulation of the aortic annular plan greater than 30 degrees from the horizontal disqualifies the right axillary approach. In contrast, the left axillary access is feasible irrespective of the native aortic plan angulation.

STEP BY STEP IMPLANTATION: NATIVE AORTIC VALVE STENOSIS

What follows is a step-by-step description of the implantation technique in a patient with senile calcific tricuspid aortic stenosis. The procedure starts with

meticulous planning. This should not only involve the operator and first assistant but also the entire TAVI team including cardiothoracic surgeon, anesthesiologist, critical care physicians, pulmonary physicians, renal physicians, and so forth. Prior to the patient coming into the catheter lab, a full and detailed assessment of the patient's comorbidities, cardiac and aortic anatomy, and peripheral vascular anatomy should have been defined. In particular, the issues surrounding vascular access should have been defined with the preferred route of access already chosen.

There should be a clear understanding of the size of the annulus, which can be clarified with immediate preprocedure TEE if required. The size of valve should have been selected, but this may be modified during the procedure depending on further information becoming available. For annulus dimensions of 20 to 23 mm, it is recommended that a small-sized (26-mm inflow) CoreValve be used. For annulus dimensions in the range of 23 to 27 mm, a large-sized (29-mm inflow) CoreValve is used. When the annulus dimension is in the intermediate range of 23 mm, it is important to use whole patient criteria to decide on the size of valve to implant. For example, is the patient is of large body habitus or small? Are the femoral arteries large or small? In general terms, if the femoral arteries are large vessels, then it is likely that a large-sized CoreValve will be required. The dimension of the aortic sinuses is also important. If the dimension is 28 mm or less, then a small-sized valve should be selected because of the risk of coronary impingement. If, however, the sinus width is 29 mm or greater, then a large-sized valve will be acceptable as the frame will still be clear of the coronary ostia.

Anesthetic practice varies widely from full general anesthesia with endotracheal intubation and TEE to light conscious sedation with local anesthesia. The choice will depend largely on local practice and preference but there may be specific patient-related issues to consider; for example, patients who require rapid mobilization and would tolerate endotracheal intubation and ventilation poorly may be best done under conscious sedation with a vigilant anesthesiologist observing the patient throughout the procedure.

The patient should be pretreated with aspirin but practice varies with respect to pretreatment with clopidogrel. Usually, patients will be fully loaded with both antiplatelet drugs prior to the procedure, but many patients undergoing TAVI suffer from gastrointestinal blood loss due to angiodysplasia or prostatic bleeding due to prostatic hypertrophy, and so on. It is usually advisable to pretreat the patient with a proton pump inhibitor and discontinue beta-blockers.

If the procedure is under general anesthesia, then TEE can be undertaken at this time with particular reference to annulus dimension and valve anatomy. Following induction of anesthesia and endotracheal intubation, an internal jugular central venous line may be placed for central venous pressure monitoring and drug administration and a right internal jugular sheath for the pacing wire. It is generally advised that the pacing wire be placed from the internal jugular vein for a number of reasons. First, it is easier to place a pacing wire atraumatically at the right ventricular apex from this approach than from the left femoral vein and, second, given that the pacing wire will remain in the patient following the procedure, it will allow early mobilization. We recommend a St. Jude 5 French balloon tip pacing wire.

The following description assumes that valve delivery will be from the right common femoral arterial approach. A 6 French sheath is inserted into the left femoral artery and a 5 French graduated pigtail catheter is advanced to the aortic bifurcation. The pigtail catheter should then be manipulated into the right common iliac artery and distally into the right common femoral artery. This cross-over technique is an important skill for the interventionist to learn because it is extremely useful for the emergent management of femoral complications.

The technique for puncturing the right common femoral artery into which the 18 French sheath will be inserted is crucial. The puncture needs to be higher than most interventional cardiologists will be familiar. It is often above the inguinal crease on the anterior abdominal wall but must still be below the inguinal ligament. An angiogram of the right common femoral artery should be taken through the graduated pigtail placed in a cross-over technique from the left femoral artery. A skin nick should be made with a scalpel, having placed the introducing needle on to the anterior abdominal wall under fluoroscopy to identify the best approach into the right common femoral artery. The loop of the pigtail catheter within the right common femoral artery can be used as a guide. Aim to puncture the vessel in the middle of the pigtail under fluoroscopic guidance and then advance a 0.035-inch J wire gently into the descending aorta. Insert a 9 French introducer sheath and, with the wire and dilator still in place, blunt dissection with Mosquito forceps is undertaken. This should ensure complete release of tissues around the sheath and a tip is to dissect all around the sheath leaving the introducer in situ to stiffen it.

The graduated pigtail should then be advanced into the noncoronary sinus of Valsalva in the most left lateral achievable position in the posterior anterior fluoroscopic projection. The arterial pressure can now be monitored from the side arm of the left femoral arterial sheath and the graduated pigtail connected to the power injector.

Typically, the femoral artery will be preclosed using the ProStar vascular closure device. The 9 French arterial sheath and dilator is removed and firm manual compression performed leaving the guidewire in place. The 10 French ProStar is then advanced along the wire into the right femoral artery until the monorail port is at the skin entry point. The wire can then be removed and the ProStar advanced slowly using gentle rotational motion. The finger and thumb pads of the device should be squeezed and the dial rotated until blood is seen to flush back through all three clear tubing ports. A Mosquito clamp can be placed on the indicator port, which should be gently pulsating with blood. Once the ProStar device is within the artery, the clear plastic ring should be rotated from a horizontal into a vertical position using a 90-degree counterclockwise rotation and the ring withdrawn to deploy the needles. Fluoroscopy can be undertaken to ensure that all four needles are deployed. Once the needles have been deployed, the table should be removed from the fluoroscopy into the spotlight and the needles harvested using a needle holder. It is best to use a long needle holder that can rest on the edge of the ProStar rim using a fulcrum-type tipping backward movement to pull the needle from the device. The needles can then be cut from the floor suture ends. It is important to respect the location of the needle and suture and the position relative to the artery must be maintained. Any slack within the sutures can be removed at this stage by gently pulling the two ends of each suture in turn simply to remove the slack rather than cheesewiring the vessel. The ProStar device is then withdrawn 10 cm and each suture is harvested and clamped into its relevant quadrant relative to its position in the vessel. The device is further withdrawn until the monorail port is 1-cm external to the skin and a 0.035-inch J wire is then advanced via the ProStar into the descending aorta. The ProStar can then be removed and the 9 French sheath readvanced over the 0.035-inch wire.

In obese patients, where there is a long track between the skin and the artery, the vessel puncture should be vertical and rather shallow to minimize the length of the track. It is also important in an obese patient to maintain forward pressure on the ProStar during needle deployment, as the pressure of the subcutaneous fat can cause the device to displace out of the vessel.

Heparin can be given at this point, 2,000 to 4,000 units, depending on weight, should be adequate. Operators vary in their practice at this point, and some elect to place the 18 French sheath at this stage. Others prefer to wait until the valve has been crossed and the Amplatzer super stiff wire is in the ventricle before placing the 18 French sheath. The advantage of inserting the 18 French sheath at this point is that bleeding around the sheath site is minimized (compared with a 9 French sheath) and, second, manipulation of the 18 French sheath into the vessel is performed with the super stiff wire tip in the descending aorta rather than in the ventricle, so the risk of the stiff wire perforating the ventricle at this point is eliminated. If it is elected to place the 18 French sheath at this point, then a diagnostic catheter should be placed into the descending aorta over the 0.035-inch J wire. The 0.035-inch J wire is removed and the super stiff wire can be safely positioned within the descending aorta through the diagnostic catheter. The diagnostic catheter and then the 9 French sheath can be removed with manual pressure applied to the vessel entry site. At this point, the 18 French sheath can be gently advanced into the femoral artery.

The importance of a good technique in advancing the 18 French sheath into the artery cannot be overestimated. It is a key tip to have a good curve on the sheath and this can be the difference between a safe smooth entry into the vessel and dissection trauma and rupture. The technique is to use gentle forward pressure with the left hand and generous rotational movement on the proximal hub of the sheath with the right hand. Once the sheath is in place, arterial pressure can be monitored from the side arm.

The next key step to the success of the procedure is to work on getting a good aortogram with clear projection of the annular plane, both fluoroscopically and into the mind's eye of the operators. It is important to obtain a clear view of the valve calcification and the image intensifier can be rotated without giving contrast prior to performing an aortogram in order to see in which plane the band of aortic calcium is narrowest. It will be in this plane that the valve lies perpendicular to the image plane. A number of methods can be used. The width of the band of calcium should be minimized. The graduated pigtail can be used to ensure that the markers on the pigtail distally are equally spaced and this implies that the aorta is in a perpendicular plane to the image. The ring of the pigtail should be seen as a complete and perfect circle rather than obliquely or as an oval. Aortography should then be performed in

a number of different projections to ensure the clearest image plane. Twenty milliliters of contrast at 15 ml per second should suffice. The key is to ensure that the three sinuses are at the same level.

The next step is to cross the aortic valve. This should be done using a 5 French Amplatzer L1 (AL1) catheter and straight soft tip wire. Start with the tip of the AL1 catheter beneath the left coronary ostium and gently advance the straight wire sequentially as the catheter is withdrawn and rotated in a clockwise fashion. Usually, it will be possible to cross even the most calcified valve fairly quickly using this technique. Once the valve is crossed, the AL1 catheter can either be advanced such that the tip of the catheter is pushed to face backward, back toward the valve, and the super stiff wire placed through this catheter. Alternatively, the AL1 catheter can simply be used to allow a 0.035-inch exchange length J wire to be placed within the ventricle. If the AL1 catheter is going to be used to lay the super stiff wire, then the tip of the catheter should be pointing backward up toward the aorta or left atrium. The straight wire can be removed, and the preshaped Amplatzer super stiff wire can then be placed within the ventricle such that the wire is looped within the ventricle with no sharp edges or shoulders impinging on the endocardium. Less-experienced operators may prefer to place the super stiff wire in the ventricle using a pigtail catheter in which case this will need to be first positioned over the exchange length J wire. It is very important to learn what type of preshaped curve should be put on to the super stiff wire because the downside of getting this part of the procedure wrong is pericardial effusion, emergency surgery, and death. It is important when preshaping the wire not to break the core of the wire and not to create any sharp corners. Ideally, the super stiff wire will lie safely coiled within the ventricle giving a stiff firm platform across the valve for valve deployment.

The next step is the aortic valvuloplasty. Typically, the Nucleus balloon will be used as previously described. Pacing should be tested at a rate of around 150 to 180 beats per minute to ensure there is adequate pressure drop during pacing and recovery afterward. The balloon should be prepared and de-aired using standard techniques and advanced on a negative vacuum. It is important to check that the assistants have fully prepared the valve prior to undertaking the valvuloplasty. The central marker of the valvuloplasty balloon should be positioned in the middle of the calcium of the aortic valve, and a full aortic valvuloplasty should be carried out under rapid ventricular pacing. It is not uncommon for the Amplatzer super stiff wire to become malpositioned prior to the valvuloplasty, particularly during the learning curve. If this is the case, then it is important to take time to reposition the wire using a pigtail catheter prior to performing the valvuloplasty.

The prepared CoreValve can now be implanted. This should be advanced over the wire, taking particular care for the second operator to ensure that the distal wire position is fixed. Usually, there will be some resistance at the entry and exit points to the sheath. The graduated pigtail should be left within the noncoronary sinus at this point. The valve should be advanced across the aortic valve using gentle forward pressure and small movements. There is no need to visualize the valve as it crosses the aortic arch—it is more important to visualize the distal wire position as the valve crosses the arch and enters the ascending aorta. The valve should be advanced across the aortic valve until the second set of reinforcements is at the midpoint of the calcium of the valve. If the blood pressure drops at this point without evidence of severe aortic regurgitation, the valve should be gently withdrawn into the ascending aorta and pressors given to raise the blood pressure. It is best to start the valve deployment with a systolic blood pressure of 100 mm Hg or greater. If the graduated pigtail catheter has become displaced from the noncoronary sinus, at this point, it is best to reposition it prior to starting valve deployment, and it may be necessary to use a guidewire to obtain this. Once the graduated pigtail catheter and valve are in position, then deployment can commence.

A further tip to ensure correct alignment of the valve within the aorta is to ensure that the distal tip of the valve delivery system is seen as a single line rather than as an oval. If the distal marker is seen as an oval, this implies that the valve delivery system lies somewhat obliquely within the aorta as it crosses the annulus, and it may be necessary to compromise on the calcium projection to ensure that the oval marker is brought into a straight line by moving the image intensifier slightly. Often, it is necessary to compromise between the two ideal positions in which the calcium is seen as the narrowest band and the distal marker is seen as a single line.

The second operator will begin deployment by small rotational movements of the microknob on the valve delivery system. A number of rotations will be required before any effect is seen at the valve tip but, gradually, the distal sheath marker will retract. As it does so, it will be necessary for the operator to gently withdraw the valve using small squeezing movements between the thumb and index finger of the right hand firmly positioned on the valve delivery system at the sheath hub. The left hand should be steadying the sheath itself. It is necessary for the assistant to stop valve deployment once one cell of the valve frame has been deployed. It will be clear whether the valve has moved forward or not. Typically, there will be a small amount of forward movement of the valve as it deploys. An aortogram can be taken at this point to ascertain valve position. If the patient is hemodynamically stable and the position is satisfactory, then further rotational movements of the microknob should be undertaken until one-third of the valve frame has been deployed. The expansion of the distal part of the frame will be seen during this maneuver; and, typically, there will again be some forward movement that should be corrected by the first operator. Forward movement of the valve is less with the Accutrak delivery catheter (Medtronic) than the original delivery catheter. Typically, hemodynamics and pressures are stable at this point.

The next step is to deploy the valve itself. The assistant should deploy up to two-thirds of the frame by further rotational movements. There should be no hesitation between the one-third and deployment points because, at this point, the valve will not be functioning and the native valve will be obstructed. There will therefore be a drop in pressure. As soon as the valve has been two-thirds deployed, the pressure should recover with the valve functioning normally. An aortogram should be obtained at this point. If it is necessary to withdraw the valve into a higher position at this point, the technique is to use gentle retraction in a sustained slow manner rather than jerky movements. Following the application of retracting pressure, the operator should pause and wait for the retracting force to be transmitted to the valve itself. If the operator is happy with the position of the two-thirds deployment point, then the graduated pigtail should be withdrawn to the aortic arch and the valve deployment completed. Following valve deployment, it is necessary to ensure that both proximal loops of the valve frame have detached from the catheter. If one loop has not released, then it will typically not be in line with the frame, but will be somewhat distorted and, as the delivery system is gently advanced, the distortion of the loop and the wire onto which the loop attaches will increase. If there is concern, then the catheter should be gently advanced and rotated. It may take several manipulations of advancing and rotating to release the loop. It may also be necessary to move the image intensifier into a lateral projection to see if the loops have fully released. Another technique will be to push on the wire, which will tend to cause the delivery system to center within the aorta, and this will also allow safe removal of the delivery system such that it does not catch on any part of the frame.

The distal wire position should be maintained and the valve delivery system retrieved into the descending aorta. The distal capsule (nose cone) of the delivery system should then be retracted into the sheath of the delivery system by advancing the macroslide (thumb control) on the delivery system. In this way, the capsule of the delivery catheter can be recaptured into the proximal catheter. If the capsule does not recapture easily, gentle rotation of the catheter should be performed. The delivery system can then be removed. The valve can be crossed by advancing the pigtail catheter over the guidewire and the gradient measured. The catheter can then be removed into the valve frame itself and an aortogram taken to identify the final position of the valve.

The next step is to perform the ProStar repair. The key tip is to pour plenty of saline over the access site so the sutures are wet and the sheath is well lubricated. Knots should be preplaced into the white and then green sutures (either the Fisherman knot or Laborde knot) and the sutures tested for free running of the knots. A tip at this point is to place the Mosquito forceps onto the end of the suture that you are going to pull. The arterial sheath should be removed slowly and completely and one or two seconds of bleeding should be allowed prior to tightening of the knots. Some operators recommend balloon compression of the proximal femoral artery to reduce the tendency to bleed at this point and other operators recommend reducing the arterial pressure at this point. Our own advice is not to undertake either of these techniques but simply to gently deploy the sutures. The sutures should not be over-tightened and it is acceptable for there to be a small amount of oozing after deployment of one or even both sutures. If there is oozing, then 5 minutes of manual compression usually deals with the majority of bleeding. Once hemostasis has been achieved, the sutures can be cut. The graduated pigtail can then be remanipulated into the right common iliac artery and an angiogram taken. In fact, the majority of operators place the pigtail catheter into the right common iliac artery prior to removal of the 18 French sheath to allow rapid access to the vessel should dissection, rupture, or hemorrhage be evident following removal of the sheath. If any of these complications are present following removal of the sheath, then a guidewire should be rapidly advanced down the femoral artery and balloon occlusion undertaken using the cross over technique.

It may be necessary to deploy a covered stent or obtain vascular surgical advice if peripheral interventional techniques cannot manage the problem satisfactorily. However, it should be possible to deal with the majority of complications using balloon occlusion peripheral angioplasty and stenting techniques.

Following aortography, aortic regurgitation may be evident. If there is grade 1 to 2 aortic regurgitation without frame distortion, then it is not necessary to undertake any balloon valvuloplasty of the newly deployed transcatheter valve. If, however, there is grade 3 aortic regurgitation or above, or there is evidence of hemodynamic compromise such as low systolic or diastolic pressure (particularly with evidence of frame underexpansion), then balloon valvuloplasty can be undertaken. Up to a 25-mm Nucleus balloon can be used for the small-sized CoreValve and a 29-mm balloon for the large-sized CoreValve. If there is evidence of severe aortic regurgitation with complete frame expansion, then it may be that the valve has been deployed too low and the techniques for dealing with this are dealt with elsewhere in this chapter.

There are some specific techniques for difficult anatomy and one of these is a horizontal aligned aorta. With this anatomy, it is easy to deploy too high and it is therefore important that the valve is not pulled back too much. It may be better to accept a low deployment and not to pull the valve after the one-third frame deployment. The valve should be deployed to the two-thirds frame deployment point and the valve repositioned at this point if necessary. It is useful to use a right anterior oblique (RAO) or posteroanterior caudal projection in this situation.

The ideal implant will be such that the lowest point of the CoreValve frame should be 4 mm below the plane of the annulus. This will be three-fourths of one full diamond cell height. This is different from the early technique in which it was recommended that the frame be deployed 12 mm (i.e., 1.5 cells) below the plane of the annulus. It is thought that low deployments more than one diamond cell height below the plane of the annulus may lead to the acquisition of heart block and, therefore, it is better to deploy somewhat higher than originally thought. It is important to understand the design of the CoreValve frame to make best use of the design in borderline anatomy. If, for example, the annulus is at the upper limit of acceptability for a given size of CoreValve, then it is best to deploy high so that the maximum width of the frame lies within the annulus. Conversely, if the valve is relatively oversized for the annulus, a low deployment (e.g., one full diamond cell height below the annulus plane) would be desirable.

The description here has outlined the step-by-step technique for deployment from the femoral artery. If the subclavian artery is being used, then it is necessary for a cardiac or vascular surgeon to cut down on to the subclavian artery and secure the vessel using vascular ties. The vessel is entered under direct vision using a needle puncture and a 0.035-inch J wire advanced to the aortic valve. It is best to use an Arrow sheath (Teleflex, Limerick, PA) initially and then change to an 18 French Cook sheath at this point. The valve should then be crossed using a 5 French AL1 diagnostic catheter with straight wire. The super stiff wire should then be placed within the ventricle using the techniques described and the 18 French sheath advanced over the stiff wire into the ascending aorta. It will be necessary for a significant portion of the sheath to be outside the artery given that the sheath tip must be 8 to 10 cm above the valve itself. The technique for deployment is identical to that for the femoral artery and, in fact, is often easier because there is a reduced tendency for the frame to move forward during deployment.

SPECIAL CASES

Aortic Regurgitation

Indications for this procedure will likely expand to include patients with aortic regurgitation who are not surgical candidates. The first key consideration is to ensure that the annulus width is within the range of acceptable annulus dimensions. The majority of cases of native valve aortic regurgitation will be associated with some degree of annulus or root dilatation and therefore may not be suitable.

There are two key considerations with regard to the implant. There may be no calcification of the valve to guide deployment and, therefore, other radiographic and echocardiographic guidance must be sought. Radiographic landmarks may include the pigtail catheter, pacing wire, or possibly sternal wires from previous coronary artery bypass surgery. It is necessary to have a clear sense of where the annulus lies from other considerations, and it may be necessary to perform aortography frequently during the valve deployment process.

The second key consideration is to consider deploying the valve during rapid ventricular pacing to reduce cardiac output. The possibility of valve displacement during deployment is higher when treating a patient with aortic regurgitation because there is no calcification on which the valve frame can anchor during partial deployment, and there may be a powerful regurgitant jet, which may cause valve displacement. Rapid ventricular pacing should be undertaken between the one-third to two-thirds deployment points to reduce cardiac output to a minimum.

Septal Hypertrophy

Discrete upper septal thickening is quite common in elderly patients with aortic stenosis, and this can represent a challenge because the bulge of septal hypertrophy can act as a step on which the lower part of the frame may incompletely expand causing superior displacement of the valve. Severe septal hypertrophy occupying a significant proportion of the outflow tract may be a contraindication to CoreValve implantation. The technique for deploying a CoreValve in a patient with severe septal hypertrophy involves ensuring that the valve deployment starts low enough within the outflow tract to effectively splint the upper septal hypertrophy. It is usual to use a left anterior oblique projection to ensure low enough deployment. It is necessary to be prepared to retrieve the valve at the two-thirds deployment step if the valve displaces superiorly. Some operators suggest deploying the valve during rapid ventricular pacing in order to reduce cardiac output and potentially reduce the risk of upward displacement.

Bicuspid Valves

The anatomy of the bicuspid aortic valve is quite different from that of the senile calcific trileaflet valve. The bicuspid valve leaflets form a dome, typically oval, in cross-section above the annulus. The principle of deploying the CoreValve in a patient with a bicuspid aortic valve is to ensure that the deployment is relatively high—that is, at the annulus or even above the annular plane. If the deployment is low, then the bicuspid valve anatomy may distort the frame and not allow complete frame expansion. This will affect the prosthetic valve function within an incompletely expanded or distorted frame.

The technique, therefore, involves starting the deployment higher than normal and effectively having only the first cell of the valve frame aligned with the calcium and withdrawing the valve as it expands such that the lower part of the frame is deployed at or even slightly above the annulus. The anatomy of a bicuspid aortic valve will anchor the CoreValve frame within the annulus, securing a stable position with satisfactory prosthetic function. The valve frame may still take on a somewhat noncircular, and possibly oval, cross-sectional profile although valve function should be satisfactory. It is appropriate to predilate with an undersized valvuloplasty balloon. Large annulus diameters such as 26 or 27 mm should be avoided with this anatomy.

Bioprosthesis

Implantation of the CoreValve into a surgical bioprosthesis is a particularly appealing application of the technology for patients who are high risk for redo surgery or nonsurgical candidates. Implanting into a xenograft can be more straightforward than implantation into a native valve so long as several important considerations are taken into account. First, there is a perfectly circular frame into which to implant the self-expanding CoreValve frame and the likelihood of paraprosthetic regurgitation is minimal. Second, because frame expansion is limited by the xenograft frame, there should be little, if any, impingement of the frame on the LVOT and atrioventricular node and the risk of heart block should be minimal. Third, the prosthetic material of the xenograft can act as a clear marker and guide as to where to place the CoreValve. Ideally, the frame of the CoreValve should lie just below the lower extent of the xenograft frame to effect a seal. A key component to the procedure is obtaining a fluoroscopic projection of the xenograft that lines up the xenograft in a plane perpendicular to the imaging plane. For the Carpentier Edwards xenograft, there will be a clear single line seen fluoroscopically when the bottom end of the frame is aligned in a perpendicular plane to the image intensifier. For the Mosaic valve (Medtronic), the three circular markers at the tips of xenograft frame should be aligned in a perfect straight line to ensure that the imaging plane is perpendicular to the alignment of the valve. For each particular xenograft, differing radiographic landmarks will be evident. It is important to know the internal diameter of the xenograft into which one is implanting and this information is available for all previously implanted xenografts. It is usual that a small-sized CoreValve will be selected for implantation in a xenograft. There are specific considerations for the particular types of xenograft; for example, in the Mitroflow (Carbomedics Inc., Arvada, CO) or a stentless xenograft (Toronto SPV valve), it is important to be aware of the possibility of coronary obstruction when deploying a valve-in-valve, and TEE is mandatory. A second important consideration when deploying within a xenograft is the fact that it is not possible to withdraw the CoreValve once deployment has started due to interaction with the xenograft frame. It is therefore necessary to commence the deployment high and aim for a high implant.

It is not uncommon to get a modest gradient across the CoreValve when deployed in a xenograft, but this should not be a particular concern. Furthermore, it is important to avoid valvuloplasty of a xenograft and simply go straight for deployment of the CoreValve. The reason for this is the leaflets of the xenograft are likely to be extremely calcified, friable, and could be severely damaged during valvuloplasty.

ASSESSMENT OF VALVE IMPLANT

Angiography

Typically, an aortogram is obtained following implantation to assess the position of the valve implant relative to the native annulus and the extent of paraprosthetic aortic regurgitation. Although some of this information is available from echocardiography, particularly periprocedural TEE, the assessment of the nature and severity of paraprosthetic leaks using echocardiography is challenging. Therefore, aortography is usually the initial assessment. The grading of aortic regurgitation angiographically should be carried out according to standard guidelines and practice but it is worth waiting several minutes as this may allow further expansion of the CoreValve frame and therefore reduce any aortic regurgitation present. The aortogram should be taken with the pigtail catheter placed just above the bioprosthetic valve within the CoreValve frame, low enough so as to fully opacify the lower part of the frame and outflow tract but high enough so as not to interfere with valve function.

A fluoroscopic projection that shows the frame in a perfect perpendicular view to the imaging plane should be selected—that is, the frame should not be seen obliquely. Furthermore, a standard amount of contrast should be used, and although this is usually 20 mL, for the procedural steps, it may be useful to use 30 to 40 mL for the final aortogram, especially if there is some doubt as to the severity of aortic regurgitation. A final useful radiographic maneuver would be to do a fluoroscopic acquisition during rotation of the image intensifier through an imaging arc so as to get a 3D sense of the CoreValve frame expansion.

Transesophageal Echocardiography

This may be available at the time of implantation if the patient is having the procedure under general anesthesia and is a very useful adjunct particularly during the learning curve. Following implantation, TEE can be used to clearly visualize the frame position within the LVOT and any impingement on the anterior mitral leaflet. TEE can also visualize the space between the frame and coronary ostia and the relationship between the frame and the aortic root. Paraprosthetic regurgitation may be difficult to assess fully because of the 3D nature of the jets, and the TEE plane may not cut through them. Continuous wave Doppler through a color jet will assist in assessment by show hemodynamic characteristics of the aortic regurgitant jet. Color Doppler can be misleading but, if a broad jet extending a long way into the outflow tract is seen, this is indicative of a severe paraprosthetic leak. TEE is also useful for assessing the relationship between the bottom of the frame and the anterior leaflet of the mitral valve and assessing any mitral regurgitation.

Hemodynamic Pressures

Following implantation of the CoreValve, the LV and aortic pressure wave forms are typically superimposable during systole with no gradient whatsoever. Two key features are useful to assess aortic regurgitation: the presence or absence of a dicrotic notch on the aortic pressure pulse and the absolute value of the diastolic pressure. Diastolic pressures following valve implantation tend to be a little low, but a pressure below 50 mm Hg should raise the possibility of hemodynamically significant aortic regurgitation.

MANEUVERS TO CORRECT UNSATISFACTORY IMPLANTATION

Operators must have an in-depth knowledge and be familiar with techniques and materials required for bail out procedures.[8]

Valve Malposition

Deployment of the CoreValve prosthesis is performed in a controlled and step-wise manner as previously described. Having said that, valve positioning remains as one of the most challenging steps of the procedure. Even after all necessary precautions have been considered, valve malposition may still occur. Only in rare instances does malposition actually jeopardize the hemodynamic status of the patient. Correct evaluation for the degree of malposition is best evaluated using either TEE or contrast angiography. A minimum of 20 mL of contrast media should be used in order to best appreciate the position of the prosthesis relative to the "aortic valve annulus" (i.e., at the level of the basal attachment line of the native aortic valve leaflets). Normally, the CoreValve prosthesis should be positioned approximately 4 mm (range 0–12 mm) below the "aortic valve annulus."

A "too low" implantation is defined as the distal edge of the valve frame positioned more than 12 mm below the annulus. This can be estimated with quantitative angiographic techniques using a graduated pigtail for calibration or by noting the number of cells that lie below the "aortic valve annulus." A "too high" implantation is defined as the inflow aspect positioned above the annulus level.

Low Implantation

Except in cases of severe LV hypertrophy, a low implantation is generally associated with moderate (grade II) to severe (grade III to IV) degrees of aortic regurgitation on contrast aortography. TEE can confirm the nature of the regurgitation (i.e., paravalvular vs. central). The anecdotal and extremely rare association between moderate-to-severe mitral regurgitation observed by postimplant TEE, and a relatively "low" implant is likely related to shifts in hemodynamic parameters (e.g., LV afterload) as opposed to anatomical considerations such as impingement of the anterior mitral valve leaflet by the inflow portion of the CoreValve prosthesis. In the case of "too low" positioning associated with significant aortic regurgitation and hemodynamic instability, the first objective would be to (1) manually reposition the valve using a "goose-neck" snare catheter. If unsuccessful, the second option to consider is (2) implantation of a second valve inside the first one (i.e., valve-in-valve technique) but positioned slightly higher.

Primary Recommendation: The "Lasso" Technique

The choice of projection on fluoroscopy is crucial and is dictated by the valve frame that should be aligned as perfectly as possible. This will provide a reliable reference line when repositioning the valve. Advance and position a 0.035-inch guidewire inside the noncoronary sinus with the use of a 5 French multipurpose catheter to serve as a landmark for the annulus, particularly in cases of poorly or noncalcified aortic valves. Advance a regular 20 to 35 mm "goose-neck" catheter alone or through a 7 French guiding catheter in order to engage one of the "loops" of the implanted valve.

The success of this maneuver is dependent on applying torsion to the frame ("unscrewing the valve"), rather than applying direct axial force (which frequently results in ejection of the valve into the ascending aorta). It is for this reason that the simultaneous use of two goose-neck catheters is strongly discouraged. The ideal position of the loops is in the anterior and posterior location on the anteroposterior projection. The worst position is when one loop lies on the external curve of the ascending aorta (almost unreachable with the goose-neck catheter). The other loop is easy to engage with the goose-neck catheter, but it is impossible to apply anything other than axial force to the valve frame. Upon loop engagement, apply gentle and slowly increasing torsion/traction to the goose-neck catheter under constant fluoroscopic guidance. At this intermediate stage, it is not rare to reach a level of traction where one feels the heart beat throughout the entire length of the catheter. Next, apply quick, short, and intermittent torsion/traction movements to the goose-neck catheter, and gradually increase force until mobilization of the valve in a more satisfactory position is achieved. Depending on the degree of visualization of the anatomy under fluoroscopy, control angiograms may need to be repeatedly performed at different stages of the process to confirm mobilization of the valve. After confirmation with hemodynamic analysis, angiogram and TEE, the goose-neck catheter is carefully detached and retrieved.

Valve-in-Valve Technique (as an Alternative)

If repositioning the valve is unsuccessful or is too dangerous due to an unfavorable position of the loops, correction of severe aortic regurgitation can still be obtained using a second CoreValve implanted inside the first one in a slightly higher position. As with the previous technique, the correct projection is crucial and the frame of the valve should be aligned as perfectly as possible. Advance the second valve into the previously implanted valve and measure the overlap distance of the two valves. While focusing on the distal (inflow) aspect, release the second valve until it is one-third deployed. Then focus on the proximal (outflow) aspect of the second valve and determine the optimal distance between the frame loops of the first and the second valve. It is important not to focus on the distal aspect (inflow) of the valves, because the "criss-cross" appearance of the struts will make it difficult to differentiate the individual valve frames. Once the optimal distance between the outflow tips is determined, deploy the remainder of the valve while maintaining the prescribed distance between the two frames. Frame loops from individual frames may serve as the most convenient markers. After complete release of the second valve, it is likely that significant aortic regurgitation will no longer be observed. When aortic regurgitation (grade ≥2) is observed, generally when tortuous anatomies challenge the implantation of the second valve, incomplete expansion and axialization of the second valve's frame should be questioned and assessed using control TEE or rotational fluoroscopy. If so, valvuloplasty postimplantation should be considered.

High Implantation

With the possibility of full valve retrieval up to four-fifths of the deployment process, such a situation should rarely occur except in cases of technical mistakes during the last steps of the procedure, such as:

1. Failure to notice incomplete disengagement of both frame loops from the delivery catheter before withdrawing the catheter.
2. Failure to manage the distal tip of the delivery catheter (i.e., nose cone) through the prosthesis after successful valve deployment resulting in tip displacement of the valve frame.
3. Postimplant dilatation without the use of rapid pacing or rapid pacing terminated to early relative to balloon inflation resulting in ejection of the balloon–valve unit into the ascending aorta.

Unfortunately, a high implantation does not offer the same attractive options for correction as a low implantation. However, it is important to first clearly define the criteria for acceptable parameters despite a "too high" implantation. To a certain extent, the sealing effect of the native calcified aortic valve around the frame (similar to a chimney above the annulus) can make a "too high" implantation perfectly compatible with a good result with none to mild or moderate aortic regurgitation. The control angiogram and the hemodynamic analysis provide the criteria for an acceptable result: (1) aortic regurgitation grade ≤2, (2) no ventricular/aortic gradient, and (3) no coronary occlusion. This last criteria may require additional aortograms in different projections and/or selective catheterization of the coronary ostia to ensure coronary flow. This also highlights the importance of evaluating a "high-implantation" option in the prescreening analysis of a patient for CoreValve implantation. In cases where valve implantation is definitively too high and incompatible with an acceptable result, the valve can be repositioned into the ascending aorta. Despite the fact that valve retrieval has been accomplished with the use of two goose-neck catheters, such a maneuver is strongly discouraged due to the high probability of arterial injury. The primary goal is to ensure a safe area for the implantation of a second valve. Repositioning of the first implanted valve high in the ascending aorta must be accomplished in order to avoid jeopardizing the functioning of the second valve by severely restricting second valve expansion or compromising coronary flow by creation of a long skirt due to two valves placed in continuity.

Because the CoreValve prosthesis measures approximately 50 to 53 mm in height depending on valve size, a safe distance of >50 mm above the annulus level is therefore optimal. The lasso technique for higher repositioning of the valve has been previously described. In small anatomies, this technique may not be feasible due to lack of space in the ascending aorta that can nullify any axial force exerted through the frame loop. In such a case, the goose-neck catheter can be advanced through the struts of the frame toward the inflow aspect, and hooking at that point. This allows for effective retrieval of the valve when pulling on the goose-neck catheter.

Next, for additional safety, the first valve should be secured in the correct position, high in the ascending aorta, with the use of the goose-neck catheter when a second valve is advanced through the first valve. This is critical in order to avoid mobilization of the first valve at the time of crossing. As a result, if a safe distance of >50 mm between the two valves has been obtained, the result of the second implantation should minimize the risk of coronary ischemia or mid- to long-term malfunction of the implanted valve as previously described when this technique is not applied.

In rare cases when the valve cannot be retrieved with the lasso technique, open surgical removal of the fully deployed prosthesis is required. If coronary flow is compromised by the tissue frame of the valve, cardiocirculatory bypass should be instituted prior to opening the chest in order to ensure adequate perfusion pressure in case of myocardial ischemia. For this, the femoral vessels are cannulated with the Seldinger technique. In all other cases, the chest is opened through a sternotomy and cardiopulmonary bypass with hypothermia is instituted by cannulating the aorta and the right atrium. The aorta is clamped, cardioplegia instituted, and the vessel incised transversely. Note that the stent frame of the prosthesis may be directly underneath the incision, so that in cases of a fairly large aorta, a longitudinal, hockey stick incision may also be considered. The supra-annular prosthesis can usually be retracted easily without applying excessive force. Retraction of the valve is facilitated by rinsing the valve frame with ice cold water. Special care must be taken if prior maneuvers with the lasso technique have led to multiple piercing of the stent frame into the adventitia. It may be necessary to cut the outflow aspect of the stent frame with wire-cutting pliers. Ascending aortic replacement may, in rare cases, be required. After removal of the malpositioned valve, standard aortic valve replacement is performed. In patients with a porcelain aorta, open retrieval of the valve may be an insurmountable challenge because the aorta cannot be clamped. The only safe option to manage these cases is the anastomosis of a Dacron prosthesis to the proximal aortic arch during a short period of hypothermic cardiocirculatory arrest. The Dacron prosthesis can then be clamped and the proximal part of the aorta, including the valve, is replaced. However, this approach bares an extremely high risk for major brain injury or multiorgan failure in the very old and considerably sick patients, so the decision has to be carefully balanced.

The rare requirement of an open surgical retrieval of a malpositioned valve prosthesis underlines the necessity of a multidisciplinary implantation team of cardiologists, cardiac surgeons, and anesthesiologists. Furthermore, it underlines the common claim of the societies of the respective medical specialties that a hybrid operation room is the ideal place for these procedures to allow for immediate intervention.

Paravalvular Regurgitation

Excluded from the discussion here is the management of paravalvular regurgitation due to too low implantation of the valve and central valvular regurgitation, which may result from technical errors. This section addresses the management of grade ≥2 aortic regurgitation following correct implantation of the valve.

Albeit not a true complication, aortic regurgitation grade ≥2 on control angiogram or TEE is not rare (>20% of overall cases). This can occur for the following reasons:

1. Low implantation of the valve
2. Underexpansion of the frame in severely calcified aortic valve
3. Underevaluation of annulus measurement

It is important to remember that due to the self-expandable nature of the frame (nitinol), there is continual frame expansion after implantation and consequently a remodeling of the annulus and the native valve may take place. As a result, in numerous occasions, where time has elapsed between the first control angiogram immediately following valve implantation and a later control aortogram taken at the end of the procedure, a distinct decrease in the degree of aortic regurgitation is observed, which validates the concept of remodeling of the anatomy after implantation of the CoreValve prosthesis. Severity of the aortic regurgitation on aortography should be evaluated carefully following minimum basic rules that include:

1. A minimum of 20 mL of contrast media injection
2. RAO projection
3. Position of the pigtail catheter slightly above the functioning portion of the implanted valve to minimize the risk of under-evaluation of the aortic regurgitation.

Despite adherence to these rules, different parameters can influence the degree of aortic regurgitation including blood pressure, heart rate, and LV dysfunction. There is the potential for underestimating the severity of the regurgitation at the time of implantation and having to face, later at follow-up, under different hemodynamic conditions, more severe aortic regurgitation. TAVI does not differ from aortic balloon valvuloplasty where grade III aortic regurgitation could be well tolerated in the presence of LV hypertrophy, and grade II aortic regurgitation not tolerated in the presence of a poor LV function. It is necessary to evaluate the severity of aortic regurgitation on TEE and aortography and undertake a hemodynamic analysis to evaluate the tolerance of aortic regurgitation. One should always measure LV and aortic pressures before and after valve implantation to better define the strategy when facing aortic regurgitation grade ≥2 post-CoreValve implantation.

Simple criteria can be proposed to predict poor hemodynamic tolerance of aortic regurgitation grade ≥2 after valve implantation that should lead to consideration of balloon valvuloplasty, including:

1. Greater than or equal to 10 mm Hg elevation of the LV end-diastolic pressure above the value prior to the implantation, or an absolute value above 25 mm Hg.
2. Greater than or equal to 10 mm Hg decrease of the diastolic pressure below the value prior to the implantation for a similar systolic pressure or an absolute diastolic pressure value below 50 mm Hg.
3. No dicrotic notch on the aortic pressure tracing.
4. Tachycardia.

The decision to perform valvuloplasty should always be evaluated carefully in regard to the potential consequences, such as dislodgement of the valve and structural damage to the valve tissue, which may not become evident before mid- or even long-term follow-up.

Coronary Obstruction

Coronary obstruction during implantation is rare, occurring in about 2% of the patients. The reasons for this potentially catastrophic event include: (a) displacement of calcium deposits or large native aortic valve leaflets in front of the coronary ostia during valve deployment, particularly in a low-lying coronary artery; (b) embolization of calcium debris into one of the coronary arteries; (c) aortic dissection with continuity of the rupture into the intima of one of the coronary ostia with resultant obstruction; and (d) a valve prosthesis that is implanted too high. In addition, coronary air embolism can lead to myocardial ischemia.

The first clinical sign of coronary obstruction is usually ST segment elevation or rhythm disturbances such as sudden third-degree atrioventricular block or ventricular fibrillation. In those cases, usually severe cardiac depression ensues and the patient may go into cardiogenic shock. A bolus angiogram of the aortic root may reveal coronary obstruction, followed by selective intubation of the coronary with balloon dilatation or stenting of the coronary ostium. If the valve is implanted too high and coronary flow is impaired by the skirt of the valve, the prostheses must be immediately retracted into the ascending aorta to relieve the obstruction. In the majority of cases, emergency cardiopulmonary bypass will have to be instituted with emergent coronary artery bypass grafting or open removal of a malpositioned valve prosthesis.

POSTOPERATIVE CARE

Postoperative care is key to the success of the procedure. Although TAVI is exacting and demanding, it is not usually the implantation itself which causes problems. These patients by their very nature have multiple comorbid pathologies and often have reduced respiratory renal and cardiac function.

Scrupulous postoperative vascular management, careful attention to detail, and close observation for several days after the procedure are necessary components to effect a successful outcome following an initially uncomplicated procedure. The areas to consider in the postoperative period are hypotension, vascular access complications, rhythm disturbances, neurological complications, renal function, pulmonary function, and infection.

Hypotension immediately following the procedure is usually due to aortic regurgitation, pericardial effusion, LV dysfunction, myocardial ischemia, bleeding, or volume depletion. It is necessary to reach the diagnosis quickly and to effect treatment as patients can deteriorate rapidly. Echocardiography should be carried out immediately and will identify aortic regurgitation, pericardial effusion, regional wall motion abnormalities, and underfilling of the ventricle. Vascular access complications may include bleeding or rupture, which should be dealt with immediately. The importance of taking angiography following the procedure has already been stressed.

Ventricular arrhythmias are uncommon, but atrial fibrillation is a not uncommon feature following TAVI and should be treated in the standard manner. A pacing wire should be left in for 24 to 48 hours because of the possibility of development of heart block following the procedure.[6] A decision regarding implantation of a permanent pacemaker should be made at an appropriate time interval following the procedure. If the patient remains pacing dependent, early pacemaker implantation is advocated to allow mobilization and discharge from hospital. New left bundle branch block is not uncommon and, when associated with development of first-degree heart block or a lengthening PR interval, consideration should be given to pacemaker implantation, recognizing that many patients who develop first-degree heart block and left bundle branch block at the time of the procedure will revert to normal conduction in due course.

Neurologic complications remain the most feared problem. Usually, a cerebrovascular event at the time of the procedure will lead to a degree of permanent neurological disability. Until carotid protection is available, the risk of embolization during aortic valvuloplasty, aortic root instrumentation, and implantation of the valve is usually unavoidable. If the patient has evidence of neurologic disability following the procedure, then an immediate consultation is required from a stroke neurologist.

Renal function should be monitored closely following the procedure. TAVI is similar to any other invasive angiographic procedure in which contrast is given and, therefore, the possibility of contrast nephropathy exists.

In patients with multiple comorbid pathologies and periods of hemodynamic instability, a deterioration in renal function should be anticipated. Daily monitoring of renal function, urine output, and fluid status is recommended for 24 to 48 hours and, in patients at risk of contrast nephropathy, standard preoperative management including fluids and other agents as per local policy should be administered. However, in our own experience, the requirement for dialysis following TAVI is very low, even in a population of patients with significantly impaired renal function preoperatively.

Postoperative chest infection is not uncommon and should be treated in the standard way. For patients who become breathless with pleuritic chest pain, pulmonary embolism should be suspected and patients are treated with standard thromboprophylaxis following the procedure during their hospital stay. Patients with multiple comorbid pathologies are prone to develop periprocedural infections, but other than chest infections, other sites of infection are in fact quite unusual. Standard antibiotic prophylaxis for valve implantation should be administered during the procedure as per local hospital protocol. It should be remembered that elevations of C-reactive protein are quite common following the procedure and may represent some inflammatory reaction to the prosthesis rather than infection.

REFERENCES

1. Flameng W, Herregods MC, Vercalsteren M, et al. Prosthesis-patient mismatch predicts structural valve degeneration in bioprosthetic heart valves. *Circulation.* 2010;121:2123–2129.
2. Piazza N, Grube E, Gerckens U, et al. Procedural and 30-day outcomes following transcatheter aortic valve implantation using the third generation (18fr) corevalve revalving system: results from the multicentre, expanded evaluation registry 1-year following ce mark approval. *EuroInterv.* 2008;4:242–249.
3. Grube E, Buellesfeld L, Mueller R, et al. Progress and current status of percutaneous aortic valve replacement: results of three device generations of the corevalve revalving system. *Circ Cardiovasc Intervent.* 2008;1:167–175.
4. Piazza N, de Jaegere PP, Schultz C, et al. Anatomy of the aortic valvar complex and its implications for percutaneous implantation of the aortic valve. *Circ Cardiovasc Interv.* 2008;1:74–81.
5. Tops LF, Wood DA, Delgado V, et al. Noninvasive evaluation of the aortic root with multislice computed tomography implications for transcatheter aortic valve replacement. *JACC Cardiovasc Imaging.* 2008;1:321–330.
6. Baan J Jr., Yong ZY, Koch KT, et al. Factors associated with cardiac conduction disorders and permanent pacemaker implantation after percutaneous aortic valve implantation with the corevalve prosthesis. *Am Heart J.* 2010;159:497–503.
7. Van Mieghem NM, Nuis RJ, Piazza N, et al. Vascular complications with transcatheter aortic valve implantation using the 18 fr medtronic corevalve system(r): the rotterdam experience. *EuroIntervention.* 2010;5:673–679.
8. Vavuranakis M, Vrachatis D, Stefanadis C. CoreValve aortic bioprosthesis: repositioning techniques. *JACC Cardiovasc Interv.* 2010;3:565; author reply 565–566.

CHAPTER 20

Transcatheter Aortic Valve Implantation: Clinical Outcomes

Philippe Généreux, Susheel K. Kodali, and Martin B. Leon

S evere aortic stenosis (AS) is well known to have a poor prognosis if treated medically.[1] For patients considered operable, surgical aortic valve replacement (sAVR) improves long-term survival and is currently the treatment of choice.[2,3] Yet, more than 30% of patients with symptomatic severe AS do not undergo aortic valve replacement (AVR), mostly because of the presence of multiple comorbidities.[4] Recently, transcatheter aortic valve implantation (TAVI) has emerged as an alternative treatment to sAVR for patients considered at high or prohibitive operative risk. Since Dr. Alain Cribier pioneered the first TAVI procedure in 2002,[5] more than 20,000 procedures worldwide have been performed. Several observational registries and cases series have been published[6-16] showing increasing evidence that TAVI is safe and viable for patients with severe AS. Recently, the first multicenter randomized control trial has been published,[17] increasing the enthusiasm for this new technology. Thus far, two different TAVI systems have advanced beyond the clinical trial stage: the balloon expandable Edwards SAPIEN transcatheter heart valve (Edwards Lifesciences Inc., Irvine, CA), suitable for a transfemoral (TF) or transapical (TA) approach; and the self-expanding Medtronic CoreValve (Medtronic, Minneapolis, MN), suitable for a TF or subclavian approach (Fig. 20-1). This chapter summarizes the current data on clinical outcomes and TAVI (Table 20-1).

INITIAL EXPERIENCE

First-in-human and Initial Reports

In 2002, Cribier and coworkers performed the first TAVI in an inoperable patient, via a transseptal antegrade approach using a balloon-expandable aortic valve prosthesis, demonstrating the feasibility of percutaneous valve implantation.[5] Two years later, Cribier and coworkers reported their series of six patients treated via antegrade TAVI, showing an immediate procedural success in five of the six patients.[18] In 2005, Grube and coworkers presented the first report of a human implantation of a self-expanding aortic valve prosthesis (CoreValve) via a retrograde approach.[19]

Soon after, two pioneers in the field reported their early work. Webb and coworkers described their initial experience using the Cribier valve (Edwards Lifesciences Inc., Irvine, CA) via an arterial retrograde approach in 18 consecutive high-risk patients.[7] The procedure was successful in 78% (14/18) of cases. No intraprocedural deaths were reported, and 89% (16/18) of the patients were alive at a mean follow-up of 75 days. Similarly, Grube and coworkers published their early-stage experience with the first generation of the CoreValve system, reporting results from 25 consecutive patients.[9] In this series, immediate procedural success was reported in 84% (21/25), whereas 20% (5/25) died in hospital.

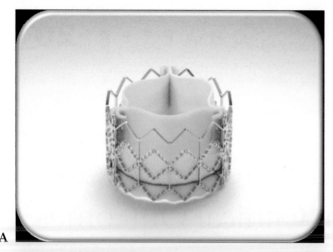

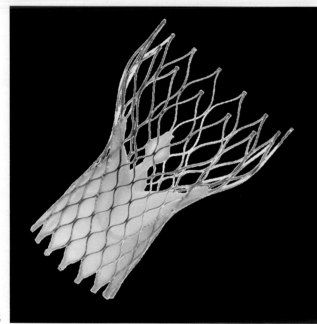

FIGURE 20-1.

A: SAPIEN transcatheter heart valve (Edwards Lifesciences Inc., Irvine, CA). **B:** CoreValve (Medtronic, Minneapolis, MN) system.

Between 2003 and 2005, there were two single-center pilot trials, I-REVIVE (Initial Registry of EndoVascular Implantation of Valves in Europe trial) and RECAST (Registry of Endovascular Critical Aortic Stenosis Treatment trial).[6] Thirty-six patients were recruited on a compassionate basis. Of them, 27 patients underwent an antegrade (transseptal) implantation, with a procedural success rate of 85% (23/27), and seven underwent an arterial retrograde implantation, with a procedural success rate of 57% (4/7). The 30-day mortality was 16.7% (6/36).

Feasibility Studies

Between 2005 and 2008, three multicenter feasibility studies using the Edwards SAPIEN device were

initiated in the United States and in Europe: The REVIVAL trial (peRcutaneousEndoVascular Implantation of VALves trial),[20,21] the TRAVERCE trial (the initial multicenter feasibility trial for TAVI),[22] and the REVIVE trial. REVIVAL enrolled 95 patients at high risk for sAVR in the United States: 40 TA[20] and 55 TF.[21] The implantation success rate of the device was 87.5% in the TA cohort and 87% in the TF cohort. The 30-day survival rate for the TA and TF populations was 82.5% and 92.7%, respectively. Similarly, the TRAVERCE trial enrolled 168 patients who underwent a TA procedure in three European centers, showing an implantation success rate of 95.8% and a 30-day mortality rate of 15%. Despite the high-risk profile of the population included, the use of first generation devices, and the early experience of the operators, these studies showed that TAVI performed by a TA or TF approach was feasible and beneficial at short term.

Similarly, Grube et al. demonstrated the safety and feasibility of the TAVI TF procedure using the 21 French or 18 French CoreValve system, with an acute procedural success rate of 74% and a 30-day mortality rate of 12%.[10]

Feasibility of Subclavian Approach

Like TA approach, a subclavian approach allows patients with unfavorable iliofemoral anatomy or extensive disease to be treated with TAVI. The data for this technique seems particularly encouraging. Indeed, Petronio et al. recently published their series of 54 patients, showing a procedural success rate of 100%, a procedural mortality of 0%, a 30-day mortality of 0%, and 6-month mortality 9.4%.[15] No specific vascular complications for subclavian access were reported. The subclavian approach is currently possible only with the CoreValve system.

Lessons Learned from the Early Experience

First-in-human cases, feasibility studies, and initial series with TAVI came from a number of single-center reports reflecting the early stages of the learning curve for TAVI operators. Lessons learned on the importance of adequate screening (annulus sizing, iliac and femoral sizing, risk stratification assessment, identification of predictors of adverse outcomes), appropriate selection of patients, and better understanding of the procedure led to a notable improvement in outcomes over time. Webb and coworkers recently reported their initial experience in their first 168 TAVI patients, highlighting

TABLE 20-1 Clinical Outcomes After TAVI According to Access Site and Device Type: Major Published Data

Authors	Type of Study	Number of Patients	STS	Logistic EuroSCORE	Follow-up	Procedural Success Rate	Death 30-day	Death 1-year	Major Access Complications	Stroke	Need for PPM
Edwards SAPIEN: TF											
Lefevre et al.[12]	Registry	61	11.3%	25.7%	12 months	95.4%	8.2%	21.3%	16.4%	3.3%	1.8%
Eltchaninoff et al.[16]	Registry	95	17.4%	25.6%	1 month	98.3%[a]	8.4%	—	6.3%	4.2%	5.3%
Himbert et al.[65]	Registry	51	15%	25%	12 months	90%	8%[b]	19%	12%	6%	6%
Rodes-Cabau et al.[11]	Registry	113	9%	—	24 months	90.5%	9.5%	25%	13.1%	3%	3.6%
Thomas et al.[14,25]	Registry	463	—	14.5%	1 month	95.2%	6.3%	18.9%	22.9%	2.4%	6.7%
Leon et al.[17]	RCT	179	11.2%	26.4%	12 months	—	6.4%[c]	30.7%[d]	16.2%	6.7%[e]	3.4%
Edwards SAPIEN: TA											
Walther et al.[22]	Feasibility study	168	—	27%	12 months	95.8%	15%	37%	1.2%	2%	2.3%
Svensson et al.[20]	Feasibilitystudy	40	13.4%	35.5%	6 months	87.5%	17.5%	—	—	5%	—
Lefevre et al.[12]	Registry	69	11.3%	33.8%	12 months	96.4%	18.8%	50.7%	5.8%[f]	1.5%	3.8%
Eltchaninoff et al.[16]	Registry	71	18.4%	26.8%	1 month	98.3%[a]	16.9%	—	5.6%[g]	2.8%	5.6%
Himbert et al.[65]	Registry	24	18%	28%	12 months	100%	16%[b]	26%	8%	0%	4%
Rodes-Cabau et al.[11]	Registry	177	10.5%	—	1 month	96.1%	11.3%	22%	13%[g]	1.7%	6.2%
Thomas et al.[25]	Registry	575	—	16.3%	1 month	95.7%	10.3%	27.9%	4.7%	2.6%	7.3%
Medtronic CoreValve: TF											
Grube et al.[10]	Registry	86	—	21.6%	1 month	88%	12%	—	—	10%	—
Piazza et al.[13]	Registry	646	—	23.1%	1 month	97.2%	8%	—	1.9%	1.9%	9.3%
Eltchaninoff et al.[16]	Registry	66	21.3%	24.7%	1 month	98.3%[a]	15.1%	—	7.5%	4.5%	25.7%
Petronio et al.[15]	Registry	460	—	19.4%	6 months	98.4%	6.1%	11.4%	2%	1.7%	16.1%
Medtronic CoreValve: SC											
Eltchaninoff et al.[16]	Registry	12	21%	24.6%	1 month	98.3%[a]	8.3%	—	8.3%	0%	25%
Petronio et al.[15]	Registry	54	—	25.3%	6 months	100%	0%	6.7%	0%	1.9%	18.5%
Zahn et al.[26i]	Registry	697	—	20.5%	1 month	98.4%	12.4%	—	19.5%	2.8%	39.3%[i]

[a]Global procedural success rate including SAPIEN TF, SAPIEN TA, and CoreValve TF and subclavian was 98.3%.

[b]In-hospital mortality.

[c]Thirty-day postprocedural mortality rate was 6.4% (11/173 patients). Thirty-day intention-to-treat mortality rate was 5% (9/179 patients).

[d]One-year intention-to-treat mortality rate.

[e]Major and minor stroke.

[f]Vascular-related complications.

[g]Apex-related complications.

[h]Outcomes reported together: 566 (81.2%) CoreValve TF, 22 (3.2%) CoreValve trans-subclavian, 106 (15.2%) SAPIEN TF.

[i]CoreValve 42.5%, SAPIEN 22%.

TAVI, transcatheter aortic valve implantation; STS, Society of Thoracic Surgeons; EuroSCORE, European System for Cardiac Operative Risk Evaluation; PPM, permanent pacemaker; TF, transfemoral; RCT, randomized controlled trial; TA, transapical; SC, subclavian.

FIGURE 20-2.

Vancouver's initial experience on 168 consecutives patients: first half versus second half 30-day mortality.

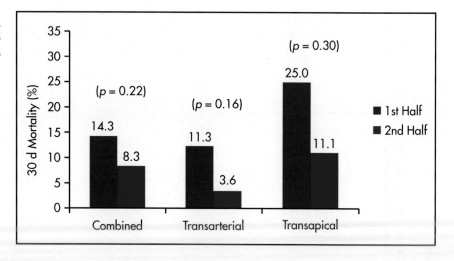

the importance of the learning curve.[23] The 30-day mortality rates of 11.3% and 25% for TF and TA, respectively, improved in the second half to 3.6% and 11.1%, respectively (Fig. 20-2). Similarly, Grube et al. reported their single-center experience with a total of 136 patients comparing the three generations of CoreValve devices (Fig. 20-3A).[24] The procedural success rate improved considerably with the smaller third-generation 18 French device (98.2%) compared to the large 25 French first-generation device (90.4%). Additionally, procedure time was reduced by almost 40% with the third-generation device compared to the first-generation device (Fig. 20-3B). Those two reports underline the importance of the operator's experience and technology improvement as the main determinants of TAVI success.

REGISTRIES

Edwards' Registries

Up to now, three major registries have been published using the Edwards SAPIEN system.[11,12,14,25] The Partner EU Registry was a pre-CE mark registry enrolling 130 patients (61 TF and 69 TA), performed in nine European centers, using the second generation bovine pericardial balloon-expandable valve.[12] All patients were determined to be high-risk operative (predicted mortality >20%) or nonoperative with a mean 30-day Society of Thoracic Surgeons (STS) risk score of 11.6%. The 30-day and 12-month survival were 91.8% and 78.7%, respectively, for the TF approach and 81.2% and 49.3%, respectively, for the TA approach. Most of the 30-day mortality was noncardiac in nature and related to patient comorbidities. One of the main limitations of this registry was the small number of patients enrolled by each site, reflecting the learning curve of most of the TAVI operators.

Similarly, Rodes-Cabau and coworkers reported the Canadian experience from six centers in 339 patients (162 TF and 177 TA) who underwent TAVI under the Canadian compassionate clinical use program.[11] The procedural success rate and the 30-day mortality rate were 90.5% and 9.5%, respectively, for the TF approach and 96.1% and 11.3%, respectively, for the TA approach. Interestingly, the survival rate at 1 year was similar for the TF group (75% [95% CI 68%–82%]) and the TA group (78% [95% CI: 53%–75%]), suggesting that a TAVI program offering TF or TA approaches to patients with comparable risk profiles could lead to similar benefits at short and long term.

The largest registry reported to date is the SOURCE (SAPIEN Aortic Bioprosthesis European Outcome) registry.[14,25] This registry was designed to assess the initial clinical results of the Edwards SAPIEN valve in consecutive patients in Europe after commercialization. Overall, 1,038 patients were enrolled in 32 European centers and were treated with either a TF (n = 463) or TA approach (n = 575). Patients treated by TA had more comorbidities at baseline than TF patients, resulting in a significantly higher EuroSCORE (29.1% vs. 25.7%; P < 0.001). Procedural success was observed in 95.2% and 92.7% of the TF and TA populations, respectively. The higher 30-day mortality observed in the TA group (10.3%) compared to the TF group (6.3%) might be explained by the higher risk profile at baseline in the TA population. The major limitation of this registry was that more than 70% of the enrolling centers had no prior experience with TAVI and enrolled more than 50% of the entire population of the registry. Moreover, all adverse events were site reported and no core laboratories were used. Recently, the one year results have been published, showing a 1-year survival of 76.1% overall, 72.1% for TA and 81.1% for TF patients. Among the surviving patients, 73.5% were in New York Heart Association class I or II at 1 year.[25]

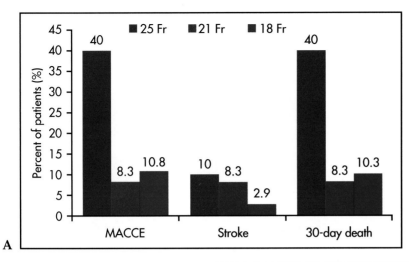

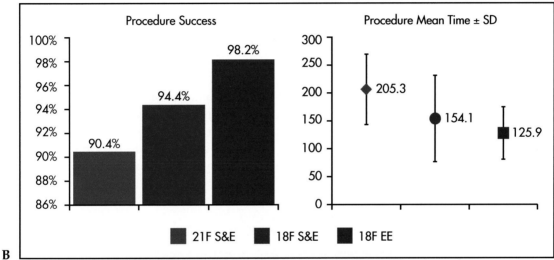

FIGURE 20-3.

A: Single center experience on 136 patients comparing three generations of CoreValve (Medtronic, Minneapolis, MN) devices. **B:** Comparison of procedural time between three generations of CoreValve devices.

CoreValve's Registries

Between April 2007 and April 2008, the multicenter expanded evaluation registry enrolled 646 patients in 51 European centers.[13] Using the third-generation 18 French CoreValve revalving system, the procedural success rate was 97.2%, procedural mortality 1.5%, 30-day all-cause mortality 8%, and the 30-day rate of stroke 1.9%. Vascular complications were remarkably low (1.9%) and the new permanent pacemaker implantation rate was also relatively low (9.3%) compared to the rate usually reported for the CoreValve device of 20% to 40% in other studies.[15,16,26] However, the conclusions of this report were limited by inconsistencies and underreporting of adverse events, as well as the absence of a core lab to collect and analyze clinical outcomes.

Recently, results from four European national registries for the CoreValve system have been presented (Euro PCR May 25–28, 2010 Paris, France)[27–30], showing 1-year survival rates ranging between 71.9% and 81.6% (Fig. 20-4).

RANDOMIZED TRIAL: PARTNER

The pivotal PARTNER (Placement of Aortic Transcatheter Valves) trial is the first multicenter, randomized clinical trial comparing TAVI with standard therapy in high-risk patients with severe AS and cardiac symptoms. The overall study design is shown in Figure 20-5. Two cohorts were prespecified: cohort A, including patients considered at high risk for conventional sAVR but deemed operable; and cohort B, including patients who were not considered suitable

FIGURE 20-4.

One-year survival in CoreValve (Medtronic, Minneapolis, MN) registries (Euro PCR May 25–28, 2010 Paris, France).[27–30]

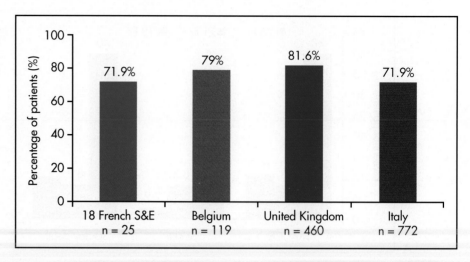

candidates for surgery. Patients were considered high risk if they had (1) a STS risk score of 10% or higher or (2) the presence of coexisting conditions that would be associated with a predicted 30-day mortality of 15% or higher or (3) those who were not considered to be suitable candidates for surgery because they had coexisting conditions that would be associated with a predicted 30-day mortality or severe morbidity of 50% or more. Exclusion criteria for this trial were patients with a bicuspid or noncalcified aortic

valve, severe renal insufficiency with a creatinine higher than 3.0 mg per dL or on dialysis, substantial coronary artery disease requiring revascularization, a left ventricular ejection fraction of less than 20%, a diameter of the aortic annulus of less than 18 mm or more than 25 mm, severe (>3+) mitral or aortic regurgitation, and/or a transient ischemic attack or stroke within the previous 6 months. For both cohorts, the primary end point was all-cause mortality over the duration of the study, and the

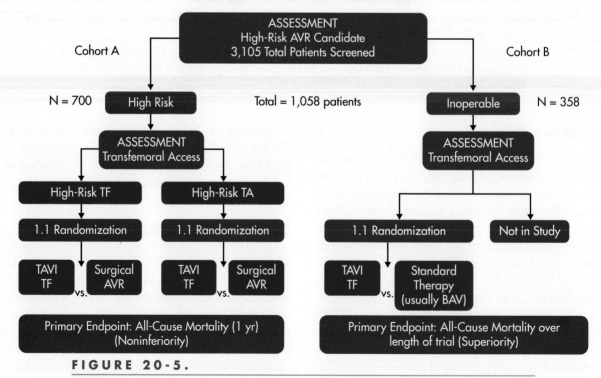

FIGURE 20-5.

PARTNER trial design. AVR, aortic valve replacement; BAV, balloon aortic valvuloplasty; TA, transapical; TAVI, transcatheter aortic valve implantation; TF, transfemoral.

coprimary end point was a composite of all-cause mortality and repeat hospitalization. Recently, the nonoperative arm (cohort B) of the PARTNER trial has been published.[17] The main findings were: TAVI was superior to standard therapy, markedly reducing the rate of all-cause mortality by 46% ($P < .0001$), cardiovascular mortality by 61% ($P < .0001$) and all-cause mortality and repeat hospitalization by 54% ($P < .0001$) (Fig. 20-6). Additionally, symptoms were significantly reduced in the TAVI group compared to the standard therapy group. At 1 year, 74.8% of surviving patients who had undergone TAVI were asymptomatic or had mild symptoms (New York

Heart Association [NYHA] class I or II), as compared with 42.0% of the surviving patients who had received standard therapy ($P < .001$). Serial echocardiographic follow-up indicated sustained reduced mean gradient and improved valve area at 1-year ($P < .0001$). However, TAVI resulted in more frequent complications at 30 days, including major vascular complications (16.2% vs. 1.1%, I < .0001), major bleeding episodes (16.8% vs. 3.9%, $P < .0001$), and major strokes (5.0% vs. 1.1%, $P = .06$). Despite an excess of vascular and neurologic complications, these results are encouraging, and improvements to current technology as well as next generation devices

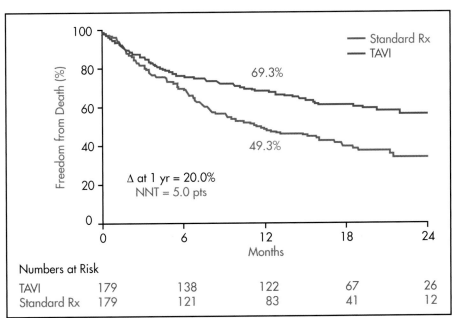

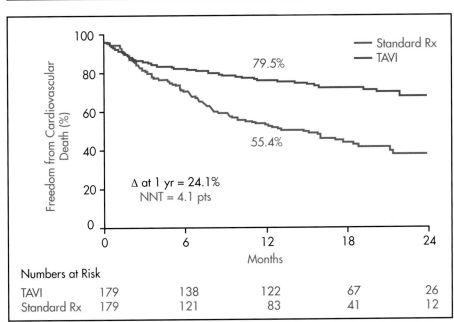

FIGURE 20-6.

A: One-year survival Kaplan-Meier curve in PARTNER trial cohort B. **B:** One-year cardiovascular death Kaplan-Meier curve in PARTNER trial cohort B. TAVI, transcatheter aortic valve implantation; NNT, number needed to treat.

(e.g., smaller device, embolic protection device) may help to reduce these events.

SPECIFIC OUTCOMES

Vascular Complications

Vascular complications remain the main limitation of TAVI performed via TF access. The use of large-diameter catheters and the high-risk characteristics of the current, treated population explains the high incidence. Small-vessel diameter, severe atherosclerotic disease, bulky calcification, and tortuosity are the main determinants of vascular complications per TAVI. The incidence of major vascular complications using the Edwards SAPIEN system (introducer sheath of 23 and 26 French, outer diameter 9 and 10 mm) vary between 8.3% and 23%[11,14,17,31,32] and between 1.9% and 14%[13,15,32,33] using the CoreValve system (18 French introducer sheath, outer diameter 7 mm). However,

use of arbitrary definitions and difficulty in identifying and systematically reporting all vascular complications make interpretation of current literature difficult. Common vascular complications include arterial dissection, closure device failure, arterial closure device-induced stenosis, and hematoma at the puncture entry point. Artery avulsion ("artery on a stick"), vessel perforation leading to retroperitoneal hematoma, aortic dissection, annulus rupture, and left ventricular perforation represent more severe complications that are fatal if not rapidly recognized and treated. Although urgent surgical intervention may be necessary in the management of major vascular complications, innovative percutaneous techniques involving proximal balloon occlusion of the iliac arteries and/or endovascular stent deployment have been suggested as useful in preventing and treating some of these issues.[34,35] An association between the occurrence of major vascular complication or major bleeding and survival has been demonstrated by several authors (Fig. 20-7).[11,17,31,32]

FIGURE 20-7.

A: Impact of major vascular complications on mortality in PARTNER trial cohort B. **B:** Impact of major bleeding on mortality in PARTNER trial cohort B.

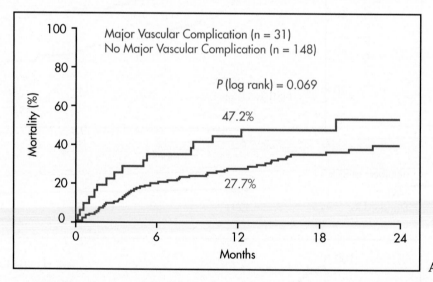

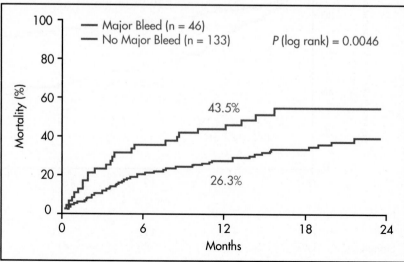

Adequate screening is therefore of the highest importance and has been shown to decrease the incidence of arterial dissection and perforation significantly. Although some vascular complications will remain unavoidable, advances in current technology with smaller delivery catheters and introducer sheaths will likely result in a decrease in vascular complication rates.

Stroke

The occurrence of clinically significant stroke during TAVI represents a tragic event. Depending on the definition used, reported incidence in the current literature varies between 1.7% and 6.7%.[11,13–17] The exact mechanism of these strokes remains unclear, and they may occur at different times during the procedure, possibly related to several factors: manipulation of a large diameter catheter through the aortic arch, retrograde crossing of a severely diseased native aortic valve, performance of balloon aortic valvuloplasty, and hemodynamic insult to the brain during rapid pacing and device deployment. Moreover, the population currently undergoing TAVI consists of very old patients in whom the incidence of atrial fibrillation and atherosclerotic disease is high, increasing the risk of periprocedural cerebrovascular events.[17,36,37] Recently, two studies reported that TAVI performed by TF access was associated with an incidence of new cerebral lesions of more than 70% following the procedure as evaluated by diffusion-weighted magnetic resonance imaging (DW-MRI).[38,39] Rodes-Cabau and coworkers also demonstrated in 60 patients that the rate of new ischemic lesions detected by DW-MRI in a TA approach (71%) is similar to the rate via the TF approach (66%), along with their patterns of distribution.[40] Although rarely associated with clinical events, the long-term consequences of these phenomena are unknown and further work is needed to determine the clinical significance of these findings. Several embolic protection devices are under investigation and early reports are encouraging and will hopefully lead to a fall in silent and clinical neurological events after TAVI.[41]

Rhythm Disturbance

Several reports have been published on conduction disturbance post-TAVI.[42–51] It is generally accepted that the self-expandable CoreValve system, because of the higher and longer-lasting radial forces as well as the deeper implantation site in the left ventricle outflow tract, has a higher rate of pacemaker requirement than the Edwards SAPIEN system. Current evidence regarding rhythm disturbance post-TAVI shows that around

20% of patients post-CoreValve implantation and 5% of patients post-Edwards SAPIEN placement will require a new permanent pacemaker.[51] However, the rates reported in the literature have varied greatly. In a series published by Zahn et al., the CoreValve system was associated with a high pacemaker implantation rate (42.5%) compared to 22% with the SAPIEN system.[26] In contrast, the recent pivotal PARTNER trial showed a lower pacemaker implantation rate, with only 3.4% of the patients requiring a permanent pacemaker post-SAPIEN valve implantation.[17] Piazza et al. published the largest experience with the CoreValve system in 646 patients, reporting a pacemaker implantation rate of 9.3% at 30 days.[13] Although fundamental differences in device structure and impact on atrioventricular conduction system exist between the two current devices, variation in practice and threshold for pacemaker implantation among physicians may also explain to a certain extent the discrepancy in new pacemaker insertion rates in current published series. Persistent new left bundle branch block has been shown to be the most prevalent electrocardiograph finding post-TAVI, being present in up to 55% of patients at 1 month post-CoreValve implantation[52] and in up to 20% of patients at 1 month post-SAPIEN implantation.[47] However, the long-term clinical signification of this finding is not well known. Interestingly, transient ST-elevation changes, mostly in the anterior and lateral leads, have been described after TA-TAVI immediately after the procedure in about 20% of patients and are probably related to incision and suturing of the apex.[42] Right bundle branch block, low level of implantation of the prosthesis, small annulus diameter compared to implanted valve size, complete atrioventricular block at the time of the procedure, and CoreValve device have been shown to be potential predictors of complete atrioventricular block post-TAVI.[43,46] According to our current knowledge, continuous postprocedural electrocardiograph monitoring should be performed for at least 72 hours in all patients after TAVI procedures and until discharge in patients with increased risk for this complication.

Paravalvular Regurgitation

Paravalvular regurgitation is a common finding after TAVI, although the clinical implications remain unknown. Aortic regurgitation is reported in 80% to 96% of TAVI cases.[17,53–56] In most cases, the degree of regurgitation is, at most, mild. Moderate and severe aortic regurgitation are found in 7% to 24% of patients.[17,53–56] Although no trial has compared the SAPIEN heart valve system and the CoreValve system, the reported

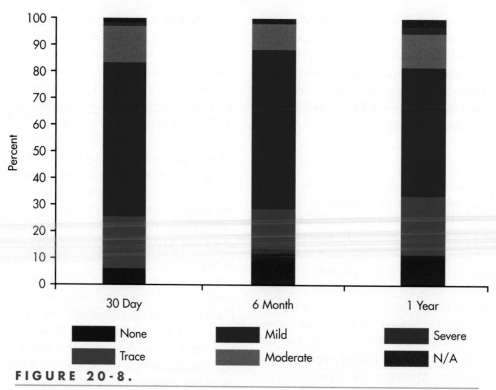

FIGURE 20-8.

Incidence and change in aortic insuffisency severity post-TAVI at 1 year in PARTNER trial cohort B.

numbers in the literature are similar for the two different approaches. There are only limited data on the long-term evolution of aortic insufficiency after TAVI. The PARTNER trial did not show an increase in the rate of moderate or severe aortic regurgitation between the 30-day and 1-year follow up with the SAPIEN valve (Fig. 20-8).[17] Similarly, Gurvitch et al. followed 30 patients over 3 years after SAPIEN implantation. They found no significant deterioration or improvement in aortic regurgitation.[53] Rajani et al. reported the evolution of the CoreValve system at 1 year. Forty-six percent of patients had an improvement in the degree of regurgitation, whereas 31% had deterioration. In most instances, the change was of 1 grade.[54] Determinants of paravalvular leakage have been proposed for the SAPIEN device. Larger annulus size, height, male sex, age, and cover index (100 × [prosthesis diameter – TEE annulus size]/prosthesis diameter) are predictors of more than mild paravalvular leakage. In this study, no aortic regurgitation of at least moderate degree was observed with a cover area >8%.[56] For the CoreValve system, greater angle of the left ventricular outflow tract is associated with a greater chance of significant regurgitation, whereas a depth of 10 mm of the device in relation to the noncoronary cusp is associated with a decreased likelihood of aortic insufficiency.[57]

Suggested treatment for acute reduction of the amount of paravalvular regurgitation may include postdilatation of the balloon expandable valve or the insertion of a second device in case of central aortic regurgitation.

Coronary Obstruction

Coronary obstruction of the left main is a rare but potentially fatal event. It might occur if a calcified native leaflet is displaced over a coronary ostium or if the valve frame or the sealing cuff is positioned directly over a coronary ostium. It could happen either at the time of balloon valvuloplasty or during the TAVI procedure. The distance between the aortic annulus and the coronary ostia, as well as the presence of bulky leaflet calcification, appears to be important risk factors. Anecdotal cases have been reported in which acute coronary obstructions have been successfully managed by immediate percutaneous angioplasty or bypass surgery.[58–61] Careful evaluation by echocardiography or computed tomography is crucial to avoid this catastrophic complication.

Symptom Improvement

Improvement in cardiac symptoms and functional class has been reported at short and medium term after

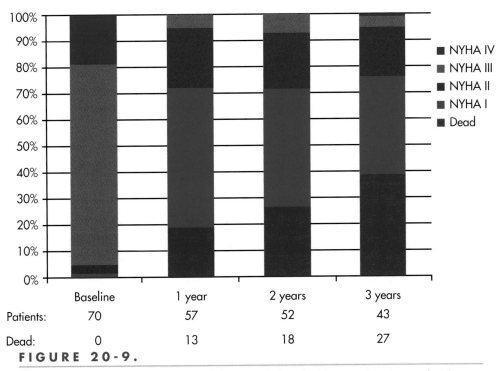

FIGURE 20-9.

New York Heart Association (NYHA) functional class incidence at baseline and at 3 years follow up.

TAVI.[13,14,17] Three-year follow up has been published and is consistent with lasting improvement in cardiac symptoms (Fig. 20-9).[53] Although 86% of patients were in NYHA III or IV at baseline, 93% of surviving patients were in NYHA class I/II at their 1-year follow up. Similarly, the pivotal randomized controlled PARTNER trial showed that patients treated with TAVI compared to patients treated with standard medical therapy have better symptom control at 1 year. Indeed, the 1-year rate of NYHA class III or IV was 25.2% for the TAVI group compared with 58.0% for the standard medical therapy group ($P < .001$).

Durability and Hemodynamic Valve Performance

TAVI has demonstrated excellent immediate- and short-term durability of the prosthesis with no evidence of structural failure at 30 days and 1 year.[11,13,14,17] Follow-up at 3 years has been recently published and revealed encouraging data, with sustained improvement in valve area and gradients (Fig. 20-10).[53] Gurvitch and coworkers evaluated 70 patients who underwent successful TF TAVI with the SAPIEN device with a minimum follow up of 3 years.[53] Transaortic mean gradient increased from 10.0 mm Hg immediately after the procedure to 12.1 mm Hg after 3 years ($P = .03$).

Valve area decreased from a mean of 1.7 ± 0.4 cm^2 after the procedure to 1.4 ± 0.3 cm^2 after 3 years ($P < .01$). Aortic incompetence after implantation was trivial or mild in 84% of cases and remained unchanged or improved over time. There were no cases of structural valvular deterioration, stent fracture, deformation, or valve migration. Ye and coworkers reported similar data at 3 years with the TA technique.[62]

CONCLUSION

Although a direct comparison between the two current devices is not available yet, both systems seem to be beneficial with regard to hemodynamic performance of the bioprosthetic valve, symptom improvement, and early and midterm survival. However, the CoreValve system has been associated with a higher rate of new pacemaker implantation, whereas vascular complications seem to be slightly higher with the first generation of the SAPIEN device, mainly because of the larger size of the current device (22 or 24 French) compared to the Corevalve System (18 French). Currently, no studies have been published directly comparing sAVR to TAVI. Cohort A of the PARTNER pivotal trial comparing sAVR to either TF or TA finished its enrollment in October 2009 and results should be published soon.

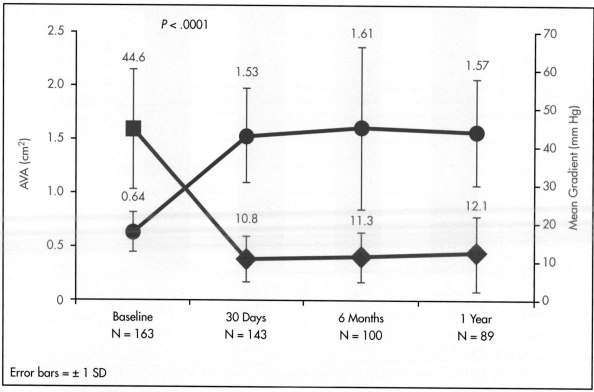

FIGURE 20-10.

Time trends in hemodynamic of prosthesis valve post TAVI in PARTNER trial cohort B.

Whereas initial reports confirmed the feasibility and the safety of TAVI, observational registries were limited by the use of older generation devices, enrollment of small number of patients, the initial learning curve of TAVI operators, self-reported outcomes, and the use of nonstandardized endpoints. Improvement of the current technology combined with the application of standardized definitions[63,64] for important clinical endpoints will enable meaningful comparisons and future well-conducted randomized trials. (See Appendix.)

REFERENCES

1. Ross J Jr, Braunwald E. Aortic stenosis. *Circulation.* 1968 Jul;38(suppl):61–7.
2. Bonow RO, Carabello BA, Kanu C, de Leon AC, Jr., Faxon DP, Freed MD, et al. ACC/AHA 2006 guidelines for the management of patients with valvular heart disease: a report of the American College of Cardiology/American Heart Association Task Force on Practice Guidelines (writing committee to revise the 1998 Guidelines for the Management of Patients With Valvular Heart Disease): developed in collaboration with the Society of Cardiovascular Anesthesiologists: endorsed by the Society for Cardiovascular Angiography and Interventions and the Society of Thoracic Surgeons. *Circulation.* 2006 Aug 1;114(5):e84–231.
3. Vahanian A, Baumgartner H, Bax J, Butchart E, Dion R, Filippatos G, et al. Guidelines on the management of valvular heart disease: The Task Force on the Management of Valvular Heart Disease of the European Society of Cardiology. *Eur Heart J.* 2007 Jan;28(2):230–68.
4. Bach DS, Siao D, Girard SE, Duvernoy C, McCallister BD, Jr., Gualano SK. Evaluation of patients with severe symptomatic aortic stenosis who do not undergo aortic valve replacement: the potential role of subjectively overestimated operative risk. *Circ Cardiovasc Qual Outcomes.* 2009 Nov;2(6):533–9.
5. Cribier A, Eltchaninoff H, Bash A, Borenstein N, Tron C, Bauer F, et al. Percutaneous transcatheter implantation of an aortic valve prosthesis for calcific aortic stenosis: first human case description. Circulation. 2002 Dec 10;106(24):3006–8.
6. Cribier A, Eltchaninoff H, Tron C, Bauer F, Agatiello C, Nercolini D, et al. Treatment of calcific aortic stenosis with the percutaneous heart valve: midterm follow-up from the initial feasibility studies: the French experience. *J Am Coll Cardiol.* 2006 Mar 21;47(6):1214–23.
7. Webb JG, Chandavimol M, Thompson CR, Ricci DR, Carere RG, Munt BI, et al. Percutaneous aortic valve implantation retrograde from the femoral artery. *Circulation.* 2006 Feb 14;113(6):842–50.

8. Webb JG, Pasupati S, Humphries K, Thompson C, Altwegg L, Moss R, et al. Percutaneous transarterial aortic valve replacement in selected high-risk patients with aortic stenosis. *Circulation*. 2007 Aug 14;116(7):755–63.

9. Grube E, Laborde JC, Gerckens U, Felderhoff T, Sauren B, Buellesfeld L, et al. Percutaneous implantation of the CoreValve self-expanding valve prosthesis in high-risk patients with aortic valve disease: the Siegburg first-in-man study. *Circulation*. 2006 Oct 10;114(15):1616–24.

10. Grube E, Schuler G, Buellesfeld L, Gerckens U, Linke A, Wenaweser P, et al. Percutaneous aortic valve replacement for severe aortic stenosis in high-risk patients using the second- and current third-generation self-expanding CoreValve prosthesis: device success and 30-day clinical outcome. *J Am Coll Cardiol*. 2007 Jul 3;50(1):69–76.

11. Rodes-Cabau J, Webb JG, Cheung A, Ye J, Dumont E, Feindel CM, et al. Transcatheter aortic valve implantation for the treatment of severe symptomatic aortic stenosis in patients at very high or prohibitive surgical risk: acute and late outcomes of the multi-center Canadian experience. *J Am Coll Cardiol*. 2010 Mar 16;55(11):1080–90.

12. Lefevre T, Kappetein AP, Wolner E, Nataf P, Thomas M, Schachinger V, et al. One year follow-up of the multi-centre European PARTNER transcatheter heart valve study. *Eur Heart J*. Nov 12.

13. Piazza N, Grube E, Gerckens U, den Heijer P, Linke A, Luha O, et al. Procedural and 30-day outcomes following transcatheter aortic valve implantation using the third generation (18 Fr) corevalve revalving system: results from the multicentre, expanded evaluation registry 1-year following CE mark approval. *EuroIntervention*. 2008 Aug;4(2):242–9.

14. Thomas M, Schymik G, Walther T, Himbert D, Lefevre T, Treede H, et al. Thirty-day results of the SAPIEN aortic Bioprosthesis European Outcome (SOURCE) Registry: A European registry of transcatheter aortic valve implantation using the Edwards SAPIEN valve. *Circulation*. 2010 Jul 6;122(1):62–9.

15. Petronio AS, De Carlo M, Bedogni F, Marzocchi A, Klugmann S, Maisano F, et al. Safety and efficacy of the subclavian approach for transcatheter aortic valve implantation with the CoreValve revalving system. *Circ Cardiovasc Interv*. Aug;3(4):359–66.

16. Eltchaninoff H, Prat A, Gilard M, Leguerrier A, Blanchard D, Fournial G, et al. Transcatheter aortic valve implantation: early results of the FRANCE (FRench Aortic National CoreValve and Edwards) registry. *Eur Heart J*. Sep 15.

17. Leon MB, Smith CR, Mack M, Miller DC, Moses JW, Svensson LG, et al. Transcatheter aortic-valve implantation for aortic stenosis in patients who cannot undergo surgery. *N Engl J Med*. Oct 21;363(17):1597–607.

18. Cribier A, Eltchaninoff H, Tron C, Bauer F, Agatiello C, Sebagh L, et al. Early experience with percutaneous transcatheter implantation of heart valve prosthesis for the treatment of end-stage inoperable patients with calcific aortic stenosis. *J Am Coll Cardiol*. 2004 Feb 18;43(4):698–703.

19. Grube E, Laborde JC, Zickmann B, Gerckens U, Felderhoff T, Sauren B, et al. First report on a human percutaneous transluminal implantation of a self-expanding valve prosthesis for interventional treatment of aortic valve stenosis. *Catheter Cardiovasc Interv*. 2005 Dec;66(4):465–9.

20. Svensson LG, Dewey T, Kapadia S, Roselli EE, Stewart A, Williams M, et al. United States feasibility study of transcatheter insertion of a stented aortic valve by the left ventricular apex. *Ann Thorac Surg*. 2008 Jul;86(1):46–54; discussion -5.

21. Kodali SK, O'Neill WW, Moses JW, Williams M, Smith CR, Tuzcu M, et al. Early and late (one year) outcomes following transcatheter aortic valve implantation in patients with severe aortic stenosis (from the United States REVIVAL trial). *Am J Cardiol*. 2011 Apr 1;107(7):1058–64.

22. Walther T, Kasimir MT, Doss M, Schuler G, Simon P, Schachinger V, et al. One-year interim follow-up results of the TRAVERCE trial: the initial feasibility study for trans-apical aortic-valve implantation. *Eur J Cardiothorac Surg*. 2010 Jul 14.

23. Webb JG, Altwegg L, Boone RH, Cheung A, Ye J, Lichtenstein S, et al. Transcatheter aortic valve implantation: impact on clinical and valve-related outcomes. *Circulation*. 2009 Jun 16;119(23):3009–16.

24. Grube E, Buellesfeld L, Mueller R, Sauren B, Zickmann B, Nair D, et al. Progress and current status of percutaneous aortic valve replacement: results of three device generations of the CoreValve Revalving system. *Circ Cardiovasc Interv*. 2008 Dec;1(3):167–75.

25. Thomas M, Schymik G, Walther T, Himbert D, Lefevre T, Treede H, et al. One-Year Outcomes of Cohort 1 in the Edwards SAPIEN Aortic Bioprosthesis European Outcome (SOURCE) Registry: The European Registry of Transcatheter Aortic Valve Implantation Using the Edwards SAPIEN Valve. *Circulation*. 2011 Jul 11.

26. Zahn R, Gerckens U, Grube E, Linke A, Sievert H, Eggebrecht H, et al. Transcatheter aortic valve implantation: first results from a multi-centre real-world registry. *Eur Heart J*. Sep 23.

27. Eltchaninoff H. TAVI French Registry, EuroPCR; May 2010; Paris, France.

28. Ludman P. TAVI United Kindom Registry; EuroPCR; May 2010; Paris, France.

29. Petronio A. TAVI Italian Registry; EuroPCR; May 2010; Paris, France.

30. Bosmans J. TAVI Belgian Registry; EuroPCR; May 2010; Paris, France.

31. Ducrocq G, Francis F, Serfaty JM, Himbert D, Maury JM, Pasi N, et al. Vascular complications of transfemoral aortic valve implantation with the Edwards SAPIEN prosthesis: incidence and impact on outcome. *EuroIntervention*. 2010 Jan;5(6):666–72.

32. Tchetche D, Dumonteil N, Sauguet A, Descoutures F, Luz A, Garcia O, et al. Thirty-day outcome and vascular complications after transarterial aortic valve implantation using both Edwards Sapien and Medtronic CoreValve bioprostheses in a mixed population. *EuroIntervention*. Jan;5(6):659–665.

33. Van Mieghem NM, Nuis RJ, Piazza N, Apostolos T, Ligthart J, Schultz C, et al. Vascular complications with transcatheter aortic valve implantation using the 18 Fr Medtronic CoreValve System: the Rotterdam experience. *EuroIntervention*. Jan;5(6):673–9.

34. Masson JB, Al Bugami S, Webb JG. Endovascular balloon occlusion for catheter-induced large artery perforation in the catheterization laboratory. *Catheter Cardiovasc Interv*. 2009 Mar 1;73(4):514–8.

35. Sharp AS, Michev I, Maisano F, Taramasso M, Godino C, Latib A, et al. A new technique for vascular access management in transcatheter aortic valve implantation. *Catheter Cardiovasc Interv*. 2010 Apr 1;75(5):784–93.

36. Kronzon I, Tunick PA. Aortic atherosclerotic disease and stroke. *Circulation*. 2006 Jul 4;114(1):63–75

37. Karalis DG, Quinn V, Victor MF, Ross JJ, Polansky M, Spratt KA, et al. Risk of catheter-related emboli in patients with atherosclerotic debris in the thoracic aorta. *Am Heart J*. 1996 Jun;131(6):1149–55.

38. Kahlert P, Knipp SC, Schlamann M, Thielmann M, Al-Rashid F, Weber M, et al. Silent and apparent cerebral ischemia after percutaneous transfemoral aortic valve implantation: a diffusion-weighted magnetic resonance imaging study. *Circulation*. Feb 23;121(7):870–8.

39. Ghanem A, Muller A, Nahle CP, Kocurek J, Werner N, Hammerstingl C, et al. Risk and fate of cerebral embolism after transfemoral aortic valve implantation: a prospective pilot study with diffusion-weighted magnetic resonance imaging. *J Am Coll Cardiol*. Apr 6;55(14):1427–32.

40. Rodes-Cabau J, Dumont E, Boone RH, Larose E, Bagur R, Gurvitch R, et al. Cerebral embolism following transcatheter aortic valve implantation comparison of transfemoral and transapical approaches. *J Am Coll Cardiol*. 2010 Dec 28;57(1):18–28.

41. Nietlispach F, Wijesinghe N, Gurvitch R, Tay E, Carpenter JP, Burns C, et al. An embolic deflection device for aortic valve interventions. *JACC Cardiovasc Interv*. Nov;3(11):1133–8.

42. Gutierrez M, Rodes-Cabau J, Bagur R, Doyle D, DeLarochelliere R, Bergeron S, et al. Electrocardiographic changes and clinical outcomes after transapical aortic valve implantation. *Am Heart J*. 2009 Aug;158(2):302–8.

43. Erkapic D, Kim WK, Weber M, Mollmann H, Berkowitsch A, Zaltsberg S, et al. Electrocardiographic and further predictors for permanent pacemaker requirement after transcatheter aortic valve implantation. *Europace*. Aug;12(8):1188–90.

44. Bleiziffer S, Ruge H, Horer J, Hutter A, Geisbusch S, Brockmann G, et al. Predictors for new-onset complete heart block after transcatheter aortic valve implantation. *JACC Cardiovasc Interv*. May;3(5):524–30.

45. Latsios G, Gerckens U, Buellesfeld L, Mueller R, John D, Yuecel S, et al. "Device landing zone" calcification, assessed by MSCT, as a predictive factor for pacemaker implantation after TAVI. *Catheter Cardiovasc Interv*. Sep 1;76(3):431–9.

46. Ferreira ND, Caeiro D, Adao L, Oliveira M, Goncalves H, Ribeiro J, et al. Incidence and predictors of permanent pacemaker requirement after transcatheter aortic valve implantation with a self-expanding bioprosthesis. *Pacing Clin Electrophysiol*. Nov;33(11):1364–72.

47. Godin M, Eltchaninoff H, Furuta A, Tron C, Anselme F, Bejar K, et al. Frequency of conduction disturbances after transcatheter implantation of an Edwards Sapien aortic valve prosthesis. *Am J Cardiol*. Sep 1;106(5):707–12.

48. Piazza N, Nuis RJ, Tzikas A, Otten A, Onuma Y, Garcia-Garcia H, et al. Persistent conduction abnormalities and requirements for pacemaking six months after transcatheter aortic valve implantation. *EuroIntervention*. Sep;6(4):475–84.

49. Haworth P, Behan M, Khawaja M, Hutchinson N, de Belder A, Trivedi U, et al. Predictors for permanent pacing after transcatheter aortic valve implantation. *Catheter Cardiovasc Interv*. Nov 1;76(5):751–6.

50. Roten L, Wenaweser P, Delacretaz E, Hellige G, Stortecky S, Tanner H, et al. Incidence and predictors of atrioventricular conduction impairment after transcatheter aortic valve implantation. *Am J Cardiol*. Nov 15;106(10):1473–80.

51. Bates MG, Matthews IG, Fazal IA, Turley AJ. Postoperative permanent pacemaker implantation in patients undergoing trans-catheter aortic valve implantation: what is the incidence and are there any predicting factors? *Interact Cardiovasc Thorac Surg*. Nov 23.

52. Piazza N, Onuma Y, Jesserun E, Kint PP, Maugenest AM, Anderson RH, et al. Early and persistent intraventricular conduction abnormalities and requirements for pacemaking after percutaneous replacement of the aortic valve. *JACC Cardiovasc Interv*. 2008 Jun;1(3):310–6.

53. Gurvitch R, Wood DA, Tay EL, Leipsic J, Ye J, Lichtenstein SV, et al. Transcatheter aortic valve implantation: durability of clinical and hemodynamic outcomes beyond 3 years in a large patient cohort. *Circulation*. 2010 Sep 28;122(13):1319–27.

54. Rajani R, Kakad M, Khawaja MZ, Lee L, James R, Saha M, et al. Paravalvular regurgitation one year after transcatheter aortic valve implantation. *Catheter Cardiovasc Interv*. May 1;75(6):868–72.

55. Godino C, Maisano F, Montorfano M, Latib A, Chieffo A, Michev I, et al. Outcomes after transcatheter aortic valve implantation with both Edwards-SAPIEN and CoreValve devices in a single center: the Milan experience. *JACC Cardiovasc Interv*. Nov;3(11):1110–21.

56. Detaint D, Lepage L, Himbert D, Brochet E, Messika-Zeitoun D, Iung B, et al. Determinants of significant paravalvular regurgitation after transcatheter aortic valve: implantation impact of device and annulus discongruence. *JACC Cardiovasc Interv*. 2009 Sep;2(9):821–7.

57. Sherif MA, Abdel-Wahab M, Stocker B, Geist V, Richardt D, Tolg R, et al. Anatomic and procedural predictors of paravalvular aortic regurgitation after implantation of the Medtronic CoreValve bioprosthesis. *J Am Coll Cardiol*. Nov 9;56(20):1623–9.

58. Stabile E, Sorropago G, Cioppa A, Cota L, Agrusta M, Lucchetti V, et al. Acute left main obstructions following TAVI. *EuroIntervention*. May;6(1):100–5.

59. Gogas BD, Zacharoulis AA, Antoniadis AG. Acute coronary occlusion following TAVI. *Catheter Cardiovasc Interv*. Dec 3.

60. Walther T, Falk V, Kempfert J, Borger MA, Fassl J, Chu MW, et al. Transapical minimally invasive aortic valve implantation; the initial 50 patients. *Eur J Cardiothorac Surg*. 2008 Jun;33(6):983–8.

61. Kukucka M, Pasic M, Dreysse S, Hetzer R. Delayed subtotal coronary obstruction after transapical aortic valve implantation. *Interact Cardiovasc Thorac Surg*. Oct 22.

62. Ye J, Cheung A, Lichtenstein SV, Nietlispach F, Albugami S, Masson JB, et al. Transapical transcatheter aortic valve implantation: follow-up to 3 years. *J Thorac Cardiovasc Surg*. May;139(5):1107–13, 13 e1.

63. Leon MB, Piazza N, Nikolsky E, Blackstone EH, Cutlip DE, Kappetein AP, et al. Standardized endpoint definitions for transcatheter aortic valve implantation clinical trials: a consensus report from the Valve Academic Research Consortium. *Eur Heart J*. Jan 6.

64. Leon MB, Piazza N, Nikolsky E, Blackstone EH, Cutlip DE, Kappetein AP, et al. Standardized endpoint definitions for transcatheter aortic valve implantation clinical trials a consensus report from the valve academic research consortium. *J Am Coll Cardiol*. Jan 18;57(3):253–69.

65. Himbert D, Descoutures F, Al-Attar N, Iung B, Ducrocq G, Detaint D, et al. Results of transfemoral or transapical aortic valve implantation following a uniform assessment in high-risk patients with aortic stenosis. *J Am Coll Cardiol*. 2009 Jul 21;54(4):303–11.

Valve Academic Research Consortium Standardized Definitions for Important Clinical Endpoints

APPENDIX TABLE 20-1 **VARC Definition of Device Success**

1. Successful vascular access, delivery, and deployment of the device and successful retrieval of the delivery system
2. Correct position of the device in the proper anatomical location
3. Intended performance of the prosthetic heart valve (aortic valve area >1.2 cm^2 and mean aortic valve gradient <20 mm Hg or peak velocity <3 m/s, without moderate or severe prosthetic valve aortic regurgitation)
4. Only one valve implanted in the proper anatomical location

VARC, Valve Academic Research Consortium.

APPENDIX TABLE 20-2 **VARC Definition of Vascular Access Site and Access-related Complications**

Major Vascular Complications

1. Any thoracic aortic dissection
2. Access site or access-related vascular injury (dissection, stenosis, perforation, rupture, arteriovenous fistula, pseudoaneurysm, hematoma, irreversible nerve injury, or compartment syndrome) leading to either death, need for significant blood transfusions (≥ 4 units), unplanned percutaneous or surgical intervention, or irreversible end-organ damage (e.g., hypogastric artery occlusion causing visceral ischemia or spinal artery injury causing neurological impairment)
3. Distal embolization (noncerebral) from a vascular source requiring surgery or resulting in amputation or irreversible end-organ damage

Minor Vascular Complications

1. Access site or access-related vascular injury (dissection, stenosis, perforation, rupture, arteriovenous fistula, or pseudoaneuysms requiring compression or thrombin injection therapy, or hematomas requiring transfusion of ≥ 2 but <4 units) not requiring unplanned percutaneous or surgical intervention and not resulting in irreversible end-organ damage
2. Distal embolization treated with embolectomy and/or thrombectomy and not resulting in amputation or irreversible end-organ damage
3. Failure of percutaneous access site closure resulting in interventional (e.g., stent graft) or surgical correction and not associated with death, need for significant blood transfusions (≥ 4 units), or irreversible end-organ damage

VARC, Valve Academic Research Consortium.

APPENDIX TABLE 20-3 **VARC Definition of Bleeding**

Life-threatening or Disabling Bleeding

1. Fatal bleeding
   OR
2. Bleeding in a critical area or organ, such as intracranial, intraspinal, intraocular, or pericardial, necessitating pericardiocentesis, or intramuscular with compartment syndrome
   OR
3. Bleeding causing hypovolemic shock or severe hypotension requiring vasopressors or surgery
   OR
4. Overt source of bleeding with drop in hemoglobin of ≥5 g/dL or whole blood or packed RBCs transfusion ≥4 units[a]

Major Bleeding

1. Overt bleeding either associated with a drop in the hemoglobin level of at least 3.0 g/dL or requiring transfusion of two or three units of whole blood/RBC
   AND
2. Does not meet criteria of life-threatening or disabling bleeding

Minor Bleeding

1. Any bleeding worthy of clinical mention (e.g., access site hematoma) that does not qualify as life-threatening, disabling, or major

[a]*Given one unit of packed RBC typically will raise blood hemoglobin concentration by 1 g/dL, an estimated decrease in hemoglobin will be calculated*
VARC, Valve Academic Research Consortium; RBC, red blood cell.

APPENDIX TABLE 20-4 **VARC Definition of Stroke**

Stroke Diagnostic Criteria

1. Rapid onset of a focal or global neurological deficit with at least one of the following: change in level of consciousness, hemiplegia, hemiparesis, numbness or sensory loss affecting one side of the body, dysphasia or aphasia, hemianopia, amaurosis fugax, or other neurological signs or symptoms consistent with stroke
2. Duration of a focal or global neurological deficit ≥24 h; OR <24 h, if therapeutic intervention(s) were performed (e.g., thrombolytic therapy or intracranial angioplasty); OR available neuroimaging documents a new hemorrhage or infarct; OR the neurological deficit results in death
3. No other readily identifiable nonstroke cause for the clinical presentation (e.g., brain tumor, trauma, infection, hypoglycemia, peripheral lesion, pharmacologic influences)[a]
4. Confirmation of the diagnosis by at least one of the following:
   Neurology or neurosurgical specialist
   Neuroimaging procedure (MR or CT scan or cerebral angiography)
   Lumbar puncture (i.e., spinal fluid analysis diagnostic of intracranial hemorrhage)

Stroke Definitions

Transient ischemic attack:
New focal neurological deficit with rapid symptom resolution (usually 1–2 h), always within 24 h
Neuroimaging without tissue injury

Stroke: (diagnosis as above, preferably with positive neuroimaging study)
Minor: Modified Rankin score <2 at 30 and 90 days[b]
Major: Modified Rankin score ≥2 at 30 and 90 days

[a]*Patients with nonfocal global encephalopathy will not be reported as a stroke without unequivocal evidence based on neuroimaging studies.*
[b]*Modified Rankin score assessments should be made by qualified individuals according to a certification process. If there is discordance between the 30- and 90-day Modified Rankin scores, a final determination of major verus minor stroke will be adjudicated by the neurology members of the clinical events committee.*
VARC, Valve Academic Research Consortium; MR, magnetic resonance; CT, computed tomography.

APPENDIX TABLE 20-5 **VARC Definition of Mortality**

Cardiovascular Mortality

Any one of the following criteria:

1. Any death due to proximate cardiac cause (e.g., MI, cardiac tamponade, worsening heart failure)
2. Unwitnessed death and death of unknown cause
3. All procedure-related deaths, including those related to a complication of the procedure or treatment for a complication of the procedure
4. Death caused by noncoronary vascular conditions such as cerebrovascular disease, pulmonary embolism, ruptured aortic aneurysm, dissecting aneurysm, or other vascular disease

VARC, Valve Academic Research Consortium; MI, myocardial infarction.

CHAPTER 21

Newer Transcatheter Aortic Valve Solutions

Joachim Schofer and Klaudija Bijuklic

Transcatheter aortic valve implantation (TAVI) is a viable therapeutic option for high surgical risk patients with severe aortic stenosis. Currently available TAVI systems are the balloon-expandable Edwards valve (Edwards Lifesciences, Irvine, CA), and the self-expandable CoreValve system (Metronic Inc., Minneapolis, MN). Both valves are attached to a stent frame, which is made of either a cobalt chromium alloy or nitinol. The risk associated with TAVI using these valves is in part related to valve misplacement, which cannot be corrected once the device has deployed. This can lead to coronary obstruction, mitral valve injury, and valve embolization. Another shortcoming of the current devices is their insufficient sealing, which in some patients results in significant aortic regurgitation. Thus, there is a need for new valve technologies, which should have the following desirable features:

- Repositionability and retrievability
- Low profile
- Good apposition to the annulus to minimize paravalvular leak and to secure the position of the prosthesis with no risk for valve embolization
- Functional assessment ability of the prosthesis before final implantation
- No interruption of blood flow during positioning and deployment of the valve in order to avoid the necessity of rapid pacing

These improvements in the properties of the second generation compared to the first generation devices should not come at the expense of function, safety, and durability of the device.

DIRECT FLOW MEDICAL

The Direct Flow Medical percutaneous aortic valve (Santa Rosa, CA) is the only nonmetallic valve among the second generation devices (Fig. 21-1).

The implant has a trileaflet valve made of bovine pericardial tissue, which is encased in a slightly tapered conformable polyester fabric cuff. The upper (aortic) and the lower (ventricular) end of the cuff consist of an independently inflatable balloon ring. The rings are interconnected by a tubular bridging system that is inflatable only via inflation of the aortic ring. The rings encircle and capture the native valve annulus ensuring axial anchoring of the device. To position and align the implant in the aortic valvular plane and to independently inflate and deflate the balloon rings, three detachable positioning/fill lumens connect the aortic ring of the implant at angular distances of 120 degrees along its perimeter. The valve is loaded in an 18 French multilumen delivery catheter (Fig. 21-2), which is introduced over 0.035-inch guidewire. An atraumatic nosecone tip allows smooth transition from the guidewire to the housing sheath. The delivery system includes an accessory recovery sheath with a nitinol mesh basket incorporated, into which the implant can be withdrawn if desired (Fig. 21-3).

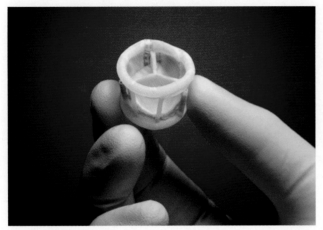

FIGURE 21-1.

Direct Flow Medical (Santa Rosa, CA) percutaneous aortic valve.

Implantation Procedure

Arterial access is achieved percutaneously with a 18 French sheath. A 5 or 6 French pigtail catheter is introduced into the contralateral femoral artery for fluoroscopic visualization of the ascending aorta and the aortic annulus. Standard balloon aortic valvuloplasty is performed to predilate the stenotic aortic valve. The delivery system is introduced over a super stiff guidewire until the implant housing is fully contained in the left ventricle. The outer sheath is retracted to expose the prosthesis. Both balloon rings are then expanded by injecting a 50:50 mixture of saline and contrast agent. Both rings are deflated, the device aligned, and the ventricle ring inflated. At this point, the valve is already fully functioning and ready for positioning without rapid pacing or cardiac support. Positioning is achieved by independently manipulating the position fill lumens to place

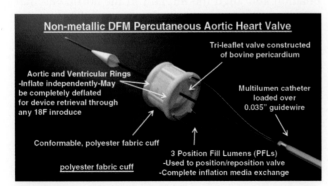

FIGURE 21-2.

Direct Flow Medical (Santa Rosa, CA) valve characteristics.

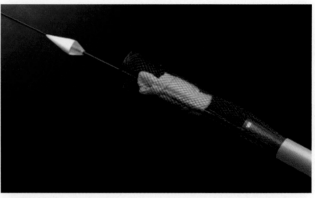

FIGURE 21-3.

Recovery sheath with a nitinol mesh basket that allows the retrieval of the Direct Flow Medical valve (Santa Rosa, CA).

the ventricular ring evenly against the ventricular aspect of the aortic annulus. The aortic ring is inflated with the same mixture of saline and contrast to fix the valve in the desired position and permit function assessment. This is done using fluoroscopy, transesophageal echocardiography, and aortography. The implant is checked for correct subcoronary position, paravalvular leakages, and complete expansion with no significant transvalvular gradient. At this point of the procedure, the implant can be easily repositioned by deflating the upper and, if necessary, the lower ring and, if a different size implant is required, it can be completely deflated and retrieved into the nitinol basket. Once the final device position and function is confirmed, the saline contrast mix is replaced by a polymer, while maintaining a pressure of 8 to 10 atmospheres. The polymer that becomes solid in less than 10 minutes and cures completely within 24 hours to keep the implant permanently in place. Contrast media added to the polymer enhances the fluoroscopic visibility of the prosthetic rings. The position fill lumens are then detached and the delivery system is removed.

Current Status

Direct Flow Medical has performed over 100 preclinical animal studies and cadaver studies. Initial clinical experience included a series of nine temporary implants performed in South America at a single center, two open heart surgical implants, and seven percutaneous implants.[1] Two transfemoral recoveries of the Direct Flow Medial valve were successfully performed. This was followed by a European prospective nonrandomized clinical trial at two centers conducted between October 2007 and August 2008.

The purpose was to determine the feasibility and safety of the device in patients with severe symptomatic aortic valve stenosis at high surgical risk (logistic EuroSCRORE ≥20%). Thirty-one patients were enrolled in the study,[2] which showed an immediate valve competence, repositionability, and retrievability and resulted in good hemodynamics in those patients in whom the device could be implanted. A new 18 French system is scheduled to be in clinical trials by the end of 2011.

THE JENAVALVE TECHNOLOGY

JenaValve Technology GmbH (Munich, Germany) was formed to develop transcatheter valve technology initially conceived by Professor Hans-Reiner Figulla and Dr. Markus Ferrari of Friedrich Schiller University (Jena, Germany). The company's current focus is on two aortic valve systems, designed for transapical and transfemoral delivery, respectively. Each system consists of a delivery catheter and self-expanding stented valve prosthesis. The prosthesis of both systems incorporates the JenaClip nitinol stent technology, with collapsible porcine valve tissue for the transapical system and collapsible pericardial tissue construction for the transfemoral system. JenaValve has focused its product development on fundamental, patented, design features:

- Low-profile prosthesis and stent design
- Feeler-guided positioning
- Unique JenaClip anchoring mechanism
- Repositioning and retrievability
- Enhanced radiopacity

These are the elemental differentiators with which the TAVI can be accomplished precisely and easily.

The JenaValve Prosthesis

The JenaClip (Fig. 21-4) comprises a double-layer system of three clips aligned in two rows, one used to affix the valve tissue onto the stent (via sutures) and the other for precise positioning and anchoring to the native diseased aortic valve annulus and leaflets. This clipping mechanism enables shortening of the stent length and reducing the radial force. As a result, atrioventricular block can be avoided. The prosthesis is available in sizes that fit native valve annulus diameters ranging from 21 to 27 mm.

The JenaValve Catheter Systems

Both delivery catheters feature an ergonomic over-the-wire design that facilitates sheathless entry. The 18

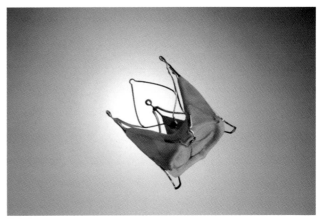

FIGURE 21-4.

The JenaValve prosthesis (Munich, Germany) for transapical application.

French equivalent transfemoral catheter has a 10 French flexible shaft to allow the catheter to navigate retrograde, even through tortuous anatomy, and to cross the aortic arch to reach the valve plane. The shorter 28 French equivalent transapical catheter has a long and flexible tip that follows the guidewire during catheter advancement and during valve deployment. Both systems are controlled through ergonomically shaped hand grips, which allow safe and deliberate positioning and release of the prosthesis (Fig. 21-5). The delivery systems for the two devices function very similarly with a simple three-step approach.

Implant Procedure

Upon advancement of the device above the aortic valve annulus, the catheter sheath is pulled back (transfemoral) or pushed forward (transapical) to release three

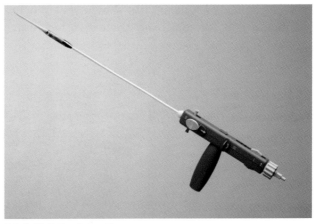

FIGURE 21-5.

The JenaValve catheter system (Munich, Germany) for transapical application.

The transapical implantation steps.

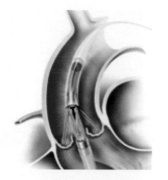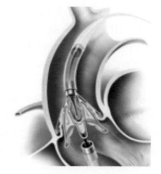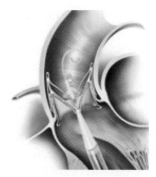

"positioning feelers" that are then maneuvered in the sinus behind the native cusps of the native aortic valve (see Figs. 21-6 and 21-7, step 1). In addition to fluoroscopic and echocardiographic visual confirmation, the feelers provide a tactile feedback to the physician for accurate positioning of the valve prosthesis.

When the feelers are properly seated and the device is in place, the native leaflets are pressed against the aortic wall and the clip mechanism captures them similar to a paperclip to provide anchoring and prevent movement of the prosthesis. Then, the catheter sheath is advanced to release the annular anchoring mechanism (step 2) followed by full release of the prosthesis (step 3).

Once temporarily released, the prosthesis fully expands, applies maximal retention force, and, at this point, the valve is immediately functional. Neither rapid pacing nor cardiac support is required during implantation, and valve retrieval and/or repositioning remain possible until final release of the prosthesis.

Current Status

First-in-human experience has shown that the implantation is a safe and easy three-step technique,

feeler-guided positioning enables precise orientation and correct positioning for safe and accurate prosthesis placement. The feelers can be advanced, rotated, repositioned or retracted into the catheter. The system takes advantage of the physician's tactile skills to locate optimal position in the "landing zone." Radial and axial fixation of the prosthesis could be accomplished due to the unique JenaClip mechanism. No coronary obstructions and atrioventricular block were observed. A feasibility and safety trial is ongoing.

HEART LEAFLET TECHNOLOGIES TRANSCATHETER AORTIC VALVE

The Heart Leaflet Technologies (HLT; Maple Grove, MN) transcatheter aortic valve is a tricuspid porcine pericardial valve, which is attached to a self-expanding and self-inverting nitinol structure that supports the valve within the native aortic annulus (Fig. 21-8). The valve is delivered through a 16 or 17 French sheath. A positioning device (backstop) facilitates the positioning of the valve without the necessity for rapid pacing. The valve can be repositioned and fully retrieved during the implant procedure.

The transfemoral implantation steps.

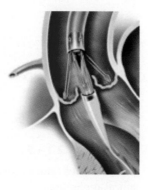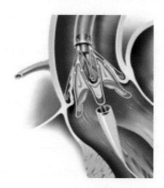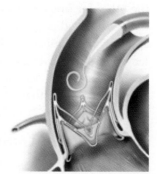

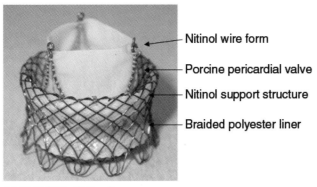

FIGURE 21-8.

Heart Leaflet Technologies (Maple Grove, MN) transcatheter aortic valve.

The HLT valve consists of four elements:

- Cross-linked tricuspid porcine pericardial tissue valve
- Superelastic nitinol wire form that supports the valve structure
- Superelastic nitinol mesh, which supports the pros-

thetic valve and keeps the valve fixed within the native valve annulus

- A braided polyester liner integrated within the support structure to prevent paravalvular leakage

The delivery system consists of six components (Fig. 21-9). These include a 16 to 17 French delivery catheter and the dilator, which is designed to provide a smooth transition from the delivery catheter tip to the guidewire (0.035 inch) and facilitates crossing the native aortic valve and the funnel catheter, which is designed to protect the porcine tissue of the valve during loading and delivery. The valve retention cables provide three attachment points to the HLT valve that are released once the proper position is achieved. The loader catheter together with the funnel catheter and valve retention cables provide a means for loading and advancing the valve into the delivery catheter. The *backstop* is a tool that is positioned against the ventricular aspect of the aortic annulus to ensure proper valve placement. Following delivery of the valve prosthesis the backstop is also used as a dilatation tool to help expand and seat the implant.

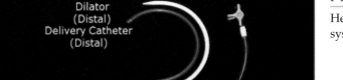

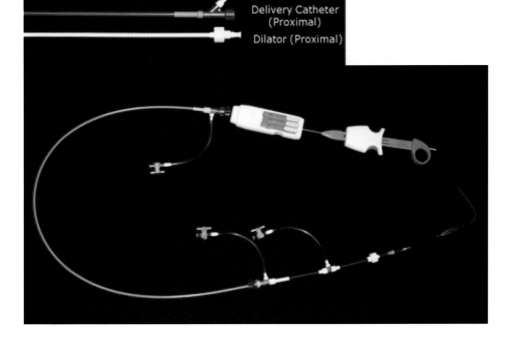

FIGURE 21-9.

Heart Leaflet Technologies (Maple Grove, MN) delivery system.

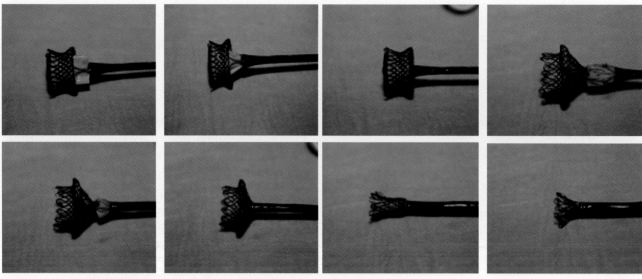

FIGURE 21-10.

Valve loading/delivery sequence of the Heart Leaflet Technologies valve (Maple Grove, MN).

This backstop is a flow-through nitinol mesh, which is not restricting blood flow and therefore eliminates the need for rapid ventricular pacing during expansion (Fig. 21-10).

Implant Procedure

The device is delivered through the femoral artery by conventional percutaneous puncture. After aortic valvuloplasty and insertion of a 5 or 6 French pigtail catheter from the contralateral site, the HLT delivery catheter and the dilator are advanced across the native aortic valve over a super stiff 0.035-inch guidewire.

The catheter is placed toward the septum in order to avoid perforation of the lateral wall when the implant is introduced. The dilator is removed and the loader catheter containing the HLT valve and the backstop is then mounted to the proximal hub of the delivery catheter. After advancement of the valve through the delivery catheter across the native aortic valve, the backstop is deployed against the ventricular aspect of the aortic annulus. The valve is pushed out of the catheter against the backstop. As soon as sufficient cuff has been deployed, it inverts on itself increasing the radial force of the implant. The valve is then completely pushed out of the catheter and correct valve position and function is verified by a transesophageal echocardiography and fluoroscopic imaging. If the valve is correctly positioned below the coronary ostia, the backstop is used for dilatation of the valve to ensure a round shape of the support

structure and sufficient sealing at the level of aortic annulus to prevent paravalvular leaks. At this point of the procedure, the valve can be retrieved if the desired results are not achieved. If the results are satisfactory, the procedure is completed by detachment of the valve retention cables.

Current Status

According to animal studies, the cuff structure is appropriately fibrosed into the native valve annulus and valve function over time is normal. The first-in-men implant was performed in Hamburg in 2009, and an improved design is scheduled to be in clinical trial end of 2011.

THE SADRA MEDICAL LOTUS VALVE SYSTEM

The Lotus valve system (Sadra Medical, Los Gatos, CA) is a fully repositionable and self-centering device designed to facilitate optimal position of the valve. The valve is functioning during deployment and can be resheathed and retrieved prior to final release.

The Lotus valve system consists of at trileaflet valve made of bovine pericardial tissue, a delivery catheter, and a delivery system for guidance and placement of the implant.

A nitinol self-expanding structure holds the valve in position (Fig. 21-11) and is adapting to the various annular geometry in the patients. Adaptive seal

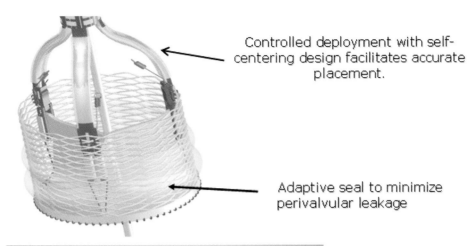

Controlled deployment with self-centering design facilitates accurate placement.

Adaptive seal to minimize perivalvular leakage

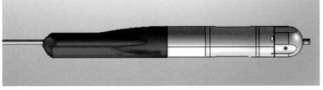

FIGURE 21-11.

Sadra Medical Lotus (Los Gatos, CA) valve system.

The handle

technology on the outer diameter of the nitinol structure is designed to minimize perivalvular leakage.

Implant Procedure

The delivery catheter is introduced using a percutaneous puncture technique via the femoral artery. The system is advanced over the aortic arch and across the aortic valve. A handle is then turned on the delivery system to control expansion of the valve. During this process, an assessment of the positioning relative to the anterior mitral leaflet and to the coronary ostia is made. At any point during valve expansion, the physician can adjust the position of the valve. Upon full expansion, flow dynamics can be assessed prior to release of the valve. If the implant needs to be

repositioned or completely retrieved and exchanged for a different size implant, it can be withdrawn partially or completely back into the sheath. When the final position is established, the release mechanism is deployed, thereby detaching the delivery system from the implant and the delivery system is removed from the patient.

Current Status

A first-in-human implantation was performed by Dr. Grube and Dr. Müller in Siegburg in July 2007. Early clinical work has confirmed the value of the accurate placement, repositionability, and retrievability of the valve. Since then, a feasibility and safety study is ongoing and several more patients have been treated.

REFERENCES

1. Low RI, Bolling SF, Yeo KK, et al. A Direct Flow Medical percutaneous aortic valve: proof of concept. *Eurointervention.* 2008;4:256–261.
2. Schofer J, Schlüter M, Treede H, et al. Retrograde transarterial implantation of a nonmetallic aortic valve prosthesis in high-surgical-risk patients with severe aortic stenosis. A first-in-man feasibility and safety study. *Circ CardiovascInterv.* 2008;2:126–133.

CHAPTER 22

Percutaneous Mitral Commissurotomy

Alec Vahanian, Dominique Himbert, Eric Brochet, and Bernard Iung

Until 1984, surgery was the only treatment for patients with mitral stenosis.[1] Since then, a large number of patients with a wide range of clinical conditions have been treated using percutaneous mitral commissurotomy (PMC), which enables the assessment of efficacy and risk.[2]

TECHNIQUE

It seems appropriate to concentrate the performance of the procedure among experienced centers in order to improve the management of the interventional procedure by decreasing the risk and improving the selection of patients.[3]

Approach

The transvenous, or antegrade, approach is the most widely used. It is performed through the femoral vein or, exceptionally, through the jugular vein. Usually, transseptal catheterization is performed under fluoroscopic guidance, ideally using several views. Continuous pressure monitoring is recommended. Echocardiography is not required during transseptal catheterization; however, it has the potential to enhance its safety, especially in the early part of the operator's experience. This has been done primarily with the transesophageal approach (transesophageal Echocardiography [TEE]). Nevertheless, the transesophageal approach is not easy in the catheterization laboratory and should probably be restricted to cases in which technical difficulties are encountered

(e.g., severe anatomic distortion). Intracardiac echocardiography (ICE) is currently considered the imaging tool of choice although the price of the device is a serious limitation in most places. Recent data suggest that real-time three-dimensional (3D) transesophageal technique may further improve the visualization of the septum and assessment of the tenting during the septal puncture.[4]

The retrograde technique without transseptal catheterization has been used with good results and no serious complications, but its use is not widespread.

Inoue Technique

The Inoue balloon, composed of nylon and rubber micromesh, is self-positioning and pressure-extensible. It is large (24–30 mm in diameter) and has a low profile (4.5 mm). The balloon has three distinct parts, each with a specific elasticity, enabling them to be inflated sequentially. This sequence allows fast, stable positioning across the valve. There are four sizes of the Inoue balloon (24, 26, 28, and 30 mm); each is pressure dependent, so its diameter can be varied by up to 4 mm as required by circumstances.

The main steps are as follows: After transseptal catheterization, a stiff guidewire is introduced into the left atrium. The femoral entry site and the atrial septum are dilated using a rigid dilator (14 French), and the balloon is introduced into the left atrium.

Inoue recommended the use of a stepwise dilation technique under echocardiographic guidance. Balloon size is chosen in accordance with the patient's height (26

313

F I G U R E   2 2 - 1 .

Percutaneous mitral commissurotomy using the Inoue technique. Sequential inflation of the
Inoue balloon across the mitral
valve.

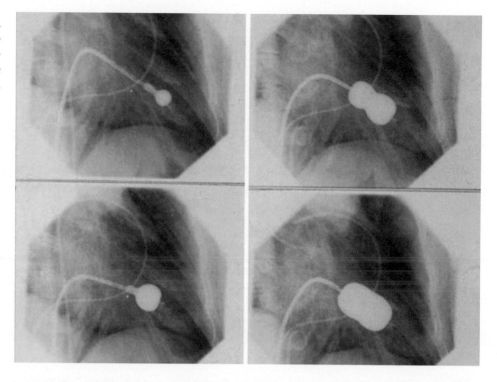

mm in very small patients or children, 28 mm in patients shorter than 1.60 m, and 30 mm in patients taller than 1.60 m). The balloon is inflated sequentially. First, the distal portion is inflated with 1 or 2 mL of a diluted contrast medium, which acts as a floating balloon catheter when crossing the mitral valve. Second, the distal part is further inflated, and the balloon is pulled back into the mitral orifice. Inflation then occurs at the level of the proximal part and finally in the central portion, with the disappearance of the central waist at full inflation (Figs. 22-1 and 22-2).[1]

The first inflation is performed 4 mm below the maximal balloon size, and the balloon size is increased in steps of 1 mm each. The balloon is then deflated and withdrawn into the left atrium. If mitral regurgitation (assessed by color Doppler echocardiography) has not increased by more than one-fourth and the valve area is less than 1 cm^2/m^2 of body surface area, the balloon is readvanced across the valve,[5] and PMC is repeated with a balloon diameter increased by 1 mm. The criteria for ending the procedure are

F I G U R E   2 2 - 2 .

Percutaneous mitral commissurotomy. Echocardiographic monitoring of the procedure using
"three-dimensional transesophageal echocardiography hands
on." The Inoue balloon is in the
left atrium facing the mitral valve
(*MV*).

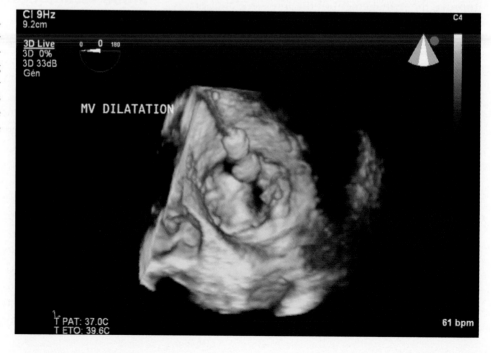

an adequate valve area or an increase in the degree of mitral regurgitation.

The Inoue technique has already become the most popular in the world, having been used in more than 10,000 patients. Finally, the stepwise technique under echocardiographic guidance certainly allows the best use of the mechanical properties of the Inoue balloon and therefore optimizes the results.

Other Techniques

The double-balloon technique using the Multi-Track system (NuMED Inc., Hopkinton, NY) and the metallic commissurotomy are currently very seldom used, if at all.

Monitoring of the Procedure

The following recommendations have been suggested for monitoring the procedure. First, use of the mean left atrial pressure and mean valve gradient can be criticized because of variations that may occur, particularly with respect to changes in the heart rate or cardiac output. Second, repeated evaluation of the valve area during the procedure by hemodynamic measurements lacks practicality and may be subject to error because of the instability of the patient's condition and the inaccuracy of Gorlin's formula in the presence of atrial shunts or mitral regurgitation. The accuracy of Doppler measurements during PMC is low, so planimetry from two-dimensional echocardiography appears to be the method of choice if it is technically feasible. Color Doppler assessment is the method of choice for sequential evaluation of changes in the degree of regurgitation. The commissural opening, which is the main parameter, is usually assessed in the parasternal short-axis view during transthoracic echocardiography (TTE). Real-time 3D echocardiography is the most accurate method for assessing the degree of opening using short-axis views (Fig. 22-3A,B).[5]

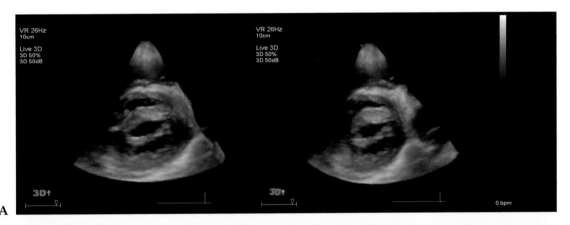

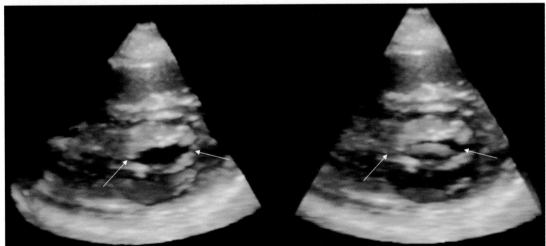

FIGURE 22-3.

A: Stepwise Inoue technique. Three-dimensional transthoracic echocardiography monitoring. Short-axis view: Opening of the anterolateral commissure after first inflation. **B:** Stepwise Inoue technique. Three-dimensional transthoracic echocardiography monitoring. Short-axis view: Opening of both commissures (as shown by *arrows*).

TABLE 22-1 **Immediate Results of Percutaneous Commissurotomy: Increase in Mitral Valve Area**

| Author | Number | Age (Yr) | Mitral Valve Area (cm²) | |
			Before PMC Technique	After PMC Technique
Chen et al.[8]	4832	37	1.1	2.1
Arora et al.[7]	4850	27	0.7	1.9
Palacios et al.[6]	879	55	0.9	1.9
Iung et al.[3]	2773	47	1.0	1.9

PMC, percutaneous mitral commissurotomy.

The following criteria have been proposed for the desired end point of the procedure: (a) mitral valve area of more than 1 cm²/m² of the body surface area; (b) complete opening of at least one commissure; or (c) appearance or increment of regurgitation greater than one-fourth. It is vital that the strategy be tailored to the individual circumstances.

After the procedure, the most accurate evaluation of valve area is achieved by echocardiography. To allow for the slight loss during the first 24 hours, this should be performed 1 to 2 days after PMC, when the valve area may be calculated by planimetry or by the half-pressure time or continuity equation method. The degree of regurgitation may be finally assessed by angiography or color Doppler flow. The most sensitive method for assessing shunting is color Doppler flow.

In experienced centers, the procedure can be performed using a single venous approach and noninvasive monitoring, which diminishes the risk, discomfort, and costs.

IMMEDIATE RESULTS

Hemodynamics

PMC usually provides an increase of more than 100% in the valve area (Table 22-1). A gradual decrease in pulmonary arterial pressure and pulmonary vascular resistance is seen.

PMC has a beneficial effect on exercise capacity. It also results in a decrease in the intensity of spontaneous echocardiographic contrast in the left atrium.

Failures

The failure rate ranges from 1% to 17%.[2,3,6-8] Most failures occur early in the investigator's experience.

Complications

Procedural *mortality* has ranged from 0% to 3% in most series (Table 22-2). The main causes of death are left ventricular perforation and poor general condition of the patient.

The incidence of *hemopericardium* has varied from 0.5% to 12.0%. Pericardial hemorrhage may be related to transseptal catheterization or to apex perforation by the guidewires or the balloon itself when exaggerated movement occurs with the over-the-wire techniques, but this latter complication is virtually eliminated with the Inoue balloon technique. If hypotension occurs during PMC, hemopericardium must be suspected and echocardiography immediately performed.

Embolism is encountered in 0.5% to 5.0% of cases. It is seldom the cause of permanent incapacitation and even more seldom the cause of death. Although the incidence of embolism is low, its potential consequences are severe, and all possible precautions must be taken to prevent it. The treatment of cerebral embolism should be in collaboration with a stroke center.

TABLE 22-2 **Severe Complications of Percutaneous Mitral Commissurotomy**

Author	Number	Age (Yr)	In-hospital Death (%)	Tamponade (%)	Embolic Events (%)	Severe Mitral Regurgitation (%)
Chen et al.[8]	4832	37	0.1	0.8	0.5	1.4
Arora et al.[7]	4850	27	0.2	0.2	0.1	1.4
Palacios et al.[6]	879	55	0.6	1.0	1.8	9.4
Iung et al.[3]	2773	47	0.4	0.2	0.4	4.1

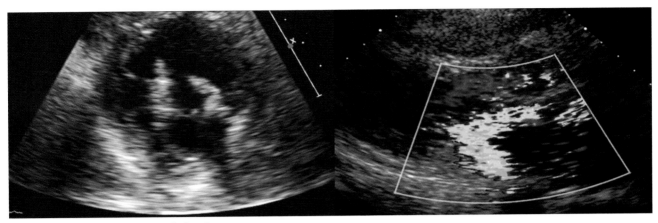

FIGURE 22-4.

Leaflet tear after percutaneous mitral commissurotomy. Transthoracic echocardiography, short-axis view. **Left:** Tear of anterior leaflet. **Right:** Diffracted jet of mitral regurgitation originating from the valvular tear.

Severe mitral regurgitation is uncommon, its frequency ranging from 2% to 19%,[2,3,6–10] and remains largely unpredictable for a given patient. Surgical findings have shown that it is related to noncommissural tearing of the posterior or anterior leaflet (Fig. 22-4). It has been suggested that the development of severe regurgitation depends more on the distribution of morphologic changes than on their severity. Severe mitral regurgitation may be well tolerated, but more often it is not, and surgery must be scheduled. In most cases, valve replacement is necessary because of the severity of the underlying valve disease.

Atrial septal defects are usually small and restrictive, with high-velocity flow. The incidence of transient, complete *heart block* is 1.5%, and it seldom requires a permanent pacemaker. After the transvenous approach, *vascular complications* are the exception. *Urgent surgery* (within 24 hours) is seldom needed for complications resulting from PMC. It may be required, however, for massive hemopericardium resulting from left ventricular perforation unresponsive to pericardiocentesis or, less frequently, for severe mitral regurgitation leading to hemodynamic collapse or refractory pulmonary edema.[9]

Overall, the incidence of failures and serious complications such as tamponade is clearly related to experience. When performed by experienced teams on properly selected patients, PMC is a relatively low-risk procedure.

Predictors of Immediate Results

The definition of good immediate results varies from series to series. The most widely accepted is a final valve area larger than 1.5 cm^2 without mitral regurgitation greater than 2/4.

Prediction of results is multifactorial. Several studies have shown that, in addition to morphologic factors, preoperative variables such as age, history of surgical commissurotomy, functional class, small mitral valve area, presence of mitral regurgitation before PMC, sinus rhythm, pulmonary artery pressure, and presence of severe tricuspid regurgitation, as well as procedural factors such as balloon size, are all independent predictors of the immediate results.[6,11]

Identification of these variables linked to outcome has enabled models to be developed with a high sensitivity of prediction. Nevertheless, the specificity is low, indicating insufficient prediction of poor immediate results. This low specificity is particularly true in regard to the lack of accurate prediction of severe mitral regurgitation.

LONG-TERM RESULTS

We are now able to analyze follow-up data up to 17 years,[6,10–16] which represents long-term results (Table 22-3).

In clinical terms, which are the most widely used, the overall mid-term results of valvuloplasty are encouraging, with an event-free survival ranging from 35% to 70% after 10 to 15 years. Prediction of long-term results is also multifactorial,[6,11,12] based on clinical variables such as age, valve anatomy as assessed by echocardiography scores, factors related to the evolutionary stage of the disease (i.e., higher New York Heart Association class before valvuloplasty), history of previous

TABLE 22-3 Late Results after Percutaneous Mitral Commissurotomy

Author	Number	Age (Yr)	Follow-Up (Yr)	Event-Free Survival (%)
Iung et al.[12]	1024	49	10	56[a]
Palacios et al.[6]	879	55	12	33[a]
Song et al.[25]	329	49	9	90[b]
Fawzy et al.[16]	493	31	13	74[a]

[a]*Survival without intervention and in New York Heart Association class I or II.*
[b]*After successful procedure.*

commissurotomy, severe tricuspid regurgitation, cardiomegaly, atrial fibrillation, high pulmonary vascular resistance, and the results of the procedure in terms of final valve area, quality of commissural opening,[14] and presence of mitral regurgitation.[10] The quality of the late results is generally considered to be independent of the technique used.

If PMC is *initially successful,* survival rates are excellent, the need for secondary surgery is infrequent, and functional improvement occurs in most cases. In most cases the improvement in valve function is stable.

Determining the incidence of restenosis is compromised by the absence of a uniform definition. Restenosis after PMC has generally been defined as a loss of more than 50% of the initial gain with a valve area less than 1.5 cm^2. After successful PMC, the incidence of restenosis is usually low, between 2% and 40%,[13,15] at time intervals ranging from 3 to 10 years. Age, mitral valve area after PMC, and anatomy are considered predictors of restenosis. The ability to perform repeat PMC in cases of recurrent mitral stenosis is one of the advantages of this nonsurgical procedure. Repeat PMC can be proposed if recurrent stenosis leads to symptoms, if it occurs several years after an initially successful procedure, and if the predominant mechanism of restenosis is commissural refusion. In such cases, immediate and midterm outcomes are good in patients with favorable characteristics. Although the results are less favorable in patients presenting with worse characteristics, repeat valvuloplasty has a palliative role in patients who are at high risk for surgery. These preliminary results are encouraging, but the exact role of re-valvuloplasty must await larger series with longer follow-up to be defined.[17]

If the immediate results are *unsatisfactory,* midterm functional results are usually poor. The prognosis of patients with severe mitral regurgitation after surgical commissurotomy or PMC is usually poor, with a lack of symptom alleviation and secondary objective deterioration. Surgical treatment is usually necessary during the following months.

In cases of an insufficient initial opening, delayed surgery is usually performed when the extracardiac conditions allow it. Here, valve replacement is necessary in almost all cases because of the unfavorable valve anatomy that was responsible for the poor initial results.

Follow-up studies also show that degree of mitral regurgitation, on the whole, remains stable or slightly decreases during follow up. Atrial septal defects are likely to close later in most cases because of a reduced interatrial pressure gradient.

PMC carries a beneficial effect on left atrial blood stasis, from which a lower risk of thromboembolism may be expected.[18] Finally, there is no direct evidence that PMC reduces the incidence of atrial fibrillation.[19] It is recommended that electric counter shock cardioversion is performed early after successful PMC if atrial fibrillation is of recent onset and in the absence of severe enlargement of the left atrium.

PERCUTANEOUS MITRAL COMMISSUROTOMY IN SPECIAL PATIENT POPULATION

Percutaneous Mitral Commissurotomy after Surgical Commissurotomy

In patients with previous surgical commissurotomy[20] the results are good, even if slightly less satisfactory than those obtained in patients without previous commissurotomy—this can probably be attributed to the less favorable characteristics observed in patients previously subjected to operation.

The indications for PMC in this subgroup of patients are similar to those for "primary PMC," but echocardiographic examination must be conducted with great care to exclude any patients in whom restenosis is due mainly to valve rigidity without significant commissural refusion. The latter mechanism should not be overlooked in the rare cases of mitral stenosis that develop in patients who have undergone mitral ring annuloplasty for correction of mitral regurgitation.

Percutaneous Mitral Commissurotomy in Patients with Severe Pulmonary Hypertension

Preliminary reports have suggested that valvuloplasty can be performed safely and effectively. In such cases, even if the valve opening is suboptimal, it may allow the decrease of pulmonary pressures and thereby the operative risk.

Percutaneous Mitral Commissurotomy in Elderly Patients

When surgery is high risk or even contraindicated but life expectancy is still acceptable, PMC is a useful option even if only palliative. In patients who still have favorable anatomy, PMC can be attempted first, resorting to surgery if results are unsatisfactory. In other patients, surgery is preferable as the first option. On the other hand, the outcome is very bad in elderly patients presenting with "end-stage" disease, who would probably be better treated conservatively.

Percutaneous Mitral Commissurotomy during Pregnancy

The experience of PMC during pregnancy represented by several hundreds of cases[21] suggests the following: From a technical point of view, during the last weeks of pregnancy, the procedure may be challenging; however, it is effective and allows for normal delivery in most cases. Regarding radiation exposure, PMC is safe for the fetus, provided that protection is provided by a shield that completely surrounds the patient's abdomen and the procedure is performed after the 20th week. In addition to radiation, PMC carries the potential risk of related hypotension and the always-present risk of complications that require urgent surgery. These data suggest that PMC can be a useful technique in the treatment of pregnant patients with mitral stenosis and refractory heart failure despite medical treatment.

Percutaneous Mitral Commissurotomy and Left Atrial Thrombosis

Left atrial thrombosis is generally considered a contraindication to PMC.[22,23] This recommendation is self-evident if the thrombus is free-floating or is situated in the left atrial cavity; it also applies when the thrombus is located on the interatrial septum. If the thrombus is located in the left atrial appendage (Fig. 22-5), it has not been shown to our satisfaction that the Inoue technique under TEE guidance precludes the risk of embolism. If the patient is clinically stable, as is the case

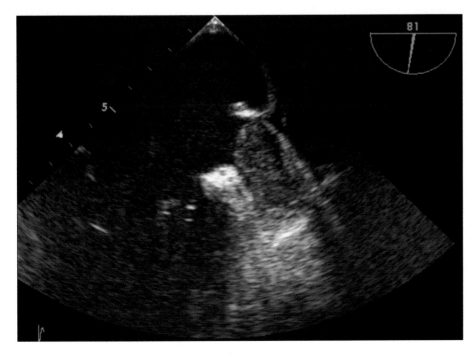

FIGURE 22-5.

Left atrial thrombus; transesophageal echocardiography.

for most patients with mitral stenosis, anticoagulant therapy can be given for 2 to 6 months[24]; then, if a new TEE shows that the thrombus has disappeared, PMC can be attempted.

SELECTION OF PATIENTS

The application of PMC depends on the patient's clinical condition and the valve anatomy.

Clinical Condition

Evaluation of the clinical condition must take into account the degree of functional disability, the presence of contraindications to transseptal catheterization, and the alternative risk of surgery as a function of the underlying cardiac and noncardiac status. Because of the small but definite risk inherent in the technique, truly asymptomatic patients with severe mitral stenosis (i.e., patients with normal physical working capacity on exercise testing) are not usually candidates for PMC, except in cases of urgent need for extra-cardiac surgery, to allow pregnancy in young women or in patients with an increased risk of embolism. Finally, PMC can be proposed in patients who are declared to be asymptomatic but who have pulmonary hypertension either at rest (systolic pulmonary pressure >50 mm Hg)[22,23] or on exercise (>60 mm Hg).[22] Under these conditions, PMC should be performed only by experienced interventionists when the anatomy is suitable, leading to a safe, effective procedure.

Contraindications to transseptal catheterization include suspected left atrial thrombosis, which must be excluded by systematic performance of TEE a few days before the procedure, severe hemorrhagic disorder, and severe cardiothoracic deformity. Increased surgical risk of cardiac origin (previous surgical commissurotomy or aortic valve replacement) or extra-cardiac origin (respiratory insufficiency, old age) makes balloon valvuloplasty preferable to surgery, at least as the first attempt, or even as the only solution in case of a strict contraindication to surgery.

Valve Anatomy

It is critical to ensure that there are no anatomical contraindications to the technique (Table 22-4). The first of these is the presence of left atrial thrombosis. The second is more than mild mitral regurgitation. PMC can however be carried out in selected patients with mitral regurgitation 2+ if the risk of surgery is high, such as in pregnant patients. Third, in cases of combined mitral stenosis and severe aortic disease, the indication

TABLE 22-4 **Contraindications to Percutaneous Mitral Commissurotomy**

Left atrial thrombosis

Mitral regurgitation >1/4

Massive or bicommissural calcification

Severe aortic valve disease, or severe tricuspid stenosis and regurgitation, associated with mitral stenosis

Severe concomitant coronary artery disease requiring bypass surgery

for surgery is obvious in the absence of contraindications. The coexistence of moderate aortic valve disease and severe mitral stenosis is another situation in which PMC is preferable to postpone the inevitable later surgical treatment of both valves.

Fourth, the presence of combined severe tricuspid stenosis and tricuspid regurgitation with clinical signs of heart failure is an indication for surgery on both valves. On the other hand, the existence of tricuspid regurgitation is not, in itself, a contraindication to the procedure even though it represents a negative prognostic factor, especially when it is associated with severe enlargement of the right atrium and atrial fibrillation.[25]

To define a threshold of valve area above which PMC should not be performed is somewhat arbitrary. In addition to measuring valve area and mean gradient, one must also take into account the stature of the patient, their functional disability, and pulmonary pressures at rest and on exercise in case of doubt. Our view regarding the performance of PMC in patients with mitral valve area >1.5 cm² is that the risks probably outweigh the benefits.

For prognostic considerations, most investigators use the Wilkins score (Table 22-5),[6] whereas others[3] use a more general assessment of valve anatomy (Table 22-6). All echocardiographic classifications have the same limitations: (a) reproducibility is difficult, because the scores are only semi-quantitative; (b) lesions may be underestimated, especially with regard to the assessment of subvalvular disease; and (c) the use of scores describing the degree of overall valve deformity may not identify localized changes in specific portions of the valve apparatus (leaflets, and especially commissures), which may increase the risk of severe mitral regurgitation.

Potential Indications

No problem of indication is presented in cases in which surgery is contraindicated or with "ideal candidates," such as young adults with good anatomy: pliable valves

TABLE 22-5 **Anatomic Classification of the Mitral Valve (Massachusetts General Hospital, Boston, MA)**

Leaflet Mobility

Highly mobile valve with restriction of only the leaflet tips

Midportion and base of leaflets have reduced mobility

Valve leaflets move forward during diastole, mainly at the base

No or minimal forward movement of the leaflets during diastole

Valvular Thickening

Leaflets near normal (4–5 mm)

Midleaflet thickening, marked thickening of the margins

Thickening extends through the entire leaflets (5–8 mm)

Marked thickening of all leaflet tissue (>8–10 mm)

Subvalvular Thickening

Minimal thickening of chordal structures just below the valve

Thickening of chordae extending up to one-third of chordal length

Thickening extending to the distal third of the chordae

Extensive thickening and shortening of all chordae extending down to the papillary muscle

Valvular Calcification

Single area of increased echocardiographic brightness

Scattered areas of brightness confined to leaflet margins

Brightness extending into the midportion of leaflets

Extensive brightness through most of the leaflet tissue

Adapted from Abascal V, Wilkins GT, O'Shea JP, et al. Prediction of successful outcome in 130 patients undergoing percutaneous balloon mitral valvotomy. Circulation. 1990;82:448–456.

TABLE 22-6 **Anatomic Classification of the Mitral Valve (Bichat Hospital, Paris)**

Echocardiographic Group	Mitral Valve Anatomy
1	Pliable noncalcified anterior mitral leaflet and mild subvalvular disease (i.e., thin chordae >10 mm long)
2	Pliable noncalcified anterior mitral leaflet and severe subvalvular disease (i.e., thickened chordae <10 mm long)
3	Calcification of mitral valve of any extent, as assessed by fluoroscopy, whatever the state of subvalvular apparatus

Adapted from Iung B, Cormier B, Ducimetiere P, et al. Immediate results of percutaneous mitral commissurotomy. Circulation. 1996; 94:2124–2130.

Western countries. For this group, some advocate immediate surgery because of the less-satisfying results of valvuloplasty, whereas others prefer valvuloplasty as an initial treatment for selected candidates, reserving the use of surgery for cases of failure or late deterioration.[30]

In this group of patients, we favor an individualistic approach that allows for the multifactorial nature of prediction. Current opinion is that surgery can be considered the treatment of choice in patients with bicommissural or heavy calcification. On the other hand, in our opinion, PMC can be attempted as a first approach in patients with extensive lesions of the subvalvular apparatus or moderate or unicommissural calcification—more so if their clinical status argues in favor of it. Surgery should be considered reasonably early if the results are unsatisfactory or there is secondary deterioration.

CONCLUSION

Large-scale use of the technique would be beneficial in developing countries, where mitral stenosis occurs frequently in patients with anatomy favorable for PMC.

In industrialized countries, the problems are different because most candidates are older, with somewhat less favorable anatomy. Careful evaluation of immediate and long-term results in this population is still needed to clearly define the respective indications for PMC and valve replacement. This process will be improved through better imaging, especially 3D echocardiography. Further improvement may be achieved through combining PMC with other interventional

and only moderate subvalvular disease (echocardiography score <8).[26] Randomized studies comparing valvuloplasty with surgical commissurotomy showed that valvuloplasty is at least comparable to surgical commissurotomy in terms of efficacy and is no doubt more comfortable for the patient.[27,28] In practice, PMC has virtually replaced surgical commissurotomy.[29] In addition, if restenosis occurs, patients treated by valvuloplasty can undergo repeat balloon catheterization or surgery without the difficulties and inherent risk resulting from pericardial adhesions and chest wall scarring.

On the other hand, much remains to be done to refine the indications for other patients, especially those with unfavorable anatomy, who are more common in procedures such as closure of left atrial appendage or ablation of the pulmonary veins, or perhaps in a more distant future percutaneous mitral valve replacement in case of failure or deterioration after PMC.

The good results that have been obtained with PMC enable us to say that, currently, this technique has an important place in the treatment of mitral stenosis and has virtually replaced surgical commissurotomy. Finally, in our opinion, when treating mitral stenosis, PMC and valve replacement must be considered not as rivals but complementary techniques, each applicable at the appropriate stage of the disease.

REFERENCES

1. Inoue K, Owaki T, Nakamura T, et al. Clinical application of transvenous mitral commissurotomy by a new balloon catheter. *J Thorac Cardiovasc Surg.* 1984;87:394–402.

2. Marijon E, Iung B, Mocumbi AO, et al. What are the differences in presentation of candidates for percutaneous mitral commissurotomy across the world and do they influence the results of the procedure? *Arch Cardiovasc Dis.* 2008;10:611–617.

3. Iung B, Nicoud-Houel A, Fondard O, et al. Temporal trends in percutaneous mitral commissurotomy over a 15-year period. *Eur Heart J.* 2004;25:701–707.

4. Silvestry FE, Kerber RE, Brook MM, et al. Echocardiography-guided interventions. *J Am Soc Echocardiogr.* 2009;22:213–231.

5. Messika–Zeitoun D, Brochet E, Holmin C, et al. Three-dimensional evaluation of the mitral valve area and comissural opening before and after percutaneous mitral commissurotomy in patients with mitral stenosis. *Eur Heart J.* 2007;28:72–79.

6. Palacios IF, Sanchez PL, Harrell LC, et al. Which patients benefit from percutaneous mitral balloon valvuloplasty? Prevalvuloplasty and postvalvuloplasty variables that predict long-term outcome. *Circulation.* 2002;105:1465–1471.

7. Arora R, Kalra GS, Sing S, et al. Percutaneous transvenous mitral commissurotomy: immediate and long-term follow-up results. *Catheter Cardiovasc Interv.* 2002;55:450–456.

8. Chen CR, Cheng TO. Percutaneous balloon mitral valvuloplasty by the Inoue technique: a multicenter study of 4832 patients in China. *Am Heart J.* 1995;129:1197–1202.

9. Varma PK, Theodore S, Neema PK, et al. Emergency surgery after percutaneous transmitral commissurotomy: operative versus echocardiographic findings, mechanisms of complications, and outcomes. *J Thorac Cardiovasc Surg.* 2005;130:772–776.

10. Kim MJ, Song JK, Song JM, et al. Long-term outcomes of significant mitral regurgitation after percutaneous mitral valvuloplasty. *Circulation.* 2006;114:2815–2822.

11. Cruz-Gonzalez I, Sanchez-Ledesma M, Martin-Moreiras J, et al. Predicting success and long-term outcomes of percutaneous mitral valvuloplasty: a multifactorial score. *Am J Med.* 2009;122:581.e11–e19.

12. Iung B, Garbarz E, Michaud P, et al. Late results of percutaneous mitral commissurotomy in a series of 1024 patients. Analysis of late clinical deterioration: frequency, anatomic findings, and predictive factors. *Circulation.* 1999;99:3272–3278.

13. Song JK, Song JM, Kang DH, et al. Restenosis and adverse clinical events after successful percutaneous mitral valvuloplasty: immediate post-procedural mitral valve area as an important prognosticator *Eur Heart J.* 2009;30:1254–1262.

14. Messika-Zeitoun D, Blanc J, Iung B, et al. Impact of degree of commissural opening after percutaneous mitral commissurotomy on long-term outcome. *JACC Cardiovasc Imaging.* 2009;2:1–7.

15. Wang A, Krasuski RA, Warner JJ, et al. Serial echocardiographic evaluation of restenosis after successful percutaneous mitral commissurotomy. *J Am Coll Cardiol.* 2002;39:328–334.

16. Fawzy ME, Shoukri M, Al Buraiki J, et al. Seventeen years clinical and echocardiographic follow up of mitral balloon valvuloplasty in 520 patients, and predictors of long-term outcome. *J Heart Valve Dis.* 2007;16:454–460.

17. Turgeman Y, Atar S, Suleiman K, et al. Feasibility, safety, and morphologic predictors of outcome of repeat percutaneous balloon mitral commissurotomy. *Am J Cardiol.* 2005;95:989–991.

18. Chiang CW, Lo SK, Ko YS, et al. Predictors of systemic embolism in patients with mitral stenosis: a prospective study. *Ann Intern Med.* 1998;128:885–889.

19. Krasuski RA, Assar MD, Wang A, et al. Usefulness of percutaneous balloon mitral commissurotomy in preventing the development of atrial fibrillation in patients with mitral stenosis. *Am J Cardiol.* 2004;93:936–939.

20. Fawzy ME, Hassan W, Shoukri M, et al. Immediate and long-term results of mitral balloon valvotomy for restenosis following previous surgical or balloon mitral commissurotomy. *Am J Cardiol.* 2005;96:971–975.

21. Esteves C, Munoz J, Braga S, et al. Immediate and long-term follow-up of percutaneous balloon mitral valvuloplasty in pregnant patients with rheumatic mitral stenosis. *Am J Cardiol.* 2006;98:812–816.

22. Bonow RO, Carabello BA, Chatterjee K, et al. ACC/AHA 2006 guidelines for the management of patients with valvular heart disease: a report of the American College of Cardiology/American Heart Association Task Force on Practice Guidelines. *J Am Coll Cardiol.* 2006;48:e1–e148.

23. Vahanian A, Baumgartner H, Bax J, et al. Guidelines on the management of valvular heart disease: The Task Force on the Management of Valvular Heart Disease of the European Society of Cardiology. *Eur Heart J.* 2007;28:230–268.

24. Silaruks S, Thinkhamrop B, Kiatchoosakun S, et al. Resolution of left atrial thrombus after 6 months

of anticoagulation in candidates for percutaneous transvenous mitral commissurotomy. *Ann Intern Med.* 2004;140:101–105.

25. Song H, Kang DH, Kim JH, et al. Percutaneous mitral valvuloplasty versus surgical treatment in mitral stenosis with severe tricuspid regurgitation. *Circulation.* 2007;116(suppl):I246–I250.

26. Gamra H, Betbout F, Ben Hamda K, et al. Balloon mitral commissurotomy in juvenile rheumatic mitral stenosis: A ten-year clinical and echocardiographic actuarial results. *Eur Heart J.* 2003;24:1349–1356.

27. Ben Fahrat M, Ayari M, Maatouk F. Percutaneous balloon versus surgical closed and open mitral commissurotomy: seven-year follow-up results of a randomized trial. *Circulation.* 1998;97:245–250.

28. Song JK, Kim MJ, Yun SC, et al. Long-term outcomes of percutaneous mitral balloon valvuloplasty versus open cardiac surgery. *J Thorac Cardiovasc Surg.* 2010;139:103–110.

29. Iung B, Baron G, Butchart EG, et al. A prospective survey of patients with valvular heart disease in Europe: The Euro Heart Survey on valvular heart disease. *Eur Heart J.* 2003;13:1231–1243.

30. Iung B, Garbarz E, Doutrelant L, et al. Late results of percutaneous mitral commissurotomy for calcific mitral stenosis. *Am J Cardiol.* 2000;85:1308–1314.

CHAPTER 23

Percutaneous Mitral Valve Repair: Edge-to-Edge Approach

Mehmet Cilingiroglu and Ted Feldman

In 1991, Alfieri and his colleagues were first to describe the surgical repair of anterior leaflet mitral valve prolapse using an edge-to-edge technique by opposing the middle scallops of the anterior and posterior leaflets with a stitch, creating a so-called dual or double-orifice mitral valve (Fig. 23-1).[1-3] The clinical success and simplicity of this technique, sometimes called edge-to-edge repair, prompted interest in development of a catheter-based technology that would enable the interventional cardiologist to perform a percutaneous, endovascular valve repair in the cardiac catheterization laboratory. During the last decade, MitraClip (Abbott Laboratories, Abbott Park, IL) has rapidly evolved as a percutaneous method of creating an edge-to-edge mitral valve repair using a transseptal approach.[4-9] The MitraClip has received CE Mark approval and has widespread use in Europe, where a high proportion of patients are at high risk for surgery. In the United States, the ultimate application of the device will depend on the results of the randomized Endovascular Valve Edge-to-edge Repair Study (EVEREST) II trial.

MITRACLIP DEVICE AND SYSTEM DESCRIPTION

The MitraClip system consists of a steerable guide catheter and a clip delivery system (CDS), which includes the detachable clip itself (Fig. 23-2). The clip is a Dacron-covered mechanical device with two arms that are opened and closed by control mechanisms on the CDS. The two arms have a span of approximately 2 cm when opened in the grasping position (Fig. 23-3); the width of the clip is 4 mm. On the inner portion of the clip is a U-shaped "gripper" that matches up to each arm and helps to stabilize the leaflets from the atrial aspect as they are captured during closure of the clip arms. Leaflet tissue is secured between the arms and each side of the gripper, and the clip is then closed and locked to effect and maintain coaptation of the two leaflets (Fig. 23-3).

The tip of the guide catheter is delivered to the left atrium (LA) using transseptal approach over a guidewire and tapered dilator. The guide catheter is 24 French proximally and tapers to 22 French at the point where it crosses the atrial septum. A steering knob on the proximal end of the guide catheter marked as $+/-$ allows for flexion and movement of the distal tip.

PROCEDURAL STEPS

The MitraClip repair procedure consists of four main steps:

1. Transseptal puncture, septal, dilatation, and steerable guide catheter insertion
2. Steering/positioning of the guide catheter and CDS
3. Leaflet grasping, leaflet insertion assessment, and clip closure
4. MitraClip deployment and system removal

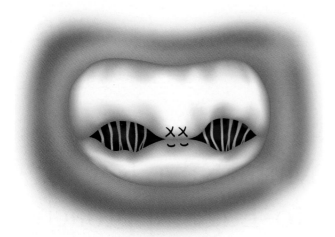

FIGURE 23-1.

Double-orifice surgical mitral valve repair with suture. Surgical repair of anterior leaflet prolapse using edge-to-edge technique by opposing the middle scallops of the anterior and posterior leaflets with a stitch creating a so-called dual- or double-orifice mitral valve.

The procedure is performed under general anesthesia using fluoroscopy and primarily transesophageal echocardiographic (TEE) guidance. It is critical that the interventional operator and the echocardiographer have a common language and understanding for the basic procedural TEE views, so that a clear communication can be maintained during the procedure.

Vascular Access

A 6 French arterial and an 8 French venous sheath are placed in the left femoral artery and vein, respectively.

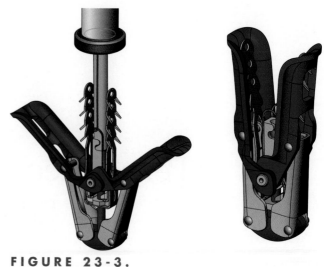

FIGURE 23-3.

Schematic drawing of the components of the clip. On the inner portion of the clip, there is a U-shaped gripper that matches up to each arm and helps to stabilize the leaflets from the atrial aspect as they are captured during closure of the clip arms. Leaflet tissue is secured between the arms and each side of the gripper, and the clip is then closed and locked to effect and maintain coaptation of the two leaflets.

A 14 French sheath is placed in the right femoral vein for transseptal access and guide catheter delivery. Using the left femoral access, a 7 French, balloon-tipped pulmonary artery catheter and a 6 French pigtail left ventricular (LV) catheter are placed. Cardiac output and baseline pulmonary capillary wedge, LV, and pulmonary artery pressures are measured. An activated clotting time (ACT) of 250 to 300 seconds is

FIGURE 23-2.

MitraClip system components (Abbott Laboratories, Abbott Park, IL). The valve repair system uses a detachable clip and a triaxial catheter system with a steerable guide catheter and a clip delivery system.

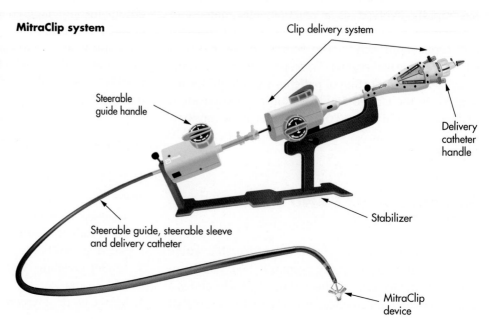

MitraClip system

Steerable guide handle

Clip delivery system

Delivery catheter handle

Steerable guide, steerable sleeve and delivery catheter

Stabilizer

MitraClip device

maintained throughout the procedure, with ACT measurements every half an hour.

Transseptal Puncture and Steerable Guide Catheter Insertion

Initially, an 8 French Mullins sheath and then a transseptal needle are advanced into the right atrium. Because of the need to approach the mitral valve at appropriate angles in all three planes of the valve (in order to assure successful and adequate grasping of the mitral leaflets), it is critical that the transseptal puncture be placed relatively posterior and relatively "high" in the fossa ovalis. This "high" puncture allows an adequate working space and distance above the mitral leaflets (ideal height from the puncture point to the plane of the mitral annulus should be 3.5–4 cm) for the delivery catheter manipulations, clip opening, and clip retraction during the grasping maneuver (Fig. 23-4A–C). If the transseptal puncture is placed too "low" in the fossa, the guide catheter tip may lie just above and too close to the mitral annular plane and subsequent orientation of the CDS, therefore, to position the clip appropriately and grasp the leaflets may not be possible because of the inadequate space in the LA above the annular plane. The transseptal puncture should also be optimally positioned from the anteroposterior perspective as posterior in the limbus of the fossa ovalis in order to enable guide tip positioning near the line of leaflet coaptation

(Fig. 23-4B). Using the TEE short-axis view at the base of the heart, position of the potential puncture site is evaluated prior to needle advancement. The "tenting" of the atrial septum can be seen as the transseptal needle is pushed against the septum (Fig. 23-4B). Using the long-axis, four-chamber view, the catheter tip should be moved to as "high" a position as possible while remaining in the fossa ovalis (Fig. 23-4C). Transseptal puncture should be only performed if such tenting is clearly seen in both of these views (Fig. 23-4B,C). IV heparin is given (50–70 units/kg) to achieve ACT ≥250 sec.

After the appropriate transseptal puncture is achieved and the LA-LV pressure is measured at baseline, a 0.035-inch, 260-cm, extra stiff, J-tipped guidewire is placed ideally in the left superior pulmonary vein or, alternatively, looped in the LA (Fig. 23-5).

After removal of Mullins sheath and the dilator, the Evalve guide catheter (Abbott Laboratories) and dilator assembly are advanced into the atrial septum and the puncture site is dilated to accommodate the 22 French guide catheter by gentle pressure and forward movement of the dilator tip, which can be visualized by echocardiography because of echogenic coils in the dilator tip (Fig. 23-6). Once the dilator tip is half to three-quarters across the septum, a few seconds wait is often useful to allow the atrial septum to stretch. Advancement of the guide catheter tip across the septum is usually easier afterward. It is important not to place guide catheter tip too far into the LA, but

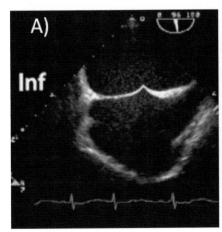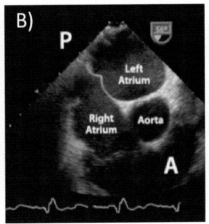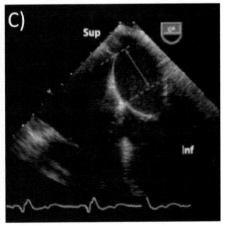

FIGURE 23-4.

Transseptal puncture guided by transesophageal echocardiography (TEE). Using TEE bi-caval **(A)** and short-axis views at the base of the heart **(B)**, position of the puncture site is evaluated, and tenting of the atrial septum can be seen as the transseptal needle is pushed against it. The tenting should be close to the posterior edge in the short-axis view and close to the superior edge of the fossa ovalis in the bicaval view. Afterward, using long-axis, four-chamber view **(C)**, the catheter tip should be moved to as high a position (at least 3 cm above the plane of the mitral valve) as possible while remaining in the fossa ovalis. Transseptal puncture should be only performed if such tenting is clearly seen in both of these views **(B,C)**.

FIGURE 23-5.

Advancement of a Mullins sheath and dilator over the guidewire into the left atrium (LA). After transseptal puncture, an 8 French Mullins sheath and dilator are advanced into the LA using a 260-cm, 0.035-inch, extra stiff, J-tipped Amplatzer guidewire (AGA Medical Corporation, Plymouth, MN) **(A)**. Ideally, the tip of the guidewire should be in the left upper pulmonary vein **(B)**.

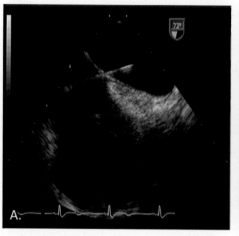
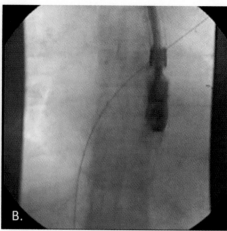

rather to aim for a position of its tip about 1 or 2 cm across the atrial septum in the short-axis view at the base (Fig. 23-7).

Steering the Guide Catheter and Clip Delivery System to the Mitral Line of Coaptation

Using the short- and long-axis atrial views by TEE, the location of the distal tip of the guide catheter tip relative to the mitral valve plane must be determined (parallel vs. perpendicular) (Fig. 23-8A). Ideally, the initial guide catheter position is perpendicular to the mitral valve plane, so that its clockwise rotation moves its tip out of the short axis on TEE. If the guide catheter tip is parallel to the mitral valve plane, tip deflection will flex the guide catheter in the short-axis plane on TEE.

It is critical to carefully de-air the guide catheter upon removal of the dilator and guide assembly once the guide catheter tip is 1 to 2 cm across the atrial septum prior to advancement of CDS. TEE and fluoroscopic guidance are both necessary as the CDS exits the guide catheter tip to ensure that the tip of the clip

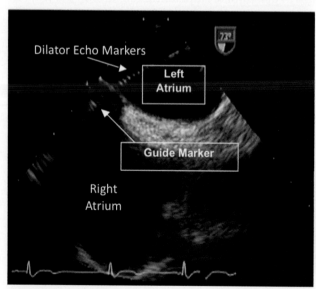

FIGURE 23-6.

Dilation of septum. The guide catheter and dilator tip are advanced slowly through the atrial septum by gradually advancing the dilator and steerable guide catheter assembly into the left atrium. The dilator is identified by its echo signature, which has a dashed or spiral appearance.

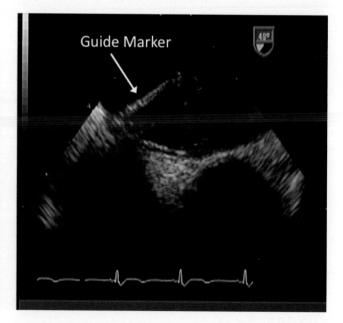

FIGURE 23-7.

Advancement of guide catheter into the left atrium (LA). It is very important not to place the guide catheter tip too far into the LA to avoid contact with LA walls, but rather to aim for a position of its tip about 1 or 2 cm across the atrial septum, in the center of LA in the short-axis view at the base.

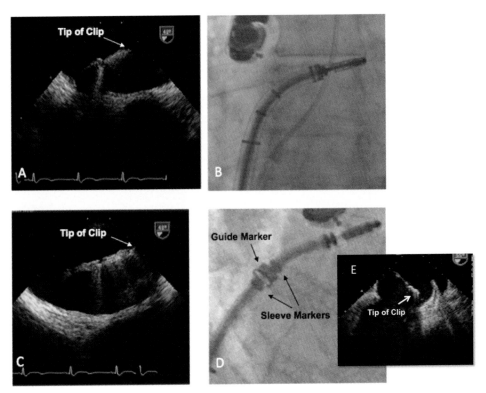

FIGURE 23-8.

A–E: Steering and positioning of MitraClip (Abbott Laboratories, Abbott Park, IL) clip delivery system (CDS) in the left atrium (LA). The CDS is advanced until its tip is even with the guide tip under fluoroscopy guidance. Then, the CDS is further advanced into the LA while observing MitraClip device in short axis at the base or two-chamber intercommissural transesophageal echocardiography views to avoid tissue contact **(A,B)**. The CDS is further advanced until the guide tip marker is centered between the sleeve markers, as determined by fluoroscopy. Afterward, the CDS is steered down toward the mitral valve **(C–E)**.

remains away from the atrial wall (Fig. 23-8A–D). The midesophageal, two-chamber, long-axis (intercommissural) view allows for evaluation of the clip location medially and laterally along the line of mitral coaptation (Fig. 23-8E). The midesophageal, long-axis, left ventricular outflow tract (LVOT) view allows for assessment of clip location anteriorly or posteriorly within the mitral orifice. The transgastric short-axis view is the best view for evaluation of clip arm orientation and supplants the intercommissural view for assessment of device position along the line of coaptation. Mitral leaflet grasping during pullback of the CDS is often best monitored in the LVOT view in order to observe the anterior and posterior leaflet capture within the open clip arms.

Once the clip and the CDS are safely outside the guide catheter tip and fluoroscopic CDS sleeve markers as seen to appropriately straddle the radiopaque marker on the guide catheter tip (Fig. 23-8D), the first adjustments in position are made to direct the clip medially toward the apex of the heart and thereby toward the mitral orifice. Typically, this can be achieved by turning the M knob (medial flexion of CDS) and modestly torquing the guide catheter clockwise (posterior) to avoid contacting either the posterior left atrial wall or the anteriorly located aortic root (Fig. 23-8C). The delivery catheter of the CDS tends to advance when deflection is applied to the steerable sheath of the CDS,

thereby requiring periodic withdrawal of the delivery catheter handle.

Fine adjustments in steering can be used incrementally to align the clip and delivery catheter parallel with the long axis of the heart and perpendicular to the mitral valve opening. Incremental medial steering changes of the CDS or modest advancement or withdrawal of guide catheter allow movement of the clip tip to a position just over the middle scallops of the anterior (A2) and posterior (P2) leaflets of the mitral valve. Using the LVOT view, further fine steering movements in the anteroposterior direction (by small amounts of rotation of the guide catheter [counterclockwise for anterior, clockwise for posterior] or using the A/P knob) are made to move the clip to the appropriate position (Fig. 23-9A,B). These views must be checked several times to be certain that movement in one plane has not changed the position of the catheter in the orthogonal plane.

The delivery catheter is then advanced 1 to 2 cm to assess the trajectory of the clip. Once in the correct position in both planes (LVOT and intercommissural views), the color flow jet is evaluated. If the orientation of the clip is correct, the clip will split the mitral regurgitation (MR) jet in both views (Fig. 23-9C). Both the guide catheter and the CDS can be advanced or pulled back slightly as one unit by pushing or pulling the stabilizing platform to help position the clip over

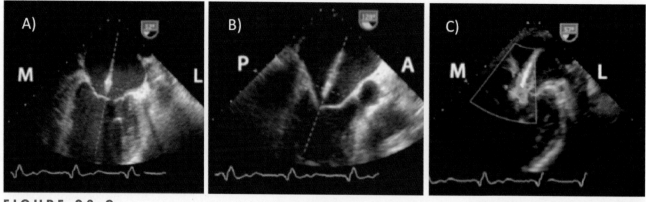

FIGURE 23-9.

A–C: Steering of clip toward the mitral valve. The MitraClip device (Abbott Laboratories, Abbott Park, IL) is steered down until the trajectory is perpendicular to the line between the annular hinge points of the mitral valve in both the left ventricular outflow tract (anteroposterior alignment) and two-chamber intercommissural (M-L alignment) imaging planes **(A,B)**. The clip is positioned over mitral regurgitation jet origin to split the jet **(C)**. ML, medial-lateral alignment.

the origin of the MR jet without significantly changing delivery catheter trajectory. While forward advancement moves the system laterally, withdrawal moves it toward the medial commissure. Clockwise and counterclockwise guide catheter manipulation helps to adjust device position anteriorly and posteriorly without significantly affecting delivery catheter trajectory. The

clip is then opened to 180 degrees, and the grippers are fully raised using fluoroscopy and TEE (Fig. 23-10A,B).

Transgastric short-axis view is used to rotate the clip so that the orientation of the clip arms is perpendicular to the line of coaptation (Fig. 23-10C,D). This step is critical as significant deviation from perpendicular alignment may result in inadequate grasp of one of the

FIGURE 23-10.

Opening of clip arms. Clip arms are opened to 180 degrees and aligned perpendicular to the line of coaptation in left ventricular outflow tract (LVOT) view. In the LVOT view, the open arms should be visible and symmetric **(A)**. Arm alignments are checked again in two-chamber intercommissural and also transgastric short axis views **(B,C)**.

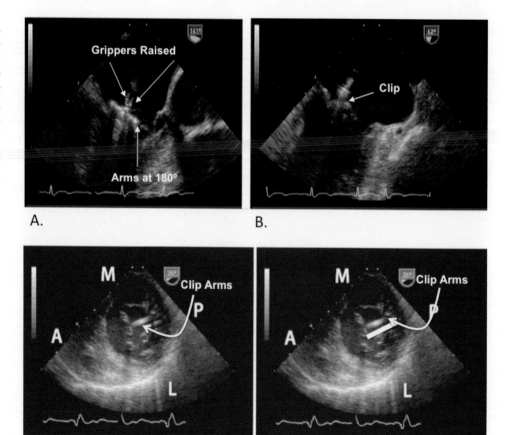

mitral leaflets. Multiple, short, to-and-fro motions are made with the delivery catheter handle during rotation of the clip to orient the clip arms and relieve the torque, which tends to be stored within the CDS. After perpendicular clip arm alignment is achieved, the clip is advanced into the LV so that the clip arms are under the free edges of the mitral leaflets (Fig. 23-11A,B). Free motion of the leaflet edges is important to note, and restriction of the leaflets by the clip arms means the clip is not far enough below the free edges to achieve a successful grasp. Generally, the most proximal portion of the gripper must be beneath the leaflets.

Using LVOT and short-axis views, a final check of the perpendicular orientation is performed with the clip in the LV to be sure that no deviation of clip arm orientation to the mitral leaflets (Fig. 23-11A,B). If there is deviation, then clip arms can be everted and the clip withdrawn into the LA, where readjustments to the

position can be made. Another passage to the LV can be made because of clip position adjustment while it is in LV is very limited and not recommended.

Leaflet Grasping, Leaflet Insertion Assessment, and Clip Closure

The leaflets are grasped by pulling back the delivery catheter in the LVOT view while the clip arms are open approximately 120 degrees (Fig. 23-12A,B). The leaflets tend to fall into the clip as the clip with this simple pullback. The pullback should be done in a slow, smooth manner to capture the leaflet edges. If atrial fibrillation is present, more than one attempt may be needed to capture both leaflets. When the open clip arms successfully immobilize the leaflets, then the grippers are quickly lowered and the clip is closed to about 60 degrees (Fig. 23-12C–E). A successful grasp captures the mitral leaflets and produces a double-orifice mitral valve with immediate reduction in the degree of MR (Fig. 23-12F). Careful interrogation in the LVOT view using slow motion frame analysis is critical to make sure that both leaflets are well captured by the clip arms (Fig. 23-12B). If there is significant motion of the mitral leaflet just as it enters the clip, the resulting grasp may not be adequate for a long-term result, with risk of escape of the leaflet from the clip. Release of the clip and repeat grasping is then necessary. If the leaflets are stable and immobile at the clip entry point, an adequate grasp has been achieved. The presence of a stable double orifice should be confirmed in the short-axis view (Fig. 23-12F).

Multiple TEE views with color and pulsed-wave Doppler should be used to evaluate the reduction in MR. Although the clip has not been completely closed at this point, a significant reduction in MR jet is expected. Once adequate leaflet insertion has been confirmed at 60 degrees of clip closure, the clip is further closed slowly until the leaflets are coapted and MR is maximally reduced. Leaflet insertion assessment is repeated using LVOT, intercommissural, and transgastric short-axis views.

MitraClip Deployment and System Removal

Prior to clip release, the patient's systolic blood pressure should be raised using an alpha agonist, and the extent of the MR jet reevaluated. An afterload challenge is important to be sure that the MR reduction will be sustained at the patient's baseline blood pressure and afterload. It is also important to remove back tension from the delivery catheter and the leaflets by slightly advancing the CDS to allow proper assessment of the

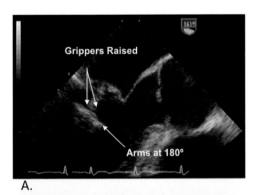

A.

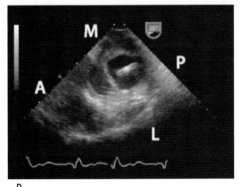

B.

FIGURE 23-11.

Crossing the mitral valve with the clip. After the proper alignment is achieved, the clip is advanced into the left ventricle so that the clip arms are under the free edges of the mitral leaflets **(A)**. Free motion of the leaflet edges is important to note, and restriction of the leaflets by the clip arms means it is not far enough below the free edges to achieve a successful grasp. Using left ventricular outflow tract and short-axis views, a final check of the perpendicular orientation is performed with the clip in the left ventricle to be sure there is no deviation of clip orientation to the mitral leaflets **(B)**.

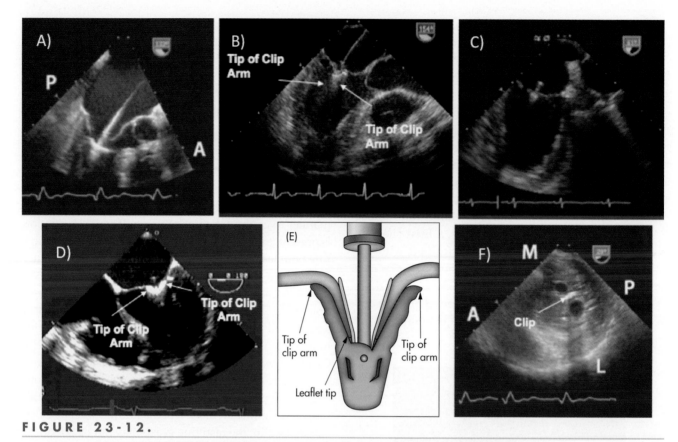

FIGURE 23-12.

Grasping of leaflets. The leaflets are grasped by retracting the delivery catheter slowly as the mitral leaflets are closing in systole in the left ventricular outflow tract view **(A,B)**. If the leaflets are successfully immobilized by the open clip arms, then the grippers are quickly lowered and clip is closed to about 60 degrees **(C–E)**. When fully inserted, the leaflets should appear to enter the center of the clip in the two-chamber intercommissural view, and leaflets should be stable medial and lateral to the clip **(C)**. This can also be confirmed in the four-chamber view **(D,E)**. Finally, the MitraClip device (Abbott Laboratories, Abbott Park, IL) is assessed in the left ventricle to confirm that the clip arms are perpendicular to the line of coaptation in transgastric short-axis view. There should also be medial and lateral contact between the anterior and posterior leaflet during diastole adjacent to the MitraClip device. **F:** The double orifice is seen on a short-axis view.

amount of residual MR. Once the desired end point is achieved, the clip is released under fluoroscopic guidance (Fig. 23-13A). Prior to release, the function of the locking mechanism is confirmed by rotation of the lock mechanism counterclockwise toward the open position to show that the clip remains closed and locked. The lock control line is then removed by pulling the line slowly, during which the operator can feel the line withdraw during each cardiac cycle. The clip is released, and then the gripper line is pulled slowly and removed in the same manner as the lock line. Removal of these two lines are the last steps, finally resulting in irreversible placement of the clip.

Right anterior oblique caudal or left anterior oblique cranial views may be used for a side view of the clip to confirm the degree of clip closure after its deployment and also to ensure that a modest space is maintained between the delivery catheter tip and the clip during lock

and gripper line withdrawal. The CDS can be removed after the clip is free and lines have been withdrawn. It is critical that the tip of the CDS is carefully retracted back into the guide catheter to avoid the damage to the LA.

Careful and reverse steering with slow retraction of the CDS back into the guide catheter is performed using TEE (Fig. 23-13B). Once the CDS is retracted, the guide catheter is withdrawn into the right atrium (Fig. 23-13C) and removed from the insertion site using figure-of-eight subcutaneous sutures, which are removed after several hours. In approximately 40% of cases, a second clip placement could be necessary for procedural success (≤2+ residual MR). If that is the case, a second CDS is advanced via the guiding catheter in the similar way as previously described, except during mitral valve crossing. The remaining steps are similar, with an important exception. While a first clip is passed from LA to LV with the clip arms open to about

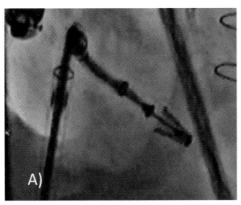
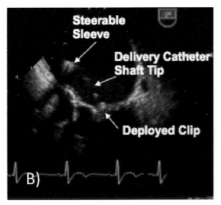
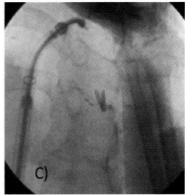

FIGURE 23-13.

MitraClip device (Abbott Laboratories, Abbott Park, IL) deployment and system removal. Once the optimal reduction in mitral regurgitation jet is achieved, the clip is released using fluoroscopy guidance **(A)**. Right anterior oblique caudal or left anterior oblique cranial views may be used for side view of the clip after deployment. It is critical that the tip of the delivery catheter must be carefully retracted back into the guide catheter to avoid damage to the left atrium. Careful and reverse steering with slow retraction of the clip delivery system back into the guide catheter is performed using transesophageal echocardiography **(B)**. Once the clip delivery system is retracted, the guide catheter is withdrawn into the right atrium and removed **(C)**. Hemodynamic measurements, mainly simultaneous left ventricle and pulmonary capillary wedge pressures, are repeated after clip placement.

180 degrees, the second clip is passed from LA to LV in a closed position, to avoid dislodging the first clip.

PATIENT SELECTION

Careful evaluation of the echocardiographic morphology of the mitral leaflets is critical for good patient selection (Fig. 23-14). Patients with either degenerative

or functional MR have been successfully treated. A coaptation length of at least 2 mm is ideal. Thus, some tissue from both leaflets should be in contact, so that there is some tissue to grasp with the clip. Although it is possible to grasp leaflets with less coaptation length, there is very little experience with longer term outcomes in this setting. With a flail mitral leaflet, a flail gap no greater than 10 mm or a flail width on short

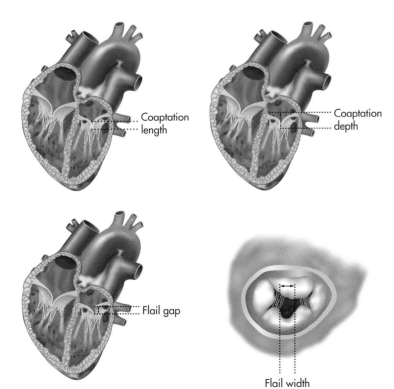

FIGURE 23-14.

Specific morphologic features of the mitral valve are required for the Evalve MitraClip (Abbott Laboratories, Abbott Park, IL) to have a good probability of success. There must be 2 mm or more coaptation length for the clip to be grasped. A flail gap larger than 10 mm makes success of adequate reduction in mitral regurgitation unlikely, as does a flail width of more than 15 mm. The need for some coaptation length effectively excludes patients with an extremely dilated mitral annulus. In these cases, left ventricular failure with chamber and annular dilatation causes the leaflet edges to be pulled apart. Annuloplasty is more likely necessary in this anatomic setting.

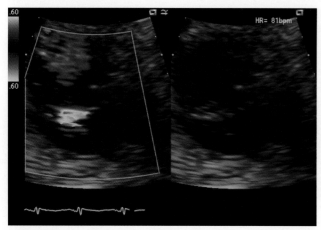

FIGURE 23-15.

The mitral regurgitation jet must arise from the central two-thirds of the line of coaptation as seen on short-axis color Doppler examination.

axis estimation less than 15 mm are also important anatomic features. The MR jet must arise from the central two-thirds of the line of coaptation as seen on short-axis color Doppler examination (Fig. 23-15). It is common for most clinical transthoracic echocardiographic exams to either omit the short-axis color Doppler interrogation of the mitral valve, or to have very little. Adequate evaluation for this therapy requires careful scanning of the mitral funnel to be sure that the jet origin is central and ideally, relatively discrete. The baseline mitral valve area should be greater than 4 cm², because placement of the clip significantly diminishes the mitral valve area and this attention to baseline mitral area is necessary to avoid the creation of mitral stenosis after clip placement. Clinically important mitral stenosis has not been created in our experience to date because of careful attention to the baseline mitral valve area during the patient screening and selection process.

MITRACLIP TRIAL OUTCOMES

The MitraClip system has been successfully evaluated in U.S. phase I and II clinical trials (EVEREST).[8-17] Patients treated to date in the Evalve EVEREST have been selected using the American Heart Association-American College of Cardiology guideline recommendations for surgical mitral valve repair. Patients with moderate to severe or severe MR (3-4+), judged by quantitative assessment of the degree of regurgitation using the American Society for Echocardiography quantitative scoring system have been included. All of

the echocardiograms were evaluated in a core laboratory. Echocardiographic anatomic inclusion criteria included specific leaflet morphologic findings to determine if adequate tissue was available and the location of the MR jet origin (from the central two-thirds of the line of coaptation). Patients were symptomatic, or if asymptomatic, had evidence of LV dysfunction for inclusion for treatment with the MitraClip.

EVEREST I, a phase I trial, has been completed in a cohort of 55 patients. Registry data from a nonrandomized group of 107 patients, 21 as well as outcomes in a high-risk cohort of 78 patients, have been reported. The primary endpoint of the EVEREST I trial was safety at 30 days. Safety was defined as freedom from death, myocardial infarction, cardiac tamponade, and cardiac surgery for failed clip or device, clip detachment, permanent stroke, or septicemia. A clip was placed successfully in about 90% of cases. Of those who achieve acute procedural success, defined as adequate reduction in MR (<2+ residual MR) without a procedural complication, two-thirds were alive and had no need for repeat procedures after 2-year follow-up. In a high-risk group of 78 patients, in addition to improvement in New York Heart Association functional class, favorable ventricular remodeling with a decrease in LV systolic and diastolic dimensions and reduction in the need for hospitalizations among high-risk patients has been demonstrated. Compared to match controls who were also considered high risk for surgery, there was improved 1-year survival.

On an intent-to-treat basis, 96 (90%) of the 107 EVEREST registry patients achieved a reduction in MR from either the clip or subsequent mitral valve surgery after attempted clip. Of the patients with acute procedure success, 64% were discharged with mild MR (1+) and 13% had MR graded as mild to moderate (1-2+). Thus, 77% had <2+ MR. About 40% of patients were treated with two clips. The composite primary efficacy end point (freedom from MR >2+, cardiac surgery for valve dysfunction, and from death for the per-protocol population at 1 year) was 66%, not including crossover to surgery. Three-year freedom from reoperation was just below 80%. Results have been similar in both degenerative and functional MR.

In-hospital and 30-day complications in the EVEREST registry included major adverse events in 9% of 107 patients. There was no procedural mortality. Bleeding requiring transfusion was the most common event, comprising almost half of the adverse events. There was one periprocedural stroke and one postprocedure death. One patient underwent reoperation for failed surgical mitral valve repair 19 days after valve repair after an unsuccessful MitraClip procedure, and one patient required ventilation for 20 days. No clip embolization has occurred at any time point. Partial clip detachment is the most important mechanical problem with the procedure. This occurred in 9% of the initial cohort and was most often detected at the protocol mandated 30-day echo exam. These partial detachments were generally not associated with symptoms. Most were treated with mitral surgery, but more recently in the registry and European experience, an additional clip has been placed. With better methods for assessment of leaflet insertion into the clip at the time of the procedure, the incidence of partial clip detachment has declined to less than 3%.

A phase II randomized trial (EVEREST II) comparing the clip with surgical repair or replacement has been completed. In this study, 279 eligible patients were prospectively randomized to percutaneous repair versus surgery using 2:1 allocation and are undergoing clinical and echocardiographic follow-up. The trial was prospective, core lab–evaluated, and event-monitored. None of the past surgical trials of mitral repair therapy have been prospective, with intention-to-treat methods or core labs. Thus, in most surgical reports, the proportion of patients for whom repair is intended but in whom replacement is ultimately performed is not clearly defined. The MR reduction results of surgical mitral repair have not been assessed using objective criteria through an echocardiography core lab with quantitative MR grading. Thus, EVEREST phase II trial is groundbreaking not only in the development of the percutaneous therapy, but also in defining the results of the mitral valve surgery in a multicenter trial. At the end of 2009, patient enrollment was completed and the 1-year follow-up time point had been reached for the entire group. The results of the trial have not yet been published, but were presented at the American College of Cardiology Annual Scientific Sessions in 2010.[17] Safety endpoints were reached in about 50% of surgery and 15% of MitraClip patients, showing superiority of safety for the percutaneous approach by intention to treat. The

1-year per protocol efficacy endpoint of the combined incidence of death, MV surgery, or reoperation for MV dysfunction was reached in about three-quarters of surgery and two-thirds of MitraClip patients, falling within the prespecified efficacy margin. A larger proportion of surgery patients had 0 to 1+ MR after 1 year. Reductions in LV volumes and dimensions were achieved in both groups after 1 year, as were improvements in New York Heart Association functional class.

The MitraClip has been approved in Europe, and early use shows a pattern weighted toward high-risk patients with about two-thirds with functional and one-third with degenerative MR. Patients treated in the initial European experience have usually been referred by surgeons.

Potential limitations of this technique include large device size (a 24 French guide catheter), technically demanding procedures and uncertainty about the long-term durability of the results since results beyond 3 years have yet to be reported. Surgical leaflet repair is almost always done in conjunction with an annuloplasty, and the surgical community sees the lack of annuloplasty as an important limitation of this approach. In addition, the feasibility and efficacy of this technique is limited to specifically suitable anatomy and is not applicable in subsets of patients with extreme pathology of leaflets including rheumatic disease or ruptured papillary muscle.

CONCLUSION

The deliberation for which treatment provides the best balance of safety and effectiveness for a given patient has long been an integral to deciding between medical management and surgery, and when surgery is an option the treatment between repair or replacement. The MitraClip procedure has recently merged as an alternative and novel percutaneous therapy for both degenerative and functional MR in selected group of patients with high surgical risk.

R E F E R E N C E S

1. Alfieri O, Maisano F, DeBonis M, et al. The Edge-to-Edge technique in mitral valve repair: a simple solution for complex problems. *J Thorac Cardiovasc Surg.* 2001;122:674–681.
2. Maisano F, Torracca L, Oppizzi M, et al. The Edge-to-edge technique: a simplified method to correct mitral insufficiency. *Eur J Cardiothorac Surg.* 1998;13:240–245.
3. Maisano F, Schreuder JJ, Oppizzi M, et al. The double orifice technique as a standardized approach to

treat mitral regurgitation due to severe myxomatous disease: surgical technique. *Eur J Cardiothorac Surg.* 2000;17:201–215.
4. Fann JI, St. Goar FG, Komtebedde J, et al. Beating heart catheter-based-edge-to-edge mitral valve procedure in a porcine model; efficacy and healing response. *Circulation.* 2004;110:988–993.
7. St. Goar FG, James FI, Komtebedde J, et al. Endovascular edge-to-edge mitral valve repair: short-term

results in a porcine model. *Circulation.* 2003;108:1990–1993.

8. Feldman T, Wasserman HS, Herrmann HC, et al. Percutaneous mitral valve repair using the edge-to-edge technique: six-month result of the EVEREST Phase-I Clinical Trial. *J Am Coll Cardiol.* 2005;46:2134–2140.

9. Feldman T, Kar S, Rinaldi M, et al. EVEREST Investigators. Percutaneous mitral repair with the MitraClip system: safety and midterm durability in the initial EVEREST (Endovascular Valve Edge-to-Edge REpair Study) cohort. *J Am Coll Cardiol.* 2009;54(8):686–694.

10. Mauri L, Garg P, Massaro J, et al. The EVEREST II Trial: design and rationale for a randomized study of the Evalve MitraClip system compared with mitral valve surgery for mitral regurgitation. *Am Heart J.* 2010;160:23–29.

11. Dang NC, Aboodi MS, Sakaguchi T, et al. Surgical revision after percutaneous mitral valve repair with a clip: initial multi-center experience. *Ann Thorac Surg.* 2005;80(6):2338–2342.

12. Argenziano M, Skipper E, Heimansohn D, et al. Surgical revision after percutaneous mitral repair with the MitraClip device. *Ann Thorac Surg.* 2010;89:72–80.

13. Herrmann H, Kar S, Siegel R, et al. Effect of percutaneous mitral repair with the MitraClip device on mitral valve area and gradient. *EuroInterv.* 2009;4:437–442.

14. Herrmann HC, Rohatgia S, Wasserman HS, et al. Effects of percutaneous edge to edge repair for mitral regurgitation on mitral valve hemodynamics. *Cathet Cardiovasc Diagn.* 2006;68:821–826.

15. Foster E, Wasserman HS, Gray W, et al. Quantitative assessment of MR severity with serial echocardiography in a multi-center clinical trial of percutaneous mitral valve repair. *Am J Cardiol.* 2007;100:1577–1583.

16. Silvestry S, Rodriguez L, Herrmann H, et al. Echocardiographic guidance and assessment of percutaneous repair for mitral regurgitation with the Evalve MitraClip: lessons learned from EVEREST I. *J Am Soc Echo.* 2007;20:1131–1140.

17. Feldman T, Mauri L, Foster E, et al. For the EVEREST II investigators: primary safety and efficacy endpoints of the EVEREST II randomized clinical trial. American College of Cardiology Scientific Sessions. Atlanta, GA; March 14–16, 2010.

CHAPTER 24

Mitral Valve Repair and Replacement: Experimental Approaches

Alexander B. Willson and John G. Webb*

T he field of transcatheter mitral valve repair and replacement excluding the MitraClip device (Abbott Laboratories, Abbott Park, IL) is yet to reach mainstream cardiology practice; however, it is an area of active research with a variety of techniques being investigated, which may potentially impact a large patient population. This field predominantly targets functional mitral regurgitation (MR) secondary to either an ischemic or nonischemic cardiomyopathy. Moderate-to-severe MR is a common problem, occurring in approximately 12% of patients postmyocardial infarction and in 20% of ischemic cardiomyopathies, where it is an independent predictor of morbidity and mortality.[1,2] The risks of surgical repair or replacement in this group is often deemed excessive and it is estimated that up to one-half of patients with severe symptomatic MR are not offered surgery due to comorbidities, notably age and impaired left ventricular function.[3]

The goal of transcatheter mitral valve therapy is to provide a less invasive, safer, and equally effective treatment option for patients at high risk of surgery. A number of transcatheter approaches to mitral valve repair have been proposed, many of which are fashioned after proven surgical therapies. Although most of these approaches to mitral repair will likely prove ineffective or have limited application, others may become viable therapeutic options. This chapter reviews the current status of experimental transcatheter mitral valve repair and replacement.

Approaches to percutaneous mitral valve repair can be categorized based on the various components of the mitral valve apparatus modified. These include the leaflets, mitral annulus, subvalvular apparatus (chordal tendineae and papillary muscles), left ventricle, and the left atrium. All are important for mitral valve function and are a potential targets for transcatheter intervention. The current status of various percutaneous therapies is presented in Table 24-1.

LEAFLET REPAIR

Complex leaflet repair is currently beyond the realm of percutaneous strategies. Surgical repair of MR due to prolapse and ruptured chords in experienced centers has high success rates with low recurrence.[4] Leaflet repair by the comparably simple Alfieri[5] approach, where the free edges of the middle anterior and posterior scallops are sutured together to create a double orifice, is, however, achievable through percutaneous approaches.

Two percutaneous leaflet repair procedures have been evaluated to date. The Mobius device (Edwards Lifesciences Inc., Irvine, CA) used a transseptal catheter to grasp the mitral leaflets using a suction port and deploy sutures. Although feasibility was demonstrated,

*Disclosure: Dr. Webb has been a consultant to Edwards Lifesciences Inc. (Irvine, CA), Guided Delivery Systems Inc. (Santa Clara, CA), Mitralign Inc. (Tewksbury, MA), Kardium Inc. (Vancouver, BC, Canada), St. Jude Medical Inc. (Minneapolis, MN), and Valtech Cardio (Tel Aviv, Israel).

TABLE 24-1 Experimental Percutaneous Mitral Valve Repair/Replacement Procedures

Mechanism	Device	Application	Vascular Approach/ Technical Aspects	Clinical Status
Edge-to-edge repair	Mobius (Edwards Life-sciences Inc., Irvine, CA)	Degenerative and functional MR	Transseptal, TEE	Not under active investigation
Coronary sinus annuloplasty	MONARC (Edwards Lifesciences Inc.)	Functional MR	Transvenous RIJ, coronary angiography	Not under active investigation
	CARILLON (Cardiac Dimensions Inc., Kirkland, WA)	Functional MR	Transvenous RIJ coronary angiography	Safety and efficacy study (TITAN)
	PTMA (Viacor Inc., Wilmington, MA)	Functional MR	Transvenous RIJ, coronary angiography	Safety and efficacy study (Ptolomeny2)
Direct mitral annuloplasty	Cardioband (Valtech Cardio, Tel Aviv, Israel)	Functional MR	Transseptal, transapical	Preclinical
	Mitralign (Mitralign Inc., Tewksbury, MA)	Functional MR	Retrograde aortic 14 French vascular access, TEE	First-in-human study
	AccuCinch (Guided Delivery Systems Inc., Santa Clara, CA)	Functional MR	Retrograde aortic 14 French vascular access, TEE	First-in-human study
Reduction in mitral orifice area	Mitral spacer (Cardiosolutions Inc., Stoughton, MA)	Functional MR	Transapical, transseptal, TEE	Preclinical
Atrial remodeling	Percutaneous septal shortening system (Ample Medical, Foster City, CA)	Functional MR	Transvenous RIJ	Not under active investigation
Left ventricular remodeling	iCoapsys (Myocor Inc., Maple Grove, MN)	Functional MR	Subxiphoid	Not under active investigation
Neochordal implantation	V Chordal adjustment system (Valtech Cardio)	Degenerative and functional MR	Transapical, transseptal, TEE	Preclinical
Percutaneous mitral valve replacement	Endovalve (Endovalve Inc., Princeton, NJ) CardiAQ (CardiAQ Valve Technologies, Inc., Irvine, CA) ValveMed	Degenerative and functional MR	Transvenous, transapical, minithoracotomy, TEE	Preclinical
Mitral valve-in-valve replacement	Edwards SAPIEN (Edwards Lifesciences Inc.)	Degenerative mitral bioprosthesis	Transapical, TEE	In clinical use

MR, mitral regurgitation; TEE, transesophageal echocardiography; RIJ, right internal jugular; PTMA, percutaneous transvenous mitral annuloplasty.

the procedure was complex and eventually abandoned.[6] In contrast, the MitraClip edge-to-edge mitral repair procedure has proven safe and often effective.[7]

Potential concerns with respect to a percutaneous edge-to-edge procedure are many. Midterm durability is established but long-term durability is not known.[7] Concomitant annular repair is thought by many to be a necessary adjunct to surgical edge-to-edge repair and, by implication, percutaneous repair.[8,9] Late implications of leaflet injury for subsequent surgical repair was an initial concern; however, repair post–MitraClip insertion has been performed.[10] This procedure has been covered in detail elsewhere in this textbook.

CORONARY SINUS ANNULOPLASTY

Surgical restrictive mitral annuloplasty using an undersized ring is a well-established method of mitral valve repair.[11] A number of percutaneous devices have attempted to reproduce the beneficial effects of surgical annuloplasty by taking advantage of the proximity of the coronary sinus to the mitral annulus. Coronary sinus annuloplasty is an indirect method of mitral annuloplasty that utilizes the close relationship of the coronary sinus to the mitral annulus. The coronary sinus and its major tributary, the great cardiac vein, parallel the annulus of the mitral valve along its

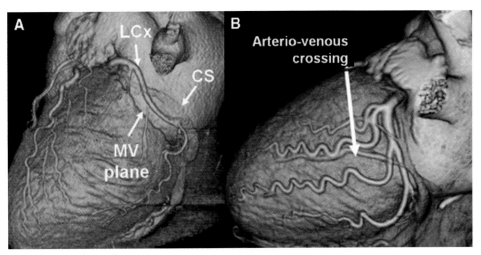

FIGURE 24-1.

Computerized tomography with three-dimensional reconstruction demonstrating the relationship of the mitral valve (*MV*), left circumflex coronary artery (*LCx*), and the coronary sinus (*CS*). **A:** The coronary sinus is on the atrial side of the mitral valve: a potential deficiency in the coronary sinus annuloplasty approaches. **B:** The close relationship between the coronary sinus and left circumflex is demonstrated—an issue with coronary artery compression in a proportion of patients undergoing coronary sinus annuloplasty.

posterior and lateral aspect (Fig. 24-1). The epicardial coronary venous system is readily accessible from the internal jugular vein as the confluence of the coronary sinus drains directly into the right atrium. Various devices (Fig. 24-2) can be introduced into the coronary sinus with the objective to displace the adjacent posterior mitral annulus toward the anterior aspect of the annulus and thereby improve coaptation of the mitral leaflets.

The coronary sinus approach is appealing for many reasons—notably, procedural simplicity with transvenous access and fluoroscopic guidance—but is also subject to several potential limitations. The coronary sinus and great cardiac vein typically lie on the atrial side of the mitral annulus rather than immediately in the plane of the annulus (Fig. 24-1). Additionally, the anatomic relationship of the sinus to the mitral annulus is highly variable.[12,13] An additional concern is that branches of the circumflex artery travel under the great cardiac vein in over one-half of the patients.[12] Coronary artery compression may occur and consequently angiographic and computed tomography anatomic screening is generally utilized.

The MONARC percutaneous transvenous annuloplasty device (Edwards Lifesciences Inc.) consists of a stent-like anchor placed in the great cardiac vein and a connecting bridge and a second anchor located proximally at the coronary sinus ostium. The compressed device can be introduced from the jugular vein utilizing

a long sheath.[14] Once positioned within the cardiac venous system, the sheath is withdrawn, thereby allowing the self-expanding nitinol alloy anchors to expand, providing fixation (Fig. 24-2B). The nitinol bridge segment is constructed like a spring with biodegradable spacers. Over a few weeks, the spacers dissolve and the bridge shortens, the anchors are drawn together, and the coronary sinus shortens further. A small feasibility study and the larger EVOLUTION I trial reported a modest reduction in MR severity and functional class in patients with functional MR; however, the benefit was small and this device is not currently being pursued.

The CARILLON mitral contour system (Cardiac Dimensions Inc., Kirkland, WA) utilizes two self-expanding helical nitinol anchors connected by a wire. The distal coronary sinus anchor is deployed, manual tension is applied to the connecting wire, and then the proximal anchor is deployed (Fig. 24-2A). Because shortening of the coronary sinus is immediate, the effect on MR and the potential for coronary compression can be readily assessed by echocardiography and angiography. If necessary, the amount of tension can be adjusted or the device can be retrieved prior to final release. Initial evaluation demonstrated a reduction in annular dimension and MR severity.[15,16] The modified CARILLON XE device was evaluated in the AMADEUS trial in 43 patients with moderate-to-severe functional MR. The device was not permanently implanted due to coronary artery compromise,

FIGURE 24-2.

Coronary sinus annuloplasty devices. **A:** CAR-ILLON XE (Cardiac Dimensions Inc., Kirkland, WA). **B:** MONARC (Edwards Lifesciences Inc., Irvine, CA). **C:** Percutaneous Transvenous Mitral Annuloplasty device (Viacor Inc., Wilmington, MA).

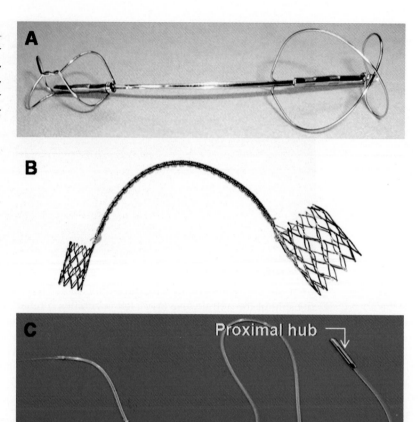

insufficient reduction in MR, or instability in 30%—and adverse events (death, myocardial infarction, coronary sinus dissection/perforation, and embolization) occurred in 15%.[17] At 6 months, there was a modest improvement in quantitative measurements of MR and functional assessment.

The Percutaneous Transvenous Mitral Annuloplasty (PTMA) device (Viacor Inc., Wilmington, MA) represents a third approach to coronary sinus annuloplasty. A catheter is inserted into the coronary sinus venous system. Metallic rods of variable length and stiffness are placed within the catheter displacing the posterior annulus anteriorly. Subsequently, rods can be exchanged through a subcutaneous implant hub positioned in a fashion similar to a pacemaker implant. Temporary implants suggested efficacy and the subsequent PTOLEMY 1 trial found a reduction of MR by at least one grade in 13 of 19 patients.[18] Unpublished results from the 29 patient PTOLEMY 2 trial (courtesy of Viacor Inc.) found a procedural success rate of 84% with a mean reduction in MR at 6 months by 1 grade in 73%.

ATRIAL REMODELING

Groups have tried to alter the direction of force applied to the mitral annulus by involving the right atrium with a coronary sinus device. The Percutaneous Septal Shortening System (PS[3]; Ample Medical Inc., Foster City, CA) utilizes transvenous access to allow placement of an anchor in the coronary sinus adjacent to the mitral P2 scallop. A transseptal puncture allows implantation of the second anchor in the interatrial septum. A magnetic catheter system facilitates placement of a wire connecting these two anchors. Tensioning this wire reduces the diameter of the mitral annulus.[19] A second similar procedure involves implanting anchors through the wall of the coronary sinus directly into the myocardium adjacent to the mitral P2 scallop and a second set of screws in the right atrium near the posteromedial trigone. Tensioning a tether between the two sets of anchors similarly remodels the mitral annulus.[20] Mitral cerclage annuloplasty is a third technique in which a guidewire is passed from the right atrium into the coronary sinus and great cardiac

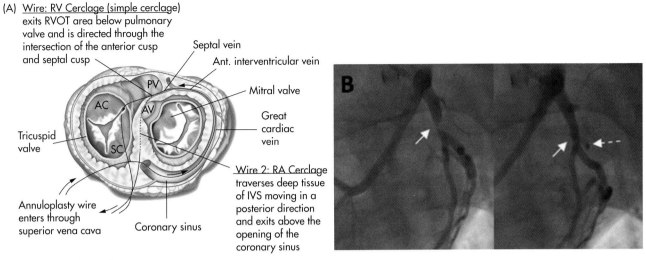

(A) <u>Wire: RV Cerclage (simple cerclage)</u> exits RVOT area below pulmonary valve and is directed through the intersection of the anterior cusp and septal cusp

Septal vein

Ant. interventricular vein

Mitral valve

Great cardiac vein

PV

AC

AV

SC

Tricuspid valve

<u>Wire 2: RA Cerclage</u> traverses deep tissue of IVS moving in a posterior direction and exits above the opening of the coronary sinus

Annuloplasty wire enters through superior vena cava

Coronary sinus

FIGURE 24-3.

Mitral cerclage annuloplasty. **A:** The guidewire can be passed into the right ventricle—however, the cerclage suture then crosses the tricuspid valve and can interfere with function—or via a more challenging pathway into the right atrium. **B:** Nitinol sleeve (*dotted arrow*) demonstrating treatment of coronary artery compression (*solid arrow*).

vein. It is then passed via a septal perforator into the right atrium where it is snared and exchanged for a suture which is fixed under tension (Fig. 24-3).[21] Animal studies have demonstrated that these techniques are feasible and may be associated with reductions in MR; however, due to complexity and modest benefit, they are not being aggressively pursued.

DIRECT ANNULOPLASTY

Direct modification of the mitral annulus aims to replicate surgical annuloplasty and avoids concern over coronary artery impingement seen in some patients undergoing indirect mitral annuloplasty. These techniques target the less fibrous posterior annulus where the majority of dilatation occurs. A reduction in the septolateral mitral annular diameter by approximately 20% is reported to be required to significantly improve the degree of MR.[22]

Percutaneous restrictive ring angioplasty has recently been achieved in animals via the transfemoral Cardioband (Valtech Cardio Ltd., Tel Aviv, Israel). The Cardioband is a partially flexible semicircular ring that can be implanted via a transseptal or transapical approach using delivery catheters (Fig. 24-4). The implant is deployed along the left atrial aspect of the posterior annulus and anchored in position using metal screws. The size of the ring can then be adjusted under echocardiography guidance to optimize reduction in MR. Human studies are anticipated.

The Mitralign percutaneous annuloplasty system (Mitralign Inc., Tewksbury, MA) involves direct suture annuloplasty. Currently, this procedure involves transesophageal echocardiographic (TEE) guidance and transarterial retrograde placement of anchors in the left ventricular aspect of the posterior annulus in two locations, at the P1 and P3 scallop which are then plicated to shorten the posterior annulus (Fig. 24-5). The AccuCinch system (Guided Delivery Systems Inc., Santa Clara, CA) also involves direct annuloplasty and requires transarterial left ventricular access and TEE guidance. Multiple anchors are placed sequentially along the left ventricular aspect of the posterior mitral annulus. The first (distal) anchor comes secured to the cinching suture. Subsequent anchors are placed over this suture. The suture is then "cinched" (similar to a belt) and locked thereby reducing the posterior mitral annulus diameter (Fig. 24-6). Both procedures have been demonstrated feasible in animals and human implants have demonstrated the potential for reductions in MR.

THERMAL ANNULAR REMODELING

Two devices have been developed to reduce mitral annular dimensions by directly applying subablative thermal energy to the annular endocardium altering the collagen framework. The ReCor device (ReCor Medical Inc., Ronkonkoma, NY) uses therapeutic ultrasound. A deflectable catheter is passed across the mitral annulus. The catheter tip contains an inflatable balloon

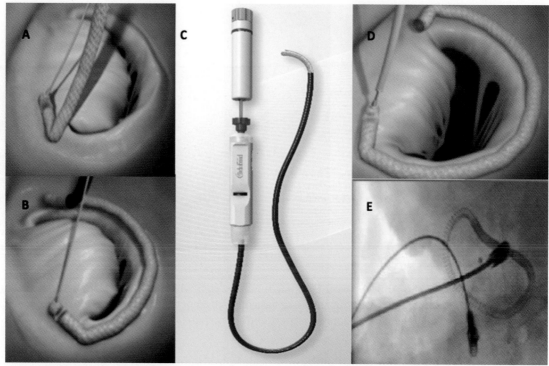

FIGURE 24-4.

Transfemoral Cardioband (Valtech Cardio Ltd., Tel Aviv, Israel). **A:** The semiflexible ring is inserted on the left atrial posterior mitral annulus. **B:** The ring is anchored with metal screws. **C:** The catheter delivery system contains the ring within its lumen. **D:** Adjustment of the ring dimensions on the beating heart. **E:** Fluoroscopic image of an earlier prototype.

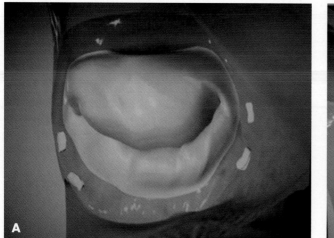

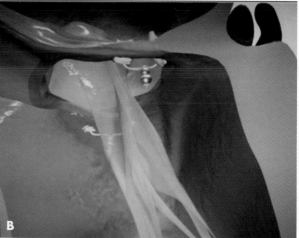

FIGURE 24-5.

Mitralign percutaneous annuloplasty system (Mitralign Inc., Tewksbury, MA). **A:** Left atrial aspect. Note each pair of pledgets have one lock. One pair of pledgets is located between the P1 and P2 scallops and the second pair between P2 and P3. **B:** Mitralign locks are located on the ventricular side. *(Continued)*

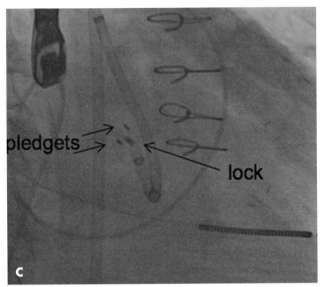

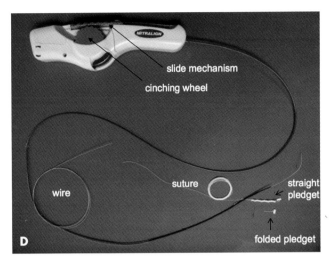

FIGURE 24-5.

(Continued) **C:** Fluoroscopic appearance. **D:** Mitralign delivery system.

which houses an ultrasound probe that is positioned in the center of the annulus. Animal models have demonstrated feasibility and first-in-human procedures have been performed. The QuantumCor device (Quantum-Cor Inc., Lake Forest, CA) uses a catheter to apply radiofrequency energy to the posterior annulus.[2] Animal models have also demonstrated feasibility.

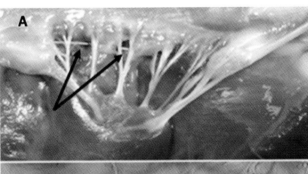

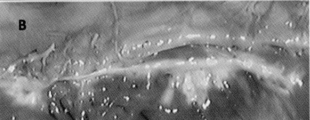

FIGURE 24-6.

AccuCinch (Guided Delivery Systems Inc., Santa Clara, CA). **A:** Acute post implant appearance in an animal model demonstrating the anchors applied to the posterior annulus with the cinching cable underneath (*arrows*). **B:** Healing appearance post implant with the mitral chords and posterior leaflet removed.

VENTRICULAR REMODELING

The iCoapsys device (Myocor Inc., Maple Grove, MN) is designed to reshape the remodeled ischemic left ventricle through external left ventricular compression and thus minimize leaflet tethering and reduce annular dimensions. The RESTOR-MV randomized control trial demonstrated that surgically implanting the iCoapsys device in patients with an ischemic cardiomyopathy and functional MR resulted in improved survival at 2 years compared to coronary artery bypass grafting plus or minus mitral valve repair (87% vs. 77%, $P < .05$). The device was also associated with a reduction in MR and left ventricular volume.[23] In the percutaneous system, subxiphoid access was utilized with a sophisticated positioning system to attach pads on the surface of the left ventricle, one anterior and one posterior. Left ventricular puncture allows a cable to connect the two pads. Tensioning the cable draws the two pads together. Although feasible and apparently effective, the somewhat complex percutaneous procedure is not currently being pursued.

MITRAL CHORDAL REPAIR

Leaflet tethering and tightening of the chordal apparatus is an important potential cause of MR (Fig. 24-7).[24] Long-term durability of surgical ring annuloplasty may be limited by adverse left ventricular remodeling with displacement of the papillary muscles resulting in leaflet tethering and incomplete leaflet

FIGURE 24-7.

Functional ischemic mitral regurgitation due to papillary muscle displacement and leaflet tethering. The effect of basal chordal cutting on leaflet coaptation is shown. Ao, aorta; LA, left atrium; LV, left ventricle; MR, mitral regurgitation.

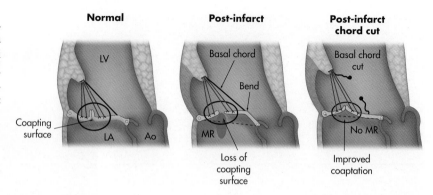

coaptation.[25] Cutting of the basal chords, while preserving the finer first order chords which attach to the leaflets tips and prevent prolapse, may increase leaflet mobility and coaptation area. Surgical data has demonstrated acute efficacy, although the potential for an adverse effect on valvular-ventricular interaction with worsening left ventricular function has not been ruled out.[24] A percutaneous option is being developed.[26]

Surgical artificial chord implantation has been utilized in the setting of prolapse secondary to ruptured chords. This is performed during cardioplegic arrest and, as such, determining the optimum chordal length can be challenging. The feasibility of real-time assessment of MR by echocardiography during transapical artificial chord implantation in animals has been demonstrated.[27] The V Chordal catheter-based system (Valtech Cardio Ltd.) involves chord implantation on the beating heart and the length of the implanted chord can be adjusted to achieve maximum MR reduction (Fig. 24-8). Intraoperative feasibility has been demonstrated and human studies using the transapical and transseptal approaches are anticipated.

REDUCTION IN MITRAL ORIFICE AREA

The mitral spacer device (Cardiosolutions Inc., Stoughton, MA) is a cylindrical-shaped balloon that floats inside the mitral annulus and is anchored via a metal rod that is secured to the left ventricular apex (Fig. 24-9). It reduces MR by reducing the regurgitant orifice area with the mitral leaflets coapting against the balloon during systole. The balloon is made from a flexible soft polymer that is filled with saline at the

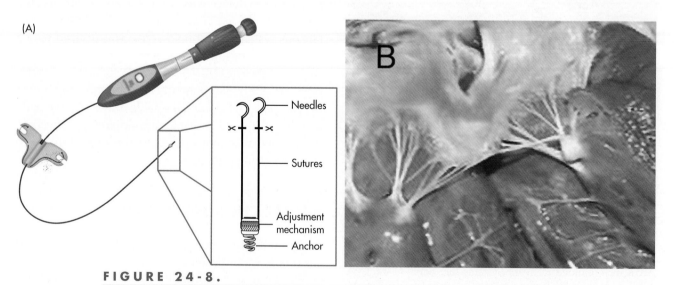

FIGURE 24-8.

The V Chordal adjustment system (Valtech Cardio Ltd., Tel Aviv, Israel) **(A)** and macroscopic appearance in an animal study **(B)**.

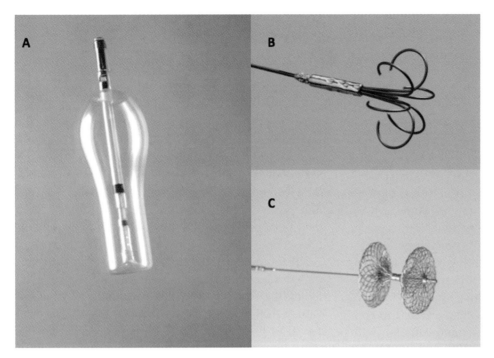

FIGURE 24-9.

The mitral spacer device consists of a balloon **(A)** that floats inside the mitral orifice and a metal anchor **(B,C)** attached to the left ventricular apex.

time of implantation. Concerns include the possibility of balloon prolapse in the left ventricle, mitral obstruction, and apical injury. Animal studies are consistent with feasibility and safety with acute reductions in MR and intraoperative transapical studies have been initiated. Because many patients with severe aortic stenosis may also have lesser degrees of MR, this might be a useful adjunct to transapical aortic valve implantation. A transseptal delivery system is also under development.

TRANSCATHETER MITRAL VALVE REPLACEMENT

Surgical repair of the mitral valve is relatively mature, and percutaneous repair is unlikely to offer the same degree of efficacy in the near future. Transcatheter mitral valve implantation may overcome some of the limitations of percutaneous mitral valve repair. Several groups[28–30] have developed transcatheter mitral valves and human studies are anticipated shortly. The mitral valve is a more challenging site for stent implantation than its aortic counterpart. TAVI uses radial force to anchor the stent within a stiff rigid aortic annulus or the ascending aorta. By comparison, the mitral annulus is saddle shaped, compliant, and dynamic during the cardiac cycle and fixation is more difficult. Although diastolic paravalvular leaks may be relatively

well tolerated in the aortic position, this may not be the case with systolic leaks in the mitral position where regurgitant gradients and mechanical stresses are higher. Additional challenges include the risk of thrombus formation in the left atrium and the possibility of interference with papillary muscles, chordal apparatus, ventricular myocardium, and the left ventricular outflow tract (LVOT).

An early version of a transcatheter mitral valve was described by Lozonschi et al.[29] Components included an atrial fixation system containing metal springs that attach around the annulus, a body consisting of a self-expanding nitinol frame containing a bioprosthetic valve, and a ventricular fixation system utilizing chords attached to the ventricular wall. A transapical approach is utilized for implantation with TEE guidance. Difficult deployment, inadequate fixation, and metal fatigue were problematic during animal evaluation.

Another group[30] developed a stentless compressible system consisting of a hollow body made from polyvinylidene fluoride with a nitinol skeleton that self expands to the contours of the left atrium. It extends from the annulus into the pulmonary veins. A porcine valve is sutured to the frame and is located within the left atrium adjacent to the annulus. Feasibility was demonstrated in an animal model. The theoretical advantage of this system is the avoidance of interference with the subvalvular apparatus and

LVOT. It also preserves and utilizes any residual function of the native mitral valve. Problems, however, are multiple, including the need to individualize development of each prosthetic left atrial body to the contours of the individual's left atrium and the inherent risk of thromboembolism.

The Endovalve device (Endovalve Inc., Princeton, NJ) incorporates a collapsible nitinol structure with integrated gripper features for fixation and bioprosthetic leaflets. A sewn fabric skirt provides perivalvular sealing. The catheter-based system is introduced through a minithoracotomy and left atriotomy. The CardiAQ Valve Technologies Inc. (Irvine, CA) transcatheter mitral valve system consists of a porcine pericardial bioprosthesis with a self-expanding frame. The system can be implanted utilizing a percutaneous transseptal antegrade approach. Animal studies with both the Endovalve and CardiAQ devices are said to confirm the feasibility of mitral valve implantation with reliable positioning, stable anchoring, and good valve hemodynamics without obstruction of the LVOT (Fig. 24-10). Other groups are also well advanced in the development of transcatheter mitral valve systems and first-in-human implantation is anticipated soon.

MITRAL VALVE-IN-VALVE REPLACEMENT

The challenge of adequate fixation of a transcatheter mitral stent within the native valve is overcome in patients with degenerative bioprosthetic mitral valves, where the prosthesis acts as a platform to secure the transcatheter heart valve by radial force and also provides a fluoroscopic landing zone. There is a growing body of evidence that TAVI within a failed bioprosthesis, a valve-in-valve procedure, is relatively safe, has high procedural success rates, and is associated with good postoperative valve function and improvements in functional class.[31]

The transseptal and retrograde approaches to the mitral valve are limited by the technical challenge of positioning the currently available balloon-expandable Edwards SAPIEN aortic valve (Edwards Lifesciences Inc.) coaxial to the mitral prosthesis. Experience so far has been with the apical access approach which facilitates coaxial positioning. Utilizing an intercostal minithoracotomy, the left ventricle is punctured and a wire advanced retrograde across the failed mitral prosthesis. The standard Ascendra Transapical delivery system (Edwards

FIGURE 24-10.

Transcatheter mitral valve replacement systems. **A:** Endovalve (Endovalve Inc., Princeton, NJ). **B,D:** Lozonschi et al. valve. **C:** CardiAQ valve (CardiAQ Valve Technologies Inc., Irvine, CA).

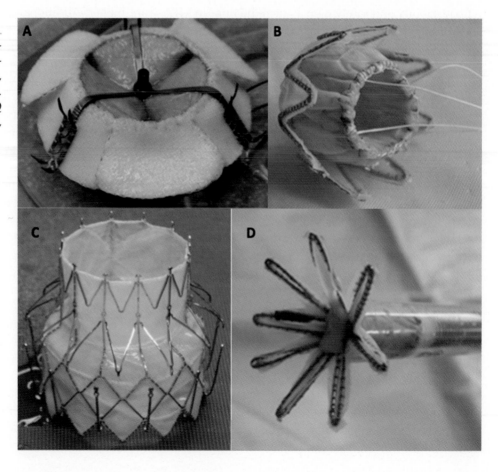

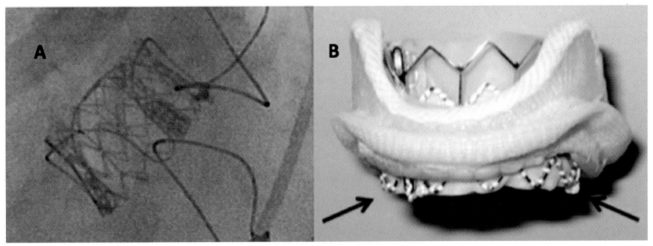

FIGURE 24-11.

Transcatheter mitral valve-in-valve deployment (SAPIEN transcatheter heart valve within a Carpentier-Edwards valve [Edwards Lifesciences Inc., Irvine, CA]). **A:** Fluoroscopic image. **B:** Correct positioning for secure fixation. The transcatheter valve overlaps the sewing ring of the surgical bioprosthesis (*arrows*).

Lifesciences Inc.) designed for aortic valve implantation is advanced over the wire and positioned under TEE and fluoroscopic guidance. Balloon expansion is performed during rapid right ventricular pacing to reduce transvalvular flow and cardiac motion (Fig. 24-11).

A thorough knowledge and understanding of the various mitral bioprosthesis designs and locations of radiopaque markers is required to ensure accurate positioning and fixation of the valve-in-valve implant. The SAPIEN valve comes in a range of sizes with external diameters of 20, 23, 26, and 29 mm. The nominal external transcatheter heart valve diameter should slightly exceed the reported internal diameter of the failed valve. With the majority of current surgical valves implanted being bioprosthetic, and the high risk associated with repeat surgery, it is expected that mitral valve-in-valve implantation will play an increasingly important role in the management of degenerative mitral bioprostheses.

CONCLUSION

Percutaneous management of mitral valve disease in clinical practice is currently limited to edge-to-edge repair utilizing the MitraClip device and also mitral valve-in-valve procedures for failed mitral surgical bioprostheses. The growing population of patients with MR provides the stimulus for continued research in this field. Several devices have reached human clinical trials but failed to progress into clinical practice due to modest reductions in MR and/or technical difficulties. The future role for these procedures remains uncertain, but this is likely to be an area of ongoing activity.

REFERENCES

1. Bursi F, Enriquez-Sarano M, Nkomo VT, et al. Heart failure and death after myocardial infarction in the community: the emerging role of mitral regurgitation. *Circulation.* 2005;111:295–301.
2. Robbins JD, Maniar PB, Cotts W, et al. Prevalence and severity of mitral regurgitation in chronic systolic heart failure. *Am J Cardiol.* 2003;91:360–362.
3. Mirabel M, Iung B, Baron G, et al. What are the characteristics of patients with severe, symptomatic, mitral regurgitation who are denied surgery? *Eur Heart J.* 2007;28:1358–1365.
4. Johnston DR, Gillinov AM, Blackstone EH, et al. Surgical repair of posterior mitral valve prolapse: implications for guidelines and percutaneous repair. *Ann Thorac Surg.* 2010;89:1385–1394.
5. Maisano F, Torracca L, Oppizzi M, et al. The edge-to-edge technique: a simplified method to correct mitral insufficiency. *Eur J Cardiothorac Surg.* 1998;13: 240–245; discussion 245–246.
6. Webb JG, Maisano F, Vahanian A, et al. Percutaneous suture edge-to-edge repair of the mitral valve. *EuroIntervention.* 2009;5:86–89.

7. Feldman T, Kar S, Rinaldi M, et al. Percutaneous mitral repair with the MitraClip system: safety and midterm durability in the initial EVEREST (Endovascular Valve Edge-to-Edge REpair Study) cohort. *J Am Coll Cardiol.* 2009;54:686–694.

8. Bhudia SK, McCarthy PM, Smedira NG, et al. Edge-to-edge (Alfieri) mitral repair: results in diverse clinical settings. *Ann Thorac Surg.* 2004;77:1598–1606.

9. Fedak PW, McCarthy PM, Bonow RO. Evolving concepts and technologies in mitral valve repair. *Circulation.* 2008;117:963–974.

10. Argenziano M, Skipper E, Heimansohn D, et al. Surgical revision after percutaneous mitral repair with the MitraClip device. *Ann Thorac Surg.* 2010;89: 72–80.

11. Savage EB, Ferguson TBJ, DiSesa VJ. Use of mitral valve repair: analysis of contemporary United States experience reported to the Society of Thoracic Surgeons National Cardiac Database. *Ann Thorac Surg.* 2003;75:820–825.

12. Tops LF, Van de Veire NR, Schuijf JD, et al. Noninvasive evaluation of coronary sinus anatomy and its relation to the mitral valve annulus: implications for percutaneous mitral annuloplasty. *Circulation.* 2007;115:1426–1432.

13. Choure AJ, Garcia MJ, Hesse B, et al. In vivo analysis of the anatomical relationship of coronary sinus to mitral annulus and left circumflex coronary artery using cardiac multidetector computed tomography: implications for percutaneous coronary sinus mitral annuloplasty. *J Am Coll Cardiol.* 2006;48:1938–1945.

14. Webb JG, Harnek J, Munt BI, et al. Percutaneous transvenous mitral annuloplasty: initial human experience with device implantation in the coronary sinus. *Circulation.* 2006;113:851–855.

15. Kaye DM, Byrne M, Alferness C, et al. Feasibility and short-term efficacy of percutaneous mitral annular reduction for the therapy of heart failure-induced mitral regurgitation. *Circulation.* 2003;108:1795–1797.

16. Duffy SJ, Federman J, Farrington C, et al. Feasibility and short-term efficacy of percutaneous mitral annular reduction for the therapy of functional mitral regurgitation in patients with heart failure. *Catheter Cardiovasc Interv.* 2006;68:205–210.

17. Schofer J, Siminiak T, Haude M, et al. Percutaneous mitral annuloplasty for functional mitral regurgitation: results of the CARILLON Mitral Annuloplasty Device European Union Study. *Circulation.* 2009;120:326–333.

18. Sack S, Kahlert P, Bilodeau L, et al. Percutaneous transvenous mitral annuloplasty: initial human experience with a novel coronary sinus implant device. *Circ Cardiovasc Interv.* 2009;2:277–284.

19. Rogers JH, Rahdert DA, Caputo GR, et al. Long-term safety and durability of percutaneous septal sinus shortening (The PS[3] System) in an ovine model. *Catheter Cardiovasc Interv.* 2009;73:540–548.

20. Sorajja P, Nishimura RA, Thompson J, et al. A novel method of percutaneous mitral valve repair for ischemic mitral regurgitation. *JACC Cardiovasc Interv.* 2008;1:663–672.

21. Kim JH, Kocaturk O, Ozturk C, et al. Mitral cerclage annuloplasty, a novel transcatheter treatment for secondary mitral valve regurgitation: initial results in swine. *J Am Coll Cardiol.* 2009;54:638–651.

22. Tibayan FA, Rodriguez F, Liang D, et al. Paneth suture annuloplasty abolishes acute ischemic mitral regurgitation but preserves annular and leaflet dynamics. *Circulation.* 2003;108 (suppl 1):II128–II133.

23. Grossi EA, Patel N, Woo YJ, et al. Outcomes of the RESTOR-MV Trial (Randomized Evaluation of a Surgical Treatment for Off-Pump Repair of the Mitral Valve). *J Am Coll Cardiol.* 2010;56:1984–1993.

24. Messas E, Yosefy C, Chaput M, et al. Chordal cutting does not adversely affect left ventricle contractile function. *Circulation.* 2006;114:I524–I528.

25. Bouma W, van der Horst IC, Wijdh-den Hamer IJ, et al. Chronic ischaemic mitral regurgitation. Current treatment results and new mechanism-based surgical approaches. *Eur J Cardiothorac Surg.* 2010;37: 170–185.

26. Slocum AH, Bosworth WR, Mazumdar A, et al. Design of a catheter-based device for performing percutaneous chordal-cutting procedures. *J Med Device.* 2009;3:25001.

27. Maisano F, Michev I, Rowe S, et al. Transapical endovascular implantation of neochordae using a suction and suture device. *Eur J Cardiothorac Surg.* 2009;36:118–122; discussion 122–123.

28. Ma L, Tozzi P, Huber CH, et al. Double-crowned valved stents for off-pump mitral valve replacement. *Eur J Cardiothorac Surg.* 2005;28:194–198; discussion 198–199.

29. Lozonschi L, Bombien R, Osaki S, et al. Transapical mitral valved stent implantation: a survival series in swine. *J Thorac Cardiovasc Surg.* 2010;140:422–426.e1.

30. Goetzenich A, Dohmen G, Hatam N, et al. A new approach to interventional atrioventricular valve therapy. *J Thorac Cardiovasc Surg.* 2010;140:97–102.

31. Webb JG, Wood DA, Ye J, et al. Transcatheter valve-in-valve implantation for failed bioprosthetic heart valves. *Circulation.* 2010;121:1848–1857.

CHAPTER 25

Pulmonic Valve Implantation in Adults

Philipp C. Lurz and Philipp Bonhoeffer*

In 2000, the first percutaneous heart valve implantation in human was performed in a 12-year-old boy. He developed dysfunction of his right ventricle (RV) to pulmonary artery (PA) conduit, which could be treated by placing a valved stent within the right ventricular outflow tract (RVOT)/pulmonary trunk and conventionally would have necessitated open-heart surgery.[1] Since this first description of a percutaneously implanted heart valve, around 2,000 percutaneous pulmonary valve implants (PPVIs) have been performed worldwide. Over the last 10 years, the Melody device (Medtronic, Minneapolis, MN) became commercially available within Europe, Canada, and the United States, making this new percutaneous strategy available to a broader population. With improvements in safety and efficacy of PPVI over the last few years,[2] this technique has been transformed from its initially pioneering nature into routine clinical care at specialized centers.

Apart from the Melody device, there is increasing experience with the Edwards SAPIEN transcatheter heart valve (Edwards Lifesciences Inc., Irvine, CA) in the pulmonary position,[3,4] which will be evaluated within a US trial.

In the following chapter, we review the indications, technical aspects, and early and late results of PPVI using the Melody device and SAPIEN transcatheter heart valve as nonsurgical treatment options for RVOT/pulmonary trunk dysfunction.

***Disclosure:** PB is consultant to Medtronic and NuMed and has received honoraria and royalties for the device described.

THE RATIONALE AND CLINICAL ROLE OF PERCUTANEOUS PULMONARY VALVE IMPLANTATION

The most common problem for adults and children late after neonatal repair of complex congenital heart disease is dysfunction of the RVOT/pulmonary trunk, either manifesting as an obstructive lesion or as pulmonary regurgitation.

Currently, surgical pulmonary valve replacement, using valved conduits (biologic valve, xenografts, homografts, etc.) has been used to treat RVOT/pulmonary trunk dysfunction. Surgical pulmonary valve replacement is a very safe procedure and can be performed with low morbidity and mortality. However, an important drawback of this treatment is the limited life span of such conduits from the RV to the PA. In the literature, this life span has been reported to be around 10 years.[5-9] As a consequence, the majority of patients have to undergo several open-heart procedures during their life. Patient management strategies have, therefore, been based on delaying surgical intervention for as long as possible, so that the number of open-heart surgeries performed on any individual patient is kept to a minimum. However, this approach bears the risk of delaying surgery beyond a theoretical point of no return when RV dysfunction, impaired exercise capacity, and increased risk for sudden death—all demonstrated consequences of chronic adverse RV loading conditions[10-13]—might be irreversible.

There is some data on RV volume thresholds as assessed on magnetic resonance imaging (MRI)[14-16] in which normalization of RV dimensions is less likely following pulmonary valve replacement. However, the impact of timing of pulmonary valve replacement on RV function, exercise performance, and, in particular, long-term survival remains undefined. This complicates the clinical decision making regarding timing of intervention in these patients.

Stenting of the RVOT/pulmonary trunk has been proposed as a feasible treatment strategy for postponing open-heart surgery,[17-20] although such "bare-metal stenting" reduces RV pressure overload at the cost of valvular incompetence. Bare-metal stenting leads to free pulmonary regurgitation in almost all cases, representing a significant drawback of this procedure.

With the introduction of PPVI, a nonsurgical technique has become available that enables treatment of both conduit obstruction and regurgitation by opening of stenotic conduits and re-valvulation of the RVOT/pulmonary trunk. This offers the potential to avoid open-heart surgery for RVOT/pulmonary trunk dysfunction in children and adults by restoring acceptable RV loading conditions.

THE MELODY TRANSCATHETER PULMONARY VALVE

Equipment and Set Up

The Melody transcatheter pulmonary valve is composed of a segment of bovine jugular vein with a central valve (Fig. 25-1). The vein is sutured inside an expanded platinum-iridium stent with a length of 34 mm that can be crimped to a size of 6 mm and re-expanded up to 22 mm. The stent, consisting of eight crown zig pattern with six segments along its length, is reinforced at each strut intersection with gold weld. The venous segment is attached to the stent by continuous sutures around the entire circumference at the inflow and outflow and also discretely at each strut intersection. The suture is clear for all points except the outflow line, which is blue to signify the outflow end of the device.

The delivery system (Ensemble, Medtronic) comprises a balloon-in-balloon deployment design at its distal end onto which the valved stent is front-loaded and crimped (Fig. 25-2). The system is available with three outer balloon diameters: 18, 20, and 22 mm. The tip of the system is blue to correspond with the outflow suture of the device and to facilitate correct orientation. The body of the system is composed of a one-piece Teflon sheath containing a braided-wire reinforced elastomer lumen. There is a retractable sheath that covers the stented valve during delivery and is pulled back

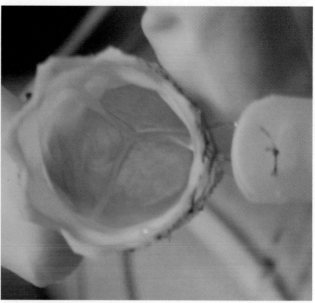

FIGURE 25-1.

Percutaneous pulmonary valve device (Melody, Medtronic, Minneapolis, MN).

just prior to deployment. Contrast can be delivered via the retracted sheath from a side port to confirm positioning of the device prior to deployment. Proximally, there are three ports: one for the guidewire (green), one to deploy the inner balloon (indigo), and one to deploy the outer balloon (orange).

We recommend performing PPVI in a catheterization laboratory with a biplane fluoroscopy set up and within a sterile environment, meeting those of surgical

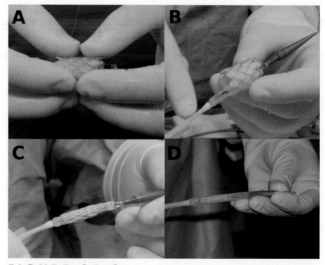

FIGURE 25-2.

A: Percutaneous pulmonary valve crimped down on a 2-mL syringe, **(B,C)** mounted the balloon-in-balloon delivery system, and **(D)** covered with the outer sheath.

valve implantations. Autotransfusion kits (pleural drainage kits, cell saver) should be available in cases of acute bleeding. Although the rate of severe complication during and post PPVI is very low, we believe that PPVI should only be performed at institution with a congenital surgical program with extracorporeal membrane oxygenation equipment and experience with this technique. Simultaneous surgical back up, however, is not part of our protocol and might not be required.

Clinical and Morphologic Criteria for Patient Selection

It is important to note that no clear-cut guidelines for when to treat RVOT/pulmonary trunk dysfunction exist. The clinical indications for PPVI outlined in the following represent our approach to timing of intervention. This approach matches the ones applied by many other institutions, but cannot be considered as first-line criteria due to limited long-term outcome data. Our indications are based on several studies assessing the physiologic acute and mid-term results post PPVI in patients with RVOT/pulmonary trunk obstruction and/or regurgitation.[2,21–23]

In the setting of RV pressure overload and RVOT/pulmonary trunk obstruction, our patients undergo PPVI if RV pressures exceed 65% of systemic pressures in the presence of symptoms. In the absence of symptoms, patients are treated if RV pressures exceed 75% of systemic pressures.[2] In the context of pulmonary regurgitation, PPVI is performed if patients have severe pulmonary regurgitation (as assessed on echocardiography or MRI) and one of the following: (a) severe RV dilatation; (b) severe RV dysfunction; (c) symptoms; or (d) impaired exercise capacity.[2,24]

To establish clinical indication criteria, all patients undergo a standardized assessment protocol. For screening, echocardiography to determine the RVOT gradient and to semiquantitatively assess the severity of pulmonary regurgitation is performed. Echocardiography is also used to estimate RV pressures (tricuspid valve regurgitant jet) and the RV to systemic pressure ratio (noninvasive blood pressure measurements). Objective exercise capacity is assessed by cardiopulmonary exercise testing on a bicycle using a ramp protocol. A peak oxygen uptake of less than 65% of predicted is considered as a significant impairment in exercise capacity. As a crucial part of our assessment, patients undergo cardiac MRI unless contraindicated. We define RV dilatation in the context of pulmonary regurgitation as severe when the indexed RV end-diastolic volume is >150 mL/m^2 or the RV

to left ventricle (LV) end-diastolic ratio is >1.7. It is of note that ventricular volume derived on MRI can differ by more than 15% depending on whether RV trabeculations are included in the volume or whether end-diastolic and end-systolic volumes are defined by the endocardial outline in each of the short-axis cine images excluding RV trabeculations. MRI also allows accurate quantification of the pulmonary regurgitation severity using PA flow measurements, providing a calculated pulmonary regurgitation fraction. Lastly, surface electrocardiograms and 24-hour Holter monitoring are performed to detect arrhythmia and define QRS duration.

Apart from clinical indications, patients have to fulfill morphological criteria to be considered suitable for pulmonary valve replacement. Suitability depends on two crucial factors, as follows.

RVOT/Pulmonary Trunk Size

The valved stent can be dilated up to 22 mm—any larger and valve leaflet coaptation may fail. This precludes PPVI in dilated anatomies. Because most native outflow tract are larger than 22 mm, PPVI is limited to conduits from the RV to the PA with very few exceptions.[2] Conduit sizes can be gathered from operative reports; however, conduits can become smaller (or larger) over time and, in order to have a full understanding of the anatomy of the outflow tract, cross-sectional imaging—in particular, MRI with three-dimensional (3D) capabilities—is crucial. It is important to realize that MRI-derived 3D reconstructions can be used to define size, but these reconstructions are performed on data acquired in diastole or from non–electrocardiogram-gated data, and thus, maximal dimensions of very distensible anatomies may be underestimated. Measurements of the RVOT/pulmonary trunk diameters are best performed on cine images in two orthogonal planes. This enables determination of the maximum diameter of the site at which PPVI may be attempted.

If results of MRI are doubtful or borderline, balloon sizing of the RVOT can be performed at the time of catheterization, which will be discussed later.

Course of the Proximal Coronary Arteries

RVOT/pulmonary trunk interventions expose the risk for coronary artery obstruction due to expansion of the RVOT.[19,25,26] In complex congenital heart disease or after surgical reinsertion into the aorta, the coronary arteries can run in close proximity to the RVOT/pulmonary trunk. It is essential to assess the course of proximal coronary arteries in relation to the RVOT/pulmonary

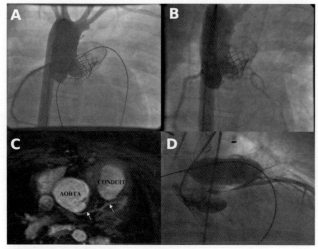

FIGURE 25-3.

A: Angiogram (left anterior oblique projection) showing compression of the left main stem coronary artery following deployment of the percutaneous pulmonary valve in a patient with very complex anatomy (double inlet left ventricle). Coronary compression led to immediate hemodynamic shock and necessitated cardiopulmonary resuscitation and manual chest compression. **B:** Reperfusion of the left coronary system following compression of the device during cardiac massage. Following decompression of the left coronary system, the patient could be stabilized and was transferred to the operating theater to undergo device removal and surgical pulmonary valve implantation. Simultaneous balloon inflation within the right ventricular outflow tract and selective coronary angiography was not performed in this patient, causing this severe complication. **C:** Three-dimensional magnetic resonance whole-heart imaging showing the left coronary artery in close proximity to the right ventricle to pulmonary artery conduit in a patient considered for percutaneous pulmonary valve implantation (the *arrows* indicate the left main respectively the left anterior descending in close proximity to the RVOT). **D:** Angiogram (left anterior oblique projection with 20 degrees of cranial angulation) showing compression of the left anterior descending coronary artery during balloon inflation in the conduit. The procedure was, therefore, abandoned in this patient and no valve implanted.

trunk prior to PPVI. On MRI 3D whole-heart images, the anatomical relationship of the coronary arteries and the proposed implantation side can be judged. In addition, aortic root angiography and, in some cases, simultaneous high-pressure balloon inflation in the implantation site and selective coronary angiography are performed at the time of catheterization and will be discussed in more detail later (Fig. 25-3).

The Catheterization

PPVI is performed under general anesthesia. Peripheral venous and arterial access are obtained. Femoral access is preferred because it allows for an easier

working position in the catheterization laboratory. However, jugular access can also be performed safely, if required.

A full aseptic technique to surgical standards is used and a single dose of broad-spectrum intravenous antibiotics is given for endocarditis prophylaxis. Fifty IU/kg heparin, or a standard dose of 5,000 IU in adults, is administered routinely at the beginning of the procedure and repeated hourly thereafter as required.

Right heart catheterization is performed according to standard techniques to assess pressures and saturations. Routinely, measurements are made in the RV, PA, and aorta. To confirm or rule out relevant pulmonary branch stenosis, additional measurements should be further acquired in the proximal and distal branch pulmonary arteries. A stiff guidewire (i.e., 0.035-inch Amplatzer ultra stiff [AGA Medical, Plymouth, MN] or 0.035-inch Back-up Meier [Boston Scientific Corp., Natick, MA]) is then positioned into a distal branch PA to provide an anchor from which to advance the delivery system.

First, biplane angiography is performed using a Multi-Track catheter (NuMed Inc., Hopkinton, NY) with the tip placed just beyond the expected position of the pulmonary valve, to allow assessment of the proposed site for device implantation and quantification of pulmonary regurgitation.

In cases with borderline large dimensions of the implantation site at MRI, these can be measured from the angiogram using a soft, sizing balloon (PTS sizing balloon catheter, NuMed).

As mentioned previously, the risk of coronary compression has to be completely ruled out. In addition to coronary assessment on MRI, we perform aortic root angiography in all patients. On biplane projection, the relationship between the coronaries and the PA can be assessed. If angiography and MRI assessment cannot fully rule out the risk for coronary compression, an additional maneuver has to be performed—simultaneous high-pressure balloon inflation in the implantation site and selective coronary angiography. It is important that the balloon is inflated up to a therapeutic diameter to assure that valve insertion is adequately mimicked by this maneuver. If this maneuver indicates a risk for coronary compression, the procedure has to be abandoned (Fig. 25-3).[25]

The Implant

Preparations prior to implantation include hand crimping and loading of the valved stent onto the delivery system. The valved stent is hand crimped over the barrel of a sterile 2-mL syringe before being front-loaded onto the delivery system. The blue stitching on the distal portion of the device is matched to the blue portion of the delivery system and verified by an independent observer to guarantee correct orientation. Further hand crimping is performed, followed by advancing the sheath over the device while a saline flush is administered via the side port to exclude air bubbles from the system (Fig. 25-2). After removal of the Multi-Track catheter, the femoral vein is dilated to 22 French and the front-loaded delivery system is advanced into the RVOT under fluoroscopic guidance.

A maneuver that can facilitate advancing the delivery system, when it is at the entrance to the conduit, is looping the system within the right atrium. This generates a forward force often overcoming resistances the system is experiencing and aiding passage into the conduit. If the delivery system has been placed too distally, forward pushing of the guidewire rather than backward pulling of the delivery system often helps to withdraw the delivery system slightly. Once the valved stent is in the appropriate position, the outer sheath is retracted uncovering the stent. There are no radiopaque markers on the sheath. This means that complete uncovering of the delivery system can only be confirmed by the marker placed on the proximal portion of the delivery system.

Partial deployment is achieved by hand inflation of the inner balloon and after final confirmation of the position the outer balloon is also hand inflated to complete deployment. The balloons are deflated and the delivery system is withdrawn. Repeat angiography and pressure measurements are made to confirm a positive outcome.

Additional Periprocedural Considerations

Predilatation

Predilatation of severely stenosed conduit can be considered in order to facilitate passage of the system. Another potential advantage of predilatation is the fact that it provides an ideal assessment of the anatomy. The location of the waist of the balloon, if present, represents the most rigid part of the implantation site and informs on the optimal landing zone for the valved stent. One could also argue that predilation of stenotic conduits optimizes the hemodynamic result, although, at present, we do not have any data to suggest so. On the other hand, predilatation potentially bears the risk of homograft rupture. Severe bleeding due to homograft rupture is rare with an incidence of ~2.5% and will be discussed later. In contrast, partial rupture of the RV to PA conduit during valve implantation is a common finding. Although clinically silent, in most cases, when occurring during valve stent implantation due to the covered nature of the stent, this could lead to severe bleeding if caused by predilatation. As so often, the decision for predilatation has to be made individually in each patient, taking the possible advantages and disadvantages into account.

Prestenting

Fractures of any type of stent placed within the RVOT/pulmonary trunk are common[19] with an incidence of around 40%. Although clinically not relevant in the majority of patients, stent fractures of the valved stent can lead to restenosis or even embolization of the stent.[27] Following PPVI, 20% of our patients have fractured their stents.[27] We previously have shown that a more dynamic RVOT, as seen in a noncalcified RVOT or noncircumferential homografts, is associated with an increased risk for stent fractures (nature and treatment of stent fracture will be discussed later in this chapter).[27] Assuming that prestenting enhances the rigidity of the implantation side, there is a potential to reduce the risk of stent fractures during follow-up by this procedure. Based on this assumption, we have changed our practice throughout the last years and have prestented the majority of patients. In a retrospective analysis, we could show that prestenting did reduce the risk of stent fractures when corrected for outflow tract type and extent of calcifications.[28] Although long-term data or prospective studies are still missing, we would recommend bare-metal stenting prior to PPVI. Also, prestenting offers a perfect landmark for correct valve positioning and potentially can lead to superior immediate hemodynamic results (Fig. 25-4).

For prestenting with bare-metal stents, we use the balloon-expandable IntraStent (Max LD, ev3, Plymouth, MN). These stents are delivered on BIB dilatation catheters (NuMED), which are chosen to have smaller nominal balloon diameters than the subsequently used PPVI delivery system and than the original outflow tract size, leaving some degree of residual outflow tract obstruction. This approach has the advantage of reducing the risk for conduit rupture during balloon dilatation with noncovered stents. In rather small conduits, which are to be dilated up to a diameter bigger than the original size, prestenting with covered stents (i.e., CP Stent, NuMED) can be performed and should reduce the clinical impact of conduit rupture.

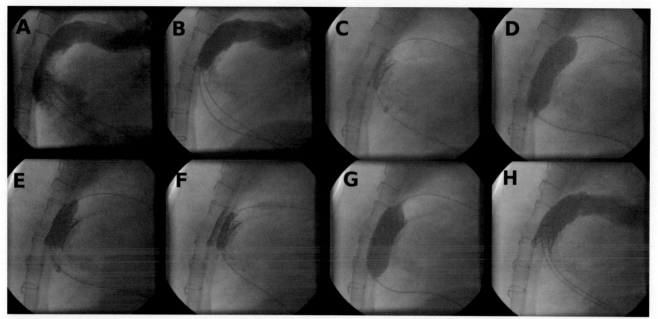

FIGURE 25-4.

Case presentation of a 22-year-old patient with pulmonary atresia, who twice underwent open heart surgery in infancy. When referred, he presented symptomatic (New York Heart Association functional class III) with significant impairment in exercise capacity (40% of predicted peak oxygen uptake). The cine angiograms are shown in lateral projection. **A:** Angiogram demonstrating severe obstruction of the 25-mm homograft in right ventricle (RV) to pulmonary artery (PA) position. Note the proximity of the conduit to the sternum/ribs; in this case, out of our early experience, primary percutaneous pulmonary valve implantation (PPVI) without prestenting was performed. **B:** Angiogram post PPVI shows good opening of the conduit and valvar competence. **C:** One year after this initial implant, this patient presented symptomatic again with suprasystemic RV pressures estimated from echocardiography. Fluoroscopy revealed severe compression of the fractured valved stent. Hemodynamic assessment revealed an RV systolic pressure of 123 mm Hg. In order to increase the radial force of the stents within the homograft, we decided to perform multiple bare-metal stenting (fluoroscopy shows an IntraStent [Max LD, ev3, Plymouth, MN]) prior to implantation positioned within the valved stent). **D:** Implantation with balloon inflation of the second IntraStent. **E:** Deflation of the balloon-in-balloon delivery system of the IntraStent reveals significant recoil when the diameter is compared to the diameter at the end of balloon inflation **(D)**. We, therefore, decided to implant a third bare-metal stent. **F:** After triple prestenting, acceptable opening of the homograft could be achieved. Therefore, we proceeded with PPVI (panel F showing the PPVI on the delivery system positioned within the previously placed stents). **G:** Postdilation of the device with a Mullins high-pressure balloon (NuMed, Hopkinton, NY). **H:** The final angiogram demonstrating good valvular competence and good acceptable opening of the homograft. Final hemodynamic assessment revealed a drop in RV systolic pressures from 123 mm Hg to 51 mm Hg. This second procedure led to complete relief of symptoms. Three years postprocedure, the patients remained asymptomatic.

Postdilatation

Previously, the adverse impact of residual RVOT/pulmonary trunk obstruction on risk of reintervention and reoperation[2] and on functional outcome[29] was demonstrated. Therefore, an aggressive approach to a residual RVOT obstruction is required in order to improve the long-term outcome post PPVI. As outlined previously, high-pressure postdilatation of the valved, and therefore covered, Melody device might be the safest option with regard to conduit rupture and represent our preferred approach. We use a Mullins high-pressure balloon (NuMed) with an Indeflator. Multiple postdilatations can be considered in the presence of any residual gradient to achieve further expansion of the device and therefore optimize the hemodynamic result (Fig. 25-4).

Procedural Complications

There is a reported complication rate of 6% both in our series of 242 patients and within the US Melody Valve Trial, including 124 patients.[30]

Major procedural complications in 366 patients included:

• Homograft rupture (n = 8) with hemodynamic compromise in 5/8 patients
• Device dislodgement (n = 2)

- Hypercarbia and elevation of LV filling pressure necessitating mechanical ventilation (n = 1)
- Compression of the main stem of the left coronary artery (n = 1) (Fig. 25-3)
- Coronary artery dissection (n = 1)
- Wide-complex tachycardia treated with cardioversion (n = 1)
- Femoral vein thrombosis (n = 1)
- Obstruction of the origin of the right PA (n = 1).
- Perforation of the left PA causing severe bleeding (n = 1).
- Bronchial bleeding (n = 3) presumably due to guidewire injury.
- Entrapment of the delivery system in the tendinous cords of the tricuspid valve (n = 2) causing significant tricuspid regurgitation

In total, bailout surgery has been required in seven patients, but none of them led to mortality. The patient with a coronary dissection had severe biventricular dysfunction before catheterization and was diagnosed during the procedure, before PPVI, with previously unrecognized occlusion of the proximal left coronary artery by the surgically placed bioprosthetic valved conduit. After coronary stenting, resuscitation, and transcatheter pulmonary valve implantation, the chronically occluded coronary was recanalized and stented. This patient was able to come off extracorporeal support but subsequently suffered an intracranial hemorrhage and died.

The cases of valve dislodgement occurred in the early phase of our experience. With increasing experience, this complication could be avoidable by appropriate pre-procedural MRI and balloon sizing. Although coronary compression should be avoidable in the vast majority of patients, it remains a complex issue and can be fatal.

Homograft rupture remains a complication, which is difficult to avoid and requires further investigations to identify patients at risk. To date, risk factors for homograft ruptures are not understood, and therefore, no recommendations regarding patient selection and risk reduction can be given. In the following, some aspects of how to deal with this severe procedural complication will be discussed.

How to Avoid or Deal with Some Complications

Bleeding Due to Homograft Rupture

Out of our experience, we recommend the following approach in the event of serious bleeding with consequent shock. As a first step, the operator should confirm bleeding. In general, there is bleeding into the pleura rather than into the pericardium. Pleural bleeding is easily suspected by fluoroscopy. If bleeding is confirmed, autotransfusion should be initiated as soon as possible. Therefore, pleural drainage and autotransfusion equipment has to be available acutely. In most cases, autotransfusion reestablishes a sufficient circulation and allows for planning of any further interventional treatment or watchful observation. A cell saver could be used during autotransfusion. However, in the very acute setting, the potential benefit of cell savers has to be counterbalanced with the loss of time and resources in such a dramatic situation. In our experience, after intensive and efficient autotransfusion, bleeding either stops or reduces to an amount, which allows safe transfer of the patient to the operating theatre. We do not recommend thoracotomy and surgical intervention acutely because this decompresses the bleed and complicates locating the source of bleeding.

Damage to the Tricuspid Valve

Significant damage to the tricuspid valve due to entrapment of the delivery system in the tendinous cords of the tricuspid valve can be avoided in most cases. Care should be taken when the tricuspid valve is crossed the first time. Especially for the less experienced operator, the tricuspid valve should be negotiated with a balloon-tipped floating catheter to minimize the risk of entrapment of any catheters or wires within the tricuspid subvalvar apparatus.

How to Handle Ultra Stiff Guidewires in the Pulmonary Arteries

The use of very stiff guidewires is needed to provide sufficient support for safe advancement of the delivery system. However, manipulation of such wires can lead to branch pulmonary arteries injury or even perforation. To avoid this complication, the operator has to ensure that the guidewire is in a stable position in one of the distal PA branches. Further, if the guidewire happens to move backward while the delivery system is pushed forward, the guidewire should be repositioned before the delivery system is advanced. The delivery system should only be advanced when the guidewire is placed correctly in one of the distal pulmonary branches. Initial positioning of the guidewire should only be performed via a luminal catheter.

Hemodynamic Outcome

The hemodynamic outcome post PPVI within the two largest published reports[2,30] is summarized in Table 25-1. Percutaneous implantation of the valved stent resulted in a significant reduction in RV systolic pressure.

TABLE 25-1 Invasively Assessed Hemodynamic Outcome Post PPVI in the Two Largest Reports for Different Primary Indications

| | The London Experience[2] (n = 151) | | | | | | | | |
| Parameter | Primary indication: pulmonary regurgitation (n = 46) | | | Primary indication: pulmonary stenosis (n = 61) | | | Primary indication: combined lesion (n = 44) | | |
	Pre	Post	P value	Pre	Post	P value	Pre	Post	P value
RV systolic pressure (mm Hg)	48 ± 13	43 ± 12	.002	72 ± 16	46 ± 13	< .001	62 ± 15	46 ± 12	< .001
PA systolic pressure (mm Hg)	31 ± 10	31 ± 9	.917	25 ± 11	26 ± 9	.373	25 ± 9	29 ± 13	.027
PA diastolic pressure (mm Hg)	11 ± 5	15 ± 6	< .001	10 ± 4	12 ± 4	.003	9 ± 4	13 ± 6	< .001
Peak RV to PA gradient (mm Hg)	20 ± 13	13 ± 9	< .001	48 ± 18	19 ± 12	< .001	37 ± 18	17 ± 8	< .001
Aortic systolic pressure (mm Hg)	94 ± 14	102 ± 16	.002	92 ± 15	98 ± 14	.004	94 ± 17	105 ± 17	.001
RV/aortic pressure (%)	52 ± 15	42 ± 11	< .001	81 ± 16	47 ± 12	< .001	67 ± 11	44 ± 15	< .001

| | The US Melody Valve Trial[30] (n = 124) | | | | | |
| Parameter | Primary indication: pulmonary regurgitation (n = 65) | | | Primary indication: pulmonary stenosis or combined lesion (n = 59) | | |
	Pre	Post	P value	Pre	Post	P value
RV systolic pressure (mm Hg)	61 ± 21	47 ± 15	.001	69 ± 13	45 ± 11	.001
PA systolic pressure (mm Hg)	35 ± 15	35 ± 13	.94	30 ± 17	32 ± 11	.9
Peak RV to PA gradient (mm Hg)	28 ± 16	13 ± 7	.001	44 ± 11	14 ± 6	.001
Aortic systolic pressure (mm Hg)	94 ± 14	113 ± 21	.001	90 ± 13	105 ± 17	.001
RV/aortic pressure (%)	65 ± 19	42 ± 12	.001	78 ± 15	43 ± 12	.001

PPVI, percutaneous pulmonary valve implantation; RV, right ventricle; PA, pulmonary artery.

Further, diastolic PA pressures have been shown to rise after deployment, indicating restoration of valvular competence. Systemic systolic pressures increase significantly post PPVI, which we postulate to be a reflection of increased systemic blood flow. Angiography prior to and after insertion shows a significant reduction in pulmonary regurgitation in the vast majority of patients.[2,31] Paravalvular leaks postprocedure are extremely rare and are seen in approximately 1 out of 50 patients.

Functional Outcome of Percutaneous Pulmonary Valve Implantation

Several studies have shown a significant improvement in New York Heart Association (NYHA) functional class post PPVI, irrespective of the treated lesion (predominantly stenosis vs. predominantly regurgitation).[29,30] In contrast, patients with a predominant stenotic lesion showed a different response to PPVI regarding to MRI and exercise testing data as compared to patients with a predominant regurgitant lesion.

MRI performed before and within 1 month after the procedure with analysis of biventricular function and calculation of great vessel blood flow has shown an improvement in effective RV stroke volume in both patients with predominant pulmonary stenosis (40.6 ± 11.0 vs. 46.8 ± 8.0 mL/m^2; $P < .001$) and predominant regurgitation (37.1 ± 6.2 vs. 44.7 ± 7.5 mL/m^2; $P < .001$).[29] In the stenotic group, this was due to decreased RV end-systolic volume and improved RV ejection fraction after marked reduction of afterload.[29] In contrast, RV ejection fraction remains unchanged in the regurgitant group, with the improvement in RV and LV effective stroke volume due to abolishment of pulmonary regurgitation (reduction in pulmonary regurgitation fraction as assessed by MRI: 39.0% ± 8.6% vs. 3.0% ± 4.7%; $P < .001$).[29] Although relief of RV volume overload resulted in a reduction in RV end-diastolic volume, the total RV stroke volume decreased in these patients with predominantly pulmonary regurgitation. These results are in line with reports on patients undergoing surgical pulmonary valve replacement for pulmonary regurgitation.[14,32] On cardiopulmonary exercise testing, only patients with a predominant stenotic lesion showed an improvement in peak oxygen uptake.[29] We speculate that significant RVOT obstruction limits the augmentation of cardiac output, which is elicited by exercise, thus reducing exercise capacity. Indeed, we were recently able to demonstrate that reduction in RVOT gradient was the only independent predictor of improved exercise capacity early after PPVI.[29] Further, we postulate that pulmonary regurgitation is reduced to a minimum (both as percentage and as absolute value) at peak exercise and is not the limiting factor for cardiac output augmentation during exercise. This is likely to be related to shortening of diastole and reduced pulmonary vascular resistance during exercise.[33] Therefore, by purely abolishing pulmonary regurgitation without

improving RV ejection fraction, peak $\dot{V}o_2$ might not be affected by PPVI acutely in this patient subgroup,[4] explaining the different behavior of the two groups in terms of exercise capacity.

Notably, when we looked at RV size and function on MRI and exercise capacity 1 year post PPVI, we found that there was no further change in any parameters from acutely post PPVI to 1 year post PPVI.[23] As mentioned previously, the ideal timing of any RVOT/pulmonary trunk intervention, whether surgical or percutaneous, remains unknown, because hard endpoints and long-term data are still missing. However, based on these results, one might suggest treating patients with pulmonary regurgitation before the onset of RV dysfunction or impaired exercise capacity.

Device Function During Follow-Up

In the cohort of patients, who did not undergo reoperation or transcatheter reintervention in this group, the peak velocity across the device increased only slightly from 1 month to 36 months after the procedure ($P = .07$). At 1, 6, 12, and 36 months, peak RVOT velocity was 2.64 ± 0.6 m/s (n = 107), 2.7 ± 0.59 m/s (n = 86), 2.66 ± 0.5 m/s (n = 83), 2.89 ± 0.74 m/s (n = 25), respectively.[2] On echocardiography, more than mild valvular incompetence was seen in patients with endocarditis only (Fig. 25-5).

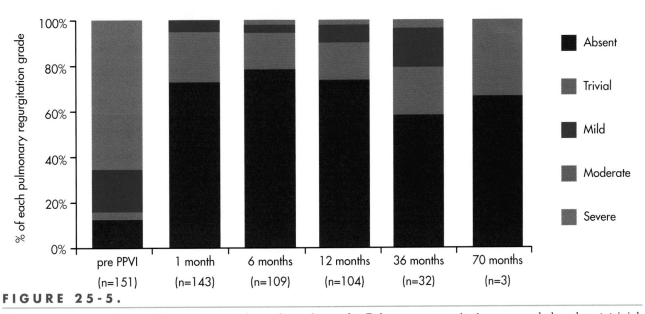

FIGURE 25-5.

Valvular competence during follow-up assessed on echocardiography. Pulmonary regurgitation was graded as absent, trivial, mild, moderate, and severe and expressed in percentage before valve implantation and at 1, 6, 12, 36, and 70 months after percutaneous pulmonary valve implantation. (Modified from Lurz P, Coats L, Khambadkone S, et al. Percutaneous pulmonary valve implantation: impact of evolving technology and learning curve on clinical outcome. *Circulation.* 2008;117:1964–1972.)

FIGURE 25-6.

Freedom from reintervention (surgical or transcatheter) during follow-up post PPVI in the US
Melody Valve Trial. (Modified from McElhinney
DB, Hellenbrand WE, Zahn EM, et al. Short- and
medium-term outcomes after transcatheter pulmonary valve placement in the expanded multicenter US melody valve trial. *Circulation.* 2010;122:
507–516.)

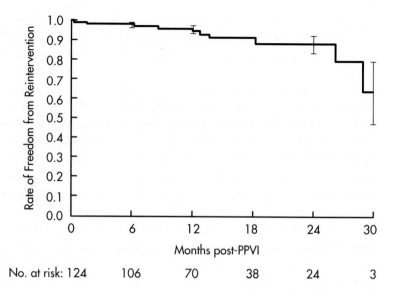

No. at risk: 124   106   70   38   24   3

Rate of Reoperation/Transcatheter Reintervention

In our assessment of the first 155 PPVI patients with a
median follow-up of 28 months, we have demonstrated
a freedom from reoperation of 93% (±2), 86% (±3), 84%
(±4), and 70% (±13), and a freedom from transcatheter r-intervention (second PPVI or balloon dilatation)
of 95% (±2), 87% (±3), 73% (±6), and 73% (±6) at 10,
30, 50, and 70 months, respectively.[2] Similar freedom
from reoperation and/or transcatheter reintervention
was achieved in the US trial (Fig. 25-6). In both patient
cohorts, restenosis was the most common reason for
reintervention, whereas this was due to stent fractures
in the majority of patients, which will be discussed further later. Within the US Melody Valve trial, independent risk factors for reintervention were the following: a
higher mean RVOT gradient on discharge echocardiography; younger age at the time of implant; and a primary implantation indication of RVOT obstruction or
mixed disease as compared to regurgitation.[30]

Stent Fractures and Valve-in-Valve Procedures

As stated before, stent fractures were and still are the
most common complications during follow-up. These
fractures are a well-known complication of RVOT
stenting with bare-metal stents with a prevalence of
43% described in the literature.[19] Following percutaneous implantation of the pulmonary valve, 20% of
our patients have fractured their stents.[27] In the majority of cases, the fractures are clinically silent, with
no increase in gradient across the valved stent. In a
small proportion of patients, stent fractures can lead

to an increase in RV pressures and gradients across
the device. In these cases, a second PPVI should be
performed. These valve-in-valve implantations have
shown to be a safe and feasible treatment option and
successfully decrease RV pressures in these patients
with stent fractures.[34] Implantation of a second stent,
however, is also advisable in all cases with loss of stent
integrity, even in the absence of stenosis to avoid late
embolization of the stent, as seen in one patient of ours.
Patients should be enrolled into a strict follow-up,
including echocardiography and bilateral chest X-ray
to detect possible stent fracture and their potential hemodynamic consequences.

From a technical point of view, second PPVI does
not differ fundamentally from the initial implant. The
first valved stent might even provide a perfect landmark for positioning of the second device, facilitating
this procedure. In the context of significant recoil and
restenosis of the implantation site, multiple prestenting can be considered to increase the radial force of the
metalwork within the RVOT, allowing for sufficient
and lasting opening of the conduit.

EDWARDS SAPIEN TRANSCATHETER HEART VALVE

The SAPIEN valve is based on the very first percutaneously implanted device in aortic position in 2002.[35] Since
then, advances in technique and device modifications
have transformed this initially pioneering approach
into a serious alternative to conventional surgical aortic valve replacement in high-risk patients.[36] Although
there are more than 5,000 aortic implants worldwide,
the experience with this device in pulmonary position

is still limited with around 80 implants, but this is most likely to increase throughout the next years.

Equipment and Set Up

The device and delivery system are equal to the one used for implants in aortic position and are described in details in the chapter on transcatheter aortic implants. Briefly, the Edwards SAPIEN valve consists of three bovine pericardial leaflets hand-sewn to a stainless steel stent. There is a fabric sealing cuff covering the lower portion of the stent to facilitate a seal with the calcified conduit and prevent paravalvular leak. Currently, the valve is available in 23- and 26-mm diameter sizes with heights of 14.5 and 16 mm, respectively.

The Retroflex II represents the latest generation of catheters for prosthesis delivery (Edwards Lifesciences Inc.). The catheter consists of a balloon catheter and a deflectable guiding catheter, and requires either 22 or 24 French hydrophilic sheaths for the 23- and 26-mm valves, respectively. The guiding catheter has a control knob on the catheter hub, which can be rotated to deflect the catheter into the tricuspid aperture and through the RV into the RVOT. The Retroflex II system also contains a retractable nose cone catheter, which facilitates atraumatic delivery of the system through the ventricle and the calcified/stenotic conduit and/or stent.

Patient Selection

Clinical indications for PPVI using the SAPIEN valve are in keeping with the ones applied for Melody implants.

Indications included right ventricular pressure overload (>75% of systemic) due to conduit obstruction, significant pulmonary regurgitation, and/or increased RV end-diastolic volume (>150 mL/m^2 as assessed on MRI). Morphological requirements were a conduit size at surgical implantation of at least 18 mm, but no larger than 30 mm, with significant discrete narrowing of the conduit.[3,4]

The Procedure

Preprocedural catheterization including assessment of the coronary artery anatomy does not differ to what has been described for Melody implants previously. Importantly, prestenting has to be performed in almost all cases. This is due to the relatively short length of the device, which would not cover the whole length of conduit obstruction in the majority of cases (Fig. 25-7).

Procedural Outcome

In a reported serious of seven implants,[3] there were no procedural complications. Prestenting was performed in all cases at the time of PPVI or during previous catheterization. Postprocedure, the RV to systemic pressure ratio decreased from 78% to 39%. The fluoroscopy time ranged from 16 to 49 min, and the procedure time ranging from 110 to 237 min.

Immediately after implantation and during a reported mean follow-up of 10 months (range 30 days to 3.5 years), there was no clinically relevant pulmonary regurgitation. Further, no stent fractures were reported.

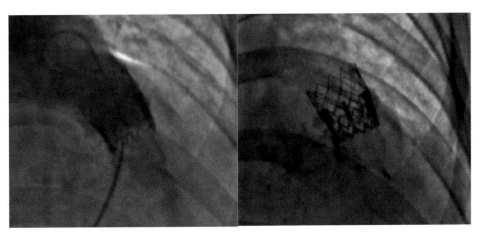

F I G U R E   2 5 - 7 .

Implantation of the SAPIEN transcatheter heart valve (Edwards Lifesciences Inc., Irvine, CA) into a stenotic pulmonary homograft conduit. Showing the final pulmonary angiogram after implantation **(left)** and the valve sitting within the previously placed bare-metal stent **(right)**. (Modified from Boone RH, Webb JG, Horlick E, et al. Transcatheter pulmonary valve implantation using the Edwards SAPIEN transcatheter heart valve. *Catheter Cardiovasc Interv.* 2010;75:286–294.)

CONCLUSION

Although data is still limited, there are encouraging results with the SAPIEN heart valve in pulmonic position. Notably, unlike what has been described after Melody implants, there are no reports of stent fractures of the SAPIEN device in pulmonic position so far. However, the rate of stent fracture during follow-up as much as safety and efficacy of this device in pulmonic position need to be assessed in further studies including more patients with a longer follow-up.

DISCUSSION

The aim of PPVI is to prolong the life span of conduits, which were surgically placed from the RV to the PA. Currently, explantation-free survival 5 years after PPVI is >70% in our patients. This prolonged conduit life span, and hence postponed surgery, should reduce the number of multiple open-heart operations over the total life span of children and young adults with congenital heart disease and potentially improve life expectancy of these patients.

Limitations still exist related to PPVI. Although significant improvement has been achieved in early and late outcomes after percutaneous implantation of pulmonary valves, the risk of stent fractures and homograft rupture are not yet sufficiently understood. Further investigations are necessary to avoid these complications.

Another limitation of the technique (whether using Melody or SAPIEN) at present is the relatively small number of patients who can benefit from this procedure (~15% of all those who would benefit from having a competent pulmonary valve). In many patients, who had repair of tetralogy of Fallot with long-standing pulmonary incompetence, the outflow tract and pulmonary trunk are dilated and distensible, precluding safe implantation of the current percutaneous device. New technology is being developed to address this patient population. Recently, we were able to achieve encouraging results in an animal model with a self-expandable device allowing for PPVI in dilated RVOTs, which has subsequently led to the first-in-human implantation of a percutaneous pulmonary valve in a dilated RVOT in January 2009.[37] This new device bears the promise to offer a nonsurgical treatment to a much broader patient population.

Ultimately, evolution of the treatment of the dysfunctional RVOT can only be achieved by continuing close cooperation between cardiologists, surgeons, specialists in imaging, and biomedical engineers.

REFERENCES

1. Bonhoeffer P, Boudjemline Y, Saliba Z, et al. Percutaneous replacement of pulmonary valve in a right-ventricle to pulmonary-artery prosthetic conduit with valve dysfunction. *Lancet.* 2000;356:1403–1405.
2. Lurz P, Coats L, Khambadkone S, et al. Percutaneous pulmonary valve implantation: impact of evolving technology and learning curve on clinical outcome. *Circulation.* 2008;117:1964–1972.
3. Boone RH, Webb JG, Horlick E, et al. Transcatheter pulmonary valve implantation using the Edwards SAPIEN transcatheter heart valve. *Catheter Cardiovasc Interv.* 2010;75:286–294.
4. Garay F, Webb J, Hijazi ZM. Percutaneous replacement of pulmonary valve using the Edwards-Cribier percutaneous heart valve: first report in a human patient. *Catheter Cardiovasc Interv.* 2006;67:659–662.
5. Boethig D, Thies WR, Hecker H, et al. Mid term course after pediatric right ventricular outflow tract reconstruction: a comparison of homografts, porcine xenografts and Contegras. *Eur J Cardiothorac Surg.* 2005;27:58–66.
6. Brown JW, Ruzmetov M, Rodefeld MD, et al. Right ventricular outflow tract reconstruction with an allograft conduit in non-ross patients: risk factors for allograft dysfunction and failure. *Ann Thorac Surg.* 2005;80:655–663; discussion 663–664.
7. Powell AJ, Lock JE, Keane JF, et al. Prolongation of RV-PA conduit life span by percutaneous stent implantation. Intermediate-term results. *Circulation.* 1995;92:3282–3288.
8. Rastan AJ, Walther T, Daehnert I, et al. Bovine jugular vein conduit for right ventricular outflow tract reconstruction: evaluation of risk factors for mid-term outcome. *Ann Thorac Surg.* 2006;82:1308–1315.
9. Tweddell JS, Pelech AN, Frommelt PC, et al. Factors affecting longevity of homograft valves used in right ventricular outflow tract reconstruction for congenital heart disease. *Circulation.* 2000;102:III130–III135.
10. Gatzoulis MA, Balaji S, Webber SA, et al. Risk factors for arrhythmia and sudden cardiac death late after repair of tetralogy of Fallot: a multicentre study. *Lancet.* 2000;356:975–981.
11. Frigiola A, Redington AN, Cullen S, et al. Pulmonary regurgitation is an important determinant of right ventricular contractile dysfunction in patients with surgically repaired tetralogy of Fallot. *Circulation.* 2004;110:II153–II157.
12. Carvalho JS, Shinebourne EA, Busst C, et al. Exercise capacity after complete repair of tetralogy of Fallot:

deleterious effects of residual pulmonary regurgitation. *Br Heart J.* 1992;67:470–473.

13. Meadows J, Powell AJ, Geva T, et al. Cardiac magnetic resonance imaging correlates of exercise capacity in patients with surgically repaired tetralogy of Fallot. *Am J Cardiol.* 2007;100:1446–1450.

14. Oosterhof T, van Straten A, Vliegen HW, et al. Preoperative thresholds for pulmonary valve replacement in patients with corrected tetralogy of Fallot using cardiovascular magnetic resonance. *Circulation.* 2007;116:545–551.

15. Buechel ER, Dave HH, Kellenberger CJ, et al. Remodelling of the right ventricle after early pulmonary valve replacement in children with repaired tetralogy of Fallot: assessment by cardiovascular magnetic resonance. *Eur Heart J.* 2005;26:2721–2727.

16. Therrien J, Provost Y, Merchant N, et al. Optimal timing for pulmonary valve replacement in adults after tetralogy of Fallot repair. *Am J Cardiol.* 2005;95:779–782.

17. O'Laughlin MP, Slack MC, Grifka RG, et al. Implantation and intermediate-term follow-up of stents in congenital heart disease. *Circulation.* 1993;88:605–614.

18. Aggarwal S, Garekar S, Forbes TJ, et al. Is stent placement effective for palliation of right ventricle to pulmonary artery conduit stenosis? *J Am Coll Cardiol.* 2007;49:480–484.

19. Peng LF, McElhinney DB, Nugent AW, et al. Endovascular stenting of obstructed right ventricle-to-pulmonary artery conduits: a 15-year experience. *Circulation.* 2006;113:2598–2605.

20. Sugiyama H, Williams W, Benson LN. Implantation of endovascular stents for the obstructive right ventricular outflow tract. *Heart.* 2005;91:1058–1063.

21. Lurz P, Puranik R, Nordmeyer J, et al. Improvement in left ventricular filling properties after relief of right ventricle to pulmonary artery conduit obstruction: contribution of septal motion and interventricular mechanical delay. *Eur Heart J.* 2009;30:2266–2274.

22. Lurz P, Nordmeyer J, Muthurangu V, et al. Comparison of bare metal stenting and percutaneous pulmonary valve implantation for treatment of right ventricular outflow tract obstruction: use of an x-ray/magnetic resonance hybrid laboratory for acute physiological assessment. *Circulation.* 2009;119:2995–3001.

23. Lurz P, Nordmeyer J, Giardini A, et al. Early versus late functional outcome after successful percutaneous pulmonary valve implantation—are the acute effects of altered right ventricular loading all we can expect? *J Am Coll Cardiol.* 2011;57:724–731.

24. Lurz P, Bonhoeffer P. Percutaneous implantation of pulmonary valves for treatment of right ventricular outflow tract dysfunction. *Cardiol Young.* 2008;18:260–267.

25. Sridharan S, Coats L, Khambadkone S, et al. Images in cardiovascular medicine. Transcatheter right ventricular outflow tract intervention: the risk to the coronary circulation. *Circulation.* 2006;113:e934–e935.

26. Maheshwari S, Bruckheimer E, Nehgme RA, et al. Single coronary artery complicating stent implantation for homograft stenosis in tetralogy of Fallot. *Cathet Cardiovasc Diagn.* 1997;42:405–407.

27. Nordmeyer J, Khambadkone S, Coats L, et al. Risk stratification, systematic classification, and anticipatory management strategies for stent fracture after percutaneous pulmonary valve implantation. *Circulation.* 2007;115:1392–1397.

28. Nordmeyer J, Lurz P, Khambadkone S, et al. Presenting with a bare metal stent before percutaneous pulmonary valve implantation: acute and 1-year outcomes. *Heart.* 2011;97:118–123.

29. Lurz P, Giardini A, Taylor AM, et al. Effect of altering pathologic right ventricular loading conditions by percutaneous pulmonary valve implantation on exercise capacity. *Am J Cardiol.* 2010;105:721–726.

30. McElhinney DB, Hellenbrand WE, Zahn EM, et al. Short- and medium-term outcomes after transcatheter pulmonary valve placement in the expanded multicenter US melody valve trial. *Circulation.* 2010;122:507–516.

31. Khambadkone S, Coats L, Taylor A, et al. Percutaneous pulmonary valve implantation in humans: results in 59 consecutive patients. *Circulation.* 2005;112:1189–1197.

32. Frigiola A, Tsang V, Bull C, et al. Biventricular response after pulmonary valve replacement for right ventricular outflow tract dysfunction: is age a predictor of outcome? *Circulation.* 2008;118:S182–S190.

33. Roest AA, Helbing WA, Kunz P, et al. Exercise MR imaging in the assessment of pulmonary regurgitation and biventricular function in patients after tetralogy of fallot repair. *Radiology.* 2002;223:204–211.

34. Nordmeyer J, Coats L, Lurz P, et al. Percutaneous pulmonary valve-in-valve implantation: a successful treatment concept for early device failure. *Eur Heart J.* 2008;29:810–815.

35. Cribier A, Eltchaninoff H, Bash A, et al. Percutaneous transcatheter implantation of an aortic valve prosthesis for calcific aortic stenosis: first human case description. *Circulation.* 2002;106:3006–3008.

36. Leon MB, Smith CR, Mack M, et al. Transcatheter aortic-valve implantation for aortic stenosis in patients who cannot undergo surgery. *N Engl J Med.* 2010;363:1597–1607.

37. Schievano S, Taylor AM, Capelli C, et al. First-in-man implantation of a novel percutaneous valve: a new approach to medical device development. *EuroIntervention.* 2010;5:745–750.

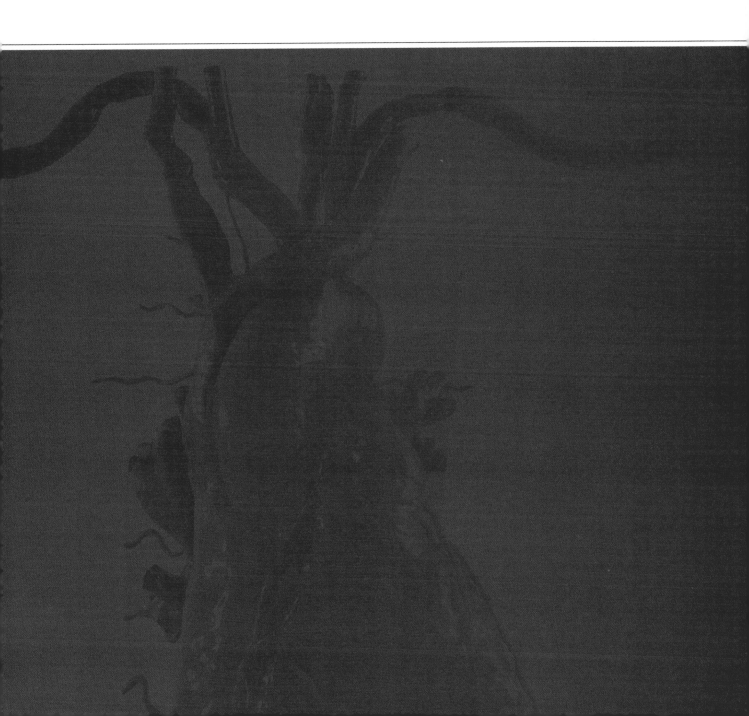

SPECIALIZED PROCEDURES

Percutaneous Treatment of Coarctation of the Aorta

Alejandro J. Torres and William E. Hellenbrand

oarctation of the aorta (CoA) is a congenital cardiac anomaly characterized by the presence of a narrowing, most commonly located at the junction of the distal aortic arch and the descending aorta, just distal to the origin of the left subclavian artery. The resulting obstruction in blood flow clinically manifests as a difference in blood pressure between the upper and lower body. Coarctation is rarely found in the ascending or abdominal aorta. CoA occurs in 0.02% to 0.06% of live births and accounts for 5% to 8% of patients with congenital heart disease.[1,2] It is more common in males, with a male to female ratio of 1.3–1.7:1, and is usually sporadic, although genetic influences can play a role (up to 35% of patients with Turner syndrome [45, XO] have CoA). The most commonly associated defects in patients who reach adulthood are bicuspid aortic valve (up to 85%); mitral valve deformities, including abnormal apposition of the papillary muscles or true parachute mitral valve; intracranial aneurysms (usually berry aneurysms of the circle of Willis in 3% to 5%); and aberrant right subclavian artery (5%).[3] The mean life expectancy of patients with CoA without intervention is approximately 35 years, with a mortality of 75% before age 46 years and 92% before age 60 years among those surviving childhood.[3] The morbidity and mortality causes are the consequence of long-term high blood pressure including left ventricular dysfunction, aortic rupture/dissection, premature coronary artery disease, and intracranial hemorrhage. The majority of adolescent and adult patients with CoA are asymptomatic and the diagnosis is usually made during hypertension evaluation. Adult patients commonly present with intermittent claudication as their only symptom. The first successful surgical repair of a CoA was described by Crafoord in 1944.[4] For the following four decades, surgery remained the only alternative for therapy, until the first balloon angioplasty was performed in a newborn in 1982 by Singer et al.[5] The introduction of endovascular stents in the early 1990s[6,7] represented an additional milestone in the transcatheter management of patients with CoA. Many studies have since demonstrated the efficacy of balloon angioplasty and stent implantation in relieving native or recurrent (postoperative) CoA in adolescents and adults and, thus, they have become the standard of care in many institutions.

CLASSIFICATION

Native Coarctation of the Aorta

The classic native CoA is described as a discrete narrowing located in the thoracic aorta distal to the left subclavian artery (Fig. 26-1). It is characterized by a ridgelike thickening of the media of the posterior and lateral aspect of the aortic wall that protrudes into the lumen opposite the insertion of the ductus arteriosus or ligamentum arteriosum. Dilatation of the aorta distal to the coarctation is common (poststenotic dilatation). The origin of the left subclavian artery can occasionally be involved within the aortic stricture. A less common form of native CoA involves a longer

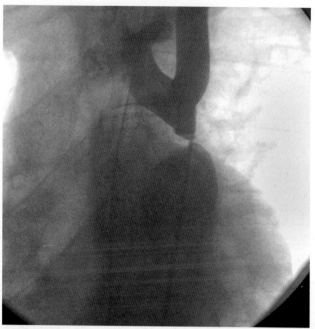

FIGURE 26-1.

Severe, discrete coarctation of the aorta. The narrowest diameter is in the classic location, distal to the left subclavian artery.

narrowed segment, also known as tubular hypoplasia of the aorta, which can involve the isthmus and part of the transverse arch (Fig. 26-2). This form occurs in conjunction with more significant left heart obstructive lesions.

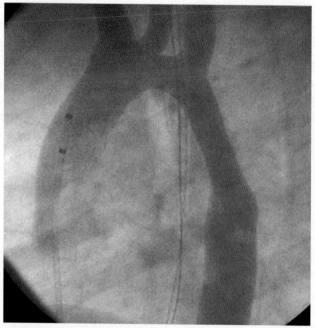

FIGURE 26-2.

Tubular hypoplasia of aorta, the transverse arch and isthmus are moderately hypoplastic.

Recurrent/Residual Coarctation of the Aorta

Recoarctation of the aorta in adult patients following a previous surgery or catheter-based intervention may be secondary to either a residual obstruction or development of restenosis. Regardless of the therapeutic approach used, the occurrence of recoarctation with isolated lesions is uncommon. The incidence of recoarctation after surgery is about 10%[8] and occurs independently of the type of surgical repair used. The causes are probably multifactorial and include technically inadequate repair, lack of growth of suture line, hypoplastic transverse arch, and so forth.

INDICATIONS FOR INTERVENTION

The presence of upper extremity systemic arterial hypertension, with an upper to lower extremity systolic blood pressure difference ≥20 mm Hg, represents the most widely accepted indication for treatment. In addition, patients with a blood pressure difference <20 mm Hg and a history of significant hypertension or abnormal blood pressure response to exercise (more than two standard deviations above the mean), in the presence of echocardiographic evidence of left ventricular hypertrophy or decreased systolic function, should also be considered for intervention. The development of better equipment, including low-profile balloons and stents that can be expanded to adult size, has lowered the age at which stent implantation can be performed without a significant risk for vascular complications. Using the currently available technology, stent implantation can be performed in patients weighing 25 to 30 kg (around 8 to 10 years of age).

IMAGING

Prior to considering endovascular management of CoA, every patient requires a detailed assessment of the anatomy and ventricular function. In adult patients, echocardiographic imaging is usually suboptimal and magnetic resonance imaging (MRI) or computed tomography (CT) scanning are the preferred noninvasive techniques to evaluate CoA. State-of-the-art MRI methods provide excellent anatomic definition of the severity and length of the CoA, the size of the adjacent segments of the aorta, as well as the anatomic relationship of the head vessels and subclavian arteries with the CoA. Discrete coarctation is arbitrarily defined as a segment ≤5 mm long, whereas a >5-mm lesion is considered a long-segment coarctation. In cases where the aortic transverse arch is involved, the narrowing is considered significant when the ratio of the diameter of the stenotic segment to the diameter of the descending aorta at the level of the diaphragm is less than 0.6.

PERCUTANEOUS TREATMENT OF COARCTATION OF THE AORTA

In adolescent and adult patients, balloon angioplasty and stent implantation have emerged as the preferred approach for the treatment of native or recurrent CoA in most centers. Surgical repair in older children and adults is associated with an extended recovery time; prolonged analgesic requirement; potential phrenic nerve and recurrent laryngeal nerve injury; and the serious, although uncommon, lower body paralysis secondary to ischemic spinal cord injury during the operation. This complication occurs in 0.5% of patients undergoing surgical CoA repair and is rare with adequate arterial collateral circulation. Intraoperative mortality rate is also higher in older patients as a consequence of degenerative aortic wall changes, coronary artery disease, and end-organ damage from chronic systemic arterial hypertension.

Balloon angioplasty produces a controlled tear of the intima and part of the media, which results in an improvement of the vessel diameter. The use of balloon angioplasty is limited to patients with discrete CoA given the high rate of reintervention in patients with isthmus hypoplasia or long tubular stenosis. Balloon angioplasty may require oversizing of the balloon to a diameter larger than the normal vessel, which may explain the high incidence of aneurysm formation reported to occur in up to 9% of cases.[9–15]

Endovascular stent implantation is now increasingly used in place of balloon dilatation for both native or recurrent coarctation in older children and adults. The use of stents provides resistance to the inward recoil force considered an important factor in recurrence following balloon angioplasty of CoA. It also minimizes the trauma to the aortic wall and the potential for aneurysm formation by limiting the dilation at the coarctation site and, at the adjacent segments of the aorta, to the diameter of the stent. Late aneurysm formation at the coarctation site may occur after stenting but seems to be less frequently encountered compared to after balloon angioplasty. The use of stents is also potentially beneficial in patients with longer segment and tubular CoA, who typically have a poor result after balloon angioplasty.

EQUIPMENT

Balloons

There is a wide variety of balloon dilation catheters currently available for stent implantation. In the past, only single large diameter balloons were available for stent implantation. These large diameter balloons expand initially at the ends, which may result in balloon rupture or wall injury by the ends of the stent at the beginning of the inflation. The development of balloon-in-balloon (BIB, NuMed, Hopkinton, NY) has been a major advance for delivery of large diameter stents. These catheters have an inner balloon and a 1-cm longer outer balloon, double the diameter of the inner balloon. They are available in outer balloon sizes of 8 to 24 mm, whereas the shaft of the catheter is either 8 or 9 French. The BIB balloon offers several advantages for stent implantation when compared to single-balloon catheters. Because the inner balloon is usually shorter than the stent, the balloon expands the stent uniformly without flaring the ends of the stent, thus decreasing the risk of balloon perforation or wall injury. The expanded inner balloon provides a better anchoring mechanism, which results in more precise control during inflation of the outer balloon. BIB catheters have a higher profile than single-balloon catheters and require larger sheaths for introduction.

Sheaths

A long sheath is required for the delivery of a hand-mounted stent via the femoral artery. There are several commercially available sheaths. The most popular is the Mullins sheath (Cook, Bloomington, IN), which has a radiopaque tip for easier visualization under fluoroscopy and a side arm that can be used for hand injection of dye to assess balloon positioning prior to stent delivery or blood pressure monitoring. Regardless of the sheath used, a large hub is required in order to avoid slippage of the stent when the balloon is introduced into the sheath. The Mullins sheaths are available in different sizes (up to 16 French) but only the ones equal to or larger than 9 French come with large-enough hubs.

Stents

There are several different endovascular stents commercially available; however, very few are expandable to the average diameter of a large adult aorta. The mean aortic arch diameter in a fully grown adult is 21.1 mm (±3.2) for women and 26.1 mm (±4.3) for men.[16] However, many patients with CoA have some degree of aortic arch hypoplasia, thus they never reach a normal diameter. In our institution, three different endovascular stents have been used for treatment of CoA over the last 10 years.

1. Palmaz XL 10-series stents (Johnson & Johnson, New Brunswick, NJ): the 3110, the 4010, and the 5010. The first two digits indicate the unexpanded stent length in millimeters (31-, 40-, and 50-mm long, respectively). The last two digits indicate the minimum diameter at which they should be expanded: 10 mm. These stents can be expanded to a maximum diameter of 25 to 28 mm. The Palmaz stent is made of stainless steel and laser-cut slots, which become diamond-shaped cells when expanded. The edges are rounded to minimize risk of balloon rupture during implantation. The main advantage of the Palmaz XL stent is the good radial strength. However, it is a rigid stent with essentially no flexibility to conform nonlinear areas and suffers significant shortening at larger diameters.

2. The Palmaz Genesis XD (Cordis, Johnson & Johnson) stent is also laser-cut from stainless steel and has a closed cell design but has a sigmoidal hinge between the cells. This property adds greater flexibility to the stent without compromising its radial strength. Elongation of the sigmoidal hinge during expansion prevents excessive foreshortening. Radial strength is good, although the rate of fracture is higher than other stents. They come in five nominal lengths (19, 25, 29, 39, and 59 mm). However, it is essential to remember that this stent cannot be expanded beyond 18 to 19 mm. Because of this limitation, the Genesis XD may be a good option for treatment of CoA in patients in whom the aorta is not expected to grow to a normal size.

3. The introduction of the IntraStent LD Max (ev3, Plymouth, MN) is a new addition to the large-sized stent category and can be dilated to 24 to 26 mm diameter. Cell edges are rounded to decrease the risk of wall injury or balloon rupture during inflation. This stent has an open-cell design that significantly reduces stent shortening and provides good radial strength at larger diameters without compromising flexibility. It is available in lengths of 16, 26, and 36 mm. Because of the open cell design and rounded edges, the risk of stent slippage over the balloon during inflation may be higher when compared to other stents.

4. The Cheatham-Platinum (CP) stent (NuMed, Hopkinton, NY) has been extensively used worldwide. Its use in the United States is currently undergoing investigation in a multicenter study. It is manufactured from wire of a platinum-iridium alloy with a zigzag design and it can be ordered to any length. The recommended minimum dilated diameter is 8 mm and the maximum diameter is 24 mm accompanied by a foreshortening of 20%, although it can be dilated to 30 mm in diameter. The CP stent is available in a covered version and has also been used outside the United States for the treatment of CoA. The stent is fitted with a covering of expanded polytetrafluoroethylene. Main indications for the use of covered stent include rescue treatment for surgical or post-transcatheter intervention aneurysms and patients with high risk of aortic wall complications due to complex CoA anatomy such as near interruption or long-segment lesions. The use of covered stents offers the potential advantage of decreasing the incidence of aortic wall complications such as aneurysms or significant intimal tears. However, covered stent misplacement can result in serious complications if accidentally implanted overlapping a main head vessels or an important descending aorta side branch.

5. Another covered stent not available in the United States is the Advanta V12 LD (Atrium Medical, Hudson, NH). This is a stainless steel, open-cell stent covered by expanded polytetrafluoroethylene that covers both the interior and exterior aspects of the stent. It comes premounted on balloons of 12-, 14-, and 16-mm diameters and can be dilated up to 22 mm with a foreshortening of about 25% at that diameter. The Advanta stent offers the advantage that can be implanted through smaller delivery systems (8 French for the 12-mm stent) than the covered CP stent, thus can be used in smaller patients.[17]

TECHNIQUE

At our institution, all procedures that involve balloon angioplasty or stent implantation for CoA are performed under general anesthesia because balloon expansion of a systemic artery produces pain at the dilation site and patient movement may compromise the success of the procedure. Access in the right or left femoral vessels is obtained in the usual fashion. Because large sheaths are used, particular attention must be paid during access of the femoral artery in order to avoid a high- or low-puncture site, which may increase the risk of vascular complications such as retroperitoneal hematoma or femoral artery occlusion. Once access is obtained, intravenous heparin is administered (100 U/kg up to 5000 U). The activated clotting time is monitored every 30 minutes and additional boluses are given in order to maintain activated clotting time levels >250 sec. After completion of the right heart catheterization, a right coronary or multipurpose catheter is advanced through the arterial sheath into the descending aorta. We usually use a soft-tip wire to carefully cross the CoA site to avoid causing a tear in the wall with a stiffer wire because the layers of the CoA wall are usually abnormal and its intima prone to injury. Once the catheter is positioned in the ascending aorta, it is replaced over a wire by a high-flow pigtail. Starting from the ascending aorta, a careful pullback is performed to obtain pressures at different levels throughout the entire aortic arch because some gradient can occasionally be found in areas other than the classic CoA site as it happens in patients with hypoplastic transverse arch. Biplane angiography is performed with the pigtail just proximal to the lesion. The first angiogram is usually taken with the X-ray cameras in the left anterior oblique and straight lateral projections (Fig. 26-3). If necessary, angiography is repeated with different angulations in order to image the lesion into its largest length. A catheter, with calibrated angiographic markers, is positioned in the field of the angiography for reliable calibration if autocalibration is not available. Whichever method is used, accurate calibration is of paramount importance because the measurements obtained will determine the size of the balloon and stent to be used, and small errors can increase the risk of complications. Once the angiographies are obtained, measurements are made at different points of the aorta in order to select the type of stent and balloon to be used. The size of the balloon should

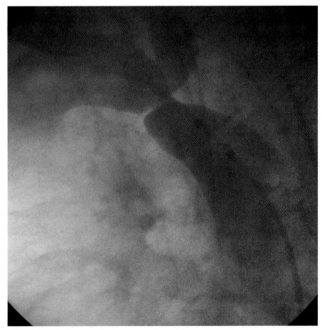

FIGURE 26-3.

Severe discrete coarctation of the aorta visualized on the lateral projection. The left subclavian artery ostium is next to the narrowest point of the coarctation.

be no more than 1 to 2 mm larger in diameter than the smallest normal aortic diameter proximal to the coarctation. Occasionally, this area is very short and involves the coarctation, thus an accurate measurement cannot be obtained. In those cases, the diameter of the transverse arch and the aorta at the level of the diaphragm are used for reference. Poststenotic dilatation of the thoracic aorta distal to the coarctation is common, and this area should not be used to size the balloon. It is our practice to test the compliance of the coarctation lesion before implanting a stent in order to decrease the risk of aortic wall complications.

In some patients, an important component of the gradient across the CoA is the result of a fold of the aortic wall at the area of the coarctation. These lesions characteristically have high compliance and can be dilated fully to the intended diameter in one procedure. Conversely, other patients with either long segment or discrete CoA have noncompliant lesions. These patients have an increased risk of aortic wall complications if higher balloon pressures are required to fully expand the stent, thus a two-staged approach is recommended for them. In order to check the CoA compliance, a balloon 2 mm smaller in diameter than the intended stent is inflated at the coarctation site to 4 to 6 atm. If a significant residual waist remains on the balloon, the stent is implanted on a slightly smaller balloon and the patient is brought back to the catheterization laboratory for full expansion of the stent 6 months later.

The selection of the stent depends on several factors and their different properties along with the anatomy of the aorta must be considered jointly. If the coarctation area has a current or is expected to reach a diameter of 20 mm or more, a large diameter stent will have to be chosen, limiting choices to the Palmaz XL or the ev3 open-cell stents. We favor the use of the stiffer Palmaz XL stent for CoA located in straight segments of the aorta and the more flexible ev3 for lesions located in curved areas. The NuMed CP stent can also be expanded to a large diameter but is not yet available in the United States. In patients in whom the aorta is not expected to grow more than 18 mm in diameter, the Genesis XD can also be used. Once the decisions for the balloon diameter and the type of stent are made, the length of the stent is chosen. Stent length selection should be based on the length of the coarctation and the estimated longitudinal shortening of the stent at the selected balloon diameter. All stents suffer progressive shortening as their diameter increases (the Palmaz XL stent shortens the most) and this should be considered when choosing a stent. Every stent manufacturer provides tables with the predicted stent length for a certain diameter. The length of the stent will also determine the length of the balloon, which should be as short as possible, but still slightly longer than the stent. A large balloon length-to-stent length ratio increases the risk of balloon perforation during inflation.

The stent is then hand-mounted on the balloon before the delivery sheath is introduced. To decrease the risk of stent migration on the balloon as it is introduced and advanced through the sheath, the stent can be tied on the balloon with a piece of sterile umbilical tape looped around the stent and balloon. The stent should not be tied at its edges as this may puncture the balloon. Another technique described is to slightly inflate the balloon to 1 to 2 atm so that it grips the stent more tightly at its edges. Although these measures may help, proper wire position, sheath selection, and careful introduction and advancement of the mounted stent through the sheath usually prevent stent slippage off the balloon.

Once the stent and balloon catheter are ready, an end-hole catheter is maneuvered retrograde across the coarctation and advanced deep into the right or left subclavian artery. A long (260 cm) super stiff wire is parked in that position, making sure that the soft end of the wire remains far from the subclavian artery origin. In lesions that involve the transverse arch, the wire positioned in the right subclavian makes a better, more gradual curve, which facilitates the stabilization of the balloon during inflation. The left subclavian artery can be used when the lesion is located more distal into the descending aorta. Whichever subclavian artery is used, the cephalic end of the balloon must be positioned distal to the origin of the vessel that holds the wire because inflation of the balloon with its tip within the subclavian artery would cause the balloon to migrate out of the vessel. The ascending aorta should not be used to position the tip of the stiff wire, as this location does not allow good fixation and stabilization, which may predispose the balloon to move back and forth during inflation. Proper wire position is absolutely crucial for the success of the procedure. The regular sheath is then exchanged for the selected long delivery sheath. In order to accommodate the balloon with the mounted stent, the delivery sheath should be one or two French larger than the indicated for the balloon catheter alone. A still frame from the aortogram showing the location of the coarctation is used as a roadmap. The long sheath is advanced retrograde until the tip of the sheath is several centimeters beyond the lesion. Proper flushing of the sheath is important because large air bubbles can be trapped within the sheath when the dilator is removed. Different maneuvers including adenosine administration and rapid right ventricular pacing[18] have been described to decrease stroke volume and blood pressure in order to prevent the stent from moving and ensure its precise placement during balloon inflation. These maneuvers should be reserved for patients with mild or moderate CoA because severe lesions have a low risk of stent migration during inflation. For ventricular pacing, a pacing catheter is placed in the right ventricle, and pacing is initiated at a rate of 180 to 200 ppm. Balloon inflation is initiated when the systolic blood pressure decreases to less than 100 mm Hg. Right ventricle pacing is continued during the inner and outer balloon inflation and terminated as soon as both balloons are deflated.

The balloon-mounted stent is advanced through the sheath to the precise position across the coarctation site; the sheath is withdrawn off the stent, making sure that the caudal end of the balloon is entirely outside the sheath. A hand angiogram can be performed through the sheath to assess the position of the balloon. If a BIB balloon is used, the inner balloon is inflated and an angiogram is repeated through the sheath to confirm the location of the stent (Fig. 26-4). At this point, the position of the balloon-stent can still be adjusted. The outer balloon is then inflated to fix the stent in the lesion, both balloons are deflated, and the catheter is removed over the wire (Fig. 26-5). If a pinpoint perforation occurs while the balloon is being inflated, the operator should continue to inflate the balloon in order to increase the pressure within the balloon and expand the stent as much as possible to decrease the risk of stent migration.

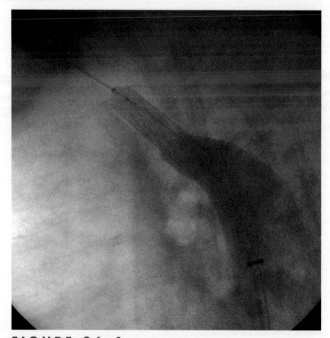

FIGURE 26-4.

Angiogram following inner balloon inflation to assess stent position.

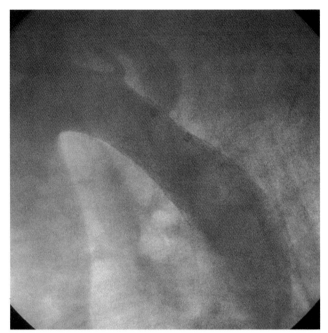

FIGURE 26-5.

Angiography following stent implantation shows resolutions of the coarctation. The stent covers the ostium of the left subclavian artery without compromising flow into the vessel.

A pullback pressure is repeated to document any residual gradient across the stent. Gentle dilatation of the stent with a larger or higher pressure balloon can be performed if a residual gradient is recorded. The caudal end of the stent may occasionally "hang" free without complete apposition against the wall of the poststenotic area of the aorta. We do not routinely recommend flaring the stent end because it offers no hemodynamic benefit and increases the risk of aortic wall injury. Overlapping of one or more brachiocephalic vessel by part of the stent is technically unavoidable in patients with hypoplastic transverse arch or CoA near the left subclavian artery ostium. The potential risk of distal embolism has been a source of concern among interventional cardiologists. However, stent overlap of a branchiocephalic vessel has not been associated to peripheral embolic events or flow disturbance of the affected vessel on early and midterm follow-up, thus should not preclude stent implantation.

RESULTS

Excellent immediate and long-term results have been unanimously reported in the majority of patients undergoing stent implantation for treatment of native or recurrent CoA since the introduction of the modality in the early 1990s.[19–23] Although previous studies of balloon angioplasty in adults consistently showed good results in the management of CoA,[11,24–26] lower gradients and larger diameters at the CoA site have been achieved with stenting as a consequence of neutralization of the elastic recoil of the vessel commonly seen after balloon angioplasty. A successful procedure is usually defined as a peak systolic residual gradient of less than 20 mm Hg and/or an increase of the CoA/descending aorta ratio to at least 0.8 in the absence of serious complications. In the Congenital Cardiovascular Interventional Study Consortium (CCISC), a recent multi-institutional study with the participation of 17, which included a total of 565 patients,[22] successful stenting of native and recurrent CoA was reported in 97.9% (553/565) of the procedures. Of the 12 patients (2.1%) in whom the procedure was unsuccessful, five had a baseline gradient of more than 60 mm Hg across the coarctation, two had undergone stent implantation in ascending to descending conduits (one patient expired secondary to aortic rupture), and another patient required emergent surgery secondary to aortic dissection. In the same study, the rate of success decreased to 92.2% (521/565) when success was defined as a residual peak systolic gradient <10 mm Hg. In this cohort, factors associated with a higher rate of success were discrete versus tunnel CoA (successful outcome in 94.6% vs. 84.6% of the patients, respectively) (Figs. 26-6 and 26-7), a larger diameter of the coarctation prior to the procedure, and a lower baseline peak systolic gradient.

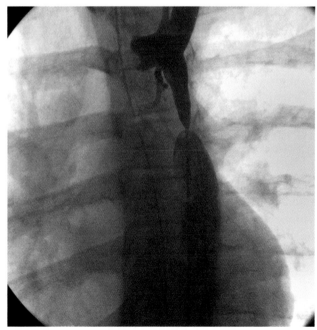

FIGURE 26-6.

Tubular coarctation of the aorta with a long-segment stenosis of the isthmus.

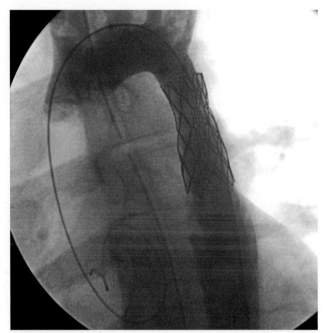

FIGURE 26-7.

Poststent implantation angiogram shows stent in good position and significant diameter increase of the isthmus.

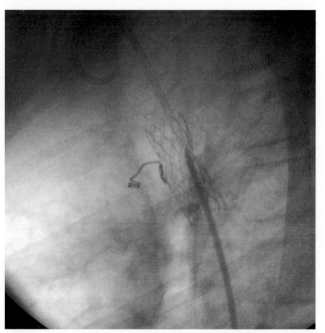

FIGURE 26-8.

Recoarctation following stent implantation secondary to circumferential fracture and partial collapse of the stent. The patent ductus artery had been coil occluded at the time of the stent implantation.

Several studies support continued good outcomes by imaging and cuff pressure or other hemodynamic evaluation on intermediate follow up.[19,20,27-29] Imaging of the aortic arch with MRI or CT scan should be performed in all patients 6 months following stent implantation, and once a year thereafter. Restenosis caused by stent fracture or intimal proliferation is rarely seen following stent implantation. The Palmaz XL stent has the lowest incidence of fracture on follow up. Localized stent fractures of one or two cell arms are occasionally seen on X-ray and have no hemodynamic significance. Circumferential stent fracture followed by stent collapse requiring reintervention has been reported in a very small percentage of patients (Figs. 26-8 and 26-9).[23] Although some degree of intimal proliferation within the stent can be visualized on follow-up angiographies, it rarely causes significant obstruction in adult patients.

Balloon redilation has been performed safely and with good results in patients with intimal proliferation or those undergoing a staged approach.[20,30] Although balloon redilation can be performed in patients with stent fracture resulting in obstruction, the implantation of a second stent is preferred.

About one-third of the patients remain hypertensive following CoA stent placement and continue to require antihypertensive medications for its control, although usually at a reduced dose. Immediate poststenting hypertension should be closely monitored, preferably

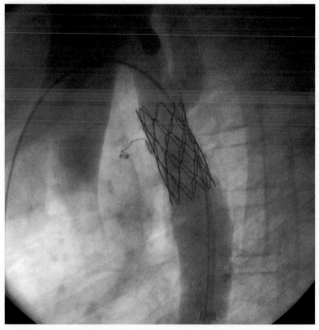

FIGURE 26-9.

Poststent angiogram shows stent in good position and resolution of the recoarctation.

in an intensive care unit, and treated to maintain systolic pressures <150 mm Hg and diastolic pressures <90 mm Hg. Nitroprusside or esmolol are the intravenous medications most commonly used until the patient can be transitioned to oral medications.

COMPLICATIONS

Because endovascular stenting of CoA can be associated with serious adverse events, it should only be performed in experienced centers with immediate cardiothoracic surgery availability. The incidence of acute complications varies among studies but has been reported in up to 14.2% of the procedures.[11,20–22,28] Complications related to CoA stent implantation are divided into three categories: aortic wall complications, technical complications, and other vascular complications.

Aortic Wall Complications

Aortic wall complications at the site of the coarctation include intimal tears, dissection, and aneurysm formation and occurred in 3.9% of the patients in the CCISC.[22] The risk of developing an aortic wall complication was higher in patients in whom high-pressure present balloon angioplasty was performed and in patients older than 40 years of age. A balloon/coarctation ratio >3.5 at the time of the procedure was also associated with a higher occurrence of aortic wall injuries at follow up, which suggests that a more conservative approach with progressive stent dilatation at different stages to achieve full expansion may be indicated in patients with severe obstruction and noncompliant lesions. Low-pressure (≤4 atm) present angioplasty to assess the compliance of the coarctation site was not associated with a higher risk of aortic wall injury.

Intimal Tears

Some degree of tearing of the intima is expected to occur within the area of the coarctation during balloon inflation and it is usually tamponaded against the wall by the stent struts. No further intervention is usually required. It was reported in eight patients (1.4%) in the CCISC study, one patient required implantation of a second stent during the same procedure, and the other one had a second stent implanted months later secondary to significant obstruction at the site of the tear.

Aortic Dissection

Aortic dissection is a serious complication, which carries a high mortality. Emergent intervention is commonly indicated in order to avoid aortic wall rupture

within the mediastinum or the potential propagation of the dissection flap into important aortic branches such as the common carotid arteries, which may result in irreversible neurologic injury. The CCISC reported nine (1.6%) cases of aortic dissection. Three patients underwent emergent surgery, two of who suffered severe neurologic injuries and died later on. Three other patients were successfully treated in the catheterization laboratory with implantation of covered stents. The last three patients were managed medically with strict control of blood pressure. One patient had resolution of the aortic dissection at 1-month follow up.

Aortic Aneurysm

Aneurysm is usually defined as a >10% dilatation of the aorta outside the stent or normal aorta that was not present prior to the procedure. Aortic aneurysms can develop at the time of the procedure or on interval follow up and usually occur at the site of the narrowest segment of the coarctation. The incidence of late aortic aneurysm following stent implantation is around 3% (Fig. 26-10).[29] Most aneurysms are small and are managed conservatively with observation. However, intervention with covered stents or surgery is indicated if an aneurysm develops during the procedure or rapid size progression is noticed during follow up (Fig. 26-11).

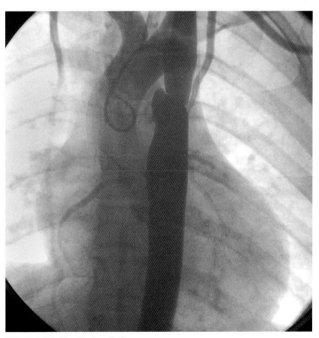

FIGURE 26-10.

Late aneurysm following balloon angioplasty. The patient presented with signs of recoarctation and the aneurysm was an incidental finding.

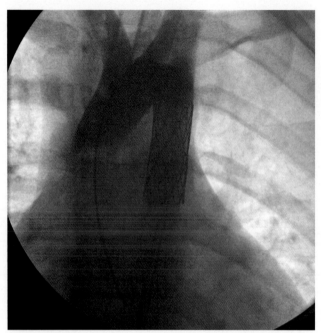

FIGURE 26-11.

Post covered stent implantation: the aneurysm has been excluded from the circulation, and there is no residual coarctation.

Technical Complications

The incidence of technical complications has decreased over the last years as a consequence of equipment design improvements. Technical complications include stent migration and/or balloon rupture during the procedure. Stent migration is associated with the use of oversized or undersized balloons or balloon rupture during inflation. The most common scenario for stent migration (14/28 of cases in the CCISC study) occurred when stents were delivered on balloons that were >2 mm larger than the aorta proximal to the coarctation. The use of undersized balloons for stent implantation in patients with a compliant lesion such as a fold or pseudocoarctation at the coarctation site are the second most common cause for stent migration. Balloon rupture is an uncommon complication and occurred in 13/565 (2.2%) in the CCISC cohort. The risk of balloon rupture is more commonly seen when very stiff stents

such as the Palmaz series or single balloon catheters are used. Migrated stents can frequently be repositioned within the coarctation site. In those patients in whom the stent cannot be repositioned, it should be expanded in the safest location available (i.e., descending thoracic aorta), trying to avoid overlapping the ostia of the abdominal aorta branches.

Vascular Complications

Femoral vessel injury occurs in 2% to 10% of the cases and includes bleeding, thrombotic complications, and vascular trauma. Procedural factors that increase the risk include large sheaths, excessive use of anticoagulants, and site of entry below the common femoral artery or above the ligamentum arteriosum. Most cases are managed conservatively. Femoral artery occlusion is very uncommon in adult patients and is usually treated with intravenous heparin infusion. Vascular surgery consult is indicated if the viability of the leg is a concern at any point. Retroperitoneal hematoma can be a life-threatening complication, which usually results from a high-femoral artery puncture. Patients who develop severe low back or abdominal pain within hours of the procedure should be evaluated for this condition with a blood count and abdominal CT scan. Cerebral vascular accidents occur in about 1% of the cases and are usually related to complications such as aortic wall injury, stent migration, balloon migration, or wire positioning. Older age also places the patients at higher risk for cerebral vascular accidents.

CONCLUSION

Intravascular stenting is a relatively safe and highly effective treatment modality in the management of CoA. It remains a technically demanding procedure, although the rate of complications has decreased—thanks to recent improvements in catheter and stent technology. For most adult patients, it represents the treatment of choice for native and recurrent CoA.

REFERENCES

1. Keith JD. Coarctation of the aorta. In: Keith JD, Rowe RD, Vlad P, eds. *Heart Disease in Infancy and Childhood*. 3rd ed. New York: Macmillan; 1978.
2. Nadas AS, Fyler DC. *Pediatric Cardiology*. 3rd ed. Philadelphia: W.B. Saunders; 1972.
3. Perloff JK, Child JS, eds. *Congenital Heart Disease in Adults*. 2nd ed. Philadelphia: W.B. Saunders; 1998.
4. Crafoord C, Nylin G. Congenital coarctation of the aorta and its surgical treatment. *J Thorac Surg*. 1945;14: 347.
5. Singer MI, Rowen M, Dorsey TJ. Transluminal aortic balloon angioplasty for coarctation of the aorta in the newborn. *Am Heart J*. 1982;103: 131–132.

6. Morrow WR, Smith VC, Ehler WJ, et al. Balloon angioplasty with stent implantation in experimental coarctation of the aorta. *Circulation.* 1994;89(6):2677–2683.

7. Grifka RG, Vick GW 3rd, O'Laughlin MP, et al. Balloon expandable intravascular stents: aortic implantation and late further dilation in growing minipigs. *Am Heart J.* 1993;126(4):979–984.

8. Midulla M, Dehaene A, Godart F, et al. TEVAR in patients with late complications of aortic coarctation repair. *J Endovasc Ther.* 2008;15(5):552–557.

9. Walhout RJ, Suttorp MJ, Mackaij GJ, et al. Long-term outcome after balloon angioplasty of coarctation of the aorta in adolescents and adults: is aneurysm formation an issue? *Catheter Cardiovasc Interv.* 2009; 73(4):549–556.

10. Fawzy ME, Awad M, Hassan W, et al. Long-term outcome (up to 15 years) of balloon angioplasty of discrete native coarctation of the aorta in adolescents and adults. *J Am Coll Cardiol.* 2004;43(6):1062–1067.

11. Pedra CA, Fontes VF, Esteves CA, et al. Stenting vs. balloon angioplasty for discrete unoperated coarctation of the aorta in adolescents and adults. *Catheter Cardiovasc Interv.* 2005;64(4):495–506.

12. Mookerjee J, Roebuck D, Derrick G. Restenosis after aortic stenting. *Cardiol Young.* 2004;14(2):210–211.

13. Golden AB, Hellenbrand WE. Coarctation of the aorta: stenting in children and adults. *Catheter Cardiovasc Interv.* 2007;69(2):289–299.

14. Ovaert C, Benson LN, Nykanen D, et al. Transcatheter treatment of coarctation of the aorta: a review. *Pediatr Cardiol.* 1998;19(1):27–44; discussion 45–47.

15. Hornung TS, Benson LN, McLaughlin PR. Interventions for aortic coarctation. *Cardiol Rev.* 2002;10(3): 139–148.

16. Garcier JM, Petitcolin V, Filaire M, et al. Normal diameter of the thoracic aorta in adults: a magnetic resonance imaging study. *Surg Radiol Anat.* 2003;25(3–4): 322–329.

17. Bruckheimer E, Birk E, Santiago R, et al. Coarctation of the aorta treated with the Advanta V12 large diameter stent: acute results. *Catheter Cardiovasc Interv.* 2010;75(3):402–406.

18. Daehnert I, Rotzsch C, Wiener M, et al. Rapid right ventricular pacing is an alternative to adenosine in catheter interventional procedures for congenital heart disease. *Heart.* 2004;90(9):1047–1050.

19. Hamdan MA, Maheshwari S, Fahey JT, et al. Endovascular stents for coarctation of the aorta: initial results and intermediate-term follow-up. *J Am Coll Cardiol.* 2001;38(5):1518–1523.

20. Suárez de Lezo J, Pan M, Romero M, et al. Immediate and follow-up findings after stent treatment for severe coarctation of aorta. *Am J Cardiol.* 1999;83(3):400–406.

21. Johnston TA, Grifka RG, Jones TK. Endovascular stents for treatment of coarctation of the aorta: acute results and follow-up experience. *Catheter Cardiovasc Interv.* 2004;62(4):499–505.

22. Forbes TJ, Garekar S, Amin Z, et al. Procedural results and acute complications in stenting native and recurrent coarctation of the aorta in patients over 4 years of age: a multi-institutional study. *Catheter Cardiovasc Interv.* 2007;70(2):276–285.

23. Forbes TJ, Moore P, Pedra CA, et al. Intermediate follow-up following intravascular stenting for treatment of coarctation of the aorta. *Catheter Cardiovasc Interv.* 2007;70(4):569–577.

24. Phadke K, Dyet JF, Aber CP, et al. Balloon angioplasty of adult aortic coarctation. *Br Heart J.* 1993;69(1):36–40.

25. Fawzy ME, Dunn B, Galal O, et al. Balloon coarctation angioplasty in adolescents and adults: early and intermediate results. *Am Heart J.* 1992;124(1):167–171.

26. Fawzy ME, Sivanandam V, Galal O, et al. One- to ten-year follow-up results of balloon angioplasty of native coarctation of the aorta in adolescents and adults. *J Am Coll Cardiol.* 1997;30(6):1542–1546.

27. Thanopoulos BD, Hadjinikolaou L, Konstadopoulou GN, et al. Stent treatment for coarctation of the aorta: intermediate term follow up and technical considerations. *Heart.* 2000;84(1):65–70.

28. Harrison DA, McLaughlin PR, Lazzam C, et al. Endovascular stents in the management of coarctation of the aorta in the adolescent and adult: one year follow up. *Heart.* 2001;85(5):561–566.

29. Suárez de Lezo J, Pan M, Romero M, et al. Percutaneous interventions on severe coarctation of the aorta: a 21-year experience. *Pediatr Cardiol.* 2005;26(2):176–189.

30. Zanjani KS, Sabi T, Moysich A, et al. Feasibility and efficacy of stent redilatation in aortic coarctation. *Catheter Cardiovasc Interv.* 2008;72(4):552–556.

Septal Ablation in Obstructive Hypertrophic Cardiomyopathy

Evan Lau and E. Murat Tuzcu

A lcohol ablation for relieving left ventricular outflow tract (LVOT) obstruction is one of several therapeutic modalities utilized in the treatment of hypertrophic obstructive cardiomyopathy. For the interventional cardiologist planning to perform an alcohol septal ablation (ASA), it is critically important to have an in-depth understanding of this complex disease with its variable clinical presentations and challenging characteristics. In this chapter, we provide a brief overview of hypertrophic cardiomyopathy (HCM) and focus on the procedural aspects of alcohol ablation.

DEFINITION

HCM is a cardiovascular disorder with a wide array of clinical presentations. Management of this disease requires appraisal of its many facets, including symptom control, risk for sudden cardiac death (SCD), implications for relatives, and more. The variety of phenotypic expressions makes the care of these patients challenging, and forces the cardiologist to apply a broad range of their skill set.

It is difficult to formulate an all-encompassing definition of HCM. From a clinical standpoint, it has generally been regarded that HCM occurs when a patient demonstrates left ventricular hypertrophy (LVH) in the absence of a primary disorder associated with myocardial hypertrophy—that is, hypertension or aortic stenosis. This type of definition fails us in a variety of ambiguous clinical circumstances, including LVH

in a well-trained athlete or in a patient with mild or well-controlled hypertension. Furthermore, a number of other genetic and infiltrative diseases may mimic HCM in rare cases. A comprehensive understanding of the genetics of HCM may ultimately provide a more precise definition. However, at present, we are only able to identify the gene mutations of 35% to 65% of patients who have clinical manifestation of this disorder.[1] Thus, there continues to be ambiguity in defining the parameters to diagnose HCM.

EPIDEMIOLOGY

The prevalence of HCM is estimated to be ~0.2% of the general population.[2] The HCM phenotype has been described in patients from infancy to advanced age. In one study, there is a 3:2 male to female predominance in patients who carry a diagnosis of HCM, but this was felt to be related to underdiagnosis in women.[3] HCM appears to be ubiquitous, being described in a multitude of ethnicities, including Caucasian, African American, Asian, and Native American populations.

NATURAL HISTORY OF THE DISEASE

Studies involving general HCM populations suggest that the vast majority of patients follow a benign course, with an annual mortality on the order of 0.6% to 1.3% per year.[4] Higher risk patients include those with risk factors for SCD, as well as patients that demonstrate advanced heart failure symptoms.[3] The presence of LVOT obstruction is an independent predictor of progression to worsening heart failure symptoms and death.[5]

PATHOPHYSIOLOGY

Several pathophysiologic mechanisms contribute to the clinical presentations associated with HCM. These include LVOT obstruction, mitral regurgitation, microvascular ischemia, diastolic dysfunction, and systolic dysfunction. The importance of each mechanism varies from patient to patient, and leads to the variety in presentations. LVOT obstruction is a unique pathophysiologic mechanism that can be demonstrated in up to 70% of patients.[6] It is the consequence of a complex interplay between the hypertrophied septum, the anterior mitral leaflet, and enlarged and/or anomalous papillary muscles, which results in systolic anterior motion (SAM) of the mitral valve. This abnormal motion of the mitral valve, primarily of the anterior mitral leaflet, encroaches upon the cross-sectional area of the LVOT, causing subvalvular obstruction. The process is dynamic and there can be fluctuations in the severity of obstruction, which tends to be exacerbated by hypovolemia, tachycardia, vasodilation, and increased contractility.

CLINICAL PRESENTATION

For those with symptomatic manifestations of HCM, there are several general categories of presentation: (a) SCD and ventricular dysrhythmia; (b) symptoms of angina, syncope, and/or dyspnea; (c) progressive heart failure due to diastolic or systolic dysfunction; and (d) atrial fibrillation (AF).[7]

Sudden Death

The most feared complication of HCM is sudden death, due to ventricular tachycardia or ventricular fibrillation. Only a small percentage of patients in a general HCM population will suffer from sudden death, and so it has been the goal of many investigators to determine those at greatest risk. The major clinical risk factors used for identifying those at highest risk include prior history of cardiac arrest, family history of sudden death, unexplained syncope, left ventricular wall thickness of greater than 30 mm, hypotensive response during exercise stress testing, and the presence of nonsustained ventricular tachycardia on Holter

monitoring.[8] The absence of any of the major risk factors has excellent negative predictive value for the risk of sudden death.[8] There are a number of other patient variables that may be taken into consideration when deciding on the need for primary prophylaxis with an implantable cardioverter defibrillator (ICD), although their exact contribution to SCD risk is still undefined: end-stage disease with goal for heart transplantation, presence of LVOT obstruction, presence of late gadolinium enhancement on magnetic resonance imaging (MRI), and the presence of apical aneurysm.[9]

Angina

Angina is a common complaint associated with HCM, occurring in up to 29% of patients.[3] In general, coronary angiography demonstrates the absence of obstructive epicardial disease.[3] Myocardial ischemia is likely a consequence of the interplay between arteriolar medial hypertrophy, impaired coronary vasodilation, and increased demand of thickened heart muscle.[10] The disruption of myocardial blood can be severe enough to cause infarction, as shown in up to 15% of patients in autopsy studies.[11]

Syncope

There are several mechanisms that may cause syncope in patients with HCM. Syncope may be a sign of a patient with the substrate for malignant ventricular tachyarrhythmia. This is oftentimes the initial consideration and may be used as a justification for the placement of an ICD. Alternatively, LVOT obstruction may be the pathophysiologic mechanism for syncope in a given patient. It may not be possible to discern between these etiologies in a given circumstance. However, although the placement of an ICD will protect against ventricular dysrhythmia, recurrent syncope does occur in patients with LVOT obstruction who are not appropriately managed.

Dyspnea

As with syncope, dyspnea may be the consequence of several mechanisms. Some patients demonstrate primarily diastolic dysfunction, with or without fluid retention. LVOT obstruction is another mechanism for dyspnea, particularly under exertional conditions. This may be unrecognized, particularly in those with little or no resting gradients, but significant provocable gradients. SAM of the mitral valve can sometimes lead to mitral regurgitation. This can be a dynamic process and is often times accompanied by subvalvular obstruction. Finally, HCM patients may develop end-stage systolic heart failure.

Congestive Heart Failure

Some patients present with congestive heart failure, due to either diastolic or systolic dysfunction. Diastolic dysfunction can range from mild diastolic heart failure to severe restrictive cardiomyopathy. Patients with HCM, presenting primarily with restrictive cardiomyopathy, account for only a small percentage of all HCM patients. The restrictive filling pattern, as seen by Doppler echocardiography, is a poor prognostic marker, with higher risk for AF, thromboembolic complications, sudden death, end-stage heart failure, and heart transplantation.[12] Some patients will progress toward a dilated cardiomyopathy as the end-stage of their HCM. The presence of systolic dysfunction also portends a worse prognosis, with greater rates of death, ICD discharge, and cardiac transplantation.[13]

Atrial Fibrillation and Thromboembolism

AF is commonly associated with HCM, with an incidence of ~2% per year and ~22% prevalence in a general HCM population.[14] HCM patients that develop AF tend to have more advanced symptoms; whether AF is a marker for more advanced disease or a contributor to worsening symptoms is unclear. The risk for thromboembolism is high for patients with combined AF and HCM, even in the absence of traditional risk factors. In one series, up to 39% of patients untreated with anticoagulation or antiplatelets suffered an ischemic stroke, as compared to 10% in warfarin-treated patients.[14] Although not related to sudden death, AF does increase the likelihood of heart failure related death.

DIFFERENTIAL DIAGNOSIS

Several disorders need to be entertained when evaluating a patient with possible HCM. In general, the diagnosis of HCM is made when there is LVH in the absence of systemic hypertension or aortic stenosis. However, HCM should be considered when the patient has hypertrophy that is disproportionate to their history of hypertension, such as if it were brief, mild, or well-controlled. Referrals for well-trained athletes with mild to moderate hypertrophy present another difficult clinical dilemma. Competitive athletes, particularly those engaging in endurance sports, may demonstrate mild increases in wall thickness (as high as 16 mm). The distinctions between "athlete's heart" and HCM are not clear cut, but echocardiographic findings supporting a pathologic diagnosis include asymmetry and focality of hypertrophy, small to normal left ventricular end-diastolic cavity size (expected to be mildly enlarged in athletic training), and Doppler findings demonstrating abnormal diastolic function. Sometimes, the distinctions are too subtle to differentiate the two, and these patients are asked to take a sabbatical from training to see if the myocardial hypertrophy regresses.[15]

There are a number of infiltrative disorders that may mimic the hypertrophy of HCM. There may even be the presence of LVOT obstruction in some of these patients. These disorders include cardiac amyloidosis, glycogen storage diseases (Pompe and Forbes diseases), Anderson-Fabry disease, mitochondrial disorders, disorders related to PRKAG2 mutations, Friederich's ataxia, Noonan syndrome, and Danon disease. These genetic disorders, involved with mutations in nonsarcomeric proteins, should be considered in patients with multisystem phenotypes.[1]

DIAGNOSTIC TESTING

Although the circumstances under which a patient receives a diagnosis of HCM are varied, generally, the diagnosis is made by echocardiography. The cardiovascular consultant must then focus their evaluation on gathering the salient information necessary for risk stratifying and managing the patient appropriately.

Electrocardiography

Electrocardiography (ECG) is limited in its ability to detect HCM. There are no highly specific findings associated with HCM. Changes consistent with LVH may be present but are not always seen. Furthermore, changes of LVH seen on ECG do not necessarily correlate with echocardiographic measurements. In the apical variant of HCM, also called Yamaguchi disease, the classic ECG findings are prominent T-wave inversions across the precordial leads.

Echocardiography

Echocardiography is the primary modality for making the diagnosis of HCM. It also provides critical information regarding prognosis and pathophysiology of the disease process. The hallmark of HCM is LVH, typically >13 mm. The pattern of hypertrophy is variable, with classic descriptions involving a thickened interventricular septum. Thickening of the septum manifests in at least three different patterns: sigmoidal (involving primarily the basal septum), reverse curve (half-moon shaped, with convexity protruding into the left ventricular cavity), and neutral (uniform thickness of the septum).[16] Other variants of HCM include apical HCM (Yamaguchi disease), as well as predominant hypertrophy of the anterolateral wall.

LVH is usually accompanied by diastolic dysfunction. In up to 82% of patients, mitral inflow velocities as assessed by pulsed wave Doppler echocardiography will demonstrate reduced maximal velocities in early diastole (E wave), and elevated velocities in late diastole (A wave).[17] This is accompanied by prolongation of deceleration times.[17] Some patients will demonstrate more severe forms of diastolic dysfunction, including restrictive patterns by pulsed wave Doppler echocardiography.[18,19] This finding can have important prognostic implications, as patients tend to have more advanced symptoms and progression of heart failure.

The physiologic phenomenon of SAM of the mitral valve, with or without LVOT obstruction, is not universal in all cases of HCM, but can be demonstrated in up to 70% of cases.[6] SAM can be identified by two-dimensional (2D) or M-mode echocardiography, which show abnormal motion of the anterior mitral leaflet toward the interventricular septum during systole (Fig. 27-1A). For some patients, anterior leaflet motion causes mitral regurgitation that is posteriorly directed. SAM may cause LVOT obstruction, which is shown as flow acceleration by color Doppler

(Fig. 27-1B) and can be quantified using continuous wave Doppler echocardiography. Dynamic, subvalvular obstruction of this nature differs from aortic stenosis by its classic, "dagger-shaped" appearance of the continuous wave Doppler profile through the aortic valve (Fig. 27-1C). Demonstration of peak subvalvular gradients of >30 mm Hg has a poor prognostic value in HCM.[20] As important as quantifying the severity of subvalvular obstruction, the clinician needs to identify the mechanisms for obstruction that predominate in a given patient, including severity of septal hypertrophy, redundancy or abnormalities of the anterior mitral leaflet, and anomalies of the papillary muscles. If intervention for LVOT obstruction is undertaken, the best modality of intervention will be informed by the mechanisms at play. For example, the presence of significant mitral regurgitation, particularly in the setting of intrinsic mitral valvular abnormalities, will favor the use of surgery over a percutaneous technique. Likewise, if papillary muscle anomalies predominate in the mechanism of SAM for a given patient, surgical correction is appropriate.

Exercise Echocardiography

Strong consideration should be given to the use of this modality in patients that are ambulatory, particularly in those patients with low or no resting subvalvular gradient.[6] SAM and LVOT obstruction may not be present on the resting examination, but may require exertional or pharmacologic provocation, using dobutamine or amyl nitrate. The advantage of an exercise test is its ability to objectively classify a patient's functional status, as well as provide the clinician with

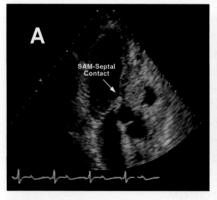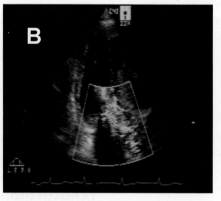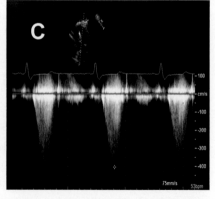

FIGURE 27-1.

A: Apical long-axis view demonstrating systolic anterior motion (SAM) of the mitral valve, with the anterior and posterior leaflets of the mitral valve making contact with the septum during systole. **B:** Same view with color Doppler demonstrates flow acceleration beginning at the point of septal-mitral contact. **C:** Continuous wave Doppler through the aortic valve in the five-chamber apical view demonstrates the classic "dagger-shaped" profile, consistent with dynamic outflow tract obstruction.

information about the presence of dynamic LVOT obstruction under physiologic conditions. For patients with high resting gradients or potential for malignant ventricular tachyarrhythmias, exercise should be avoided or used with caution.

Cardiac Magnetic Resonance Imaging

Cardiac MRI provides information about the morphology, physiology, and tissue characteristics in HCM patients. Cine imaging accurately shows the presence of hypertrophy, its location, and morphology. Compared to echocardiography, it is able to identify hypertrophy that may be otherwise missed, such as in the anterolateral wall of the left ventricle. The superiority of image quality also provides more accurate assessment of wall thickness. Cine imaging is able to identify the presence of SAM and LVOT obstruction. Although it lacks the ability to quantify the severity of obstruction, the improvement in tissue characterization allows for more precise determination of mechanisms of obstruction. This can be particularly useful in identifying anomalies of the papillary muscle. Delayed-enhancement imaging can provide evidence for the presence of scar. Significant attention has been paid to the prognostic value of this, particularly as it relates to ventricular tachyarrhythmia and risk for sudden death.[21,22]

Routine use of cardiac MRI in patients with HCM is controversial. Proponents would argue that it provides diagnostic and prognostic information above that obtained by echocardiography alone. This would include accurate measurements of hypertrophy, precise determination of hypertrophy location, as well as presence of scar. Arguments against routine use include overlap of information provided by the two modalities, increased cost, and unclear benefit in prognostication.

Holter Monitoring

Routine Holter monitoring should be considered for most patients with HCM. The presence of nonsustained ventricular tachycardia is an important risk factor for the risk of sudden death, and should be used in consideration for ICD placement.

Genetic Testing

Although HCM is a genetic disorder, genetic testing currently has a limited role in the management of patients. Only 35% to 65% of patients with HCM have a gene mutation that is identifiable by today's commercially available tests.[1] There is limited data that links particular genotypes to clinical outcomes. The prognosis of any given patient with a particular genotype is unclear, given the variability of penetrance. Currently, the most important role of genetic testing is identifying the responsible gene in index cases and, subsequently, testing family members to determine the presence of that mutation.

For the majority of patients, the genetic underpinning of HCM is a mutation in a sarcomeric protein, including beta-myosin heavy chain, myosin-binding protein C, troponin T and I, as well as others. It has been recognized that mutations involving Z-disc and calcium-handling genes of the cardiomyocyte may also lead to the HCM phenotype.[1]

Managing the implications for family members is a multistep process. Consideration should be given toward identifying the genetic mutation of the index patient. If one is identified, family members at risk can be screened for the presence of a mutation. Those identified as carriers of the mutation can be screened with periodic echocardiograms to look for the emergence of the HCM phenotype. In families where the genetic mutation has not been determined, members at risk should be screened with periodic echocardiograms.

Cardiac Catheterization

With the sophistication of today's imaging modalities, cardiac catheterization is infrequently used to make a diagnosis of HCM. The role of invasive catheterization is usually limited to planning/performance of ASA and as preoperative testing prior to septal myectomy. In limited circumstances, cardiac catheterization is used to confirm and quantitate subvalvular obstruction. The hemodynamic findings of HCM include the demonstration of a pressure gradient below the aortic valve. This is best done by continuous pressure measurement during pullback of an end-hole catheter (Judkins right or multipurpose catheters) from the ventricular apex to the aortic valve. This maneuver is most helpful when the gradients by imaging modality are inadequate, or for monitoring success at time of ASA. Another hemodynamic finding is the Brockenbrough-Morrow-Braunwald sign (Fig. 27-2), which is the demonstration of an increase in LVOT gradient after a premature ventricular contraction accompanied with a narrowing of the systemic pulse pressure.[23] In rare situations, this may help in differentiating aortic stenosis from subvalvular obstruction; in patients with aortic stenosis, the gradient will increase, but there will also be an increase in the systemic pulse pressure.

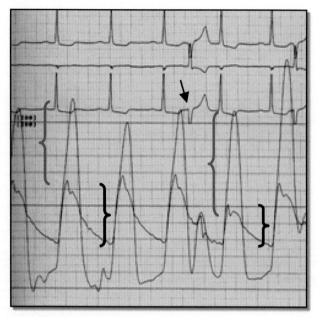

FIGURE 27-2.

Simultaneous aortic and left ventricular pressure tracings demonstrate the Brockenbrough-Morrow-Braunwald sign, whereby the beat following a premature ventricular contraction (*black arrow*) produces a greater aortic–left ventricle gradient (*red brackets*) and a narrowed aortic pulse pressure (*black brackets*).

The role for angiography in patients with HCM is multifold. The rate of concomitant coronary artery disease in a general HCM population is low, but angiography may be warranted in selected patients. There are some characteristic appearances of the epicardial and intramural coronary vessels in HCM patients, but these are generally insensitive and not part of the diagnostic algorithm. In those patients with significant LVOT obstruction, the most important role for coronary angiography is characterization of the septal perforator anatomy, focusing on the patient's candidacy for ASA.

MANAGEMENT

Several important facets of the disease should be considered for each patient evaluated for HCM: (a) risk of sudden death, (b) symptom management with evaluation for the presence of LVOT obstruction, and (c) implications for family members. We focus our following discussions on the basic management issues of patients with HCM. Outside of what has been previously mentioned, we do not provide an in-depth discussion on genetic counseling and the management of a patient's family members. Likewise, we will not address those

patients with advanced heart failure, who have failed medical therapy, and are not candidates for interventional procedures. These HCM patients with severe systolic or diastolic dysfunction should be considered for cardiac transplantation.

The principles of managing LVOT obstruction deserve special consideration. Maneuvers that decrease left ventricular dimensions tend to exacerbate the severity of LVOT obstruction. These include hypovolemia, tachycardia, and vasodilation—situations promoting these phenomena should be avoided or treated appropriately (i.e., bleeding, dehydration, rapid AF, sepsis, etc). This also means that diuretics should be used judiciously in patients with LVOT obstruction. Likewise, pure vasodilators should be used cautiously. In situations where there is severe LVOT obstruction and critical illness, medications with positive inotropic effects should be avoided. Hypotension in these settings should be treated with pure vasoconstrictors. In patients with LVOT obstruction and cardiogenic shock, maneuvers that are contraindicated in left ventricular systolic dysfunction, such as beta-blockade, volume resuscitation, and vasoconstriction, are indicated.

Sudden Death Risk

Implantable Cardioverter-Defibrillators

The principal modality for primary and secondary prevention of sudden death in HCM patients is the use of ICDs. Every patient with a diagnosis of HCM should be evaluated for sudden death risk factors, including prior cardiac arrest, non-sustained ventricular tachycardia on monitoring, massive septal hypertrophy (>30 mm), hypotensive response to exercise, family history of sudden death, and prior unexplained syncope. As such, clinical history and testing, including Holter monitoring, echocardiography, and exercise testing, should be focused to address these risk factors. In general, the presence of one of these risk factors places the patient in a high-risk category and warrants the implantation of an ICD. In some cases, alternative factors may help to determine the candidacy for ICD implantation, including the presence of LVOT obstruction, prior or planned ASA, the presence of a ventricular aneurysm, the presence of scar on MRI imaging, and listing for cardiac transplantation. In addition to considerations for ICD implantation, the general recommendation for all patients with HCM, with or without sudden death risk factors, is to abstain from competitive sports. Even for patients that receive an ICD, this recommendation should stand.

Angina, Dyspnea, and Left Ventricular Outflow Tract Obstruction

Pharmacotherapy

For the management of anginal and dyspnea symptoms, there are three agents that are in use for patients with HCM: beta-blockers, calcium channel blockers, and disopyramide. Most studies evaluating these agents have been small scale studies with physiologic or symptomatic outcomes; there is a dearth of large scale studies demonstrating superiority of one agent in terms of mortality or other hard endpoints.

Many of the studies evaluating beta-blockade in patients with HCM have involved nonselective beta-blockers such as nadolol and propanolol; many clinicians have extrapolated their benefits to selective beta-blockers which are in routine use. Beta-blockers have been shown to improve exercise tolerance, decrease anginal symptoms, and decrease the severity of LVOT obstruction.[24,25] Verapamil has also been studied and demonstrated to improve symptoms of dyspnea and exercise tolerance.[26,27] There have been head-to-head comparisons of verapamil to nadolol, and it appears that there may be more benefit in subjective reports of functional capacity, but no clear benefit in objective measures.[24] The role of verapamil in the management of LVOT obstruction is controversial. Some studies suggest an improvement in LVOT gradients, however, there is theoretic concern that vasodilatory effects may worsen obstruction and adverse outcomes have been reported with its use in patients with severe gradients.[28] Disopyramide has negative inotropic and vasoconstrictive properties that make it an attractive alternative for patients with severe LVOT obstruction. Several studies have demonstrated that ~50% reduction of gradients can be achieved in patients who are managed without invasive septal reduction techniques.[29–31] Given the data in total, it is reasonable to use beta-blockers as a first-line agent in patients with mild angina or dyspnea. In patients where anginal symptoms predominate, verapamil may be a more effective choice, but it should probably be avoided in patients with severe LVOT obstruction. Finally, disopyramide is an attractive option in patients whose symptoms are primarily due to LVOT obstruction, oftentimes in combination with beta-blockade.

Septal Myectomy

Invasive septal reduction is indicated in patients with New York Heart Association (NYHA) class III to IV symptoms in the presence of LVOT obstruction with gradients >50 mm Hg at rest or with provocation. Septal myectomy has become the gold standard for septal reduction. It involves removal of the muscular septum, guided by visualization and palpation from the aortic side of the aortic valve. Resection is carried out from the most basal portion of the septum to the area of the cavity involved with septal-mitral contact, sometimes extending to the base of the posteromedial papillary muscle.[32] Nonrandomized studies show consistent reduction in LVOT gradients, with concomitant improvement in functional capacity.[33–35] Observational data suggests that patients undergoing septal myectomy may have mortality benefit when compared to those who did not undergo the procedure.[34] For some patients, the mechanism of LVOT obstruction is not completely relieved by septal myectomy due to abnormalities of the mitral valve or subvalvular apparatus. A number of surgical techniques have been described to address a variety of these issues, including mitral valve repair/plication and papillary muscle realignment/resection. In cases where there is significant intrinsic mitral valve abnormality, mitral valve replacement is carried out with a low profile prosthesis.

Alcohol Septal Ablation

PATIENT SELECTION AND OUTCOMES

Since its first description in 1995, ASA has emerged as an important tool in the treatment of HCM patients with LVOT obstruction.[36] This procedure involves the injection of ethanol into a septal perforator to create a controlled infarction of the portion of hypertrophied septum causing LVOT obstruction (Fig. 27-3). Candidates for the procedure include patients with symptoms of NYHA class III to IV symptoms. Symptoms should be attributed to peak LVOT gradients of >50 mm Hg at rest or with provocation, in the setting of a basal septum that is at least 1.8 cm thick. The patient must have adequate septal perforator anatomy with at least one proximal septal perforator of ≥1.0 mm in diameter (Table 27-1). Attention should be paid toward the angle of the septal perforator takeoff from the left anterior descending (LAD) artery; an angle >90 degrees will make the procedure technically challenging (Fig. 27-4). Preprocedural evaluation should also focus on the mechanism of LVOT obstruction for a given patient. In ideal candidates, the hypertrophied septum is the dominant pathology in the physiology of LVOT obstruction. However, select patients will have other mechanisms contributing to LVOT obstruction, including redundancy of the anterior mitral leaflet or subvalvular apparatus,

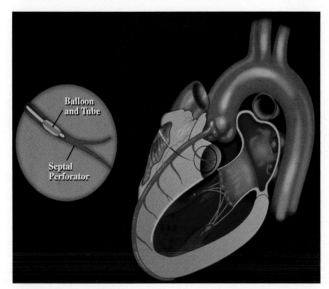

FIGURE 27-3.

Graphical depiction of alcohol septal ablation. Alcohol is injected via a balloon catheter into the septal perforator that supplies the portion of septum involved with septal-mitral contact and left ventricular outflow tract obstruction.

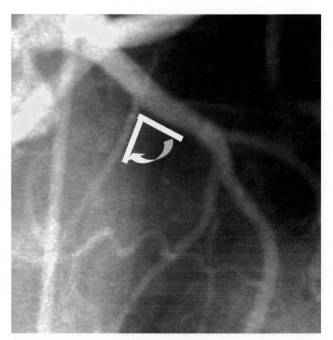

FIGURE 27-4.

Posteroanterior cranial view of the left anterior descending and septal perforators. The size and take-off angle of the septal perforator from the left anterior descending artery is critical in selecting the target branch.

anterior angulation of the papillary muscle head, or direct insertion of the papillary muscle into the mitral valve. Dynamic mitral regurgitation is common, but some patients will have moderate to severe mitral regurgitation that is independent of SAM and would not be corrected by ASA alone. For patients with these physiologic and anatomic concerns, surgical myectomy should be considered before proceeding toward ASA. Another important consideration involves the risk of sudden death. There has been a theoretic concern that the scar created by ASA will leave a substrate for ventricular tachyarrhythmias. This theoretic risk has not been clearly demonstrated in patients undergoing ASA.[37–40]

There are no randomized comparisons between surgical myectomy and ASA. There have been several nonrandomized studies that have attempted comparisons, but these are confounded by selection bias as the groups referred for surgical myectomy differ from those undergoing ASA. A meta-analysis compiling data from these studies showed that in these two highly selected groups, there were few differences in postprocedural outcomes.[41] The data does demonstrate statistically significant differences in postprocedural pacemaker implantation and LVOT gradient reduction, both in favor of surgical myectomy. Both techniques resulted in similar functional class improvement. With regard to short- and long-term mortality, and ventricular arrhythmias, there were no statistically significant differences (Table 27-2). Still, there are divided camps that tout surgical myectomy or ASA as the superior procedure and this controversy is unlikely to be resolved in the near future. Ultimately, the choice for any particular patient falls on clinician/institutional bias, mechanism of LVOT obstruction, and patient characteristics and preferences.

TABLE 27-1 Patient Selection Criteria for Alcohol Septal Ablation

Severe heart failure symptoms (i.e., NYHA class III–IV) despite maximal medical therapy

Septal thickness >18 mm

Subaortic gradient >50 mm Hg (resting or with provocation) due to SAM

Absence of papillary muscle or mitral valvular anomalies (i.e., anomalous papillary muscle insertion)

Absence of significant coronary arterial disease

Compatible septal perforator branch arterial anatomy

Relative contraindications to surgical myectomy (i.e., age, comorbidity)

NYHA, New York Heart Association; SAM, systolic anterior motion of the mitral valve.

TABLE 27-2 Pooled Effect Estimates for Outcomes Comparing Alcohol Septal Ablation with Septal Myectomy

Outcome	Estimate Used	Pooled Estimate	95% CI	P Value[b]
Short-term mortality	RD	0.01[a]	−0.01–0.03	.35
Long-term mortality	RD	0.02[a]	−0.05–0.09	.55
Pacemaker implantation	OR	2.57	1.68–3.93	< .001
Ventricular arrhythmia	OR	1.34	0.54–3.32	.52
NYHA class	SMD	0.30[a]	−0.03–0.63	.08
LVOT gradient reduction	SMD	0.45[a]	0.13–0.77	< .01

[a]*Negative values favor alcohol septal ablation, positive values favor septal myectomy.*
[b]*P < .05 is considered significant.*
CI, confidence interval; NYHA, New York Heart Association class; LVOT, left ventricular outflow tract obstruction; OR, odds ratio; RD, risk difference; SMD, standardized mean difference.
Adapted from Agarwal S, Tuzcu EM, Desai M, et al. Updated meta-analysis of septal alcohol ablation versus myectomy for hypertrophic cardiomyopathy. J Am Coll Cardiol. 2010;55(8):823–834.

PROCEDURAL TECHNIQUE

The procedure begins with a hemodynamic assessment of the LVOT gradient. This is performed by placing an end-hole catheter into the left ventricular apex with measurement of the ventricular and aortic pressures during gradual withdrawal through the LVOT and into the aorta. Alternatively, simultaneous measurements of aortic and left ventricle pressures can be performed with the use of a long-sheath in the descending aorta and an end-hole catheter in the left ventricle. For predominantly latent gradients, the use of isoproterenol, dobutamine, or amyl nitrate may be necessary to appreciate the severity of obstruction. Hemodynamic confirmation is critical, both to confirm the diagnosis and determine the success of intervention.

The proceduralist should then turn attention toward coronary angiography, looking for concomitant obstructive atherosclerotic lesions, as well as performing a detailed assessment of the septal perforator anatomy. The presence of obstructive coronary artery disease, particularly in proximal locations, should alert the operator for increased risk of complications and prompt consideration for revascularization. The ideal septal perforator should be located in the basal septum and possess a diameter of 1.0 to 2.0 mm. Smaller arteries would be difficult to cannulate with a balloon; larger arteries may subtend too large an area of myocardium. As previously mentioned, the angle of take-off is another critical feature, as perforators that are >90 degrees will pose a challenge for balloon placement. These issues are usually well demonstrated by right anterior oblique cranial and posteroanterior cranial views. For septal perforators with large enough subdivisions, the operator should determine the branches that supply the left and right portions of the septum—those supplying the left ventricular portion of the septum would be optimal. To adequately examine this anatomy, a left anterior oblique cranial view may be necessary.

The next step involves placement of a temporary transvenous pacemaker wire, to protect the patient against postprocedural heart block. This is best placed from the internal jugular veins as it will remain in the patient for a minimum of 48 hours. Because of the proclivity for passive fixation wires to migrate over time, we generally opt for placement of an active fixation pacemaker.

Once the septal anatomy has been determined, and the temporary pacemaker wire inserted, a guide catheter (such as a 6 or 7 French XB3.5) is used to engage the left main coronary artery. A 0.014-inch guidewire is placed into the septal perforator of interest (Fig. 27-5A). The subsequent steps are undertaken to confirm the area of myocardium supplied by the septal perforator. An over-the-wire angioplasty balloon, usually 1.0 to 2.0 mm in diameter, 10 mm in length, is passed into the septal perforator. If the take-off of the artery is >90 degrees, it may prove difficult to advance the balloon from the LAD into the septal perforator. If this is the case, a stiffer guidewire may be used to provide extra support. With the balloon in the intended artery, it is then inflated to 10 to 12 atm to completely occlude the septal artery (Fig. 27-5B). Complete occlusion of the septal perforator branch is confirmed by coronary angiography. Angiographic contrast is slowly injected through the balloon and into the artery at a rate similar to the intended rate of ethanol injection (Fig. 27-5C). The operator looks to see that no contrast refluxes into the LAD or travels by way of collaterals to another

A: A 0.014-inch guidewire is introduced into the target septal perforator. **B:** A 2.0 × 15 mm over-the-wire balloon is placed over the guidewire into the septal perforator; the balloon is inflated and there is no contrast flow from the left anterior descending (LAD) artery into the septal branch. The over-the-wire balloon is inflated and contrast is injected into the septal perforator, confirming complete occlusion and lack of contrast flow into the LAD artery, confirming the safety of injecting ethanol **(C).** **D:** Following ethanol injection, there is distal loss of the septal perforator branch.

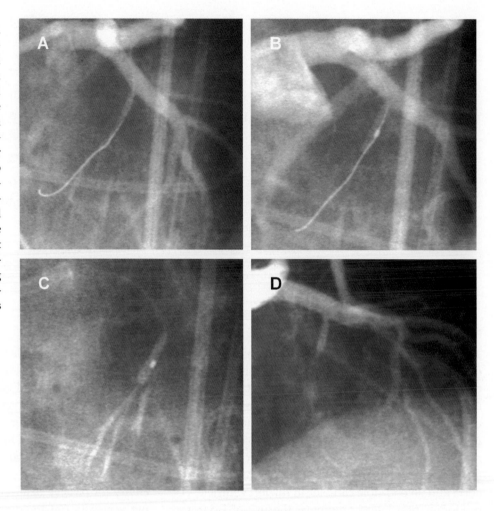

artery (i.e., posterior descending artery), suggesting the possibility of ethanol damage to unintended arteries. The contrast blush will provide some reference as to the size and location of the myocardium that will be infarcted. The speed of wash-out of the contrast will also suggest the amount of collateral blood flow to the myocardium; robust collaterals from a different source will negatively impact the operator's ability to infarct that segment of myocardium. Echocardiographic myocardial contrast is then used to further delineate the segment of myocardium subtended by the artery. Surface echocardiography should be performed in the

A: Apical long-axis view demonstrating the point of septal-mitral contact. **B:** Myocardial contrast is injected into the septal perforator selected for ethanol injection, with subsequent enhancement of the portion of the septum involved with septal-mitral contact. Care is taken to ensure that there is no contrast enhancement in other territories. SAM, systolic anterior motion of the mitral valve.

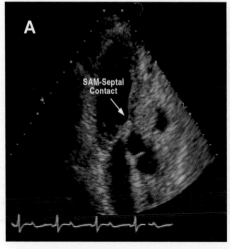
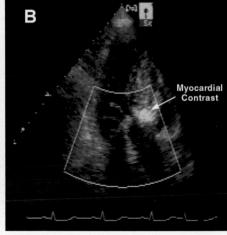

standard parasternal long-axis, apical five-chamber, and apical long-axis views, with focus on the basal septum. In the past, Albumex (Mallinckrodt Medical, St. Louis, MO), a first generation echocardiographic contrast, was injected into the septal artery and then imaged by surface echocardiography (Fig. 27-6). Unfortunately, Albumex is no longer available in many countries. Instead, second- and third-generation agents are used, which has proven to be problematic because rapid transmission through capillary beds causes ventricular opacification and "shadowing" that makes interpretation difficult. In our laboratory, we decrease the potency of the contrast agents by opening the contrast bottles 10 to 15 minutes prior to use. We also dilute the agent in a 1:5 or 1:10 mixture with saline prior to injection. The mechanical index of the ultrasound beam should be decreased to avoid rapid destruction of the microbubbles in the contrast agent. Once the agent is injected, the operator should look for the area of enhancement. Ideally, the portion of the septum involved with septal-mitral contact during SAM is the only segment that should demonstrate enhancement. Enhancement of areas outside of this region, including the right ventricle, the left ventricular inferior wall, or the left ventricular papillary muscles would suggest the possibility of infarction to unintended areas. Thus, careful transthoracic echocardiographic imaging is necessary to ensure proper septal artery selection. A third and final check involves measurement of the LVOT gradient during prolonged balloon inflation in the septal artery. Generally, a reduction of >30% is considered confirmation of appropriate septal selection. Less gradient reduction by balloon inflation alone does not necessarily indicate that the procedure will be unsuccessful.

Immediately before ethanol injection, a final visual confirmation that the balloon has not migrated should be made. Also, the temporary pacemaker wire should be confirmed to have a suitable capture threshold. Once these are verified, 1 to 3 mL of ethanol is injected into the septal artery over a 1- to 5-minute period. If there was rapid wash-out of contrast blush from collateral vessels, the rate of injection should be slowed. After ethanol injection, 0.3 to.5 mL of saline should be instilled through the balloon to flush out remaining ethanol. The balloon should be left inflated for an additional 10 minutes, to prevent ethanol reflux into the LAD and provide enough time for ethanol contact with the myocardial tissues. The gradient should be retested: a resting gradient of <30 mm Hg or a greater than 50% reduction in the provocable gradient is considered to be a technical success (Fig. 27-7). If there is inadequate gradient reduction, some operators

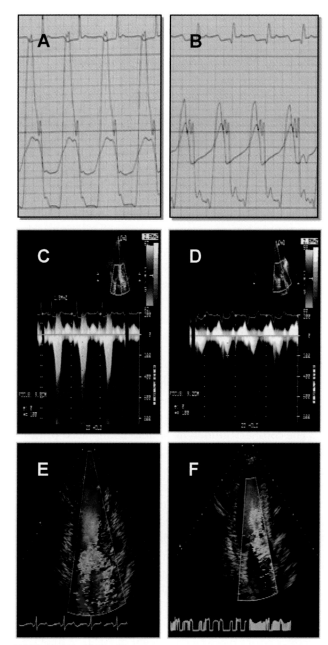

FIGURE 27-7.

Left ventricular outflow tract (LVOT) gradient reduction during septal ablation. During the procedure, progress is demonstrated by serial, simultaneous measurements of the left ventricle and aortic pressures. **A:** Preprocedural gradients, with marked reduction after injection of ethanol **(B)**. Serial measurements of continuous wave Doppler in the apical long-axis view show a similar finding, with high velocity of blood flow through the LVOT before the procedure **(C)** and a significant reduction afterward **(D)**. This is also seen by color Doppler, which demonstrates flow acceleration in the LVOT as well as posteriorly directed mitral regurgitation **(E)**; both findings are attenuated following alcohol septal ablation **(F)**.

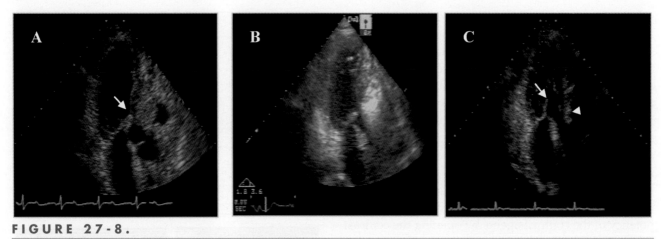

FIGURE 27-8.

Apical long-axis views taken at different time points. **A:** Before ablation, there is severe systolic anterior motion (SAM) with septal-mitral contact (*arrow*). Immediately following ablation, there is marginal reduction in SAM; reduction in LVOT obstruction is largely related to stunning of the septal myocardium (**B**). **C:** Three months following the procedure, there is significant reduction in SAM (*arrow*). In addition, there has been maturation of infarction and reduction in the thickness of the septum (*arrowhead*).

recommend repeating the procedure with another septal perforator, if a suitable one exists. Others are in favor of waiting 3 months before making a decision as long as alcohol is applied to the desired area.

The coronary guidewire should be replaced prior to removal of the balloon. It is recommended to perform coronary angiography with the guidewire in place to maintain access to the left main and LAD artery, should any complications of the procedure be detected. The septal perforator is often occluded at time of final angiography, but continued patency of the artery with diminished flow can be seen (Fig. 27-5D).

Immediate postprocedural care should take place in an intensive care setting for 48 hours, monitoring for complications that may be seen after myocardial infarction. Typically, the creatine phosphokinase levels postprocedure rise to a peak level of 700 to 2,100 U/L, correlating with the size of the infarction created.[42] In the absence of significant heart block or bradyarrhythmia, the temporary pacemaker wire can be removed after 48 hours. The patient generally spends an additional 48 to 72 hours on a regular nursing floor for continued observation. Although rare, there can be late ventricular arrhythmias.

The physiologic changes in LVOT obstruction following ASA occur in several steps (Fig. 27-8). There is an immediate response in LVOT gradient while in the catheterization laboratory due to stunning of the myocardium. In the early period after the procedure, the LVOT gradient may recur, because significant tissue edema in the basal septum contributes to worsening obstruction. Finally, over a period of weeks, the

process of infarction completes, with tissue regression and scar formation (Figs. 27-8 and 27-9).[43] It is in this period that the overall success of ASA can be determined. Although the mechanisms of LVOT obstruction relief differ from the immediate compared to the late postprocedural period, acute relief of the gradient predicts lasting success.[44] Conversely, the presence of residual gradient at the end of the procedure, predicts failure in the long term. Overall, the gradient reduction seen by echocardiography 3 months following ASA represents the long-term gradient reduction to be expected.[43]

Serious complications related to ASA are rare. Procedure-related mortality ranges from 1% to 4%

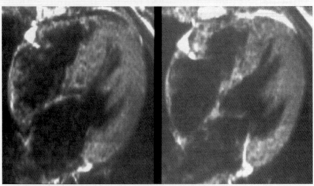

FIGURE 27-9

Cardiac magnetic resonance images in the four-chamber view. The patient has severe hypertrophy of the interventricular septum (**A**). Three months following the septal ablation, there has been a significant reduction in the thickness of the upper septum (**B**).

depending on the center.[44] A right bundle branch block is common and can be observed in up to 36% of patients.[45] Patients with preexisting left bundle branch block are at high risk for complete heart block following this procedure.[46] Rapid ethanol injection is also associated with more advanced degrees of heart block.[46] The requirement for permanent pacemaker placement ranges from 10% to 33% of patients.[41] Recently, the risk of needing a pacemaker has declined to <15%, paralleling the reduction in the volume of the alcohol used by most operators. Rare but catastrophic complications include coronary dissection, ethanol extravasation into the LAD, cardiac perforation with tamponade, and ventricular septal rupture. Ventricular dysrhythmia can occur during the procedure and in the immediate postprocedural period (48 hours). As previously mentioned, the long-term risk for sudden death after ASA is unknown.

Management of HCM patients requires a comprehensive evaluation and involves the use of various medications, restriction of some activities and, when necessary, ICD implantation. When relief of LVOT obstruction is needed, surgical and percutaneous approaches should not be seen as competing modalities, but rather as complementary techniques. Many factors should be taken into account in choosing the appropriate procedure for a given patient: patient's age and comorbidities; the morphology of the septum, mitral valve, and papillary muscles; capabilities of the center; and preferences of the patients. In properly selected patients, alcohol ablation can be performed safely with excellent results.

REFERENCES

1. Bos JM, Towbin JA, Ackerman MJ. Diagnostic, prognostic, and therapeutic implications of genetic testing for hypertrophic cardiomyopathy. *J Am Coll Cardiol*. 2009;54(3):201–211.
2. Maron BJ, Gardin JM, Flack JM, et al. Prevalence of hypertrophic cardiomyopathy in a general population of young adults. Echocardiographic analysis of 4111 subjects in the CARDIA Study. Coronary Artery Risk Development in (Young) Adults. *Circulation*. 1995;92(4):785–789.
3. Olivotto I, Maron MS, Adabag AS, et al. Gender-related differences in the clinical presentation and outcome of hypertrophic cardiomyopathy. *J Am Coll Cardiol*. 2005;46(3):480–487.
4. Maron BJ, Casey SA, Poliac LC, et al. Clinical course of hypertrophic cardiomyopathy in a regional United States cohort. *JAMA*. 1999;281(7):650–655.
5. Maron MS, Olivotto I, Betocchi S, et al. Effect of left ventricular outflow tract obstruction on clinical outcome in hypertrophic cardiomyopathy. *New Engl J Med*. 2003;348(4):295–303.
6. Maron MS, Olivotto I, Zenovich AG, et al. Hypertrophic cardiomyopathy is predominantly a disease of left ventricular outflow tract obstruction. *Circulation*. 2006;114(21):2232–2239.
7. Maron BJ. Hypertrophic cardiomyopathy: a systematic review. *JAMA*. 2002;287(10):1308–1320.
8. Elliott PM, Poloniecki J, Dickie S, et al. Sudden death in hypertrophic cardiomyopathy: identification of high risk patients. *J Am Coll Cardiol*. 2000;36(7):2212–2218.
9. Maron BJ. Contemporary insights and strategies for risk stratification and prevention of sudden death in hypertrophic cardiomyopathy. *Circulation*. 2010;121(3):445–456.
10. Maron BJ, Wolfson JK, Epstein SE, et al. Intramural ("small vessel") coronary artery disease in hypertrophic cardiomyopathy. *J Am Coll Cardiol*. 1986;8(3):545–557.
11. Basso C, Thiene G, Corrado D, et al. Hypertrophic cardiomyopathy and sudden death in the young: pathologic evidence of myocardial ischemia. *Hum Path*. 2000;31(8):988–998.
12. Biagini E, Spirito P, Leone O, et al. Heart transplantation in hypertrophic cardiomyopathy. *Am J Cardiol*. 2008;101(3):387–392.
13. Thaman R, Gimeno JR, Murphy RT, et al. Prevalence and clinical significance of systolic impairment in hypertrophic cardiomyopathy. *Heart*. 2005;91(7):920–925.
14. Olivotto I, Cecchi F, Casey SA, et al. Impact of atrial fibrillation on the clinical course of hypertrophic cardiomyopathy. *Circulation*. 2001;104(21):2517–2524.
15. Maron BJ, Pelliccia A, Spirito P. Cardiac disease in young trained athletes. Insights into methods for distinguishing athlete's heart from structural heart disease, with particular emphasis on hypertrophic cardiomyopathy. *Circulation*. 1995;91(5):1596–1601.
16. Lever HM, Karam RF, Currie PJ, et al. Hypertrophic cardiomyopathy in the elderly. Distinctions from the young based on cardiac shape. *Circulation*. 1989;79(3):580–589.
17. Maron BJ, Spirito P, Green KJ, et al. Noninvasive assessment of left ventricular diastolic function by pulsed Doppler echocardiography in patients with hypertrophic cardiomyopathy. *J Am Coll Cardiol*. 1987;10(4):733–742.
18. Kubo T, Gimeno JR, Bahl A, et al. Prevalence, clinical significance, and genetic basis of hypertrophic cardiomyopathy with restrictive phenotype. *J Am Coll Cardiol*. 2007;49(25):2419–2426.
19. Biagini E, Spirito P, Rocchi G, et al. Prognostic implications of the Doppler restrictive filling pattern in hypertrophic cardiomyopathy. *Am J Cardiol*. 2009;104(12):1727–1731.
20. Maron MS, Olivotto I, Betocchi S, et al. Effect of left ventricular outflow tract obstruction on clinical

outcome in hypertrophic cardiomyopathy. *New Engl J Med.* 2003;348(4):295–303.

21. Adabag AS, Maron BJ, Appelbaum E, et al. Occurrence and frequency of arrhythmias in hypertrophic cardiomyopathy in relation to delayed enhancement on cardiovascular magnetic resonance. *J Am Coll Cardiol.* 2008;51(14):1369–1374.

22. Kwon DH, Setser RM, Popovi ZB, et al. Association of myocardial fibrosis, electrocardiography and ventricular tachyarrhythmia in hypertrophic cardiomyopathy: a delayed contrast enhanced MRI study. *Int J Cardiovasc Imaging.* 2008;24(6):617–625.

23. Brockenbrough EC, Braunwald E, Morrow AG. A hemodynamic technic for the detection of hypertrophic subaortic stenosis. *Circulation.* 1961;23:189–194.

24. Gilligan DM, Chan WL, Joshi J, et al. A double-blind, placebo-controlled crossover trial of nadolol and verapamil in mild and moderately symptomatic hypertrophic cardiomyopathy. *J Am Coll Cardiol.* 1993;21(7):1672–1679.

25. Harrison DC, Braunwald E, Glick G, et al. Effects of beta-adrenergic blockade on the circulation with particular reference to observations in patients with hypertrophic subaortic stenosis. *Circulation.* 1964;29:84–98.

26. Spicer RL, Rocchini AP, Crowley DC, et al. Chronic verapamil therapy in pediatric and young adult patients with hypertrophic cardiomyopathy. *Am J Cardiol.* 1984;53(11):1614–1619.

27. Rosing DR, Kent KM, Maron BJ, et al. Verapamil therapy: a new approach to the pharmacologic treatment of hypertrophic cardiomyopathy. II. Effects on exercise capacity and symptomatic status. *Circulation.* 1979;60(6):1208–1213.

28. Epstein SE, Rosing DR. Verapamil: its potential for causing serious complications in patients with hypertrophic cardiomyopathy. *Circulation.* 1981;64(3):437–441.

29. Sherrid MV, Barac I, McKenna WJ, et al. Multicenter study of the efficacy and safety of disopyramide in obstructive hypertrophic cardiomyopathy. *J Am Coll Cardiol.* 2005;45(8):1251–1258.

30. Pollick C. Muscular subaortic stenosis: hemodynamic and clinical improvement after disopyramide. *New Engl J Med.* 1982;307(16):997–999.

31. Pollick C, Kimball B, Henderson M, et al. Disopyramide in hypertrophic cardiomyopathy. I. Hemodynamic assessment after intravenous administration. *Am J Cardiol.* 1988;62(17):1248–1251.

32. Dearani JA, Danielson GK. Septal myectomy for obstructive hypertrophic cardiomyopathy. *Semin Thorac Cardiovasc Surg Pediatr Card Surg Annu.* 2005:86–91.

33. Smedira NG, Lytle BW, Lever HM, et al. Current effectiveness and risks of isolated septal myectomy for hypertrophic obstructive cardiomyopathy. *Ann Thorac Surg.* 2008;85(1):127–133.

34. Ommen SR, Maron BJ, Olivotto I, et al. Long-term effects of surgical septal myectomy on survival in patients with obstructive hypertrophic cardiomyopathy. *J Am Coll Cardiol.* 2005;46(3):470–476.

35. Merrill WH, Friesinger GC, Graham TP, et al. Long-lasting improvement after septal myectomy for hypertrophic obstructive cardiomyopathy. *Ann Thorac Surg.* 2000;69(6):1732–1735; discussion 1735–1736.

36. Sigwart U. Non-surgical myocardial reduction for hypertrophic obstructive cardiomyopathy. *Lancet.* 1995;346(8969):211–214.

37. Noseworthy PA, Rosenberg MA, Fifer MA, et al. Ventricular arrhythmia following alcohol septal ablation for obstructive hypertrophic cardiomyopathy. *Am J Cardiol.* 2009;104(1):128–132.

38. Cuoco FA, Spencer WH, Fernandes VL, et al. Implantable cardioverter-defibrillator therapy for primary prevention of sudden death after alcohol septal ablation of hypertrophic cardiomyopathy. *J Am Coll Cardiol.* 2008;52(21):1718–1723.

39. Leonardi RA, Kransdorf EP, Simel DL, et al. Meta-analyses of septal reduction therapies for obstructive hypertrophic cardiomyopathy: comparative rates of overall mortality and sudden cardiac death after treatment. *Circ Cardiovasc Interv.* 2010;3(2):97–104.

40. Klopotowski M, Chojnowska L, Malek LA, et al. The risk of non-sustained ventricular tachycardia after percutaneous alcohol septal ablation in patients with hypertrophic obstructive cardiomyopathy. *Clin Res Cardiol.* 2010;99(5):285–292.

41. Agarwal S, Tuzcu EM, Desai MY, et al. Updated meta-analysis of septal alcohol ablation versus myectomy for hypertrophic cardiomyopathy. *J Am Coll Cardiol.* 2010;55(8):823–834.

42. Hage FG, Aqel R, Aljaroudi W, et al. Correlation between serum cardiac markers and myocardial infarct size quantified by myocardial perfusion imaging in patients with hypertrophic cardiomyopathy after alcohol septal ablation. *Am J Cardiol.* 2010;105(2):261–266.

43. Yoerger DM, Picard MH, Palacios IF, et al. Time course of pressure gradient response after first alcohol septal ablation for obstructive hypertrophic cardiomyopathy. *Am J Cardiol.* 2006;97(10):1511–1514.

44. Chang SM, Lakkis NM, Franklin J, et al. Predictors of outcome after alcohol septal ablation therapy in patients with hypertrophic obstructive cardiomyopathy. *Circulation.* 2004;109(7):824–827.

45. Talreja DR, Nishimura RA, Edwards WD, et al. Alcohol septal ablation versus surgical septal myectomy: comparison of effects on atrioventricular conduction tissue. *J Am Coll Cardiol.* 2004;44(12):2329–2332.

46. Chang SM, Nagueh SF, Spencer WH, et al. Complete heart block: determinants and clinical impact in patients with hypertrophic obstructive cardiomyopathy undergoing nonsurgical septal reduction therapy. *J Am Coll Cardiol.* 2003;42(2):296–300.

Page numbers followed by an "*f*" denote figures; those followed by a "*t*" denote tables.